The Unofficial Guide to PASSING OSCEs

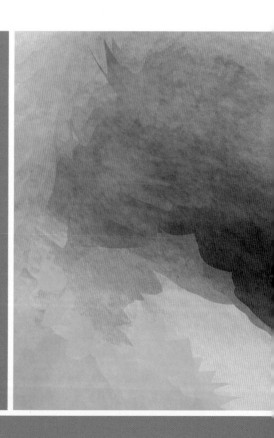

Series Editor

Zeshan Qureshi, BM, BSc (Hons), MSc, MRCPCH, FAcadMEd, MRCPS(Glasg)
Paediatric Registrar
London Deanery
United Kingdom

Editor

Emily Hotton, MBChB (Dist), BSc (Hons) PhD, MRCOG
Women's and Children's Research Southmead Hospital;
Translational Health Sciences University of Bristol, Bristol
United Kingdom

Associate Editor

Sammie Mak, MBChB
Junior Doctor
NHS England, Manchester
United Kingdom

ELSEVIER

Notices

Practitioners and researchers must always rely on their own experience and knowledge in evaluating and using any information, methods, compounds or experiments described herein. Because of rapid advances in the medical sciences, in particular, independent verification of diagnoses and drug dosages should be made. To the fullest extent of the law, no responsibility is assumed by Elsevier, authors, editors or contributors for any injury and/or damage to persons or property as a matter of products liability, negligence or otherwise, or from any use or operation of any methods, products, instructions, or ideas contained in the material herein.

ISBN: 978-0-3239-3654-5

Content Strategist: Jeremy Bowes
Content Project Manager: Shubham Dixit
Design: Miles Hitchen
Illustration Manager: Akshaya Mohan
Marketing Manager: Deborah Watkins

Printed in India by Replika Press Pvt. Ltd.

Last digit is the print number: 9 8 7 6 5 4 3 2 1

The Unofficial Guide to PASSING OSCEs

Series Editor Foreword

The Unofficial Guide to Medicine is not just about helping students study, it is also about allowing those that learn to take back control of their own education. Since its inception, it has been driven by the voices of students, and through this, democratised the process of medical education, blurring the line between learners and teachers.

Medical education is an evolving process, and the latest iteration of our titles has been rewritten to bring them up to date with modern curriculums, after extensive deliberation and consultation. We have kept the series up to date, incorporating new guidelines and perspectives from a wide range of students, junior doctors, and senior clinicians. There is greater consistency across the titles, more illustrations, and through these and other changes, I hope the books will now be even better study aids.

These books though are a process of continual improvement. By reading this book, I hope that you not only get through your exams but also consider contributing to a future edition. You may be a student now, but you are also the future of medical education.

I wish you all the best with your future career and any upcoming exams.

Zeshan Qureshi
November 2022

OSCE Hints and Tips

For years now the OSCE has become a fundamental way of examining medical students, especially in the final years of training. These exams not only examine knowledge but focus on other key elements such as communication skills, empathy, quick thinking and adaptability.

This textbook aims to equip you with the comprehensive knowledge to ace these exams. Together with our mark scheme book (*Unofficial Guide to Passing OSCEs: Candidate Briefings, Patient Briefings and Mark Schemes*), our goal is to provide you with as much exposure to OSCE topics as we can, providing useful tips along the way. Written by a range of authors from medical students, fresh graduates to established doctors, we hope this book empowers you in your preparation for your OSCEs.

This chapter outlines general hints and tips for before, during and after your OSCE. We also discuss sitting OSCE exams in the midst of a global pandemic.

PREPARING FOR YOUR OSCES

- Revise in a group. You can try to set a fixed date and time for which a group of people can get together to do OSCE revision. This can be 2 h in the evening or a lunchtime during the weekend. If there is a definitive date, then it is more likely to happen, and people are less likely to procrastinate.
- Practise stations that are already written and can be accessible online or in books, e.g. our *Candidate Briefing, Patient Briefing and Mark Scheme* book. However, if you have the time, try writing your own OSCE stations along with the mark scheme. This allows you to put yourself in the shoes of an examiner and you realise what can easily be tested and what may be more difficult to assess.
- Choose the people you practise with. It is good for you to practise with other medics as they will know what is expected of you and can give you tips on how to improve. Practising with non-medic friends is also helpful, especially for communication skill stations, because you need to ensure that you do not use medical jargon and speak clearly and succinctly.
- When you are practising, remember to set a timer for the length of time that the station will last in the real examination. This gives you an impression of how long you spend on various sections and will help you improve your time management. Even if the alarm rings when the time is up, continue with what you had in mind so that you can get an idea of how much longer you would have needed.

- Speak to your senior colleagues about their experience. They would have had their OSCEs very recently so their advice is likely to be specific to you and can give you valuable insight, especially if this is your first OSCE.
- When you want to brush up on your clinical skills, visit your university's clinical skills laboratory. This can usually be self-booked so that you have a time slot during which you can practise skills on mannequins; for example, venepuncture, cannulation.
- Take time during your placements to get used to using common medical equipment. You don't want to be using a tendon hammer or tuning fork for the first time during an OSCE examination!
- When you are on placement, practise taking histories from real patients and then present back to a clinician who can give feedback. Though this can be daunting at first, the more you do it, the better you become and your summary at the end of an OSCE station will also come across as more concise.
- There's a wide variety of resources that you can use to prepare for OSCEs, including: OSCE books, YouTube videos, flashcards and question banks. See what works for you.
- When you have prepared a lot, then you have a general expectation of the day and can hopefully reduce any exam nervousness which would directly impact on your performance.

DURING THE OSCES

- Dress as if you are going into placement; therefore general rules apply. For example, be bare below the elbow and wear your identity badge.
- Act confidently. It makes the patient feel less anxious and gives the impression to the examiner that you are in control.
- When you walk into the station, be sure to look around the room and table for any equipment that may have been left out for you. This can give you helpful reminders and prompts as to what you may need to use.
- Wash your hands at least before and after every station.
- Always introduce yourself to the patient, including your name, role and why you are here today.

- Confirm the patient's identity at the beginning and gain consent before proceeding to do anything.
- Smile! A smile can go a long way.
- If an examiner asks you to re-read the instructions, do so. It may be that you had misread them and are performing the wrong task.
- Don't lie. If you don't know an answer to a question that the patient or the examiner asks, then admit that you don't know but that you will try and find out. Treat it as you would do in real life so if in reality you would consult a senior, then do that in an OSCE station as well. It is vital that you show that you will be a safe doctor.
- Listen. Give your patient that 'golden minute' for them to speak and express all that they want to. If they stop talking, ask another open question; for example, 'Can you tell me a bit more about that?'
- Don't be put off if the examiner looks unimpressed. They are meant to be impartial and not expose themselves too much.
- If you have made a mistake, don't panic. Continue with the station and try to score as many points elsewhere as you can.
- ICE. Explore the patient's *ideas*, *concerns* and *expectations*. These communication skills can get you many points and if you have a blank moment or run out of questions during a history, this gives you some good discussion points as well as showing empathy.
- Be organised and manage your time effectively throughout.
- Do keep an open mind. Even if you think that you have got the correct diagnosis from the start, remember still to ask all other relevant questions to ensure that important differentials have been safely ruled out. It is more important to show your systematic thinking rather than to get the correct diagnosis.
- Thank the patient for their time at the end of the station.
- If you have time to spare at the end of your station, think about whether you may have missed something or would like to add more. It's not too late to mention it now.
- Do it your way. Use a structure or format that you are comfortable with. Everyone will have their own ways of doing something and a cardiovascular examination can be done in 20 different ways.
- Know your structure to history taking, especially for the different specialties; for example, psychiatry, obstetrics and gynaecology, paediatrics.
- Explain what you are doing in a physical examination station as you go along. Sometimes you may be blocking the examiner's view and if they can't see that you've done something – for example, looked at the fingernails for signs of clubbing – then they will assume that you haven't done so and you won't be rewarded the points.
- Work with the patient. If it is a paediatric patient, then you will need to adapt your mannerisms and language to make it easier for the child to understand.

AFTER THE OSCES

- Relax! The examination is over and now it's time for you to have your well-deserved rest.
- If you would like to, you can try and record what stations came up and review it later when you need to prepare for OSCEs again.
- It's down to the individual but some people find it useful to discuss the stations with their peers. This might help them to learn from mistakes, but don't dwell too much on what others have done as there is no single way of doing a station.
- If you write down the mistakes that you think you have made, then later you can reflect on these, especially if you know that similar topics will be retested in later years.

SITTING THE OSCE EXAM DURING A GLOBAL PANDEMIC

During the creation of this textbook we have sadly lived through the Covid-19 pandemic. This has altered the way that we practise medicine but also how learning, education and training are provided. Different countries and regions will adapt exams depending on local rules and restrictions; however, we hope to give you an overview of the ways that OSCE exams are to be adapted.

- More frequent OSCEs throughout the year: Increasing the frequency of OSCEs means that they can be smaller, limiting the number of students, staff and actors in any one place together.
- Virtual OSCEs: This method will remove examiners from the room and instead OSCEs will be recorded and watched by examiners. The actors will help in timekeeping and there will be timers at each station.
- Patient OSCEs: This method requires students to perform OSCEs whilst on clinical placement. The examiners will be their tutors on that placement.

Additionally, there will almost certainly be a requirement for everyone present at an OSCE station to wear a facemask. Wearing a facemask adds additional complexity to an OSCE station:

- Masks muffle the sound of your voice. It will be more important than ever to speak up and to speak clearly.
- They muffle the sound of the patient's voice. You will need to ensure that you listen to your patient very carefully.
- They reduce the ability for non-verbal communication. We communicate a lot with our faces. You

will need to make sure that you increase other ways of non-verbal communication, such as nodding or shaking your head and hand gesticulation.

- Consider the facemask when examining the patient. Many examinations require you to look inside the patient's mouth or nose. This may now be prohibited. If the station you are sitting requires this, state to the examiner, 'I would now like to examine the patient's mouth'. The examiner will let you know whether to proceed or not.

We appreciate that OSCEs are often the most stressful of the medical exams and we hope this book helps you to feel prepared to sit the exam with confidence. We wish you all the best in your upcoming examinations.

Contributors

Ali Abdaal
West Suffolk NHS Foundation Trust
United Kingdom

Steph Connaire, MBBCh
Cardiology Registrar, Wales
United Kingdom

Carys Flemming, MBChB, MRCP
GPST1, Crawley and East Surrey Hospital Programme
East Surrey Hospital, Redhill
United Kingdom

Ruth Harrison, MbChB, MRCPsych
Psychiatry Specialist Registrar
Avon and Wiltshire Mental Health Partnership NHS
    Trust
United Kingdom

Elewys Hearne, BMedSci, MBChB, MSc, FEBO
Severn Deanery
United Kingdom

Stacey Kelly, MB Bch BAO, BSc Hons
Institute of Pathology
Royal Victoria Hospital, Belfast
United Kingdom

**Selina Khan, MB, BSc (Hons), MSc, FRCOphth,
PGCert, ChB**
Bristol Eye Hospital
Lower Maudlin Street, Bristol
United Kingdom

Lisa Kirk, MBChB, MRCOG, PG Cert
Southmead Hospital, Bristol
United Kingdom

Louise Lynch
Medical Student
The University of Edinburgh
United Kingdom

Christopher Moseley, BM BSc (Hons) FACEM
Sir Charles Gairdner Hospital, Perth
Australia

**Emma Price, MBBS, MRCPH, MSc Health
Professional Ed**
Child Health, QEQM Hospital
East Kent Hospitals NHS Foundation Trust
United Kingdom

Ella Quintela, BMBS
Department of Anaesthesia
Sheffield Teaching Hospitals Trust;
School of Health and Related Research
University of Sheffield
United Kingdom

Contents

History Taking

Content Outline

Eliciting a history from a patient is an essential skill necessary for any doctor, regardless of specialty.

Taking a history is more than just working down a checklist of symptoms and, despite what you may interpret from textbooks, does not always need to be done in a set order. The doctors who are most effective in history taking often adapt their questioning so that it naturally follows the conversation with their patient.

It is important to remember that history taking is more than just information gathering. It involves two-way communication with the patient, in which active listening and non-verbal communication are key.

Study Action Plan

- Practise history taking in small groups
- Take turns to be the patient, doctor and assessor. Ask your colleagues to take the time to get into character and to think of a specific disease and how it might present. This is good clinical revision as well!
- Ask your assessor to provide constructive feedback and reflect on this feedback
- Work towards being observed by more experienced clinicians, whether in role play scenarios or on the wards with real patients
- If possible, go to acute medical admission wards. Ask to clerk patients and then discuss them with senior staff. This stimulates both a real-life role and the role you might expect an actor to take on in an OSCE

When in doubt or under stress, go back to the basics. The simple history-taking format and SOCRATES (site, onset, character, radiation, associated symptoms, timing, exacerbating and relieving factors, severity) should never be forgotten and always remember the importance of communication.

STATION 1.1: TIREDNESS

SCENARIO

You are a junior doctor in primary care and have been asked to see Yvonne Paisley, a 48-year-old woman, who has presented feeling tired all the time. She has noticed a significant amount of unintentional weight loss and her partner reports that she seems paler than usual. Additionally, she has felt some lumps in her neck. Please take a history from Mrs Paisley, present your findings and formulate an appropriate management plan.

Cardinal Symptoms

Weight loss
Night sweats
Reduced appetite
Pallor
Bleeding
Low mood
Daytime sleepiness
Polyuria or nocturia
Lymphadenopathy
Anaemia

HISTORY OF PRESENTING COMPLAINT

ANAEMIA FIG 1.1

- Tiredness: Especially on exertion, or at the end of the day
- Syncope: May feel light-headed or faint, especially on standing up or after exertion
- Breathlessness: A compensatory mechanism for reduced oxygen carriage in the blood
- Palpitations: These increase cardiac output and compensate for reduced total oxygen carriage
- Bleeding: Epistaxis, haematuria, blood blisters, gastrointestinal (GI) bleeding, excessive menorrhagia, bruising or petechiae
- Worsening of pre-existing ischaemic conditions: For example, angina or claudication. Commonly, anaemia can have an additive effect on ischaemic conditions, as it further reduces delivery of oxygen to tissues. This means angina will be symptomatic on less exertion than without anaemia

WEIGHT LOSS

- Degree of weight loss: Quantify the exact amount of weight lost over a specified period of time or subjectively; for example, clothes seem to be looser compared to last year
- Intent: Intentional or unintentional weight loss, change in diet or appetite

NECK LUMPS

- Location: A central location could point to a thyroid goitre or a lymphoma
- When were they first noticed? Some neck lumps are congenital (for example, branchial cyst) whereas others are acquired (for example, lymphoma)
- Characteristic: Enlarging, tender, mobility.

TIREDNESS

- Clarification: Clarify what the patient means by 'tired'
- Onset: Particular events that happened at the time of onset
- Duration of symptoms: How long has the symptom been present?
- Pattern of tiredness: On exertion, in the morning, constant
- Exercise: Enquire about the patient's usual level of functioning
- Sleep patterns: Night shifts, frequent travel, early-morning wakening (suggestive of depression), daytime sleepiness (suggestive of sleep apnoea)

ASSOCIATED SYMPTOMS

Other symptoms to enquire about include:
- Fever
- Night sweats
- Malaise
- Depression

PAST MEDICAL AND SURGICAL HISTORY

In this scenario, it is also important to enquire about:
- General: Ask about any known medical conditions, relevant treatments and any hospital admission
- Vaccination history: Important as infections, for example, measles, may occur in unvaccinated populations
- Malignancy: Specifically, lymphoma is important, both in the personal and family history
- Infections: Recent illness, Epstein–Barr virus (EBV), cytomegalovirus (CMV) and risk factors for chronic infection; for example, tuberculosis (TB), human immunodeficiency virus (HIV) and hepatitis
- Chronic medical conditions: Diabetes mellitus, hypothyroidism
- Psychiatric history: Low mood, depression, anxiety

MEDICATION HISTORY

Enquire about prescribed medications (including any recent changes) and over-the-counter medications. Allergies should be included, with the specific reaction noted. In this scenario be aware of medications that:
- Increase bleeding risk: Warfarin, direct oral anticoagulants (DOACs)
- Cause bone marrow failure: Chemotherapy
- Cause tiredness as a side effect: Antihistamines, codeine, tramadol, opiates

SOCIAL HISTORY

Social history includes enquiring about occupation, residence, lifestyle (diet, exercise, smoking, alcohol, substance abuse) and recent travel. Additionally in this scenario, consider:
- Smoking: Document pack years, calculated as the number of packs per day multiplied by the number of years smoked
- Alcohol and illicit drug use: Document units of alcohol consumed per week. Alcohol may be the cause of symptoms or may give a clue to diagnosis; for example, liver disease, depression
- Exercise: Establish baseline level of functioning and effect of tiredness on activities of daily living (ADL)
- Occupation: Ask about shift work, long working hours
- Recent travel abroad: Consider tropical infection
- Risk assessment for HIV and other blood-borne viruses: Ask about sexual history, intravenous (IV) drug use, tattoos or piercings and blood transfusions

FAMILY HISTORY

Many chronic diseases run in families and may account for the presenting features above. Ask about any significant family history, including:
- Malignancy

- Diabetes
- Thyroid disorders
- Coeliac disease

SYSTEMS REVIEW

On systems review, particularly pertinent questions to the above case may include questions regarding:

- Fever: Relating to infection and malignancy
- Jaundice or itching: Relating to liver disease
- Bone pain: There may be a primary or secondary bone malignancy
- Anaemia: Pallor, light-headedness, palpitations, breathlessness, worsening of pre-existing ischaemic conditions, bleeding
- Cardiorespiratory: Snoring, apnoeic episodes and excessive daytime sleepiness or sleep apnoea, chronic cough at night (seen in asthma), peripheral oedema, orthopnoea, paroxysmal nocturnal dyspnoea (seen in cardiac failure)
- GI: Jaundice, itching, diarrhoea, GI bleeding
- Diabetes: Polyuria, nocturia
- Psychiatric: Low mood, early-morning wakening, anhedonia, anxiety, stress

Risk Factors for Lymphoma

HODGKIN LYMPHOMA	NON-HODGKIN LYMPHOMA
HIV	Age
EBV	Immunodeficiency
	Exposure to certain chemicals
	Autoimmune disease
	EBV

Differential Diagnosis

DISEASE	CLINICAL PRESENTATION	INVESTIGATIONS	MANAGEMENT
Lymphoma	• Lymphadenopathy, which may be painful or painless • Weight loss • Night sweats	• Full blood count (FBCs) • Blood film • Chest X-ray (CXR) • Ultrasound of neck • Lymph node biopsy	• Chemotherapy (mostly)
Infectious mononucleosis	• Fever • Pharyngitis • Lymphadenopathy	• Monospot blood test	• No specific treatment required
Anaemia of chronic disease	• Insidious onset • Fatigue • Pallor • Shortness of breath	• FBCs • Blood film • Further investigations depend on the underlying disease	• Symptomatic management of anaemia • Treating the underlying disease; for example, malignancy
Diabetes	• Polyuria • Polydipsia • Fatigue • Recurrent infections	• Blood glucose • Haemoglobin A_{1c} (HbA$_{1c}$)	• Education • Lifestyle advice: Diet and exercise • Oral hypoglycaemic agents • Insulin
Obstructive sleep apnoea	• Snoring and apnoeic episodes • Unrefreshing sleep • Excessive daytime sleepiness	• Sleep studies	• Weight loss • Smoking cessation • Avoid alcohol and sedatives • Continuous positive airways pressure (CPAP) mask
Depression	• Low mood • Anhedonia • Loss of appetite • Sleep disturbance	• Consider thyroid function tests (TFTs)	• Psychosocial interventions • Antidepressants
Chronic fatigue syndrome	• Unexplained persistent fatigue not explained by other conditions	• Investigations to rule out other causes	• Support and reassurance • Avoid exacerbating factors • Regular graded exercise • Rehabilitation programmes • Medications; for example, amitriptyline, selective serotonin reuptake inhibitors (SSRIs)

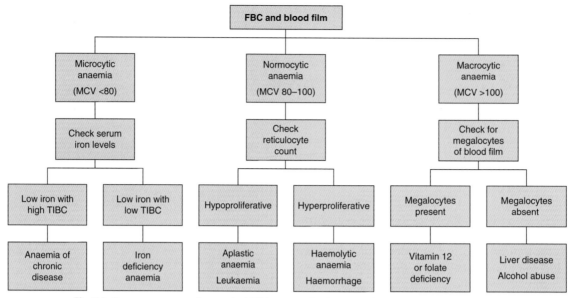

Fig. 1.1 Common causes of anaemia. MCV, mean cell volume; TIBC, total iron-binding capacity.

 Present Your Findings

Mrs Paisley is a 48-year-old woman who has presented with feeling tired all the time, weight loss, pallor and neck lumps. These symptoms are also associated with severe, drenching night sweats. Mrs Paisley is normally fit and well with no significant past medical history or family history.

The most likely diagnosis is lymphoma, with possible differential diagnoses of infectious mononucleosis or anaemia.

I would like to examine Mrs Paisley fully and request further investigations, including: FBCs, urea and electrolytes (U&Es), coagulations screen, lactate dehydrogenase, blood film, a CXR and an ultrasound of her neck.

QUESTIONS AND ANSWERS FOR CANDIDATE

How is a lymph node biopsy performed?
There are several ways to perform a lymph node biopsy. The underlying diagnosis and location of the lymph node often dictate the method used. These include:
- Open biopsy, under local or general anaesthetic
- Sentinal node biopsy, using a radioactive tracer to detect the sentinel node
- Needle biopsy

What are the possible neurological complications of infectious mononucleosis?
- Bell's palsy
- Encephalitis or viral meningitis
- Guillain–Barré syndrome

Give three common causes of a normocytic anaemia.
- Renal failure
- Bone marrow failure
- Chronic inflammation

A Case to Learn From

We had an elderly woman who was admitted confused, and we were not able to take a full history from her. Her routine admission bloods showed she was anaemic. It was not until we requested a blood film that she was diagnosed with a haematological malignancy. Always check the blood film in an anaemic patient.

Top Tip

When presented with a patient who has a lump, it is vital to examine the whole lymphoreticular system and not just the area the patient is concerned about.

STATION 1.2: WEIGHT LOSS

SCENARIO

You are a junior doctor in primary care and have been asked to see Aysha Patel, a 64-year-old woman, who has presented with weight loss. She has lost 13 kg over the last 6 weeks and is very concerned by this. She has a history of hypertension, angina and gastro-oesophageal reflux disease (GORD). Please take a history from Mrs Patel, present your findings and formulate an appropriate management plan.

> **🏃 Cardinal Symptoms**
>
> Loss of appetite
> Fever
> Dysphagia
> Change in bowel habit
> Cough
> Breathlessness
> Polydipsia or polyuria

HISTORY OF PRESENTING COMPLAINT

WEIGHT LOSS

- Quantify: Amount of weight loss and the period of time it was lost over
- Cause: Intentional or unintentional
- Diet: Number, size and content of meals, snacks and fluid intake (Table 1.1)

ASSOCIATED SYMPTOMS

Other symptoms to enquire about include:
- Fever
- Night sweats
- Malaise
- Fatigue

PAST MEDICAL AND SURGICAL HISTORY

- Any chronic medical conditions; for example:
  - Heart failure
  - Chronic obstructive pulmonary disease (COPD)
  - Chronic kidney disease
  - Inflammatory bowel disease
  - Rheumatoid arthritis
  - Diabetes
  - Chronic pancreatitis
  - Coeliac disease
  - HIV
- Previous surgeries; for example, GI surgery may lead to malabsorption

MEDICATION HISTORY

Enquire about prescribed medications (including any recent changes) and over-the-counter medications. Allergies should be included, with the specific reaction noted. In this scenario it is also important to note:

- Appetite suppressants: Metformin, antidepressants, levodopa, theophylline, digoxin
- Dry mouth: Anticholinergics
- Nausea: Antidepressants, digoxin, metformin, antibiotics
- Dysphagia: Non-steroidal anti-inflammatory drugs (NSAIDs), bisphosphonates
- Laxatives: For example, senna or lactulose

SOCIAL HISTORY

Social history includes enquiring about occupation, residence, lifestyle (diet, exercise, smoking, alcohol, substance abuse) and recent travel. Additionally in this scenario, consider:

- Smoking: Document pack years, calculated as the number of packs per day multiplied by the number of years smoked
- Alcohol and illicit drug use: Units of alcohol consumed per week, use of illicit drugs; for example, cocaine and amphetamines
- Diet: Nutritional intake and any changes in diet to account for weight loss
- Exercise: Enquire about level of physical activity and whether this has changed
- Recent travel abroad: Tropical infections and chronic GI infections; for example, *Giardia*

FAMILY HISTORY

Enquire about any significant family history, including:

- Malignancy
- Infections; for example, TB

SYSTEMS REVIEW

On systems review, particularly pertinent questions to the above case may include:
- GI: Nausea and vomiting, early satiety, dysphagia, abdominal pain, change in bowel habit, bleeding per rectum (PR), poor appetite
- Respiratory: Cough, breathlessness, haemoptysis, chest pain
- Endocrine: Polyuria and polydipsia, symptoms of hyperthyroidism; for example, heat intolerance, palpitations and tremor

> **⚠ Risk Factors for Colorectal Cancer**
>
> - Increased age
> - Chronic inflammatory bowel disease
> - Diabetes
> - Family history
> - History of polyps
> - Obesity
> - Diet; for example, excess consumption of red and processed meat

Differential Diagnosis

DISEASE	CLINICAL PRESENTATION	INVESTIGATIONS	MANAGEMENT
Malabsorption	• Weight loss • Fatigue • Steatorrhoea • Anaemia	• FBCs • U&Es • Liver function tests (LFTs) • Amylase • C-reactive protein (CRP) • Anti-tissue transglutaminase (TTG) antibody or endomysial antibodies	• Management dependent on cause; for example, gluten-free diet in coeliac disease, Creon for pancreatitis • Refer to dietician
HIV	• Fever • Fatigue • Lymphadenopathy • Opportunistic infections in acquired immune deficiency syndrome (AIDS)	• HIV blood test or point-of-care test (POCT)	• Antiretroviral drugs
Tuberculosis	• Fever • Night sweats • Anorexia • Cough • Haemoptysis • Erythema nodosum	• Sputum culture (acid-fast bacilli) • CXR • Tuberculin test	• Medications, including rifampicin, isoniazid, pyrazinamide and ethambutol
Diabetes	• Polyuria • Polydipsia • Fatigue • Recurrent infections	• Blood glucose • HbA$_{1c}$	• Education • Diet and exercise • Oral hypoglycaemic agents • Insulin
Hyperthyroidism	• Weight loss • Tremor • Palpitations • Heat intolerance • Menstrual disturbance	• TFTs	• Beta-blockers • Carbimazole • Radioactive iodine • Thyroidectomy
Anorexia nervosa	• Body mass index (BMI) <17.5 • Intense fear of gaining weight • Restricted diet	• Electrolytes	• Support and information • Refer to specialist eating disorders clinic or mental health team
Depression	• Low mood • Anhedonia • Loss of appetite • Sleep disturbance	• Dependent on associated symptoms, e.g. TFTs	• Psychosocial interventions • Antidepressants
Malignancy	• Weight loss • Cachexia • Fatigue • Symptoms dependent on site	• FBCs • U&Es • LFTs • Bone profile • Tumour markers • Staging computed tomography (CT) scan	• Surgery • Chemotherapy • Radiotherapy • Palliative care

Table 1.1   **Differential diagnosis for weight loss with reduced and preserved appetites**

WEIGHT LOSS WITH REDUCED APPETITE	WEIGHT LOSS WITH PRESERVED APPETITE
• Malignancy • GI disease • Oesophageal disease • Severe cardiac or respiratory failure • Any chronic inflammatory disease • HIV	• Diabetes mellitus • Hyperthyroidism • Malabsorption • Phaeochromocytoma

Present Your Findings

Mrs Patel is a 64-year-old woman who has presented with 13 kg weight loss over a period of 6 weeks. This is associated with a loss of appetite, general malaise and a change in bowel habit with diarrhoea. There is no history of fever or other infective symptoms. She has a past medical history of hypertension, angina and gastro-oesophageal reflux. There is no significant smoking or alcohol history and she has not travelled abroad recently.

I feel the most likely diagnosis is colorectal cancer, with differentials being malabsorption or hyperthyroidism.

I would like to examine Mrs Patel fully and request bloods, including FBCs, U&Es, LFTs, CRP and TFTs. Given Mrs Patel's age and 6-week history of loose stools, I would like to investigate further for a possible colorectal malignancy with a colonoscopy.

? QUESTIONS AND ANSWERS FOR CANDIDATE

What are the clinical features of anorexia nervosa?
- Body weight <85% of expected or BMI <17.5
- Intense fear of gaining weight
- Restricted calorie intake
- Often a misperception of body shape
- Women may have amenorrhoea

How might a patient with a new diagnosis of diabetes mellitus present?
- Ketoacidosis or hyperosmolar non-ketotic coma
- Weight loss
- Polydipsia and polyuria
- Recurrent infections
- Complications; for example, neuropathy, nephropathy or retinopathy

What is the definition of significant unintentional weight loss?
- Unintentional weight loss of more than 5% of body weight over a period of 12 months

A Case to Learn From

I saw a 55-year-old man who presented with significant unintentional weight loss. There were no other red-flag symptoms and initial investigations were normal. I took a further detailed history, asking specifically about diet and nutritional intake. This revealed that the patient, in fact, had a very poor diet, consisting largely of cereal and crackers, but he didn't identify this as an issue. I provided further information of healthy eating and education and offered a follow-up appointment to monitor progress. It is often important to gain more information on a patient's lifestyle and to educate and empower patients to take responsibility for their own health.

 Top Tip

Weight loss in the elderly should not be ignored. It can be caused by both underlying medical pathology and social factors such as social isolation and poor mobility, leading to difficulty shopping and cooking.

STATION 1.3: CHEST PAIN

SCENARIO

You are a junior doctor working in the emergency department (ED) and you have been asked to see Amy Jones. She is a 60-year-old woman who presented with a 2-h history of central chest pain, shortness of breath and sweating. Please take a history, present your findings and formulate an appropriate management plan.

Cardinal Symptoms

Chest pain
Breathlessness
Nausea and vomiting
Sweatiness or clamminess
Palpitations
Syncope or pre-syncope
Cough

HISTORY OF PRESENTING COMPLAINT

PAIN

When a patient presents with pain, you can use the acronym SOCRATES to remember the questions that you should ask:
- *Site*: Central, retrosternal or left-sided pain is typical of cardiac pain
- *Onset*: Sudden or gradual
- *Character*: For example, heavy, crushing, tearing, pleuritic or burning
- *Radiation*: Determine the location of radiation; for example, to the jaw, arm or back
- *Associated symptoms*: See below
- *Timing*: Duration of symptom, for current and any previous episodes
- *Exacerbating and relieving factors*: Whether it is exacerbated by exertion, deep inspiration, movement, eating, position. Whether it is relieved by rest, glyceryl trinitrate (GTN) spray, antacids, simple analgesics, bronchodilators
- *Severity*: Score out of 10

ASSOCIATED SYMPTOMS

Other symptoms to enquire about include:
- Cardiac:
  - Ischaemia: Nausea and vomiting, sweating, pallor, breathlessness
  - Arrhythmias: Palpitations, dizziness, syncope
  - Heart failure: Paroxysmal nocturnal dyspnoea (PND), orthopnoea, peripheral oedema
- Constitutional: Fever, malaise, weight loss

PAST MEDICAL AND SURGICAL HISTORY

In this scenario, it is also important to enquire about:
- Cardiovascular risk factors:
  - Previous myocardial infarction (MI) (and any previous cardiac procedures)
  - Hypertension
  - Hypercholesterolaemia
  - Diabetes mellitus
  - Peripheral vascular disease
  - Stroke
- Respiratory risk factors:
  - Asthma or COPD
  - Previous pneumothorax
- GI risk factors:
  - Peptic ulcer disease

MEDICATION HISTORY

Enquire about prescribed medications (including any recent changes) and over-the-counter medications. Allergies should be included, with the specific reaction noted. In this scenario it is also important to note:
- Cardiovascular medications: For example, angiotensin-converting enzyme inhibitors (ACEi), beta-blockers and GTN spray
- GI medications: Antacids, NSAIDs, steroids indicated in gastritis, peptic ulcer disease
- Respiratory medications: Bronchodilators
- Oral contraceptive use: Increases thromboembolic risk

SOCIAL HISTORY

Social history includes enquiring about occupation, residence, lifestyle (diet, exercise, smoking, alcohol, substance abuse) and recent travel. Additionally in this scenario, consider:
- Smoking: Document pack years, calculated as the number of packs per day multiplied by the number of years smoked
- Alcohol and illicit drug use: Calculate weekly units
- Diet and exercise: An unhealthy diet and physical inactivity are risk factors for ischaemic heart disease

- Occupation: For example, heavy goods vehicle (HGV) driver, airline pilot

FAMILY HISTORY

Ask about any significant family history, including:
- Ischaemic heart disease
- Thrombophilia

SYSTEMS REVIEW

On systems review, particularly pertinent questions to the above case may include questions regarding:
- Respiratory:
  - Pneumonia: Cough, sputum, fever
  - Pulmonary embolism (PE): Haemoptysis, calf pain and swelling
  - Asthma or COPD: Wheeze
- GI:
  - GORD: Heartburn, acid regurgitation
  - Peptic ulcer disease: Epigastric pain, haematemesis, melaena
- Trauma:
  - Any recent chest trauma

Risk Factors for Acute Coronary Syndrome (ACS)

- Hypertension
- Smoking
- Previous MI (Table 1.2)
- Diabetes
- Obesity
- Increased age
- Hypercholesterolaemia

Table 1.2   Details on the artery and ECG leads affected by different types of MI

	ARTERY	ECG LEADS
Inferior MI	Right coronary	II, III, aVF
Anteroseptal MI	Left anterior descending	V1–V4
Anterolateral MI	Left anterior descending or left circumflex	V4–V5, I, aVL
Lateral MI	Left circumflex	I, aVL, V5–V6
Posterior MI	Left circumflex or right coronary	Dominant R wave in V1–V2, ST depression

Differential Diagnosis

DISEASE	CLINICAL PRESENTATION	INVESTIGATIONS	MANAGEMENT
ACS	• Central chest pain • Pain radiating to jaw/left arm • Nausea • Sweating • Breathlessness • Symptoms last >20 min	• Electrocardiogram (ECG) • Cardiac markers, i.e. troponin	• Oxygen • Morphine • Antiemetic • Aspirin and clopidogrel/ ticagrel /prasugrel or • Urgent percutaneous coronary intervention (PCI) or • Thrombolysis if ST elevation MI (STEMI)
Angina	• Chest pain on exertion • Pain radiating to the jaw or left arm • Symptoms typically last < 20 min • Symptoms are relieved by rest or GTN spray	• ECG • Cardiac markers, i.e. troponin	• Rest • GTN spray
Aortic dissection	• Sudden, severe, tearing interscapular pain	• ECG • CXR • CT angiography or conventional angiography	• Oxygen • IV access and cross-match 6 units of red cells • Analgesia • Urgent vascular review
Pericarditis	• Pleuritic chest pain • Relieved by sitting forwards	• FBCs • U&Es • CRP • Troponin • ECG • CXR • Echocardiogram	• NSAIDs
PE	• Breathlessness • Pleuritic chest pain • Haemoptysis • Venous thromboembolic (VTE) risk factors	• FBCs • U&Es • D-dimer • Arterial blood gas (ABG) • ECG • CXR • CT pulmonary angiography (CTPA)	• Oxygen • Anticoagulation
Pneumonia	• Productive cough • Pleuritic chest pain • Breathlessness • Fever	• FBCs • CRP • U&Es • Blood cultures • Sputum microscopy, culture and sensitivity (MC&S) • Legionella and pneumococcal antigens • CXR	• Oxygen • Antibiotics
Pneumothorax	• Pleuritic chest pain • Breathlessness • May have a history of trauma	• CXR	• Oxygen • Chest drain or aspiration
Oesophageal reflux or spasm	• Burning retrosternal discomfort • Worse on lying down and after certain foods • Waterbrash, acid reflux	• FBCs • U&Es • Troponin • ECG • CXR	• Avoid precipitants; for example, spicy food • Antacids for reflux • Muscle relaxants for spasm; for example, nifedipine
Musculoskeletal chest pain	• Pain worse on palpation or movement • May be pleuritic	• FBCs • U&Es • Troponin • ECG • CXR	• Reassurance • Analgesia

Present Your Findings

Mrs Jones is a 60-year-old woman with a background of hypertension and diabetes, who presented with a 2-h history of central chest pain. She describes the pain as crushing in nature and radiating to her jaw. It was associated with nausea, sweating and breathlessness and not relieved by GTN spray.

I think that the most likely diagnosis would be ACS with a differential diagnosis of GORD.

I would like to get an ECG urgently and take bloods, including troponin. If there are ECG changes or a raised troponin level, I would ensure that the patient receives the appropriate management for ACS, including oxygen, 300 mg aspirin, 300 mg clopidogrel, analgesia, antiemetics and GTN spray and refer to cardiology. If the ECG shows ST elevation, I would contact cardiology urgently for primary percutaneous coronary intervention.

❓ QUESTIONS AND ANSWERS FOR CANDIDATE

What are the indications for PCI or thrombolysis?
- PCI is the treatment of choice in a STEMI. However, if PCI cannot be performed within 120 min of first medical contact and there are no contraindications, thrombolysis is an alternative. Thrombolysis is not indicated in patients with symptoms for over 12 h
- The indications for PCI or thrombolysis are any one of the following:
  - ST elevation of >1 mm in two limb leads
  - ST elevation of ≥ 2 mm in two or more contiguous chest leads
  - Left bundle branch block (LBBB) in the presence of a typical history of acute MI

Name three complications that can occur after an MI.
- Arrhythmias
- Heart failure
- Mitral regurgitation (secondary to papillary muscle dysfunction or chordal or papillary muscle rupture)
- Ventricular septal defect
- Dressler's syndrome
- Left ventricular aneurysm

What is the pathogenesis of atherosclerosis?
- Endothelial dysfunction leads to the accumulation of oxidised lipoproteins which are taken up by macrophages to form foam cells. This can be seen on the endothelium as a 'fatty streak'
- Release of cytokines leads to further accumulation of macrophages and smooth-muscle cell migration and proliferation
- Collagen is produced by the smooth muscle and this results in the formation of a fibrolipid plaque

- This plaque may grow slowly, causing a narrowing of the coronary vessel, or may undergo thrombosis and cause obstruction

A Case to Learn From

A 60-year-old woman presented to the ED feeling generally unwell. She looked pale and clammy. She had type 2 diabetes and had started nitrofurantoin 2 days previously for a urinary tract infection. She was initially treated for presumed urosepsis; however, her ECG showed ST depression. Her troponin level came back at > 4000 ng/mL and her white cell count and CRP were not significantly raised. She was subsequently commenced on treatment for ACS and referred to cardiology. It is important to remember that not all patients with ACS have chest pain, particularly elderly patients, women and those with diabetes (or any other disease associated with neuropathy).

Top Tip

Do not be falsely reassured by a normal ECG and examination. The ECG may be normal in patients with cardiac chest pain, particularly in unstable angina.

STATION 1.4: PALPITATIONS

SCENARIO

You are a junior doctor working in the ED and are asked to see Jane Porter, a 29-year-old woman, who has presented with palpitations. She has had a number of previous similar episodes, lasting a few minutes each time. Please take a history from Miss Porter, present your findings and formulate an appropriate management plan.

🏃 Cardinal Symptoms

Breathlessness
Chest pain
Syncope

HISTORY OF PRESENTING COMPLAINT

PALPITATIONS
- Onset: Sudden or gradual; ask the patient what she was doing at the time of onset
- Frequency: Given as number of occurrences over a specified time range; for example, a day or week
- Duration of episode: The average length of an episode so far and the longest
- Character: Fast or slow, regular or irregular, sensation that the heart has momentarily stopped
- Exacerbating factors: Caffeine, alcohol, prescribed medication, illicit drugs, anxiety

- Termination: Spontaneous, with exercise, Valsalva manoeuvre

ASSOCIATED SYMPTOMS

Other symptoms to enquire about include:
- Breathlessness
- Light-headedness
- Syncope
- Chest pain
- Constitutional symptoms; for example, fever, night sweats, malaise, weight loss

PAST MEDICAL AND SURGICAL HISTORY

In this scenario, it is also important to enquire about:
- Cardiovascular risk factors:
  - Previous MI (and any previous cardiac procedures)
  - Hypertension
  - Hypercholesterolaemia
  - Diabetes mellitus
  - Peripheral vascular disease
  - Stroke
- Acute illnesses; for example, pneumonia.
- Known cardiovascular disease; for example, previous MI, arrhythmias, structural heart disease
- Hyperthyroidism or hypothyroidism
- Anxiety

MEDICATION HISTORY

Enquire about prescribed medications (including any recent changes) and over-the-counter medications. Allergies should be included, with the specific reaction noted. In this scenario it is also important to note:
- Beta agonists: Arrhythmias are known side effects
- Levothyroxine: Arrhythmias are known side effects
- Antiarrhythmics: If given too much, they can have the opposite effect and induce arrhythmias
- Theophylline: Arrhythmias are known side effects

- Drugs that can prolong QT interval: For example, antipsychotics, antidepressants, macrolide antibiotics

SOCIAL HISTORY

Social history includes enquiring about occupation, residence, lifestyle (diet, exercise, smoking, alcohol, substance abuse) and recent travel. Additionally in this scenario, consider:
- Smoking: Document pack years, calculated as the number of packs per day multiplied by the number of years smoked
- Alcohol and illicit drug use: Document units of alcohol consumed per week, any use of cocaine, amphetamines
- Diet: Caffeine consumption
- Occupation: Type of tasks carried out at work, specifically anything strenuous

FAMILY HISTORY

Ask about any significant family history, including:
- Cardiovascular disease: Ischaemic heart disease, congenital heart disease, hypertrophic cardiomyopathy, long QT syndrome
- Sudden death: Especially if at a young age, < 50 years old

SYSTEMS REVIEW

On systems review, particularly pertinent questions to the above case may include questions regarding:
- Endocrine: Increased heat intolerance, tremor, weight loss, loose stools and diarrhoea

Risk Factors for Supraventricular Tachycardia (SVT)

- Congenital heart disease
- Coronary artery disease
- Problems with thyroid glands
- Smoking
- Illicit drugs; for example, cocaine

Differential Diagnosis

DISEASE	CLINICAL PRESENTATION	INVESTIGATIONS	MANAGEMENT
Atrial fibrillation	• Palpitations • Breathlessness • Light-headedness • ± Chest pain	• FBCs • U&Es • TFTs • Magnesium • Calcium • CRP • ± D-dimer • Troponin • ECG • CXR • Echo	• Direct-current (DC) cardioversion if haemodynamically compromised • Treatment of precipitant • Rate control • Rhythm control • Anticoagulation
SVT	• Palpitations • Breathlessness • Light-headedness • ± Chest pain	• ECG	• Vagal manoeuvres • Adenosine

Continued

🏠 Differential Diagnosis—cont'd

DISEASE	CLINICAL PRESENTATION	INVESTIGATIONS	MANAGEMENT
Ventricular tachycardia (VT)	• Palpitations • Breathlessness • Light-headedness • ± Chest pain • Cardiac arrest	• U&Es • Magnesium • Calcium • ECG	• DC cardioversion if haemodynamically compromised • Amiodarone • Pulseless VT: • Call the arrest team!
Complete heart block	• Palpitations • Breathlessness • Light-headedness • ± Chest pain	• FBCs • U&Es • TFTs • Magnesium • Calcium • ECG	• Acute treatment: Atropine, consider external pacing • Chronic treatment: Pacemaker
Hyperthyroidism	• Weight loss • Tremor • Palpitations • Heat intolerance • Menstrual disturbance	• TFTs	• Beta-blockers • Carbimazole • Radioactive iodine • Thyroidectomy
Anxiety	• Palpitations • Breathlessness • Chest discomfort • Sweating • Light-headedness • Tremor	• TFTs	• Psychological therapies • Antidepressants

ADDITIONAL INFORMATION

CAUSES OF ATRIAL FIBRILLATION

The below causes can be remember using the acronym PIRATES:
- *Pulmonary* disease or *phaeochromocytoma*
- *Ischaemia*
- *Rheumatic* heart disease
- *Anaemia* or *atrial* myxoma or *acid*–base disturbance
- *Thyrotoxicosis*
- *Ethanol* or *electrolyte* disturbance or *endocarditis*
- *Sepsis* or *sympathomimetics*

🔍 Present Your Findings

Miss Porter is a 29-year-old woman who presented to the ED with palpitations. The palpitations were sudden-onset and were present for around 15 min. They felt fast and regular in character and were associated with shortness of breath and light-headedness. Jane has had three previous similar episodes, lasting around 5 min. She is otherwise fit and well and has no other significant past medical history. She does drink coffee and had had four cups of coffee today.

The most likely diagnosis is SVT, precipitated by caffeine.

I would like to examine Jane fully and request bloods, including electrolytes and a 12-lead ECG.

❓ QUESTIONS AND ANSWERS FOR CANDIDATE

How do you assess haemodynamic stability in a patient with an SVT?
- Check capillary refill centrally and peripherally
- Measure blood pressure (BP)
- Monitor levels of confusion and Glasgow Coma Scale (GCS)
- Keep on continuous monitoring

Describe the typical ECG changes of atrial fibrillation.
- Irregular narrow-complex tachycardia with no clear P waves

What is the mechanism of action of adenosine?
- Adenosine temporarily blocks electrical conduction through the atrioventricular node. This can both terminate re-entrant tachycardias and may unmask other arrhythmias such as atrial fibrillation

A Case to Learn From

While working in the ED I saw a 60-year-old female patient who presented with a 24-h history of palpitations. An ECG on presentation showed atrial fibrillation with a fast ventricular response. Further assessment revealed an underlying diagnosis of community-acquired pneumonia. The atrial fibrillation settled with treatment of the pneumonia. This is a reminder always to look for an underlying cause of new-onset atrial fibrillation.

Top Tip

Ask the patient to tap the pattern of their palpitations. This will help to determine characteristic features such as whether the palpitations are slow or fast, regular or irregular, or whether the patient is experiencing missed beats.

STATION 1.5: COUGH

SCENARIO

You are a junior doctor in primary care and have been asked to see Gerald Gordon, a 60-year-old man, who has presented with a 3-day history of a productive cough and has been finding it increasingly difficult to sleep and get around his house. He is a lifelong cigarette smoker. Please take a history from Mr Gordon, present your findings and formulate an appropriate management plan.

HISTORY OF PRESENTING COMPLAINT

 Cardinal Symptoms

Dry or productive cough
Chest pain
Breathlessness
Wheeze
Haemoptysis
Fever
Weight loss

COUGH

- Onset: Whether there was anything else going on when it started; for example, infection
- Duration: How long the cough has been present
- Productive or non-productive: If productive, describe the colour and consistency, whether there is any haemoptysis
- Pattern: For example, cough worse at night is often seen in asthma
- Exacerbating factors: For example, cold weather, exercise, dust

SLEEPING DIFFICULTY

- Duration: How long has the sleeping difficulty been going on?
- Frequency: Establish whether it happens every night or occasionally
- Stress: Find out if the patient is going through any personal stresses or difficulties

ASSOCIATED SYMPTOMS

Other symptoms to enquire about include:
- Weight loss
- Fever
- Night sweats

PAST MEDICAL AND SURGICAL HISTORY

In this scenario, it is also important to enquire about:
- Respiratory:
  - Asthma or COPD: Any previous hospital admissions or admissions to intensive therapy/treatment unit (ITU)
  - Childhood asthma, wheeze or bronchiolitis
  - Bronchiectasis
  - It can also be useful to find out whether the patient has had any previous respiratory investigations; for example, lung function tests, CT scans or allergen testing
- Malignancy
- Infections; for example, TB, pneumonia
- Thromboembolic disease
- Gastro-oesophageal reflux

MEDICATION HISTORY

Enquire about prescribed medications (including any recent changes) and over-the-counter medications. Allergies should be included, with the specific reaction noted. In this scenario it is also important to note:
- Use of inhalers: Compliance and inhaler technique
- Steroids: Number of courses in the last year
- ACEi: Cough is a side effect
- Aspirin and NSAIDs: May exacerbate asthma

SOCIAL HISTORY

Social history includes enquiring about occupation, residence, lifestyle (diet, exercise, smoking, alcohol, substance abuse) and recent travel. Additionally in this scenario, consider:
- Smoking: Document pack years, calculated as the number of packs per day multiplied by the number of years smoked
- Alcohol and illicit drug use: Calculate weekly units
- Exercise: Baseline functional status and exercise tolerance
- Recent travel: Could indicate atypical infections and long-haul flights are a risk factor for PE
- Occupation: For example, asbestos exposure, coal mining, paint spraying, farming, baking
- Pets: For example, birds

FAMILY HISTORY

Ask about any significant family history, including:
- Atopy: Asthma, hay fever, eczema
- Venous thromboembolism
- Lung cancer
- Tuberculosis

SYSTEMS REVIEW

On systems review, particularly pertinent questions to the above case may include questions regarding:

🏠 Differential Diagnosis

DISEASE	CLINICAL PRESENTATION	INVESTIGATIONS	MANAGEMENT
Pneumonia	• Productive cough • Pleuritic chest pain • Shortness of breath • Fever	• FBCs • U&Es • LFTs • CRP • Blood cultures • Sputum MC&S • Legionella and pneumococcal antigens • CXR	• Oxygen • Antibiotics
Asthma	• Shortness of breath • Wheeze • Cough • Chest tightness	• Peak expiratory flow rate (PEFR) • FBCs • U&Es • CRP • ABG • CXR • Spirometry	• Oxygen • Salbutamol ± ipratropium nebulisers • Prednisolone or hydrocortisone • Aminophylline • Magnesium • Antibiotics (if infection)
COPD	• Shortness of breath • Cough • Chest tightness • Increased sputum production • Reduced exercise tolerance	• FBCs • CRP • U&Es • ABG • CXR • Sputum MC&S • Spirometry	• Oxygen (via a Venturi mask) • Salbutamol ± ipratropium nebulisers • Prednisolone or hydrocortisone • Antibiotics (if infection) • Aminophylline • Non-invasive ventilation (NIV)
Lung cancer	• Weight loss • Shortness of breath • Chest pain • Smoking history	• FBCs • CRP • U&Es • LFTs • Bone profile • CXR • CT thorax and abdomen	• Chemotherapy • Radiotherapy • Surgery
Interstitial pulmonary fibrosis	• Gradual onset • Exertional breathlessness • Chronic dry cough	• FBCs • CRP • U&Es • LFTs • Spirometry • CXR • High-resolution CT (HRCT) • Lung biopsy	• Oxygen • Pulmonary rehabilitation • Steroids in acute exacerbation • Antifibrotic agents • Lung transplantation
Postnasal drip	• Feeling of needing to clear the throat • Nasal congestion • History of upper respiratory tract infection	• Not usually required	• Nasal steroid spray • Antihistamines
Gastro-oesophageal reflux	• Cough worse on lying flat and after heavy meals • Dyspepsia	• Trial of treatment • 24-h pH monitoring • Oesophageal manometry	• Protein pump inhibitor; for example, omeprazole • H_2 antagonist; for example, ranitidine

• Constitutional: Weight loss, fever, night sweats
• Respiratory: Breathlessness, wheeze, chest pain, hoarse voice
• Nasal: Nasal discharge, congestion, 'dripping' sensation at the back of the throat
• GI: Retrosternal burning discomfort

Risk Factors for Lung Cancer

- Smoking
- Asbestos exposure
- Air pollution
- Radon gas exposure
- Increased age
- Other respiratory problems; for example, COPD, tuberculosis

ADDITIONAL INFORMATION

CATEGORISING COUGHS

Cough can be categorised according to duration:
- Acute: Less than 3 weeks
- Subacute: 3–8 weeks
- Chronic: More than 8 weeks: all patients with a chronic cough should have a CXR

 Present Your Findings

Mr Gordon is a 60-year-old man who presents with a 3-day history of a gradually worsening cough, productive of purulent sputum. He reports breathlessness at rest, wheeze and decreased exercise tolerance. Occasionally there is also haemoptysis. He has lost 3 kg in the last 2 months and is increasingly reliant on his wife for support with ADLs. He has a 50-pack year smoking history and was diagnosed with COPD 5 years ago.

I think that the most likely diagnosis would be malignancy, with differentials being acute exacerbation of COPD and community-acquired pneumonia.

I would like to perform a full physical examination and request bloods, an ECG, send a sputum sample, perform an ABG and get a CXR.

❓ QUESTIONS AND ANSWERS FOR CANDIDATE

How can you grade the severity of community-acquired pneumonia?

Using the CURB-65 score, one point is given for each of the following:
- *Confusion*
- *Urea* >7 mmol/L
- *Respiratory* rate >30 breaths/min
- *BP* <90 mmHg systolic or <60 mmHg diastolic
- *Age* >65

A higher score equates with a greater mortality.
- 0–1: Patient may be treated in the community
- 2: Admit to hospital
- 3–5: Assess for ITU admission

What are the common organisms causing community-acquired pneumonia?
- *Streptococcus pneumoniae*
- *Legionella pneumophila*
- *Staphylococcus aureus*
- *Influenza*
- *Mycoplasma pneumoniae*

What are the features of life-threatening asthma?
- PEFR <33%
- SaO_2 <92%
- PaO_2 <8 kPa
- Normal $PaCO_2$ (4.6–6 kPa)
- Silent chest
- Cyanosis
- Exhaustion
- Poor respiratory effort
- Hypotension
- Bradycardia

 A Case to Learn From

In the high dependency unit a patient was reviewed who had been admitted with a diagnosis of infective exacerbation of COPD. This was a new COPD diagnosis. Respiratory failure persisted despite the use of bilevel positive airway pressure (BiPAP). ITU were called for consideration of airway intubation. No one had recorded baseline functional status in the clerking. The patient was now too sick to find out and the team were unable to contact the next of kin. As the deterioration was caused by infection (which was likely reversible), good pre-morbid function would have provided further evidence for intubation. Without knowing baseline function, the decision was very difficult!

 Top Tip

It is important to take a detailed occupational history to determine if there are any potential triggers for the cough, such as exposure to fumes or dusts. Remember to ask about previous occupations too, not just the most current or most recent.

STATION 1.6: SHORTNESS OF BREATH

SCENARIO

You are a junior doctor on the acute medical ward and have been asked to see Sophie Stark, a 59-year-old woman, who was referred by her primary care doctor with a 3-day history of worsening shortness of breath (SOB). This is associated with a productive cough, wheeze and difficulty walking up the stairs. Please take a history from Mrs Stark, present your findings and formulate an appropriate management plan.

Cardinal Symptoms

Shortness of breath
Wheeze
Cough
Fever
Orthopnoea
PND
Chest pain
Palpitations
Reduced exercise tolerance

HISTORY OF PRESENTING COMPLAINT

SHORTNESS OF BREATH

- Duration: How long has the SOB has been present?
- Onset: Gradual or acute
- Character: Constant or intermittent
- Exercise: Baseline function and exercise tolerance compared to current
- Exacerbating and relieving factors: For example, worse on exertion, lying down, medications. Relieved by inhalers, rest, use of pillows to sit up at night

ASSOCIATED SYMPTOMS

Other symptoms to enquire about include:
- Fever
- Reduced appetite
- Weight loss
- Night sweats
- Cough
- Wheeze
- Pleuritic chest pain

PAST MEDICAL AND SURGICAL HISTORY

In this scenario, it is also important to enquire about:
- Respiratory disease:
  - Asthma
  - COPD
  - Other chronic respiratory diseases; for example, bronchiectasis and pulmonary fibrosis
- Cardiac disease:
  - Ischaemic heart disease
  - Heart failure
  - Arrhythmias
  - Valvular heart disease
  - Enquire about cardiovascular risk factors; for example, hypertension, high cholesterol and diabetes
- Risk factors for VTE:
  - Immobility
  - Recent surgery
  - Long-haul flight
  - Known thrombophilia
  - Previous history of VTE
  - Malignancy
  - Use of combined oral contraceptive pill

MEDICATION HISTORY

Enquire about prescribed medications (including any recent changes) and over-the-counter medications. Allergies should be included, with the specific reaction noted. In this scenario it is also important to note:
- Inhalers: Compliance and technique
- NSAIDs and beta-blockers: May exacerbate asthma
- Oral contraceptive use: Increased risk of PE
- Cardiac medications: For example, ACEi, beta-blockers and diuretics

SOCIAL HISTORY

Social history includes enquiring about occupation, residence, lifestyle (diet, exercise, smoking, alcohol, substance abuse) and recent travel. Additionally in this scenario, consider:
- Smoking: Document pack years, calculated as the number of packs per day multiplied by the number of years smoked
- Alcohol: Document units of alcohol consumed per week
- Occupation: Jobs worked across lifetime, particularly asking about exposure to smoke and asbestos. Enquire about occupational lung diseases, including occupational asthma, asbestosis, silicosis and coal worker's pneumoconiosis
- Travel: Particularly in the last 3 months
- Impact of symptoms on daily life: For example, on shopping, exercising, employment and associated mood
- Contact with infectious diseases: For example, TB, pneumonia
- Pets: Important in asthma and hypersensitivity pneumonitis

FAMILY HISTORY

Ask about any significant family history, including:
- Family history of atopy: Asthma, hay fever, eczema, food allergies
- Ischaemic heart disease
- Thrombophilia, increasing risk for PE
- Cystic fibrosis: Autosomal-recessive inheritance

SYSTEMS REVIEW

On systems review, particularly pertinent questions to the above case may include questions regarding:
- Cardiac: Orthopnoea, PND, chest pain, palpitations, leg swelling

Differential Diagnosis

DISEASE	CLINICAL PRESENTATION	INVESTIGATIONS	MANAGEMENT
Asthma	• SOB • Wheeze • Cough • Chest tightness	• PEFR • FBCs • CRPs • U&Es • ABG • CXR • Spirometry	• Oxygen • Salbutamol ± ipratropium nebulisers • Prednisolone or hydrocortisone • Aminophylline • Magnesium • Antibiotics (if infection)
COPD	• SOB • Cough • Chest tightness • Increased sputum production • Reduced exercise tolerance	• FBCs • CRP • U&Es • ABG • CXR • Sputum MC&S • Spirometry	• Controlled oxygen therapy • Salbutamol ± ipratropium nebulisers • Prednisolone or hydrocortisone • Antibiotics (if infection)
Acute heart failure	• SOB • Orthopnoea • PND • Frothy sputum • Peripheral oedema	• FBCs • U&Es • Troponin • ABG • ECG • CXR • Echocardiogram	• Oxygen • IV furosemide • Morphine • GTN spray or infusion if systolic BP >100 mmHg
Pneumonia	• Productive cough • Pleuritic chest pain • SOB • Fever	• FBCs • CRP • U&Es • Blood cultures • Sputum MC&S • CXR • Legionella and pneumococcal antigens	• Oxygen • IV fluids • Antibiotics
Pneumothorax	• SOB • Pleuritic chest pain	• FBCs • CRP • U&Es • ABG • CXR	Primary: • Monitor if small • Aspiration or chest drain if large Secondary: • Aspiration or chest drain
Pleural effusion	• SOB • Cough • Pleuritic chest pain	• FBCs • U&Es • CRP • LFTs • ABG • CXR • Pleural ultrasound and aspiration	• Depends on likely cause • Therapeutic aspiration or chest drain if large and causing compromise
PE	• SOB • Pleuritic chest pain • Haemoptysis	• D-dimer • CXR • CTPA	• Anticoagulation

Risk Factors for Pneumonia

- Children < 2 years old and adults > 65 years old
- Smoking
- Chronic disease; for example, COPD
- Immunosuppressed
- Recent visits to or stay in healthcare settings; for example, care homes, hospitals

ADDITIONAL INFORMATION

GRADING BREATHLESSNESS

The Medical Research Council (MRC) dyspnoea scale can be used to grade breathlessness in relation to exertion for patients with COPD (Table 1.3).

Table 1.3 MRC dyspnoea scale

SEVERITY	GRADE	IMPACT
Mild	1	Breathless only with strenuous exercise
Moderate	2	Breathless when hurrying on a flat surface or walking up an incline
	3	Has to walk slower than people of the same age or has to stop for breath when walking at own pace
Severe	4	Stops for breath after walking 100 m or after a few minutes of walking
	5	Too breathless to leave the house or breathless on (un)dressing

Present Your Findings

Mrs Stark is a 59-year-old woman with known COPD who has presented with a 3-day history of worsening shortness of breath associated with wheeze and a productive cough. She is usually able to walk up the stairs at home but has been struggling over the last few days due to her breathlessness. She lives at home with her husband and is usually independently mobile. She reports regular use of her inhalers and does not have home oxygen or home nebulisers. She is a smoker with a 50-pack year history.

I think that the most likely diagnosis would be an infective exacerbation of COPD with a differential diagnosis of community-acquired pneumonia.

I would like to examine Mrs Stark fully and request bloods, including FBCs, U&Es and CRP, and perform an ABG. I would also like to request a CXR, ensure adequate hydration and start broad-spectrum oral antibiotics.

❓ QUESTIONS AND ANSWERS FOR CANDIDATE

How would you manage an acute exacerbation of COPD?
- Controlled oxygen via Venturi mask, aiming for saturations of 88–92%
- Salbutamol nebuliser 2.5–5 mg ± ipratropium nebuliser 500 mcg 4–6-hourly (run with air, not oxygen)
- Prednisolone 30 mg or hydrocortisone 200 mg IV
- Antibiotics if infective exacerbation
- Chest physiotherapy
- If not improving with nebulisers, involve a senior and consider IV aminophylline infusion
- If there is worsening hypoxia or hypercapnia despite the above measures (pH ≤7.3, hypoxia, hypercapnia), involve a senior and consider NIV

How is COPD severity categorised?
Spirometry is used to predict severity:
- Stage 1 (mild): forced expiratory volume in 1 s (FEV_1) ≥80%
- Stage 2 (moderate): FEV_1 50–80% predicted
- Stage 3 (severe): FEV_1 30–49% predicted
- Stage 4 (very severe): FEV_1 ≤30% predicted

Name the two types of COPD.
- Bronchitis: Chronic inflammation of the airways (trachea, bronchi and bronchioles)
- Emphysema: Gradual destruction of the alveoli

🗨 A Case to Learn From

An elderly man presented to the ED with breathlessness and low oxygen saturations, with a known diagnosis of COPD. He was acutely put on high-flow oxygen to maintain his saturations ≥94%, but a repeat ABG was not done. He remained on high-flow oxygen for a long period of time, after which he became increasingly confused and drowsy. On doing an ABG it was found that, although his oxygenation had improved, he was retaining carbon dioxide. Be vigilant for signs of carbon dioxide retention in patients with COPD and monitor response to oxygen with an ABG. Remember that oxygen is a drug and should be prescribed appropriately.

💡 Top Tip

It is the duty of every doctor to highlight the importance of stopping smoking and signpost patients to appropriate services for nicotine replacement therapy or smoking cessation services. Stopping smoking at any age can give extra years of life and slows decline in lung function, as well as reducing risk to those around the patient, including unborn children. All patients with COPD who smoke should be offered advice on smoking cessation.

STATION 1.7: ABDOMINAL PAIN

SCENARIO

You are a junior doctor in the ED and are asked to see Sophie Angelman, a 23-year-old female, who has presented with abdominal pain. The pain started this morning but has now moved to the right side and became more severe. Please take a history from Sophie, present your findings and formulate an appropriate management plan.

Cardinal Symptoms

Weight loss
Anorexia
Dysphagia
Nausea and vomiting
Reflux/dyspepsia
Rectal bleeding/melaena
Haematemesis
Altered bowel habit
Rectal bleeding
Jaundice

HISTORY OF PRESENTING COMPLAINT

PAIN

When a patient presents with pain, you can use the acronym SOCRATES to remember the questions that you should ask:

- *Site*: Ask the patient if they can point to a specific site where the pain is
- *Onset*: Sudden or gradual. What the patient was doing at the time of onset
- *Character*: Constant, cramping, sharp, stabbing, dull ache
- *Radiation*: For example, through to the back, from loin to groin
- *Associated symptoms*: See below
- *Timing*: Duration and any similar previous episodes
- *Exacerbating and relieving factors*: Ask if worse on eating, coughing, movement. Or if relieved by eating, defecation, analgesia
- *Severity*: Pain score out of 10, currently and at its worst

ASSOCIATED SYMPTOMS

Other symptoms to enquire about include:
- Fever
- Sweatiness
- Reduced appetite
- Diarrhoea
- Nausea and vomiting
- Weight loss
- Dysphagia
- Dyspepsia
- Jaundice
- Abdominal distension
- Change in bowel habit
- Rectal bleeding or haematemesis

PAST MEDICAL AND SURGICAL HISTORY

- Medical: Diabetes mellitus, ischaemic heart disease, inflammatory bowel disease, jaundice, haematological conditions
- Surgical: Previous surgery, gallstones, pancreatic disease

MEDICATION HISTORY

Enquire about prescribed medications (including any recent changes) and over-the-counter medications. Allergies should be included, with the specific reaction noted. In this scenario it is also important to note:

- NSAIDs: Gastritis, peptic ulcer
- Steroids: Peptic ulcer, pancreatitis
- Bisphosphonates: Oesophageal reactions, peptic ulcer
- Azathioprine: Pancreatitis
- Others: Analgesia and antispasmodics

SOCIAL HISTORY

Social history includes enquiring about occupation, residence, lifestyle (diet, exercise, smoking, alcohol, substance abuse) and recent travel. Additionally in this scenario, consider:

- Smoking: Document pack years, calculated as the number of packs per day multiplied by the number of years smoked
- Alcohol and illicit drug use: Alcohol is an important cause of liver disease and pancreatitis
- Diet: Fatty foods typically exacerbate pain from gallstones. Spicy foods and caffeine can exacerbate gastro-oesophageal reflux symptoms. Diet may also be relevant in coeliac disease and irritable bowel syndrome
- Travel history: Important to elicit in patients with diarrhoea and vomiting
- Occupation: Impact of symptoms on daily life

FAMILY HISTORY

Enquire about any significant family history, including:
- Colorectal cancer
- Hereditary bowel disease; for example, familial adenomatous polyposis (FAP), hereditary non-polyposis colorectal cancer (HNPCC)

SYSTEMS REVIEW

On systems review, particularly pertinent questions to the above case may include:
- Renal: Dysuria, frequency, haematuria, prostatic symptoms
- Gynaecological: Last menstrual period (LMP), vaginal bleeding, discharge, dysmenorrhoea, dyspareunia

Risk Factors for Appendicitis

- Chronic inflammatory bowel disease
- Family history of appendicitis
- Teenage years and young adult age of 15–30 years old

Differential Diagnosis

DISEASE	CLINICAL PRESENTATION	INVESTIGATIONS	MANAGEMENT
Perforation	• Severe abdominal pain • Peritonitis	• FBCs • U&Es • CRP • LFTs • Venous blood gas (VBG) • Erect CXR • Consider urgent CT	• Nil by mouth (NBM) • IV fluids • Oxygen • Analgesia • IV antibiotics • Cross-match bloods • Emergency laparotomy
Appendicitis	• Initially central colicky pain, then constant right iliac fossa pain • Anorexia • Nausea and vomiting	• FBCs • U&Es • CRP • VBG • CT if > 65 years old or diagnosis unclear • Ultrasound scan (USS)	• NBM • IV fluids • Oxygen • Analgesia • Cross-match bloods • Open or laparoscopic appendicectomy • IV antibiotics for perforation
Bowel obstruction	• Abdominal pain • Distension • Nausea and vomiting • Constipation	• FBCs • U&Es • CRP • LFTs • VBG • Abdominal X-ray (AXR) • Erect CXR	If small-bowel obstruction: • NBM • Nasogastric (NG) tube • IV fluidsIf large-bowel obstruction: • NBM • IV fluids • Surgery is usually required
Acute pancreatitis	• Epigastric pain, radiating to the back • Anorexia • Vomiting	• FBCs • U&Es • CRP • LFTs • Amylase • Glucose • Calcium • VBG • USS abdomen	• NBM • IV fluids • Oxygen • Analgesia • NG tube • Catheter • May need endoscopic retrograde cholangiopancreatography (ERCP) if gallstones
Peptic ulcer disease/ gastritis	• Dyspepsia • Epigastric pain • Haematemesis/melaena	• FBCs • U&Es • CRP • LFTs • VBG • Erect CXR • Endoscopy.	• Lifestyle changes; for example, tackling smoking, alcohol, diet • Antacids • Triple therapy if Helicobacter pylori
Gallstones	• Right upper-quadrant pain • Nausea and vomiting	• FBCs • U&Es • CRP • LFTs • VBG • USS abdomen	• Analgesia • Dietary advice • Antibiotics if cholecystitis • Cholecystectomy
Diverticulitis	• Pain • Change in bowel habit • PR bleeding	• FBCs • U&Es • CRP • LFTs • VBG • Erect CXR • CT or colonoscopy	• NBM • Analgesia • IV fluids • Antibiotics
Ruptured abdominal aortic aneurysm (AAA)	• Abdominal pain • Back pain • Collapse • Tender pulsatile abdominal mass	• FBCs • U&Es • CRP • LFTs • Coagulation screen • VBG • Urgent USS or CT	• Oxygen • Analgesia • Antiemetic • IV fluids • Catheter • Cross-match • Urgent vascular surgery

Differential Diagnosis—cont'd

DISEASE	CLINICAL PRESENTATION	INVESTIGATIONS	MANAGEMENT
Renal colic	• Loin to groin colicky pain • Nausea and vomiting • Haematuria • Dysuria • Strangury	• FBCs • U&Es • CRP • LFTs • Calcium • Urate • VBG • CT kidneys, ureters and bladder (KUB)	• Analgesia; for example, diclofenac PR • Antiemetic • Antibiotics if infection • Stones <5 mm should pass spontaneously • Referral to urology if persistent pain, hydronephrosis or infection
Ectopic pregnancy	• Abdominal pain • Per vaginam (PV) bleeding • Recent amenorrhoea • Collapse • Shock • Peritonitis if rupture	• FBCs • U&Es • CRP • Urine or serum beta-human chorionic gonadotrophin (beta-hCG) • Pelvic USS	If stable: • Analgesia • Referral to gynaecologylf unstable: • NBM • Cross-match • Analgesia • IV fluids • Urgent referral to gynaecology

Present Your Findings

Miss Angelman is a 23-year-old woman who presented with a 1-day history of initially vague, central abdominal pain which subsequently localised to the right iliac fossa. The pain is worse on coughing and moving and is associated with nausea, vomiting and anorexia. There are no gynaecological or urinary symptoms of note. She is otherwise fit and well, has no recent travel history and has not been in contact with anyone unwell.

I feel the most likely diagnosis is acute appendicitis. However, I would like to rule out a gynaecological cause for Sophie's symptoms.

I would perform a full physical examination and request bloods, including FBCs, U&Es, LFTs, amylase, CRP, VBG, beta-hCG, and perform a urine dip. I would also request an erect CXR to look for air under the diaphragm if I was concerned about perforation.

QUESTIONS AND ANSWERS FOR CANDIDATE

What are the potential complications of acute appendicitis?
* Perforation
* Appendix mass
* Abscess

Name three common causes of peritonitis.
* Acute perforated appendicitis
* Acute perforated diverticular disease
* Upper GI perforation; for example, peptic ulcer disease
* Perforated colonic or gastric tumour
* Postsurgical intervention; for example, anastomotic leak

* Ruptured ectopic pregnancy

Name three differential diagnoses for right-upper-quadrant pain (Fig. 1.2).
* Biliary colic
* Cholecystitis
* Cholangitis
* Hepatitis
* Right lower-lobe pneumonia

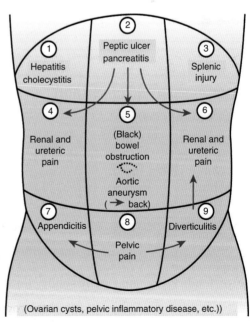

Fig. 1.2 The causes of abdominal pain shown by site.

A Case to Learn From

When I was working in the ED an 86-year-old patient presented with central abdominal discomfort and vague back pain. She was noted to be bradycardic and with a systolic BP of 100 mmHg on admission, and therefore the consultant asked me to see her. On examination, she had central abdominal tenderness. As I was finishing my assessment, the consultant appeared around the curtain with the ultrasound machine, and a bedside scan showed a leaking abdominal aortic aneurysm! Don't forget this as an important cause of abdominal pain.

 Top Tip

You should always consider pregnancy as a cause for symptoms in a woman of reproductive age.

STATION 1.8: DYSPHAGIA

SCENARIO

You are a junior doctor in primary care and have been asked to see Melody Jones, a 72-year-old woman, who has had difficulty swallowing over the last 2 months. She is finding it difficult to swallow both solid foods and liquids. She has also lost 7 kg in weight. Please take a history from Mrs Jones, present your findings and formulate an appropriate management plan.

 Cardinal Symptoms

Dysphagia (Table 1.4)
Odynophagia
Vomiting or regurgitation
Dyspepsia
Weight loss
Neurological symptoms

HISTORY OF PRESENTING COMPLAINT

DIFFICULTY SWALLOWING

* Clarification: Ask the patient to describe specifically what she means by 'difficulty swallowing'
* Onset: Did anything in particular happen at onset of the symptom; for example, trauma to the head or neck?
* Duration: How long has the symptom been present?
* Progression: For example, symptoms getting progressively worse or intermittent and non-progressive
* Type of food: Dysphagia with solids, liquids or both
* Site: Ask the patient to point to where she feels food gets stuck

ASSOCIATED SYMPTOMS

Other symptoms to enquire about include:
* Difficulty with the initiation of swallowing
* Coughing or choking while eating
* Nasal regurgitation
* Feeling of a lump in the throat
* Weight loss
* Reduced appetite
* Fever

PAST MEDICAL AND SURGICAL HISTORY

In this scenario, it is also important to enquire about:
* Recurrent pneumonia, suggesting aspiration
* Gastro-oesophageal reflux, causing peptic stricture
* Barrett's oesophagus
* Neurological disease; for example, stroke, Parkinson's disease, myasthenia gravis, multiple sclerosis
* Rheumatological disease; for example, systemic sclerosis, Sjögren's disease
* Immunosuppression increases the risk of oesophageal infection
* Previous radiotherapy to the thorax
* GI surgery

MEDICATION HISTORY

Enquire about prescribed medications (including any recent changes) and over-the-counter medications. Allergies should be included, with the specific reaction noted. In this scenario it is also important to note:
* Medications which are associated with increasing the risk of oesophagitis: For example, NSAIDs, bisphosphonates, steroids

SOCIAL HISTORY

Social history includes enquiring about occupation, residence, lifestyle (diet, exercise, smoking, alcohol, substance abuse) and recent travel. Additionally in this scenario, consider:
* Smoking: Document pack years, calculated as the number of packs per day multiplied by the number of years smoked
* Alcohol and illicit drug use: Document units of alcohol consumed per week
* Diet: Ask what the patient has been managing to eat and drink
* Occupation: Ask about current and previous occupations

FAMILY HISTORY

Ask about any significant family history, including:
* History of malignancy

SYSTEMS REVIEW

On systems review, particularly pertinent questions to the above case may include questions regarding:

- GI: Dry mouth, halitosis, nausea and vomiting, regurgitation, acid reflux, odynophagia, retrosternal pain, abdominal pain, change in bowel habit
- Neurological: Tremor of Parkinson's disease, dysarthria, dysphonia, weakness

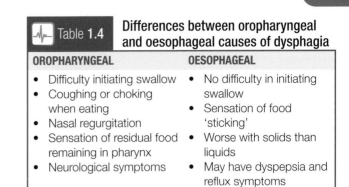

Table 1.4 Differences between oropharyngeal and oesophageal causes of dysphagia

OROPHARYNGEAL	OESOPHAGEAL
• Difficulty initiating swallow • Coughing or choking when eating • Nasal regurgitation • Sensation of residual food remaining in pharynx • Neurological symptoms	• No difficulty in initiating swallow • Sensation of food 'sticking' • Worse with solids than liquids • May have dyspepsia and reflux symptoms

Risk Factors for Oesophageal Cancer

- Barrett's oesophagus
- GORD
- Obesity
- Smoking
- Increased age
- Excess alcohol consumption

Differential Diagnosis

DISEASE	CLINICAL PRESENTATION	INVESTIGATIONS	MANAGEMENT
Oesophageal stricture	• Dysphagia after a long history of gastro-oesophageal reflux	• Endoscopy with biopsy	• Endoscopic dilatation
Oesophageal cancer	• Rapidly progressive dysphagia • Weight loss	• Endoscopy with biopsy • Staging CT scan	• Chemotherapy • Radiotherapy • Surgery • Endoscopic stenting
Achalasia	• Gradually progressive dysphagia to solids and then liquids • Regurgitation	• Barium swallow • Oesophageal manometry • Endoscopy	• Endoscopic botulinum toxin injection • Endoscopic dilatation • Surgery
Eosinophilic oesophagitis	• Typically a young patient • Intermittent dysphagia • History of atopy	• Endoscopy with biopsy	• Steroid inhaler
Oesophageal candidiasis	• Odynophagia • Immunocompromised or recent antibiotics	• Endoscopy and biopsy	• Fluconazole
Diffuse oesophageal spasm	• Intermittent retrosternal pain • Dysphagia	• Barium swallow • Oesophageal manometry • Endoscopy	• Avoid precipitants; for example, hot or cold food • Calcium channel blocker; for example, diltiazem
Pharyngeal pouch	• Halitosis • Bulge in the neck • Regurgitation • Coughing and aspiration	• Barium swallow	• Surgery
Bulbar or pseudobulbar palsy	• Difficulty initiating swallow • Neurological symptoms and signs	• Barium swallow	• Speech and language therapy (SALT) review • Thickened fluids • NG tube or percutaneous endoscopic gastrostomy (PEG)

Present Your Findings

Mrs Jones is a 72-year-old woman with a 2-month history of progressive dysphagia. She initially had difficulty swallowing solids, but this has progressed to liquids as well. She describes retrosternal discomfort and the sensation of food 'sticking'. These symptoms are associated with significant weight loss.

My differential diagnosis includes oesophageal cancer or peptic stricture.

I would like to perform a full physical examination and arrange an endoscopy to investigate these symptoms further.

❓ QUESTIONS AND ANSWERS FOR CANDIDATE

What are the three phases of swallowing?

1. Oral phase: Food is chewed and mixed with saliva to form a bolus, which the tongue then pushes to the back of the mouth
2. Pharyngeal phase: As the bolus reaches the pharynx, sensory receptors activate the involuntary phase of swallowing, which pushes the food bolus further back into the pharynx. The vocal cords close and the epiglottis covers the larynx to protect the airway
3. Oesophageal phase: The bolus moves into the oesophagus where muscle contractions push it into the stomach

What is achalasia?

- Achalasia is an oesophageal motility disorder where there is failure of the lower oesophageal sphincter to relax and a loss of peristalsis in the oesophagus. This causes an obstruction to the passage of food into the stomach

Explain Barrett's oesophagus and the recommendations for its surveillance.

- Barrett's oesophagus is a condition where the squamous mucosa of the oesophagus undergoes metaplastic change to columnar mucosa, secondary to chronic GORD. It confers an increased risk of oesophageal adenocarcinoma, therefore it is recommended that patients undergo surveillance with regular endoscopy every 2 years

A Case to Learn From

An elderly woman presented to her primary care doctor with difficulty swallowing. A thorough history revealed that this patient was actually experiencing xerostomia (a dry mouth) which was making it difficult to swallow food, rather than dysphagia. This case highlights the importance in establishing exactly what the patient means by 'difficulty swallowing'.

Top Tip

It is important to establish whether the dysphagia is worse with solid foods or liquids and if there has been progression in dysphagia from solids to more liquid consistencies. These points in the history are very helpful in subsequently narrowing down the differential diagnoses.

STATION 1.9: NAUSEA AND VOMITING

SCENARIO

You are a junior doctor in primary care and have been asked to see Jack Fawn, a 28-year-old man, who presented with a 2-day history of nausea and vomiting. He feels generally unwell and is struggling to hold down any food. Please take a history from Jack, present your findings and formulate an appropriate management plan.

Cardinal Symptoms

Abdominal pain
Abdominal distension
Diarrhoea
Fever
Headache

HISTORY OF PRESENTING COMPLAINT

NAUSEA AND VOMITING

- Onset: Any particular event when the symptoms came on; for example, attended a party
- Duration: Length of time the symptoms have been present
- Clarification: Clarify that patient is vomiting rather than experiencing regurgitation, expectoration or haemoptysis
- Timing: Any patterns, cyclical vomiting syndrome, relationship to eating and to medications
- Frequency: How often in a certain time period; for example, number of vomiting episodes per day
- Character and colour of vomitus: Undigested food, bilious, fresh red blood, coffee-ground, faeculent
- Volume: Small or large volume
- Exacerbating factors: Worse on waking up, movement
- Nutrition: Ability to retain food and fluids

ASSOCIATED SYMPTOMS

Other symptoms to enquire about include:
- Any unwell contacts with similar symptoms
- Fever
- Weight loss
- Loss of appetite
- Malaise

PAST MEDICAL AND SURGICAL HISTORY

In this scenario, it is also important to enquire about:
- Pregnancy
- Malignancy
- Diabetes
- Renal stones
- Head trauma
- Migraine
- Chronic liver disease and any known oesophageal varices
- Previous abdominal surgery

MEDICATION HISTORY

Enquire about prescribed medications (including any recent changes) and over-the-counter medications. Allergies should be included, with the specific reaction noted. In this scenario it is also important to note:

- Any overdose(s)
- Medications causing nausea and vomiting as a side effect: Chemotherapy, antibiotics, opioids, digoxin
- Increased risk of upper GI bleeding: NSAIDs, steroids, warfarin, DOACs

SOCIAL HISTORY

Social history includes enquiring about occupation, residence, lifestyle (diet, exercise, smoking, alcohol, substance abuse) and recent travel. Additionally in this scenario, consider:

- Smoking: Document pack years, calculated as the number of packs per day multiplied by the number of years smoked
- Alcohol and illicit drug use: Document units of alcohol consumed per week. Both excess alcohol consumption and acute withdrawal may cause vomiting
- Diet: Any potential culprits for food poisoning; for example, poultry or eggs
- Unwell contacts: Infectious gastroenteritis may spread rapidly in a communal setting; for example, schools and hospitals

- Recent travel abroad: Ask about the areas travelled to (including brief stopovers) and duration of travel
- Occupation: Working with food, children, in a hospital

FAMILY HISTORY

Ask about any significant family history, including:

- GI disease
- Disorders of metabolism

SYSTEMS REVIEW

On systems review, particularly pertinent questions to the above case may include questions regarding:

- GI: Jaundice, dysphagia, early satiety, abdominal pain, abdominal distension, change in bowel habit, blood or mucus in stool, melaena
- Neurological: Headache, vertigo, hearing loss, neck stiffness, photophobia
- Genitourinary: Pregnancy, delayed menstrual period, loin pain, dysuria, haematuria
- Ears, nose and throat (ENT): Vertigo, tinnitus, deafness

Risk Factors for Bowel Obstruction

- Previous abdominal surgery
- Radiation to the abdomen or pelvis
- Colorectal cancer
- Inflammatory bowel disease
- Hernias
- Volvulus
- Diverticulitis

Differential Diagnosis

DISEASE	CLINICAL PRESENTATION	INVESTIGATIONS	MANAGEMENT
Gastroenteritis	• Vomiting • Diarrhoea • Fever	• FBCs • U&Es • CRP • Stool MC&S	• Fluids • Oral rehydration solution • Bland diet • Antibiotics are not routinely indicated
Bowel obstruction	• Vomiting (may be faeculent) • Abdominal distension • Colicky abdominal pain • Absolute constipation	• FBCs • U&Es • CRP • Lactate • AXR	• NBM • NG tube • IV fluids • Refer to surgeons
Acute abdomen	• Severe abdominal pain	• FBCs • U&Es • CRP • Amylase • Lactate • Erect CXR • AXR • CT abdomen and pelvis	• Urgent referral to surgeons
Upper GI bleed	• Haematemesis • Epigastric pain • Melaena	• FBCs • U&Es • CRP • Lactate • G&S • Cross-match	• NBM • IV fluids or blood • Endoscopy

Continued

🏠 Differential Diagnosis—cont'd

DISEASE	CLINICAL PRESENTATION	INVESTIGATIONS	MANAGEMENT
Labyrinthitis	• Vertigo • Nausea and vomiting	• May not be required	• Labyrinthine sedatives; for example, prochlorperazine or cyclizine
Migraine	• Aura • Visual disturbance • Headache (often unilateral) • Nausea and vomiting	• May not be required	• Avoid known triggers. If an acute attack: • Triptan and simple analgesia. If recurrent and severe: • Propranolol
Pregnancy	• Known pregnancy or delayed menstrual period	• Beta-hCG • U&Es	• Pharmacological intervention not usually required • Antiemetics if severe • IV fluids if dehydrated
Raised intracranial pressure	• Headache • Focal neurological symptoms	• FBCs • U&Es • CRP • CT or magnetic resonance imaging (MRI) head	• Dependent on cause • Refer to neurosurgeons
Diabetic ketoacidosis	• Vomiting • Abdominal pain • Polyuria • Polydipsia • May or may not have known diagnosis of diabetes	• Blood glucose • Ketones • FBCs • U&Es • CRP • VBG	• IV fluids • Fixed-rate insulin infusion

ADDITIONAL INFORMATION

CAUSES OF VOMITING

The acronym VOMITING can be used to remember the common causes of vomiting:
- *Vestibular*
- *Opiates* or *obstruction*
- *Metabolic* or *migraine*
- *Infection*
- *Toxins* or *tumour*
- *Increased* intracranial pressure
- *Neurogenic*
- *GI* or *gestation*

🔍 Present Your Findings

Mr Fawn is a 28-year-old man with a 2-day history of nausea and vomiting. He has vomited six times today and yesterday and is unable to hold down any food, but he is managing regular sips of water. There is no blood or bile in the vomitus and it is not faeculent. It is associated with a fever, diarrhoea and cramping abdominal pains. Jack did go to a street food festival 3 days ago and his friend is also suffering from similar symptoms.

I think the most likely diagnosis is gastroenteritis.

I would advise Jack to keep well hydrated with fluids and oral rehydration solution. If I was concerned about dehydration, I would consider admission of IV fluids.

❓ QUESTIONS AND ANSWERS FOR CANDIDATE

Name three common causative organisms of bacterial gastroenteritis.
- *Campylobacter*
- *Shigella*
- *Salmonella*
- *Escherichia coli* (*E. coli*)
- *Yersinia enterocolitica*
- *Vibrio cholerae*

How might you assess the hydration status of a vomiting patient?
- BP
- Heart rate
- Mucous membranes
- Skin turgor

What are the side effects of the commonly used antiemetics cyclizine, metoclopramide and ondansetron?
- Cyclizine: Anticholinergic side effects, including urinary retention, dry mouth and blurred vision
- Metoclopramide: Extrapyramidal side effects
- Ondansetron: Constipation, flushing, headache

Table **1.5**	Common antiemetics and their sites of action	
ANTIEMETIC	**RECEPTOR SITES**	**ACTION**
Metoclopramide	Dopamine antagonist	• Acts centrally and on the gut • Prokinetic antiemetic
Ondansetron	$5HT_3$ antagonist	• Acts centrally and on gut
Cyclizine	Histamine and acetylcholine antagonist	• Acts on the vestibular system and the vomiting centre
Haloperidol	D_2 dopamine antagonist	• Acts centrally
Domperidone	Dopamine antagonist	• Acts on the gut • Prokinetic antiemetic • Poor penetration of the blood–brain barrier
Levomepromazine	$5HT_2$, dopamine, acetylcholine and histamine antagonist	• Acts centrally • Broad spectrum of action

A Case to Learn From

When I was working in oncology I was asked to review a patient with significant nausea and vomiting despite regular antiemetics. She was receiving chemotherapy for metastatic breast cancer and after taking a history, I felt the most likely diagnosis was nausea and vomiting secondary to chemotherapy. However, after examining the patient, I found she was unsteady on her feet and displayed some cerebellar signs. Imaging revealed multiple new cerebral and cerebellar brain metastases. Her symptoms improved with regular dexamethasone and her oncologist arranged brain radiotherapy. If I hadn't thoroughly examined this patient I may have missed this diagnosis!

Top Tip

Don't just prescribe antiemetics blindly. Try to establish the cause of nausea and vomiting and prescribe the most appropriate. If you prescribe a patient domperidone, but they have bowel obstruction, for example, you will make things worse! (Table 1.5)

STATION 1.10: DIARRHOEA

SCENARIO

You are a junior doctor in primary care and have been asked to see Danielle Sanderson, a 60-year-old woman, who has been experiencing severe abdominal pain and diarrhoea for the past 4 days. She was recently discharged from hospital following an appendicectomy. Please take a history from Mrs Sanderson, present your findings and formulate an appropriate management plan.

Cardinal Symptoms

Nausea and vomiting
Abdominal pain
Rectal bleeding
Fever
Weight loss

HISTORY OF PRESENTING COMPLAINT

DIARRHOEA

• Amount: Quantify the bowel movements
• Frequency: Number of bowel movements in a given period of time; for example, 1 day or week, and establish whether there is the need to open bowels at night
• Stool character: Consistency, colour, greasy, difficult to flush, blood or mucus in stool
• Exacerbating and relieving factors: For example, worsened by certain food

ASSOCIATED SYMPTOMS

Other symptoms to enquire about include:
• Fever
• Malaise
• Weight loss
• Anorexia
• Mouth ulcers
• Nausea and vomiting
• Dysphagia
• Abdominal pain
• Tenesmus
• Rectal bleeding

PAST MEDICAL AND SURGICAL HISTORY

In this scenario, it is also important to enquire about:
• Diabetes
• Inflammatory bowel disease
• Irritable bowel syndrome
• Abdominal surgery
• History of constipation
• Hyperthyroidism
• Immunosuppression; for example, transplant, HIV, chemotherapy

MEDICATION HISTORY

Enquire about prescribed medications (including any recent changes) and over-the-counter medications. Allergies should be included, with the specific reaction noted. In this scenario it is also important to note:

- Recent antibiotics: *Clostridium difficile*
- Chemotherapy: Diarrhoea is a common side effect
- Laxatives: Do not miss this iatrogenic cause!
- Iron supplements: Both diarrhoea and constipation are common side effects
- Protein pump inhibitor (PPI): Diarrhoea is a known side effect

SOCIAL HISTORY

Social history includes enquiring about occupation, residence, lifestyle (diet, exercise, smoking, alcohol, substance abuse) and recent travel. Additionally in this scenario, consider:

- Smoking: Document pack years, calculated as the number of packs per day multiplied by the number of years smoked
- Alcohol and illicit drug use: Chronic pancreatitis may cause diarrhoea
- Diet: Specifically fibre intake

- Occupation: As a potential cause but also may have implications for return to work (healthcare, food)
- Travel abroad: Traveller's diarrhoea

FAMILY HISTORY

Ask about any significant family history, including:
- Inflammatory bowel disease
- Coeliac disease
- Malignancy

SYSTEMS REVIEW

On systems review, particularly pertinent questions to the above case may include questions regarding:
- Extraintestinal: Arthralgia, rash, eye symptoms

Risk Factors for *Clostridium difficile* Infection
- Increased age
- Use of antibiotics, especially cephalosporins, fluoroquinolones and clindamycin
- Use of PPI
- Exposure to healthcare settings; for example, hospital

Differential Diagnosis

DISEASE	CLINICAL PRESENTATION	INVESTIGATIONS	MANAGEMENT
Gastroenteritis	• Sudden onset of diarrhoea • ± Vomiting • Cramping abdominal pains	• FBCs • U&Es • CRP • LFTs • Stool MC&S	• Encourage oral fluids • Oral rehydration solutions • IV fluids if not tolerating oral • Antiemetics • Antibiotics may be indicated if bacterial cause
Clostridium difficile	• Abdominal pain • Diarrhoea • Recent antibiotics	• FBCs • U&Es • CRP • LFTs • Stool analysis • AXR	• Barrier nursing • Oral metronidazole or vancomycin • Faecal transplantation
Inflammatory bowel disease	• Weight loss • Abdominal pain • Bloody diarrhoea • Extraintestinal symptoms	• FBCs • U&Es • CRP • LFTs • Stool MC&S • AXR • Colonoscopy	• IV, oral or topical steroids • 5-aminosalicylic acid (5-ASA) tablets • Suppositories or enemas • Infliximab or ciclosporin • Refer to surgeons if severe flare
Diverticular disease	• Bloody diarrhoea • Pain in left iliac fossa	• FBCs • U&Es • CRP • LFTs • Stool MC&S • Barium enema or colonoscopy	• Antibiotics if diverticulitis • High-fibre diet • Stool softeners

Differential Diagnosis—cont'd

DISEASE	CLINICAL PRESENTATION	INVESTIGATIONS	MANAGEMENT
Colorectal cancer	• Weight loss • Anorexia • Change in bowel habit • Rectal bleeding	• FBCs • U&Es • CRP • LFTs • Stool MC&S • Colonoscopy or CT colonography	• Surgical resection when possible • Chemotherapy • Radiotherapy
Overflow diarrhoea	• History of constipation	• FBCs • U&Es • CRP • LFTs • Stool MC&S • AXR	• Laxatives
Coeliac disease	• Weight loss • Chronic diarrhoea • Abdominal pain • Symptoms of malabsorption	• FBCs • U&Es • CRP • LFTs • Haematinics • Endomysial antibody (EMA) or TTG antibody • Stool MC&S • Duodenal biopsy	• Gluten-free diet
Irritable bowel syndrome	• Abdominal pain and bloating, relieved by defecation • Often fluctuates between diarrhoea and constipation	• FBCs • U&Es • CRP • LFTs • Stool MC&S • Coeliac antibodies	• Dietary and lifestyle advice • Mebeverine • Loperamide • Laxatives

ADDITIONAL INFORMATION

TRAVELLER'S DIARRHOEA

- High-risk areas include most of Asia, Africa, the Middle East and Latin America
- The commonest route of infection is through the ingestion of contaminated foods
- Causative organisms include:
  - *E. coli*
  - *Salmonella*
  - *Shigella*
  - *Campylobacter*
  - Giardiasis
  - Amoebic dysentery
  - Cholera
  - Tropical sprue

Present Your Findings

Mrs Sanderson is a 60-year-old woman who presents with a 4-day history of severe lower abdominal pain. This is associated with the passage of foul-smelling watery stools, approximately eight times a day. She has been feeling nauseous and feverish and was recently discharged from hospital after completing a 7-day course of clindamycin. There is no blood or mucus in the stool. She is otherwise well.

This is consistent with a diagnosis of infective diarrhoea, possibly *Clostridium difficile* given the recent antibiotic course.

I would readmit Mrs Sanderson to hospital for IV fluids, stool analysis and, if indicated, antibiotic therapy.

QUESTIONS AND ANSWERS FOR CANDIDATE

What is *Clostridium difficile* and how is it treated?
- *Clostridium difficile* is a Gram-positive spore-forming anaerobic bacillus which colonises the GI tract via the faeco-oral route
- It is facilitated by disruption of the normal gut flora by antibiotics
- This can lead to diarrhoea and pseudomembranous colitis
- Treatment consists of oral metronidazole or oral vancomycin, with barrier nursing, in the first instance. IV antibiotics may be used if the patient fails to improve

What are the key differences that distinguish ulcerative colitis and Crohn's disease?
- Please see Table 1.6 for answers

What are the extraintestinal manifestations of inflammatory bowel disease?
- Please see Table 1.7 for answers

Table 1.6   Key differences between ulcerative colitis and Crohn's disease

FEATURE	ULCERATIVE COLITIS	CROHN'S DISEASE
Symptoms	• Diarrhoea with blood or mucus in the stool • Lower abdominal pain • Faecal urgency • Tenesmus	• Diarrhoea with blood or mucus in the stool (less commonly) • Abdominal pain • Mouth ulcers • Malabsorption • Weight loss
GI involvement	• Involvement of the colon only, with proximal extension from the rectum (though may have a 'backwash' ileitis)	• From 'mouth to anus', the terminal ileum is commonly involved
Histology	• Mucosal and submucosal inflammation • Goblet cell depletion • Glandular distortion • Mucosal ulcers • Crypt abscesses	• Patchy transmural inflammation with skip lesions • Granulomas

Table 1.7   Extraintestinal manifestations of inflammatory bowel disease

SITE	MANIFESTATION
Eye changes	Iritis, uveitis, episcleritis
Musculoskeletal	Seronegative arthritis, osteoporosis
Dermatological	Erythema nodosum, pyoderma gangrenosum, aphthous mouth ulcers
Other	Autoimmune haemolytic anaemia, finger clubbing, growth failure, primary sclerosing cholangitis, interstitial lung disease (rare)

A Case to Learn From

A 54-year-old man was admitted with diarrhoea six times a day over the previous 3 days which was associated with some cramping abdominal pain. The diagnosis of gastroenteritis was initially made but a thorough drug history revealed this patient was receiving an immunotherapy treatment for metastatic melanoma. The team subsequently contacted the acute oncology service who explained that the immunotherapy treatment can cause colitis and advised to commence IV methylprednisolone and for an urgent gastroenterology review.

Top Tip

Always ask patients to explain what they mean by 'diarrhoea', as patients may use this term to describe many different symptoms such as an increase in frequency of normal stool or faecal incontinence. Always establish what the patient's usual bowel habit is as this is very variable between individuals.

STATION 1.11: OLIGURIA

SCENARIO

You have been asked to review 72-year-old Mr Kaur during your ward cover shift. He was admitted under the medical team yesterday following a fall. The nursing staff are concerned as he has passed very little urine since admission. Please take a history from Mr Kaur, present your findings and formulate an appropriate management plan.

Cardinal Symptoms

Abdominal pain
Poor stream
Hesitancy
Urgency
Haematuria
Fever
Poor oral intake
Diarrhoea and vomiting

HISTORY OF PRESENTING COMPLAINT

OLIGURIA

- Duration of symptoms: Length of time the symptom has been present
- The last time of micturition: Including volume if possible
- Amount of urine passed: Determine if it is oliguria (defined as a urine output of less than 0.5 mL/kg/h) or anuria
- History of fluid loss: For example, diarrhoea, vomiting, stoma output, haemorrhage, leaking wounds, burns
- Quantify amount of oral fluid intake: Including the type of fluid
- Urine character: Enquire about haematuria, clots, obstructions

ASSOCIATED SYMPTOMS

Other symptoms to enquire about include:
- Abdominal pain
- Fever
- Malaise
- Night sweats
- Weight loss

PAST MEDICAL AND SURGICAL HISTORY

In this scenario, it is also important to enquire about:
- Benign prostatic hypertrophy
- Prostate cancer
- Renal failure
- Infection or sepsis
- Recent surgery
- Constipation

MEDICATION HISTORY

Enquire about prescribed medications (including any recent changes) and over-the-counter medications. Allergies should be included, with the specific reaction noted. In this scenario it is also important to note:
- Alpha-adrenoreceptor antagonist and 5 alpha-reductase inhibitors: Treatment for prostatic hypertrophy
- Nephrotoxic drugs: For example, NSAIDs, gentamicin, ACEi, metformin, which may cause acute kidney injury (AKI)
- Contrast: Contrast-induced nephropathy
- Anticholinergics: Urinary retention

SOCIAL HISTORY

Social history includes enquiring about occupation, residence, lifestyle (diet, exercise, smoking, alcohol, substance abuse) and recent travel. Additionally in this scenario, consider:
- Smoking: Document pack years, calculated as the number of packs per day multiplied by the number of years smoked
- Alcohol and illicit drug use: Document units of alcohol consumed per week
- Occupation: Increased risk of bladder cancer if working in textile or rubber industry

FAMILY HISTORY

Ask about any significant family history, including:
- History of renal disease

SYSTEMS REVIEW

On systems review, particularly pertinent questions to the above case may include questions regarding:
- Cardiovascular: Breathlessness, orthopnoea, PND
- Endocrine: Weight change, hair and skin changes, heat or cold intolerance, change in bowel habit, palpitations, menorrhagia or amenorrhoea
- Respiratory: Cough, wheeze, pleuritic chest pain
- Lower urinary tract symptoms (LUTS): Urgency, frequency, hesitancy, dribbling, incontinence
- Uraemic symptoms: Lethargy, anorexia, nausea, vomiting, pruritus, lethargy

Risk Factors for AKI

- Poor oral intake
- Increased age
- Diabetes
- Peripheral vascular disease
- Hypertension
- Pre-existing kidney disease
- Heart failure

Differential Diagnosis

DISEASE	CLINICAL PRESENTATION	INVESTIGATIONS	MANAGEMENT
Acute urinary retention	• Suprapubic pain • Urge to urinate • Palpable bladder	• Bladder scan	• Catheterise
AKI	• Acute deterioration in renal function	• U&Es • VBG • Urine dip • Urine MC&S • Renal tract USS	• Stop nephrotoxics • IV fluids • Treat complications; for example, hyperkalaemia
Chronic kidney disease (CKD)	• Often no symptoms • Nausea • Anorexia • Lethargy • Itch	• U&Es • Urine dip • Urine MC&S • Renal tract USS	• Control BP and diabetes • Avoid nephrotoxics • Dialysis if end-stage
Hypovolaemia	• Low fluid input • High fluid output • Excess losses	• Calculate fluid balance • U&Es	• IV fluids
Septic shock	• Pyrexia • Hypotension • Tachycardia • Tachypnoea	• FBCs • U&Es • CRP • LFTs • CXR • Urine dip ± MC&S	• Oxygen • IV fluids • IV antibiotics

ADDITIONAL INFORMATION

RENAL REPLACEMENT THERAPY (RRT)

If conservative management is insufficient, a patient with severe AKI may require urgent RRT. This will require either admission to intensive care or transfer to a renal unit for haemofiltration or dialysis.

RRT is commonly carried out in intensive care using a type of venous central line called a vascath. A vascath will be sited in a large central vein; for example, the internal jugular vein or subclavian vein. It allows blood to be taken from the patient to the machine and returned back to the patient.

 Present Your Findings

Mr Kaur is a 72-year-old man who was admitted to hospital following a fall. He is currently being treated for a likely urinary tract infection and his U&Es on admission showed an AKI. He has passed only 320 mL of urine over the previous 24 h and his oral intake has been poor for the last few days. There is no history of excessive fluid loss and he denies any abdominal pain.

The most likely causes for Mr Kaur's oliguria are poor oral fluid intake and an AKI.

I would like to take repeat U&Es, review the drug chart and prescribe IV fluids. I would ask the nursing staff to continue to monitor fluid balance closely and I would consider inserting a urinary catheter.

 QUESTIONS AND ANSWERS FOR CANDIDATE

What are the indications for dialysis or haemofiltration in AKI?
- Persistent or intractable:
  - Refractory hyperkalaemia
  - Pulmonary oedema
  - Severe metabolic acidosis
  - Uraemic symptoms; for example, encephalopathy, pericarditis

Name three causes of acute urinary retention.
- Prostatic obstruction
- Constipation
- Drugs; for example, anticholinergics
- Clot retention
- Urethral stricture
- Bladder stone

How do you manage hyperkalaemia?
- Stop any medications that may be contributing; for example, spironolactone
- Repeat U&Es if the result is a surprise, as the blood sample may have haemolysed
- ECG to look for changes associated with hyperkalaemia. If there are ECG changes or $K^+ > 6.5$ mmol/L:
  - 10 mL calcium gluconate 10%
  - 10 units of Actrapid insulin in 50 mL 50% glucose
  - Consider 5 mg salbutamol nebuliser

 A Case to Learn From

I saw a patient in the ED who presented with symptoms of acute urinary retention with suprapubic pain and inability to pass urine. I initially thought the patient might have a urinary tract infection; however, further questioning revealed a history of loin pain suggestive of a renal stone. Following discussion with my senior, I requested a CT KUB which in fact showed a large stone causing obstruction at the bladder neck. This was the cause for this patient's urinary retention. Don't always trust your first instinct.

 Top Tip

Remember constipation as a common cause for acute urinary retention.

STATION 1.12: HEADACHE

SCENARIO

You are the junior doctor on call and have been asked to review Anna Hart, a 25-year-old patient, who has presented to the ED with a new and severe headache. Please take a history from Ms Hart, present your findings and formulate an appropriate management plan.

 Cardinal Symptoms

Head trauma
Focal neurological deficit
Reduced GCS
Confusion
Fever
Neck stiffness
Photophobia

HISTORY OF PRESENTING COMPLAINT

HEADACHE

When a patient presents with pain, you can use the acronym SOCRATES to remember the questions that you should ask:
- *Site*: Specific location, unilateral or bilateral
- *Onset*: Sudden or gradual, what the patient was doing at the time of onset
- *Character*: For example, throbbing, stabbing, tight
- *Radiation*: For example, to the face, eye or neck
- *Associated symptoms*: See below
- *Timing*: Duration that the pain lasts for, previous episodes, whether there is a temporal pattern to the headaches
- *Exacerbating and relieving factors*: Headache worse on lying down or coughing is a red-flag symptom for raised intracranial pressure. Known triggers for migraine include cheese, chocolate and red wine and sleep deprivation. Migraines may be relieved by

simple analgesia, sitting in a quiet and dark room, sleep
- *Severity*: Score out of 10

ASSOCIATED SYMPTOMS

Other symptoms to enquire about include:
- Nausea and vomiting
- Scalp tenderness
- Watering of the eye or nasal congestion
- Weight loss

PAST MEDICAL AND SURGICAL HISTORY

In this scenario, it is also important to enquire about:
- Any recent head injury or neck trauma
- Recent illnesses; for example, sinusitis or otitis media
- Coagulopathy
- Immunosuppression

MEDICATION HISTORY

Enquire about prescribed medications (including any recent changes) and over-the-counter medications. Allergies should be included, with the specific reaction noted. In this scenario it is also important to note:
- Analgesics: May suggest medication overuse headache
- Anticoagulants: To determine the patient's bleeding or clotting risk
- Oral contraceptive pill: In some patients can be associated with an increased clotting risk
- Nitrates: Cause vasodilation which can trigger headaches

SOCIAL HISTORY

Social history includes enquiring about occupation, residence, lifestyle (diet, exercise, smoking, alcohol, substance abuse) and recent travel. Additionally in this scenario, consider:
- Smoking: Document pack years, calculated as the number of packs per day multiplied by the number of years smoked

- Alcohol and illicit drug use: Document units consumed per week. Cocaine abuse is a risk factor for subarachnoid haemorrhage
- Unwell contacts: Meningitis
- Recent travel abroad: Malaria, cerebral TB
- Occupation: Enquire about any stresses at work, impact of headaches on work
- Lifestyle: Ask about home life and any stresses or financial worries

FAMILY HISTORY

Ask about any significant family history, including:
- Any history of headaches, particularly migraines
- Subarachnoid haemorrhage
- Kidney disease: Autosomal-dominant polycystic disease is associated with berry aneurysms
- Thromboembolism

SYSTEMS REVIEW

On systems review, particularly pertinent questions to the above case may include questions regarding:
- Cardiorespiratory: Snoring, apnoeic episodes and excessive daytime sleepiness or sleep apnoea
- Neurological: Aura, loss of consciousness, confusion, motor or sensory deficit, gait, disturbance in vision, speech or hearing, incontinence
- Meningism: Fever, neck stiffness, photophobia and rash
- Psychiatric: Low mood, early-morning wakening, anhedonia, anxiety, stress

Risk Factors for Meningitis
- Age: Newborns to young adults, and those over 65 years old
- Travel abroad
- Recent contact with meningococcal meningitis or septicaemia
- Unvaccinated against meningitis
- Immunosuppressed
- Living with others in a communal setting; for example, student accommodation

Differential Diagnosis

DISEASE	CLINICAL PRESENTATION	INVESTIGATIONS	MANAGEMENT
Subarachnoid haemorrhage	• 'Thunder-clap' headache • May have neck stiffness	• CT head • Lumbar puncture (LP) if CT normal	• Analgesia • Antiemetics • Refer urgently to neurosurgery
Meningitis	• Fever • Photophobia • Neck stiffness • Rash	• FBCs • U&Es • CRP • CT head • LP	• Ceftriaxone stat

Continued

Differential Diagnosis—cont'd

DISEASE	CLINICAL PRESENTATION	INVESTIGATIONS	MANAGEMENT
Encephalitis	• Fever • Confusion • Reduced GCS	• FBCs • U&Es • CRP • CT head • LP	• Aciclovir
Space-occupying lesion	• Headache worse on waking/coughing • Focal neurological signs	• CT or MRI brain	• Referral to neurosurgery • May advise mannitol or dexamethasone
Migraine	• Aura • Visual disturbance • Often unilateral headache • Nausea and vomiting	• May not be required	• Avoid known triggers • Triptan and simple analgesia in acute attacks • Prophylaxis with propranolol if recurrent and severe
Temporal arteritis	• Unilateral headache • Scalp tenderness • Jaw claudication	• FBCs • U&Es • LFTs • Erythrocyte sedimentation rate (ESR) • Temporal artery biopsy	• High-dose prednisolone
Tension headache	• Sensation of a tight band around the head • Stress • Low mood	• May not be required	• Reassurance • Measures to alleviate stress
Sinusitis	• History of upper respiratory tract symptoms • Purulent nasal discharge • Tenderness over sinuses	• May not be required	• Simple analgesia • Decongestants • Steroid nasal spray • Consider antibiotics if severe or persisting symptoms
Trigeminal neuralgia	• Stabbing pain in distribution of trigeminal nerve	• May not be required	• Carbamazepine • Pregabalin ± amitriptyline
Cluster headache	• Severe headache focused around one eye • Watery eyes • Runny or blocked nose • Sweating, usually at night	• CT or MRI brain	If acute attack: • High-flow oxygen, triptan Prophylaxis: • Verapamil

ADDITIONAL INFORMATION

⚠ Cerebrospinal fluid (CSF) characteristics differentiating likely cause of meningitis

	NORMAL	VIRAL	BACTERIAL	TUBERCULOSIS
Appearance	Clear	Clear/turbid	Turbid/purulent	Turbid/viscous
Predominant cell type	Lymphocytes	Lymphocytes	Polymorphs	Lymphocytes
White cell count ($\times 10^6$/L)	<5	5–1000	100–50,000	<500
Protein (g/L)	0.2–0.4	0.4–1	>1	1–5
Glucose	⅔–½ blood glucose	> ½ blood glucose	< ½ blood glucose	< ½ blood glucose

Present Your Findings

Ms Hart is a 25-year-old woman who has presented with a 6-h history of generalised headache that was gradual in onset, aching in character and 9/10 in severity. There is no radiation, but the pain is associated with fever, general malaise, photophobia and neck stiffness. Bright lights intensely aggravate the pain, and nothing seems to make it better. She has never had this before. There are no associated rashes. She has no significant past medical history and is on no regular medication. There are no unwell contacts of note, but there has been a recent outbreak of meningococcal meningitis in the community.

This is consistent with a diagnosis of meningitis.

Following a full examination, I would request bloods including FBCs, U&Es and CRP. I would order a CT scan before an LP and prescribe a stat dose of IV ceftriaxone.

QUESTIONS AND ANSWERS FOR CANDIDATE

Name three potential complications of meningitis.
- Raised intracranial pressure
- Hydrocephalus
- Seizures
- Focal neurological deficit
- Stroke from arterial or venous thrombosis
- Cerebral abscess or empyema

Name three common causative organisms in encephalitis.
- Viral:
  - Herpes simplex virus (most common)
  - Varicella zoster virus
  - Enterovirus (echovirus, coxsackievirus, poliovirus)
  - Mumps, measles
  - Arboviruses
- Bacterial:
  - TB
  - *Listeria*
  - *Streptococcus pneumoniae*
  - *Neisseria meningitidis*
- Other:
  - *Cryptococcus neoformans*
  - *Toxoplasma gondii*

How can a subarachnoid haemorrhage be graded?
- See Table 1.8 for answers

 A Case to Learn From

A 30-year-old patient presented to her primary care physician with a headache. She had a long history of migraines which had been managed with simple analgesia and sumatriptan. The patient had felt her headache had changed recently and was worried about this. Subsequent assessment and further investigation revealed a diagnosis of venous sinus thrombosis. This case is a reminder to be cautious of a change in usual headache and to take separate histories if the patient presents with more than one type of headache.

 Table 1.8 **Grading of a subarachnoid haemorrhage**

GRADE	DESCRIPTION
1	Asymptomatic, mild headache, slight nuchal rigidity
2	Moderate to severe headache, nuchal rigidity, no neurological deficit except cranial nerve palsy
3	Drowsy or confused, mild focal neurological deficit
4	Stupor, moderate to severe hemiparesis
5	Coma, decerebrate posturing

 Top Tip

In relation to subarachnoid haemorrhage, the truly sudden onset of the headache is critical: how long it took from the very first moment of the headache to its peak intensity. This is a vital indicator of whether a subarachnoid haemorrhage has to be considered.

STATION 1.13: COLLAPSE

SCENARIO

You are a junior doctor working on the medical assessment unit and have been asked to see Mr Jones, a 65-year-old man, who has been referred by his primary care doctor following three episodes of collapse over the last 4 days. Each episode lasted a few minutes with full recovery. He has a history of diabetes and had an MI 5 years ago. Please take a history from Mr Jones, present your findings and formulate an appropriate management plan.

Cardinal Symptoms

Prodromal symptoms
Loss of consciousness
Seizure activity
Tongue biting
Loss of consciousness
Time to recovery
Postictal symptoms

HISTORY OF PRESENTING COMPLAINT

COLLAPSE

- What happened before the collapse?
  - Prodromal symptoms; for example, flushing, light-headedness, blurred vision
  - Aura
  - Sudden-onset headache
  - Chest pain, dyspnoea or palpitations
  - Ask about potential triggers or precipitants; for example, hot environment, prolonged standing, fasting

- Antecedent head trauma
- What happened during the episode (remember to take a collateral history from any witnesses to the event)?
  - Loss of consciousness
  - Seizure activity
  - Duration of episode
  - Colour of patient; for example, pale, cyanosed
  - Presence of a pulse during the episode
- How was the patient after the episode?
  - Time to recovery
  - Postictal symptoms; for example, confusion, drowsiness, headache, limb weakness and nausea
  - Evidence of tongue biting and incontinence suggests seizure
  - Any injury sustained

ASSOCIATED SYMPTOMS

Other symptoms to enquire about include:
- Fever
- Tiredness
- Malaise
- Night sweats
- Weight loss

PAST MEDICAL AND SURGICAL HISTORY

In this scenario it is also important to note a history of:
- Epilepsy
- Structural or ischaemic cardiac disease
- Diabetes
- Postural hypotension
- Parkinson's disease
- Anxiety disorders

MEDICATION HISTORY

Enquire about prescribed medications (including any recent changes) and over-the-counter medications. Include allergies and the specific reaction. In this scenario it is also important to note:
- Antihypertensives and diuretics: Postural hypotension
- Beta-blockers: Bradycardia
- Insulin and oral diabetes medications: Hypoglycaemia
- Antiepileptic medications: Compliance

SOCIAL HISTORY

Social history includes enquiring about occupation, residence, lifestyle (diet, exercise, smoking, alcohol, substance abuse) and recent travel. Additionally in this scenario, consider:
- Smoking: Document pack years, calculated as the number of packs per day multiplied by the number of years smoked
- Alcohol and illicit drug use: Whether there is a history of substance abuse
- Occupation: Impact of symptoms; for example, HGV driver, operates heavy machinery
- Lifestyle: Salt intake, fluid intake, exercise

FAMILY HISTORY

Ask about any significant family history, including:
- History of sudden death

SYSTEMS REVIEW

On systems review, particularly pertinent questions to the above case may include questions regarding:
- Cardiovascular: Palpitations, dizziness, syncope, postural hypotension
- Respiratory: Haemoptysis, calf pain and swelling, pleuritic chest pain
- Gynaecological: LMP and possibility of pregnancy, whether there is a coil in situ

Risk Factors for Cardiac Syncope
- Increased age
- Male
- Presence of heart disease
- Positive family history
- Previous episodes

Differential Diagnosis

DISEASE	CLINICAL PRESENTATION	INVESTIGATIONS	MANAGEMENT
Seizure	• Aura • Limb jerking • Incontinence • Postictal phase	• FBCs • U&Es • LFTs • Glucose • Calcium • Magnesium • Anticonvulsant levels • Beta-hCG • CT head • Electroencephalogram (EEG) • MRI	• Oxygen • IV lorazepam if over 5 min. Buccal midazolam and rectal diazepam are alternatives • ITU support and IV phenytoin if seizures continue • Thiopental or propofol if ongoing

Differential Diagnosis—cont'd

DISEASE	CLINICAL PRESENTATION	INVESTIGATIONS	MANAGEMENT
Arrhythmia	• Sudden loss of consciousness • Usually with no prodromal symptoms • Pallor • Quick recovery	• FBCs • U&Es • Calcium • Magnesium • 12-lead ECG • 24-h tape	• Treatment of arrhythmia • Correct electrolyte disturbances • May need a pacemaker if heart block
Hypoglycaemia	• Known diabetes • Preceding hunger and sweating	• Blood glucose	• Glucose tablets/gel or fruit juice if conscious, followed by long-acting carbohydrate • IV glucose (200 mL 10% or 100 mL 20%) if unconscious or low GCS
Vasovagal syncope	• Preceding precipitant • Nausea • Sweating • Darkening of vision	• May not be necessary	• Reassurance
Cerebrovascular accident (CVA)	• Sudden-onset neurological symptoms	• FBCs • U&Es • Lipid profile • Glucose • Coagulation screen • CT head • ECG • Carotid Doppler	If ischaemic: • Thrombolysis if <4.5 h, or aspirin If haemorrhagic: • Refer to neurosurgeons
Aortic stenosis	• Syncope on exercise • Angina • Breathlessness	• Echocardiogram	• Valve replacement
Postural hypotension	• Sudden loss of consciousness after standing up from sitting or lying down	• Lying and standing BP	• Review medications • Support stockings • Fludrocortisone or midodrine
Carotid sinus syncope	• Syncope on turning head	• Carotid Doppler scan	• Aspirin • Surgical referral if >70% stenosis
PE	• Sudden-onset breathlessness • Pleuritic chest pain • Presence of risk factors for venous thromboembolism	• D-dimer • CTPA	• Thrombolysis if large or bilateral PE with hypotension or collapse • Otherwise, treatment dose low-molecular-weight heparin then warfarin

Distinguishing between seizures and syncope

	SEIZURE	SYNCOPE
Before	Aura May have no warning	There may be an obvious precipitant; for example, hot environment, prolonged standing Prodromal symptoms
During	Tonic-clonic movements Tongue biting Incontinence Cyanosis Irregular breathing Longer duration	Pallor Myoclonic jerks may be a feature Shorter duration
After	Slower to recover Postictal symptoms; for example, confusion, headache, limb weakness	Quick recovery

Present Your Findings

Mr Jones is a 65-year-old man who has experienced several episodes of collapse over the past 4 days. Each episode came without warning and lasted for a few minutes. His wife has witnessed these and noted he became pale and cold to touch and on one occasion his body started to shake. There is no history of incontinence or tongue biting and Mr Jones recovered quickly from the events with no postictal symptoms.

The most likely diagnosis would be cardiac syncope, given the history and Mr Jones' past medical history of ischaemic heart disease.

I would like to admit Mr Jones to a monitored bed for further assessment and observation.

? QUESTIONS AND ANSWERS FOR CANDIDATE

How would you assess and manage a patient who presented following a first fit?
- Detailed history from the patient and any witnesses
- General examination with full and comprehensive neurological and cardiovascular examinations
- Bloods, including FBCs, U&Es, glucose, calcium, magnesium
- ECG
- CT head if focal neurological signs, head injury, low GCS or known bleeding disorder
- Discharge home accompanied by a responsible adult and refer to first fit clinic if full recovery, normal examinations and normal bloods and ECG. Admit if patient does not satisfy these criteria or if more than one seizure
- Advise patient not to drive or operate heavy machinery

What are the causes of postural hypotension?
- Medications such as antihypertensives and diuretics
- Hypovolaemia
- Autonomic dysfunction; for example, diabetes, Parkinson's disease

Name three triggers that can induce carotid sinus hypersensitivity.
- Head turning
- Wearing a tight collar around the neck
- Shaving

A Case to Learn From

A 52-year-old woman was brought into the ED by ambulance after being found collapsed on the street. According to witnesses at the scene she was seen to fall to the ground and start shaking violently and this lasted around 5 min. The diagnosis of seizure was made and further investigations revealed that this patient was severely hyponatraemic, despite not taking any sodium-lowering medications. The cause of hyponatraemia was subsequently investigated, but this case is a reminder that seizures can be provoked by many causes, including electrolyte disturbances. Severe symptoms such as seizures are relatively common in patients with an acute and marked reduction in sodium level.

Top Tip

Always remember to get a collateral history when there has been a witness to the event. This can provide further key information to narrow down the differential diagnosis.

STATION 1.14: WEAKNESS

SCENARIO

You are a junior doctor in primary care and have been asked to see James Harper, a 67-year-old man, who has presented with right-leg weakness. His past medical history includes hypertension and hypercholesterolaemia. Please take a history from Mr Harper, present your findings and formulate an appropriate management plan.

Cardinal Symptoms

Distribution of weakness
Sensory disturbance
Back pain
Sphincter disturbance
Dysarthria or dysphasia
Disturbed gait

HISTORY OF PRESENTING COMPLAINT

WEAKNESS

- Clarification: Establish exactly what the patient means by weakness
- Distribution of weakness: Generalised or localised, symmetrical or asymmetrical, distal or proximal
- Onset: Acute or gradual onset
- Duration: Length of time the symptom has been present
- Progression and pattern of symptoms: Progressive or intermittent with periods of relapse and remission
- Exacerbation and relieving factors: For example, fatigability seen with myasthenia gravis

ASSOCIATED SYMPTOMS

Other symptoms to enquire about include:
- Fever
- Night sweats
- Weight loss
- Malaise
- Rash
- Sphincter disturbance
- Sensory loss
- Difficulty walking
- Back pain

PAST MEDICAL AND SURGICAL HISTORY

In this scenario, it is also important to enquire about:
- Vascular risk factors: For example, stroke, transient ischaemic attack (TIA), MI, angina, diabetes, hypertension, hypercholesterolaemia
- Atrial fibrillation
- Seizures
- Multiple sclerosis
- Malignancy
- Recent viral illness: For example, gastroenteritis, upper respiratory viral tract infection
- Endocrine disease: Hypothyroidism, Cushing's syndrome, Addison's disease
- Depression

MEDICATION HISTORY

Enquire about prescribed medications (including any recent changes) and over-the-counter medications. Allergies should be included, with the specific reaction noted. In this scenario it is also important to note:
- Anticoagulants: Increased risk of intracranial haemorrhage
- Steroids: Myopathy
- Statins: Myopathy
- Antiepileptics: History of seizures, postictal weakness

SOCIAL HISTORY

Social history includes enquiring about occupation, residence, lifestyle (diet, exercise, smoking, alcohol, substance abuse) and recent travel. Additionally in this scenario, consider:
- Smoking: Document pack years, calculated as the number of packs per day multiplied by the number of years smoked
- Alcohol and illicit drug use: Document units of alcohol consumed per week, enquire about use of recreational drugs; for example, cocaine, amphetamines
- Occupation: Driving regulations, heavy machinery, HGV driver
- Impacts on ADLs: Social and work life

FAMILY HISTORY

Ask about any significant family history, including:
- Subarachnoid haemorrhage
- Stroke or MI
- Muscle dystrophies
- Periodic paralysis
- Charcot–Marie–Tooth

SYSTEMS REVIEW

On systems review, particularly pertinent questions to the above case may include questions regarding:
- Neurological: Headache, nausea and vomiting, dysphasia, dysarthria, visual disturbance, facial weakness and numbness
- Musculoskeletal: Back pain, joint pain, swelling, stiffness, deformity

Risk Factors for Stroke

- Hypertension
- Diabetes
- Smoking
- Ischaemic heart disease
- Hypercholesterolaemia
- Brain aneurysms or arteriovenous malformations
- Increased age

Differential Diagnosis

DISEASE	CLINICAL PRESENTATION	INVESTIGATIONS	MANAGEMENT
Stroke	• Sudden onset • Focal neurology	• FBCs • U&Es • LFTs • Serum glucose level • Serum lipids level • Clotting screen • CT head	If ischaemia: • Thrombolysis if indicated. or aspirin 300 mg • Nil by mouth • SALT review. If haemorrhage: • Referral to neurosurgeon
TIA	• Sudden onset • Focal neurology • Resolves completely within 24 h	• FBCs • U&Es • LFTs • Serum glucose level • Serum lipids level • Clotting screen • CT or MRI head • Carotid Dopplers	• Treatment of risk factors • Medications; for example, clopidogrel • Refer to TIA clinic

Continued

Differential Diagnosis—cont'd

DISEASE	CLINICAL PRESENTATION	INVESTIGATIONS	MANAGEMENT
Todd's paresis	• History of seizure and postictal symptoms	• FBCs • U&Es • LFTs • Serum glucose level • Calcium • Magnesium • Anticonvulsant levels • Beta-hCG • CT head • EEG • MRI	• Supportive • The paralysis will resolve
Myasthenia gravis	• Diplopia • Ptosis • Limb weakness • Symptoms worsened by exercise	• Anti-acetylcholine receptor (AChR) antibodies • Muscle-specific tyrosine kinase (MuSK) antibodies • Neurophysiology • CT thymus	• Anticholinesterase; for example, pyridostigmine or neostigmine • Thymectomy
Guillain–Barré syndrome	• Progressive • Symmetrical • Ascending weakness • Often a few weeks after an infection	• LP • Nerve conduction studies	• IV immunoglobulin
Multiple sclerosis	• Neurological deficits distributed in time and space	• MRI	• High-dose steroids for acute relapses • Disease-modifying drugs; for example, beta-interferon and glatiramer, natalizumab, fingolimod

ADDITIONAL INFORMATION

ABCD² SCORE

The ABCD^2 score is used to estimate the risk of stroke after a suspected TIA (Table 1.9).

 Present Your Findings

Mr Harper is a 67-year-old man with a history of hypertension and hypercholesterolaemia, who has presented with a 2-h history of right-leg weakness. This was sudden in onset and associated with weakness and numbness of the right arm. He has had no previous similar episodes in the past.

The most likely diagnosis is an ischaemic stroke.

I would like to assess and examine Mr Harper rapidly and then request an urgent CT head to rule out an intracranial haemorrhage. If there is no intracranial haemorrhage, I would consider thrombolysis for ischaemic stroke.

❓ QUESTIONS AND ANSWERS FOR CANDIDATE

Explain the immediate management of a patient with a stroke.
- CT head
- If intracranial haemorrhage ruled out on CT scan:
  - Thrombolysis, i.e. alteplase if within 4.5 h of onset of symptoms
  - Aspirin 300 mg if thrombolysis not indicated
  - NBM

- IV fluids
- Request SALT assessment

Name three risk factors for stroke.
- Age
- Hypertension
- Diabetes
- Atrial fibrillation
- Previous stroke, TIA or MI
- Smoking
- Obesity and physical inactivity
- Hyperviscosity syndromes

When would a carotid endarterectomy or carotid stenting typically be performed?
- Patients with >70% carotid artery stenosis

 A Case to Learn From

A 70-year-old man was brought into the ED by ambulance after being found collapsed on the floor in his bedroom by his carers. He was unable to speak or comprehend simple commands and examination revealed that he had significant left-sided weakness. A CT scan was arranged which confirmed a right middle cerebral artery infarct. He was not eligible for thrombolysis as he presented >4.5 h from the onset of symptoms; therefore he was commenced on aspirin and transferred to the stroke ward for rehabilitation. It is vital to know the time of symptom onset to assess eligibility for thrombolysis.

Table 1.9	ABCD² scoring system: A score of ≥4 is considered high risk	
RISK FACTOR		**POINTS**
Age	≥ 60 years old	1
BP	Systolic ≥ 140 mmHg or Diastolic ≥ 90 mmHg	1
Clinical features of TIA (choose one)	Unilateral weakness with or without speech impairment or Speech impairment without unilateral weakness	2 / 1
Duration	TIA duration ≥ 60 min or TIA duration 10–59 min	2 / 1
Diabetes		1
Total ABCD² score 0–7.		

> **Top Tip**
>
> Hypoglycaemia can mimic a stroke!

STATION 1.15: HYPOTHYROIDISM

SCENARIO

You are a junior doctor in primary care and have been asked to see Mr Long, a 45-year-old man, who noticed a lump in his neck 2 weeks ago. He thinks the lump has grown and he is worried about what is causing it. He is a smoker with a 20-pack year history and drinks around 30 units of alcohol each week. He has no other medical history. Please take a history from Mr Long, present your findings and formulate an appropriate management plan.

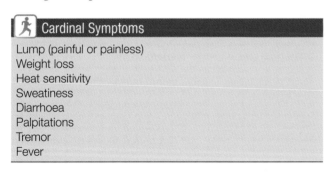

Cardinal Symptoms

Lump (painful or painless)
Weight loss
Heat sensitivity
Sweatiness
Diarrhoea
Palpitations
Tremor
Fever

HISTORY OF PRESENTING COMPLAINT

NECK LUMP

- Onset: Sudden or gradual
- Duration: Length of time the symptoms have been present
- Site: Down the midline or on the lateral side of the neck. If located laterally, the site in relation to the posterior and anterior triangles
- Size: Including change in size over time
- Number: Single or multiple neck lumps

- Skin changes: For example, erythema
- Character: For example, painful or painless. Shape
- Exacerbating and relieving factors: Pain during or before eating occurs in disease of salivary glands; for example, stones or malignancy

ASSOCIATED SYMPTOMS

Other symptoms to enquire about include:
- Weight loss
- Loss of appetite
- Fever
- Night sweats
- Malaise

PAST MEDICAL AND SURGICAL HISTORY

- Thyroid disease: Hyperthyroidism or hypothyroidism
- Malignancy: Haematological malignancy or metastatic spread
- Infection: For example, infectious mononucleosis (usually caused by EBV), streptococcal sore throat, TB, dental abscess

MEDICATION HISTORY

Enquire about prescribed medications (including any recent changes) and over-the-counter medications. Allergies should be included, with the specific reaction noted. In this scenario it is also important to note:
- Phenytoin
- Amiodarone
- Lithium
- Levothyroxine
- Carbimazole

  The above medications all have the potential to affect the thyroid gland.

SOCIAL HISTORY

Social history includes enquiring about occupation, residence, lifestyle (diet, exercise, smoking, alcohol, substance abuse) and recent travel. Additionally in this scenario, consider:
- Smoking: Document pack years, calculated as the number of packs per day multiplied by the number of years smoked
- Alcohol and illicit drug use: Document units of alcohol consumed per week
- Diet: Increased risk of head and neck cancer with a poor diet, particularly if deficient in vitamins A and C

FAMILY HISTORY

Ask about any significant family history, including:
- Malignancy
- Tuberculosis

SYSTEMS REVIEW

On systems review, particularly pertinent questions to the above case may include questions regarding:

- Thyroid: Weight change, hair and skin changes, heat or cold intolerance, change in bowel habit, palpitations, menorrhagia or amenorrhoea
- ENT: Sore throat, ear pain or discharge, white or red patches in the mouth, non-healing ulcers, unexplained loosening of teeth, dysphonia
- GI: Dysphagia secondary to compression of the oesophagus, symptoms suggestive of underlying malignancy causing lymphadenopathy; for example, change in bowel habit
- Respiratory: Breathlessness or stridor due to compression of the trachea, symptoms of underlying malignancy causing lymphadenopathy; for example, cough, haemoptysis

Risk Factors for Head and Neck Cancer

- Smoking
- Alcohol
- Diet: Increased risk with poor diet, particularly if deficient in vitamins A and C
- Human papillomavirus infection
- EBV infection
- Chronic syphilis infection

ADDITIONAL INFORMATION

CAUSES OF LYMPHADENOPATHY

- Infection: Upper respiratory tract infection, infectious mononucleosis (usually caused by EBV), TB, HIV

- Malignant: primary or secondary
- Other: Sarcoid, connective tissue disease, drugs

Present Your Findings

Mr Long is a 45-year-old man who has presented with a 2-week history of a lump in the neck. The lump is around 2 cm in diameter, firm and non-mobile and situated to the left lateral side of the neck. There are no overlying skin changes. Mr Long thinks that he has lost weight recently as his clothes feel looser and he has become intolerant to heat. He is a long-term smoker and drinks around 30 units of alcohol each week. He has no other medical problems and no significant past medical history.

My differential diagnoses include a toxic thyroid nodule, possibly malignant in aetiology, a thyroglossal cyst or cervical lymphadenopathy.

I would like to examine the neck and request TFTs and an USS.

QUESTIONS AND ANSWERS FOR CANDIDATE

What is a thyroglossal cyst?

- A painless, smooth, cystic midline swelling that develops from a remnant of the thyroglossal cyst
- It rises as the patient swallows or protrudes their tongue

Name three symptoms of hypothyroidism.

- Tiredness
- Weight gain
- Constipation
- Cold intolerance
- Dry skin
- Hair loss, especially to the outer one-third of the eyebrows
- Depression
- Bradycardia

Differential Diagnosis

DISEASE	CLINICAL PRESENTATION	INVESTIGATIONS	MANAGEMENT
Cervical lymphadenopathy	• Acute onset of tender, mobile lump • Often concurrent infection	• FBCs • U&Es • CRP	• Depends on cause • Reassurance if reactive lymphadenopathy
Goitre	• Generalised neck swelling • May have symptoms of hyper- or hypothyroidism	• TFTs • USS	• Reassurance if simple goitre • Otherwise treat the cause
Thyroid nodule	• Solitary neck lump in the region of thyroid gland	• TFTs • USS	• Refer to thyroid surgeon or endocrinology
Thyroglossal cyst	• Painless • Smooth, cystic midline swelling • Usually in a young adult	• TFTs • USS	• May require drainage before excision if infected
Salivary gland disease	• Pain and swelling on eating	• X-ray • Sialography	• Refer to ENT • May require surgical removal
Acute parotitis	• Pain and swelling at the angle of the jaw • Fever	• FBCs • U&Es • CRP • Swab any pus for MC&S • USS	• Good oral hygiene • Rehydration • Antibiotics • May require surgery

Describe the treatment of hyperthyroidism.
- Beta-blockers: Useful for symptom control until antithyroid medication takes effect
- Carbimazole: Inhibits the synthesis of thyroid hormones
- Radioactive iodine
- Surgery: Partial or total thyroidectomy

 A Case to Learn From

I was asked to see a patient in the ED during my medical on-call as a junior doctor. The patient was a 49-year-old woman who presented with a short history of generalised neck swelling. She was otherwise well with no previous medical history. Her neck was obviously swollen on examination with no discrete palpable lumps. I was unsure what this represented and wondered if this might be superior vena cava obstruction, so I asked for senior advice. Further investigation revealed that this patient had a large toxic goitre. I had not even considered this diagnosis due to the apparent acuteness of symptoms.

 Top Tip

Remember to discern whether the patient has experienced any symptoms or has any signs of tracheal compression such as stridor or breathlessness. This will require admission and urgent referral to a thyroid surgeon.

STATION 1.16: INTERMITTENT CLAUDICATION

SCENARIO

You are a junior doctor in primary care and have been asked to see Mr Brown, a 63-year-old man who presents with worsening leg pain on exertion. He is a long-term cigarette smoker and has type 2 diabetes, with a recent HbA$_{1c}$ of 9%. Please take a history from Mr Brown, present your findings and formulate an appropriate management plan.

 Cardinal Symptoms

Cramping leg pain on walking
Relief with rest
Cold feet
Skin changes
Ulcers

HISTORY OF PRESENTING COMPLAINT

PAIN

When a patient presents with pain, you can use the acronym SOCRATES to remember the questions that you should ask:
- *Site*: Location of the pain. The site is suggestive of ischaemic territory, and therefore if the pain is vascular, the culprit artery can be predicted
- *Onset*: Sudden or gradual. Sudden-onset pain is suggestive of an embolic event rather than a thrombotic event. Ask the patient what they were doing when the pain came on
- *Character*: For example, cramping, dull ache, stabbing, sharp
- *Radiation*: If so, ask the patient to delineate the area. If this is in a dermatomal distribution, consider nerve compression
- *Associated symptoms*: See below
- *Timing*: Duration of pain and any previous episodes
- *Exacerbating and relieving factors*: Pain worse with increasing level of exercise, or relieved by rest
- *Severity*: Score out of 10

ASSOCIATED SYMPTOMS

Other symptoms to enquire about include:
- Foot ulcers
- Numbness
- Cold feet
- White skin
- Weakness
- Impotence

PAST MEDICAL AND SURGICAL HISTORY

In this scenario, it is also important to enquire about:
- Vascular risk factors; for example, angina, MI, stroke, TIA, hypertension, hypercholesterolaemia
- Diabetes

MEDICATION HISTORY

Enquire about prescribed medications (including any recent changes) and over-the-counter medications. Allergies should be included, with the specific reaction noted. In this scenario it is also important to note:
- Analgesia: To assess the severity of leg pain
- Antihypertensives: To assess how much medication is required to control the patient's BP
- Statins: Also note the dosage to assess if it is for primary or secondary prevention
- Oral hypoglycaemic agents: For example, insulin
- Aspirin: An antiplatelet

SOCIAL HISTORY

Social history includes enquiring about occupation, residence, lifestyle (diet, exercise, smoking, alcohol, substance abuse) and recent travel. Additionally in this scenario, consider:
- Smoking: Document pack years, calculated as the number of packs per day multiplied by the number of years smoked
- Alcohol and illicit drug use: Document units of alcohol consumed per week
- Exercise: Physical inactivity and obesity are risk factors for peripheral vascular disease. Establish distance walked for onset of symptoms

FAMILY HISTORY

Ask about any significant family history, including:
- Ischaemic heart disease
- Peripheral vascular disease
- Stroke

SYSTEMS REVIEW

On systems review, particularly pertinent questions to the above case may include questions regarding:
- Neurological: Limb weakness, sensory disturbance, gait disturbance
- Cardiovascular: Leg swelling, hypercholesterolaemia, hypertension
- Respiratory: Haemoptysis, calf pain and swelling, pleuritic chest pain

Risk Factors for Peripheral Vascular Disease

- Smoking
- Hypercholesterolaemia
- Hypertension
- Obesity
- Diabetes
- Chronic kidney disease
- Increased age

ADDITIONAL INFORMATION

FINDINGS IN ACUTE LIMB ISCHAEMIA

Examination findings in acute limb ischaemia can be remembered as the 6 Ps:
- Pain
- Pallor
- Pulselessness
- Paralysis
- Paraesthesia
- Perishingly cold

PATTERN OF PAIN AND SITE OF STENOSIS:

- Buttock or thigh pain: Aortoiliac disease
- Calf pain: Femoropopliteal disease

CLASSIFICATION OF LOWER-LIMB ISCHAEMIA

The Fontaine classification of lower-limb ischaemia

CLASS	SYMPTOMS AND SIGNS
I	Asymptomatic
II	Intermittent claudication
III	Rest pain[a]
IV	Ulcers/gangrene[a]

[a]Grades III and IV indicate critical limb ischaemia.

Present Your Findings

Mr Brown is a 63-year-old man with poorly controlled type 2 diabetes mellitus. He presents with gradual-onset, cramping left calf pain on exertion. This comes on predictably after walking 30 m. It is relieved on resting for 5 min and by simple analgesia. He does not have any rest pain. He has a 20-pack year smoking history and is otherwise fit and well. He is on metformin, but no other regular medications.

This is consistent with a diagnosis of intermittent claudication.

I would like to examine Mr Brown fully and request bloods, an ABPI and a duplex ultrasound to determine the site of disease.

Differential Diagnosis

DISEASE	CLINICAL PRESENTATION	INVESTIGATIONS	MANAGEMENT
Chronic lower-limb ischaemia	• Cramping lower-limb pain on walking • Relieved by rest	• FBCs • U&Es • Lipids • Blood glucose or HbA_{1c} • Ankle brachial pressure index (ABPI) • Duplex USS	• Aspirin 75 mg OD • Exercise • Reduce risk factors; for example, stop smoking, lose weight, control BP, statins
Critical limb ischaemia	• Deteriorating claudication • Nocturnal rest pain	• Duplex USS • Angiography	• Analgesia • Urgent referral to vascular surgeon for revascularisation
Spinal stenosis	• Pain in lower back, buttocks or legs on walking • Relieved by forward flexion	• MRI	• Analgesia • Physiotherapy • Steroid injection • Surgery
Sciatica	• Pain radiating from the buttock down the back of the leg	• May not be required	• Analgesia • Physiotherapy

QUESTIONS AND ANSWERS FOR CANDIDATE

What clinical features would be suggestive of acute embolism?

- Sudden onset of symptoms
- Known embolic source; for example, atrial fibrillation, mural thrombus post-MI
- Absence of other symptoms of intermittent claudication; for example, leg pain on exertion, but eases with rest
- Cold legs because there has been no time for collateral blood supply to develop
- Normal vascular exam in the other leg

What investigations might be done in a patient with intermittent claudication?

- Resting Doppler pressure indexes
- Urinalysis (may find glycosuria)
- BP
- ECG
- Bloods: FBCs (may find polycythaemia, anaemia), U&Es (may reveal renovascular disease), lipid profile, fasting glucose
- Exercise testing: Foot pressure normally rises with exercise but is reduced in the presence of occlusive arterial disease
- Non-invasive imaging: Doppler ultrasonography, magnetic resonance angiography (MRA) and computed tomography angiography (CTA)
- Echocardiography: Detect cardiac disease, if concerned about cardiac emboli

What management options are there for a claudication?

- Medical therapy:
  - Risk factor management: Stop smoking, lose weight, modify diet and treat hypertension and diabetes
  - Exercise: To open and develop the collateral circulation
  - Take care not to injure the leg, since healing is generally poor
  - Aspirin and BP control
- Revascularisation:
  - Percutaneous balloon angioplasty and stent insertion
  - Bypass surgery; for example, aortoiliac bypass or femoropopliteal bypass
  - Amputation

A Case to Learn From

An elderly woman presented to her primary care doctor with reduced mobility. She had been finding it difficult to walk for months but had put this down to getting old and general aches and pains. She was a long-term smoker with a 40-pack year history. Examination of the legs revealed cold feet and pallor with loss of foot pulses bilaterally and absent popliteal pulse in the left leg. Further investigations confirmed a diagnosis of chronic peripheral ischaemia. It is easy for elderly patients to put a lot of things down to old age, so we must make sure that we rule out the important causes first!

Top Tip

Be vigilant for signs of critical limb ischaemia. It often progresses to limb loss or progressive tissue loss if left untreated.

STATION 1.17: SWOLLEN CALF

SCENARIO

You are a junior doctor in primary care and have been asked to see Mrs Maynard, a 70-year-old woman, who presented with a 3-week history of leg swelling. The swelling has become progressively worse and is affecting her mobility. She has a history of angina, hypertension, recurrent urinary tract infections and COPD. Please take a history from Mrs Maynard, present your findings and formulate an appropriate management plan.

Cardinal Symptoms

Unilateral or bilateral swelling
Skin changes
Pain
Trauma
Risk factors for VTE

HISTORY OF PRESENTING COMPLAINT

SWELLING

- Onset: Acute or gradual onset
- Duration: Length of time the symptom has been present
- Pattern: Unilateral or bilateral leg swelling, symmetrical or asymmetrical
- Timing: Constant or intermittent; dependent oedema is typically worse at the end of the day
- Exacerbating and relieving factors: For example, worsen on immobility, relieved by elevation of legs or diuretics
- Recent trauma or insect bites: Portal of entry for cellulitis
- Risk factors for VTE: For example, recent surgery, immobility, pregnancy

ASSOCIATED SYMPTOMS

Other symptoms to enquire about include:
- Fever
- Malaise
- Weight loss
- Night sweats
- Calf pain
- Localised tenderness over swelling
- Skin changes; for example, redness, brown haemosoderin discoloration, ulcers

PAST MEDICAL AND SURGICAL HISTORY

In this scenario, it is also important to enquire about:
- Heart failure or other cardiovascular disease
- VTE risk factors
- Previous history of deep-vein thrombosis (DVT) or varicose veins, which may cause venous insufficiency
- Malabsorption; for example, inflammatory bowel disease, coeliac disease
- Chronic lung disease
- Renal disease
- Chronic liver disease
- Hypothyroidism
- Lymphoedema

MEDICATION HISTORY

Enquire about prescribed medications (including any recent changes) and over-the-counter medications. Allergies should be included, with the specific reaction noted. In this scenario it is also important to note:
- Calcium channel blockers: For example, amlodipine, as leg swelling is a common side effect
- Steroids, NSAIDs: Can cause fluid retention
- Oral contraceptives and hormone replacement therapy (HRT): Increased risk of VTE
- Nephrotoxic medications: For example, NSAIDs, ACEi, gentamicin, which can cause potential damage to the kidneys

SOCIAL HISTORY

Social history includes enquiring about occupation, residence, lifestyle (diet, exercise, smoking, alcohol, substance abuse) and recent travel. Additionally in this scenario, consider:

- Smoking: Document pack years, calculated as the number of packs per day multiplied by the number of years smoked
- Alcohol and illicit drug use: Document units of alcohol per week
- Exercise: Level of mobility, impact of symptoms on ADLs

FAMILY HISTORY

Ask about any significant family history, including:
- Ischaemic heart disease
- Thrombophilia

SYSTEMS REVIEW

On systems review, particularly pertinent questions to the above case may include questions regarding:
- Heart failure: Breathlessness, orthopnoea, PND
- DVT: Calf pain and tenderness
- Cellulitis: Fever, redness, tenderness
- Cor pulmonale: Symptoms of chronic respiratory disease such as chronic cough and breathlessness
- Renal disease: Oedema in nephrotic syndrome, uraemic symptoms and reduced urine output in renal failure
- Malabsorption: Weight loss, diarrhoea
- Hypothyroidism: Fatigue, lethargy, weight gain, constipation, dry skin, dry hair, goitre

Risk Factors for Heart Failure

- Hypertension
- Coronary artery disease
- Previous MI
- Diabetes
- Congenital heart defects
- Obesity
- Smoking
- Increased age

Differential Diagnosis

DISEASE	CLINICAL PRESENTATION	INVESTIGATIONS	MANAGEMENT
Congestive cardiac failure	• Bilateral pitting lower-leg oedema • Breathlessness • Orthopnoea • PND	• Brain natriuretic peptide (BNP) • CXR • Echocardiogram	• ACEi • Beta-blocker • Diuretic; for example, furosemide
DVT	• Acute onset • Unilateral calf pain • Swelling • Redness	• D-dimer • US Doppler	• Anticoagulation
Cellulitis	• Unilateral leg swelling • Redness • Tenderness • Fever	• FBCs • U&Es • CRP	• Antibiotics; for example, flucloxacillin
Hypoalbuminaemia	• Bilateral leg swelling	• FBCs • U&Es • LFTs, including albumin	• Treat the cause • Oral nutritional supplements; may require NG feeding or total parenteral nutrition (TPN)
Lymphoedema	• Gradual onset • Bilateral non-pitting oedema		• Leg elevation • Compression stocking

ADDITIONAL INFORMATION

WELL'S SCORE

The Well's score to assess for the likelihood of DVTs can be calculated as per Table 1.10.

Clinical probability simplified score:

- 2 points or more – DVT 'likely'
- 1 point or less – DVT 'unlikely'

 Present Your Findings

Mrs Maynard is a 70-year-old woman who presented with a 3-week history of bilateral and symmetrical lower-leg swelling. There is no associated fever, pain or redness. She has a history of angina and hypertension and was recently prescribed amlodipine. Her mobility is usually limited due to breathlessness, but this has reduced over the last few weeks.

The possible differential diagnoses include peripheral oedema secondary to heart failure, leg swelling as a side effect of the recently prescribed calcium channel blocker and cor pulmonale.

There are a number of potential diagnoses in this case and I would like to examine Mrs Maynard fully and request further investigations, including bloods and a BNP to help narrow these down.

 Table 1.10 **Well's score for DVTs**

CLINICAL FEATURE	POINTS
Active cancer (treatment ongoing, within 6 months, or palliative)	1
Paralysis, paresis or recent plaster or immobilisation of the lower extremities	1
Recently bedridden for more than 3 days or major surgery within 12 weeks requiring general or regional anaesthesia	1
Localised tenderness along the distribution of the deep venous system	1
Entire leg swollen	1
Calf swelling 3 cm larger than asymptomatic side	1
Pitting oedema confined to the symptomatic leg	1
Collateral superficial veins (non-varicose)	1
Previously documented DVT	1
An alternative diagnosis is at least as likely as DVT	1

❓ QUESTIONS AND ANSWERS FOR CANDIDATE

Describe the management of lymphoedema.

- Leg elevation
- Compression stocking
- Exercise
- Antibiotics if infection is present
- Manual lymph drainage
- Surgery

What is cor pulmonale?

- Cor pulmonale is right-sided heart failure due to chronic pulmonary hypertension

What are the potential causes of a raised D-dimer?

- DVT
- Infection
- Malignancy
- Following trauma
- Postsurgery

 A Case to Learn From

I reviewed a patient on the ward who had significant bilateral lower-leg swelling due to lymphoedema. The patient explained how she had previously been independently mobile and able to perform all ADLs independently. However, the lymphoedema made it extremely difficult for her to walk and she subsequently spent the majority of her time now sat in an armchair or in bed. This had significantly affected her mood and she had started to feel depressed. This case demonstrates the huge impact such symptoms can have on patients' lives.

💡 **Top Tip**

Don't forget to auscultate the lungs in a patient with leg swelling. A patient with pulmonary oedema due to congestive heart failure will likely have bibasal crackles.

STATION 1.18: BACK PAIN

SCENARIO

You are a junior doctor in primary care and have been asked to see Mrs Fletcher, a 60-year-old woman who presented with back pain. She has also become incontinent and is feeling unsteady on her feet. Please take a history from Mrs Fletcher, present your findings and formulate an appropriate management plan.

HISTORY OF PRESENTING COMPLAINT

PAIN

When a patient presents with pain, you can use the acronym SOCRATES to remember the questions that you should ask:

- *Site*: Ask the patient if they can point to a specific site
- *Onset*: Sudden or gradual, what the patient was doing at the time of onset

🏃 **Cardinal Symptoms**

Constitutional symptoms: Fever, night sweats, weight loss
Thoracic pain
Night pain
Leg weakness, numbness or paraesthesia
Bladder or bowel dysfunction
Saddle anaesthesia

- *Character*: For example, a tight band, dull, sharp, electric shock
- *Radiation*: For example, down the buttock and thigh, or all the way down to the foot
- *Associated symptoms*: See below
- *Timing*: Including duration of symptoms, any previous episodes, constant or intermittent
- *Exacerbating and relieving factors*: Worsened or eased by exercise, rest, movement, sitting or bending forwards, heat therapy
- *Severity*: score out of 10

ASSOCIATED SYMPTOMS

Other symptoms to enquire about include:
- Weight loss
- Fever
- Night sweats
- Sphincter disturbance
- Sensory loss
- Difficulty walking
- Leg weakness

PAST MEDICAL AND SURGICAL HISTORY

In this scenario, it is also important to enquire about:
- Cancer
- Osteoporosis
- Arthritis
- Previous spinal problems or spinal surgery
- Involvement of physiotherapists, osteopaths, chiropractors or other professionals

MEDICATION HISTORY

Enquire about prescribed medications (including any recent changes) and over-the-counter medications. Allergies should be included, with the specific reaction noted. In this scenario it is also important to note:
- Analgesia: To gauge severity
- Steroids: Risk of osteoporosis

SOCIAL HISTORY

Social history includes enquiring about occupation, residence, lifestyle (diet, exercise, smoking, alcohol, substance abuse) and recent travel. Additionally in this scenario, consider:
- Smoking: Document pack years, calculated as the number of packs per day multiplied by the number of years smoked
- Alcohol and illicit drug use: Document units of alcohol per week
- Exercise: Reduced mobility
- Occupation: Manual labour, heavy lifting

FAMILY HISTORY

Ask about any significant family history, including:
- History of joint or back problems

SYSTEMS REVIEW

On systems review, particularly pertinent questions to the above case may include questions regarding:
- Neurological: Weakness or paraesthesia in the lower limbs. Urinary retention or incontinence, faecal incontinence, saddle anaesthesia
- Musculoskeletal: Previous muscle injury, sprains or ligament tears
- Mobility: Reduced mobility, difficulty walking

Risk Factors for Cauda Equina Syndrome

- Spinal stenosis
- Degenerative disc disease
- Birth defects; for example, spina bifida
- Previous spinal surgery
- Haemorrhages affecting the spinal cord

ADDITIONAL INFORMATION

RED-FLAG SYMPTOMS FOR BACK PAIN

- History of malignancy or immunosuppression
- Age <20 years or >55 years
- Constitutional symptoms: Fever, night sweats, weight loss
- Thoracic pain
- Night pain
- Progressive neurological deficit
- Saddle anaesthesia or sphincter disturbance

BONE METASTASIS

The mnemonic 'LP Thomas Knows Best' can be used to remember cancers that commonly metastasise to the bones:
- Liver
- Prostate
- Thyroid
- Kidney
- Breast

Present Your Findings

Mrs Fletcher is a 60-year-old woman who has presented with back pain. She has recently been diagnosed with breast cancer. She has been experiencing new-onset, gradually progressive, lower-back pain over the last 2 days. It radiates down both legs and is associated with urinary and faecal incontinence. Her legs feel weak and she is unsteady on her feet.

This is consistent with a diagnosis of cauda equina syndrome secondary to lumbar spine metastases.

This is a medical emergency, requiring an urgent MRI, steroid therapy and consideration for further neurosurgical or oncological intervention.

Differential Diagnosis

DISEASE	CLINICAL PRESENTATION	INVESTIGATIONS	MANAGEMENT
Spinal cord compression	• Back pain • Weakness • Loss of sensation below the level of the lesion	• MRI spine	• High-dose steroids • Neurosurgery • Radiotherapy
Cauda equina syndrome	• Leg weakness • Pain (often bilateral) • Bladder and/or bowel dysfunction • Saddle anaesthesia.	• MRI spine	• High-dose steroids • Neurosurgery • Radiotherapy
Mechanical back pain	• Pain worse on movement • May be chronic	• Rarely indicated	• Early mobilisation • Analgesia • Benzodiazepine for muscle spasm • Physiotherapy
Vertebral compression fracture	• Sudden onset • Pain • Reduced range of movement • Elderly	• Spinal X-ray	• Analgesia • Treatment of osteoporosis
Spinal stenosis	• Back pain with neurogenic claudication	• MRI spine	• Analgesia • Physiotherapy • Surgery

❓ QUESTIONS AND ANSWERS FOR CANDIDATE

What is ankylosing spondylitis?
• Ankylosing spondylitis is a seronegative spondylitis affecting the spine and sacroiliac joints. It is most common in young males. The primary symptoms include back pain and stiffness, usually worse in the morning or after periods of inactivity

How is ankylosing spondylitis managed?
• Conservative:
  • Regular exercise and physiotherapy
• Medical:
  • NSAIDs and analgesia for pain
  • Sulphasalazine and tumour necrosis factor-alpha antagonists may also be used

What are some risk factors for vertebral fractures?
• Prolonged steroid use
• Osteoporosis
• Trauma

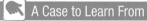

A Case to Learn From

A 69-year-old man with prostate cancer presented with back pain and leg weakness and was treated for suspected malignant spinal cord compression. He was in significant pain and required a number of analgesics and substantial amounts of morphine. The medical team therefore referred him to palliative care who provided invaluable advice on medications for better pain control and psychological support. Specialist psychological support can often reduce the requirement of analgesics. The palliative care team are an invaluable source of help and support when managing pain and polypharmacy.

💡 Top Tip

X-rays are not routinely recommended for people with lower-back pain and no red-flag features.

STATION 1.19: INHERITED DISEASE

SCENARIO

You are a doctor in cardiology clinic and have been asked to see Mr Jones, a 42-year-old man, who has been referred to outpatient clinic by his primary care doctor who recently diagnosed a heart murmur. His primary care doctor has noted that Mr Jones is very tall with long extremities and hyperextensible joints. He has a family history of cardiac problems and wonders whether this may be genetic. Please take a history from Mr Jones, present your findings and formulate an appropriate management plan.

Cardinal Symptoms

Tall
Slender
Disproportionately long arms, legs and fingers
Chest deformities
High arched palate
Heart murmurs
Visual problems
Flexible joints

HISTORY OF PRESENTING COMPLAINT

- Establish why the patient presented to his primary care doctor initially and whether the patient is symptomatic

MURMUR

- Take a cardiac history in view of the murmur:
  - Chest pain
  - Difficulty in breathing
  - Palpitations
  - Exercise tolerance
  - Syncope

ASSOCIATED SYMPTOMS

- Enquire into any further signs or symptoms of Marfan's syndrome, which appears to be the diagnosis in question:
  - Tall with long extremities
  - Arachnodactyly
  - Hyperextensible joints
  - High-arched palate
  - Scoliosis

PAST MEDICAL AND SURGICAL HISTORY

In this scenario, it is also important to enquire about:
- Requirement for spectacles or previous eye surgery
- Previous cardiac surgery or chest drains (pneumothorax)
- Any previous cardiac screening or surveillance
- Hypertension (associated with coarctation of the aorta)
- Thyroid disease (in review of murmur)

MEDICATION HISTORY

Enquire about prescribed medications (including any recent changes) and over-the-counter medications. Allergies should be included, with the specific reaction noted. In this scenario it is also important to note:
- Beta-blockers and angiotensin receptor blockers: Can slow aortic root dilatation

SOCIAL HISTORY

Social history includes enquiring about occupation, residence, lifestyle (diet, exercise, smoking, alcohol, substance abuse) and recent travel. Additionally in this scenario, consider:
- Smoking: Document pack years, calculated as the number of packs per day multiplied by the number of years smoked
- Alcohol and illicit drug use: Document units of alcohol per week
- Occupation: Cardiac problems may have implications

FAMILY HISTORY

If there is a history of inherited disease in the family or there is clinical suspicion that a condition in the affected individual may be genetic, it is important to be able to take a detailed family history. This involves asking a series of questions about the individual's first- and second-degree relatives and depicting the information as a pedigree.

Pertinent questions to ask include:
- Name of the condition(s) reported in affected family members
- Relationship of the affected individual to the patient
- Family's origin and ethnicity
- Any consanguinity
- Age of family members at onset of condition
- Pregnancy outcomes of the patient and relatives, including any miscarriages

This information can then be represented in a pedigree diagram

SYSTEMS REVIEW

On systems review, particularly pertinent questions to the above case may include questions regarding:
- Cardiovascular: Chest pain, hypertension, heart failure
- Respiratory: Breathlessness, cyanosis
- Visual: Impaired vision, glasses or contact lens wearer
- Musculoskeletal: Loss of function, deformity, instability, locking

ADDITIONAL INFORMATION

DRAWING A PEDIGREE DIAGRAM

Pedigree diagrams are used to depict the family history of a genetic condition and to work out the pattern of inheritance (Fig. 1.3). Symbols represent each member of the family, their gender and their disease state.

A pedigree diagram should be started with the affected individual who presented with symptoms.

Autosomal-Dominant Conditions (e.g. Huntington's Disease)

An autosomal-dominant inheritance pattern will show family members affected in each successive generation (Fig. 1.4). Any child born will have a 50% chance of inheriting the condition.

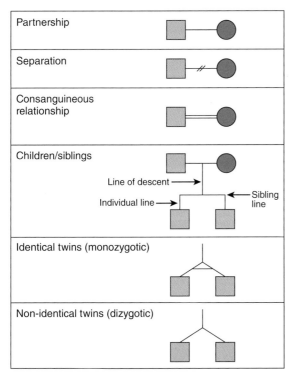

Fig. 1.3 Pedigree diagram symbols and their meanings.

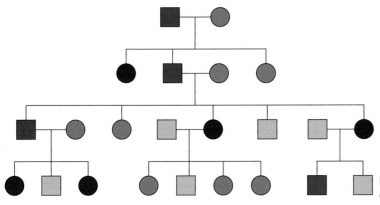

Fig. 1.4 A pedigree diagram showing a pattern of autosomal-dominant inheritance.

Autosomal-Recessive Conditions (e.g. Cystic Fibrosis)

An autosomal-recessive condition needs two copies of a gene, one inherited from each parent (Fig. 1.5). The risk of a child being affected by an autosomal-recessive condition is increased in consanguinity.

X-Linked Recessive Conditions (e.g. Duchenne and Becker Muscular Dystrophy)

A gene alteration occurs on the X chromosome. As males have only one X chromosome, they will develop the condition. The gene alteration can be transmitted from female carriers to their sons, but affected males cannot transmit the condition to their sons (Fig. 1.6).

Present Your Findings

Mr Jones is a tall 42-year-old man, with long extremities, arachnodactyly and hyperextensible joints, who has recently been diagnosed with a heart murmur. He also reports a previous history of pneumothorax. Mr Jones has a family history of cardiac problems and his father has had aortic root repair surgery. A detailed family history and pedigree diagram show an autosomal-dominant inheritance pattern and therefore point to a diagnosis of Marfan's syndrome.

I would like to perform a full physical examination and use the Ghent criteria to help confirm my diagnosis. I will refer Mr Jones to a cardiologist and ensure family members are screened for Marfan's syndrome.

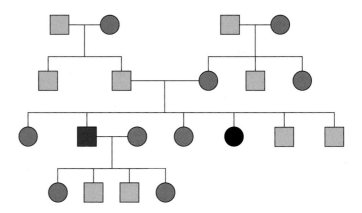

Fig. 1.5 A pedigree diagram showing a pattern of autosomal-recessive inheritance.

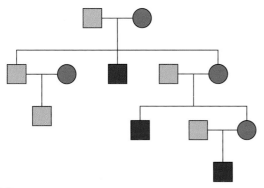

Fig. 1.6 A pedigree diagram showing a pattern of X-linked recessive inheritance.

❓ QUESTIONS AND ANSWERS FOR CANDIDATE

What is Mendelian inheritance?
- Mendelian inheritance patterns describe inheritance of disorders caused by errors on one specific gene. The main modes of Mendelian inheritance are:
  - Autosomal-dominant
  - Autosomal-recessive
  - X-linked dominant
  - X-linked recessive

Name three autosomal-recessive conditions.
- Cystic fibrosis
- Sickle cell anaemia
- Phenylketonuria
- Medium-chain acyl-CoA dehydrogenase deficiency (MCADD)

What is the genetic mutation and inheritance pattern that causes Down syndrome?
- Down syndrome is the most common chromosomal abnormality in humans
- It is a disorder of chromosomal inheritance, also known as trisomy 21, as there are three copies of chromosome 21. This is due to aneuploidy

- Aneuploidy describes a condition where cells do not have the expected number of chromosomes. The commonest cause is meiotic non-disjunction during oogenesis or spermatogenesis, leaving a gamete with zero or two copies of a particular chromosome. When the gamete is fertilised, the resulting embryo will have one or three copies of the affected chromosome, instead of the expected two

🐘 A Case to Learn From

Always remember the key questions you need to ask your patient, even if you find them challenging. Whilst taking a genetic history, I made an incorrect assumption and failed to discuss consanguinity. This is a sensitive but important topic to discuss and may be key to understanding whether there is a risk of a condition being inherited from both sides of the family.

💡 Top Tip

If you are unsure regarding the nature of inheritance for a condition, draw a family tree and ask the patient to describe who is affected. Doing this together can be a useful exercise.

STATION 1.20: JOINT PAIN

SCENARIO

You are a junior doctor in the ED and have been asked to see Jack Hassall, a 30-year-old man, who presented with a 2-day history of pain and swelling in his right knee. He is fit and well with no significant medical history. Please take a history from Jack, present your findings and formulate an appropriate management plan.

Cardinal Symptoms

Redness
Deformity
Loss of function
Mono-/oligo-/polyarthritis
Symmetrical or asymmetrical joint involvement
Fever
Malaise

HISTORY OF PRESENTING COMPLAINT

PAIN

When a patient presents with pain, you can use the acronym SOCRATES to remember the questions that you should ask:
- *Site*: Establish distribution of symptoms, including number of joints involved, symmetrical or asymmetrical joint involvement, large or small joints affected
- *Onset*: Ask the patient what they were doing at the time of onset, if there is any obvious trigger or recent trauma, sudden or insidious onset
- *Character*: Ask the patient to describe the pain
- *Radiation*: For example, from the hip to the knee
- *Associated symptoms*: See below
- *Timing*: Duration of symptoms and any previous episodes. Also ask whether symptoms are worse in the morning, which is suggestive of inflammatory arthritis
- *Exacerbating and relieving factors*: Worsened by exercise and trauma and relieved by rest, analgesia, NSAIDs
- *Severity*: Score out of 10

ASSOCIATED SYMPTOMS

Other symptoms to enquire about include:
- Fever
- Night sweats
- Malaise
- Weight loss
- Joint deformity/loss of function
- Skin changes

PAST MEDICAL AND SURGICAL HISTORY

In this scenario, it is also important to enquire about:
- Known joint problems such as arthritis
- Psoriasis: Psoriatic arthritis
- Gout
- Inflammatory bowel disease: Enteropathic spondyloarthropathy
- Sexually transmitted infection: Reactive arthritis
- Gastroenteritis: Reactive arthritis
- Immunocompromise: Septic arthritis
- Haemophilia: Haemarthrosis
- Previous fractures or orthopaedic surgery, including prosthetic joints

MEDICATION HISTORY

Enquire about prescribed medications (including any recent changes) and over-the-counter medications. Allergies should be included, with the specific reaction noted. In this scenario it is also important to note:
- NSAIDs: Could point towards an inflammatory disease if the joint pain is eased by NSAIDs
- Steroids: Immunosuppressant
- Disease-modifying antirheumatic drugs (DMARDs): Immunosuppressant
- Anticoagulants: Risk of haemarthrosis
- Diuretics: Increased risk of gout

SOCIAL HISTORY

Social history includes enquiring about occupation, residence, lifestyle (diet, exercise, smoking, alcohol, substance abuse) and recent travel. Additionally in this scenario, consider:
- Smoking: Document pack years, calculated as the number of packs per day multiplied by the number of years smoked
- Alcohol and illicit drug use: Document units of alcohol consumed per week
- Diet: High-purine diet is a risk factor for gout
- Exercise: Sport and hobbies, impact of symptoms on mobility and ADLs
- Occupation: Manual labour, repetitive use of joint, excess kneeling causing prepatellar bursitis

FAMILY HISTORY

Ask about any significant family history, including:
- Musculoskeletal problems; for example, rheumatoid arthritis, psoriatic arthritis
- Inflammatory bowel disease

SYSTEMS REVIEW

On systems review, particularly pertinent questions to the above case may include questions regarding:
- Musculoskeletal: Swelling, redness, stiffness, loss of function, deformity, instability, locking
- Rheumatological: Rash, ulcers, Raynaud's, dry eyes and mouth, alopecia
- GI: Symptoms suggestive of inflammatory bowel disease or gastroenteritis
- Genitourinary: Symptoms suggestive of sexually transmitted infections; for example, dysuria and discharge

Risk Factors for Septic Arthritis

- Joint problems; for example, arthritis or gout
- Previous joint surgery
- Open wounds or active infection
- Intravenous drug user
- Immunocompromised
- Smoking
- Diabetes

ADDITIONAL INFORMATION

CAUSES OF JOINT PAIN

ARTHRITIS is a useful mnemonic to remember causes of joint pain:
- *Arthritis* (rheumatoid arthritis, osteoarthritis)
- *Reactive* arthritis
- *Trauma*
- *Hyperuricaemia* (gout)

Differential Diagnosis

DISEASE	CLINICAL PRESENTATION	INVESTIGATIONS	MANAGEMENT
Septic arthritis	• Fever with tender, swollen and red single joint	• FBCs • U&Es • CRP • ESR • Blood culture • Joint aspiration • X-ray	• Urgent referral to orthopaedics • Antibiotics • Analgesia
Rheumatoid arthritis	• Usually symmetrical • Peripheral joint involvement • Pain • Stiffness • Swelling • Early deformity	• FBCs • U&Es • CRP • ESR • Rheumatoid factor • X-ray	• Analgesia • NSAIDs • Physiotherapy • Steroids • DMARDs • Biological therapies
Osteoarthritis	• Joint pain • Worse with activity • Stiffness	• FBCs • U&Es • CRP • ESR • X-ray	• Analgesia • Exercise • Physiotherapy • Weight loss • Walking aids • Joint replacement
Gout	• Acute onset • Pain • Swollen • Joint affected is usually first metatarsal joint (big toe)	• FBCs • U&Es • CRP • ESR • Urate • Joint aspiration • X-ray	• Exclude infection • Rest • NSAIDs or colchicine • Steroid joint injection • Allopurinol if recurrent attacks
Pseudogout	• Gradual onset • Single joint pain • Attacks are less severe than gout attacks	• FBCs • U&Es • CRP • ESR • Urate • Joint aspiration • X-ray	• Treat acute attacks like gout
Reiter's syndrome	• Joint pain associated with urethritis and conjunctivitis • Typically in a young patient	• FBCs • U&Es • CRP • ESR • Rheumatoid factor • Chlamydia swab and urine sample • Joint aspiration if effusion	• Rest • Analgesia • Antibiotics if for infection; for example, Chlamydia
Psoriatic arthritis	• Arthritis with a history or evidence of psoriasis	• FBCs • U&Es • CRP • ESR • Rheumatoid factor • X-ray	• Analgesia • NSAIDs • Immunosuppressants

Differential Diagnosis—cont'd

DISEASE	CLINICAL PRESENTATION	INVESTIGATIONS	MANAGEMENT
Haemarthrosis	• Acutely swollen and painful joint • History of trauma	• FBCs • U&Es • CRP • ESR • X-ray • Joint aspiration	• Analgesia • Joint aspiration

- *Referred* pain
- *Infection* (septic arthritis)
- *Connective* tissue disease (systemic lupus erythematosus (SLE), Sjögren's syndrome, systemic sclerosis)
- *Inflammatory* bowel disease
- *Spondyloarthropathies* (ankylosing spondylitis, psoriatic arthritis)

Present Your Findings

Mr Hassall is a 30-year-old man who presented to the ED with a 2-day history of pain and swelling in his right knee. It has become increasingly difficult to weight bear due to the pain. He is a keen football player, but there is no history of trauma. There are no other affected joints. He feels systemically well; however, he did suffer from diarrhoea and vomiting 2 weeks ago after he returned home from a holiday in Spain. He is otherwise fit and well with no other medical conditions and there is no family history of joint problems.

My main differential diagnoses would include septic arthritis, reactive arthritis and gout.

I would like to examine Jack's knee, including the joint above and below, and I would like to request bloods and an X-ray and arrange a joint aspiration.

❓ QUESTIONS AND ANSWERS FOR CANDIDATE

What are the treatment options for osteoarthritis?
- Analgesia; for example, paracetamol, NSAIDs
- Exercise and physiotherapy
- Weight loss if overweight
- Walking aids
- Steroid injection
- Total or partial knee replacement

Which conditions typically cause a monoarthritis?
- Septic arthritis
- Trauma
- Haemarthrosis
- Osteoarthritis
- Crystal arthropathy: Gout, pseudogout
- Reactive arthritis
- Psoriatic arthritis
- Rheumatoid arthritis

How is disease activity measured in rheumatoid arthritis?
- The DAS28 score, whereby DAS stands for Disease Activity Score, and 28 refers to the 28 joints that are examined in the assessment

- To calculate the DAS28, the healthcare professional will count the number of swollen joints and the number of tender joints (out of the 28), take bloods to measure ESR or CRP and ask the patient to make an assessment of his health
- All of the results will then produce a score and DAS28 can be interpreted as below:
  - > 5.2: Active disease
  - < 3.2: Low disease activity
  - < 2.6: Remission

A Case to Learn From

I saw a patient during my primary care rotation with knee pain. I took a history and examined his knee fully and subsequently organised an X-ray of the knee. No abnormality was detected on the knee X-ray. I therefore discussed this case with my supervisor who suggested that the patient's knee pain could be radiating from the hip. This case reminded me always to examine the joint above and below.

💡 Top Tip

Always consider septic arthritis. A failure to recognise the diagnosis can quickly lead to irreversible joint damage, so have a low threshold for checking a CRP.

STATION 1.21: BREAST LUMP

SCENARIO

You are a junior doctor in primary care and have been asked to see Mrs Patterson, a 45-year-old woman, who has noticed a lump in her left breast. Please take a history, present your findings and formulate an appropriate plan.

Cardinal Symptoms

Pain
Skin changes
Nipple discharge
Nipple changes
Changes with menstrual cycle

HISTORY OF PRESENTING COMPLAINT

BREAST LUMP

- Site: Location of the lump
- Onset: When the lump was first noticed, presence of preceding trauma
- Size: Including any changes over time
- Consistency: Including any changes over time
- Character: Painful or painless, mobility
- Appearance: Including breast or nipple changes; for example, nipple inversion or distortion, eczema
- Nipple discharge: For example, blood, pus, milk
- Skin changes: For example, dimpling, oedema, ulceration, erythema, eczema
- Relation to hormonal changes: Changes throughout the menstrual cycle; for example, cyclical breast pain
- Relevant breast history: Previous lumps or history of other breast problems in the past

ASSOCIATED SYMPTOMS

Other symptoms to enquire about include:
- Whether currently breastfeeding or not
- Fever
- Malaise
- Weight loss
- Night sweats

PAST MEDICAL AND SURGICAL HISTORY

In this scenario, it is also important to enquire about:
- Pregnancy and breastfeeding: Galactocoele, mastitis, breast abscess
- Previous breast lumps or breast problems
- Cancer
- Exposure to ionising radiation: Increased risk of breast cancer

MEDICATION HISTORY

Enquire about prescribed medications (including any recent changes) and over-the-counter medications. Allergies should be included, with the specific reaction noted. In this scenario it is also important to note:
- Oral contraceptive pill: Small increased risk of breast cancer
- HRT: Increased risk of breast cancer following the use of unopposed oestrogen in HRT for 10–15 years

SOCIAL HISTORY

Social history includes enquiring about occupation, residence, lifestyle (diet, exercise, smoking, alcohol, substance abuse) and recent travel. Additionally in this scenario, consider:

- Smoking: Document pack years, calculated as the number of packs per day multiplied by the number of years smoked
- Alcohol: Risk factor for breast cancer
- Occupation: Occupational exposures to potential carcinogens

FAMILY HISTORY

Ask about any significant family history, including:
- Cancer, in particular breast cancer and ovarian cancer. Some of the features of familial breast cancer include:
  - Several family members affected
  - Early age of presentation
  - Bilateral breast involvement is common
  - History of related cancers; for example, ovary, endometrial, colorectal

SYSTEMS REVIEW

On systems review, particularly pertinent questions to the above case may include questions regarding:
- Pregnancies: Parity and most recent pregnancy
- Menstruation: Date of LMP

Risk Factors for Breast Cancer

- Increased age
- Early menarche
- Late menopause
- Nulliparity
- Smoking
- Positive family history
- Exogenous oestrogen; for example, oral contraceptive pill, HRT
- Previous exposure to ionising radiation

ADDITIONAL INFORMATION

TRIPLE ASSESSMENT

The breast triple assessment is a 'one-stop' hospital clinic that allows rapid assessment of breast problems and early detection of breast cancer. The combined approach to assessment has >90% sensitivity and specificity. It has three key components:
1. History and examination:
   - Table 1.11 outlines the signs and symptoms of breast cancer
2. Imaging:
   - Mammography (low-dose X-rays to the breast tissues): To detect mass lesions or microcalcifications
   - Ultrasound scan: A better form of imaging in women <35 years old and men due to density of breast tissue
3. Biopsy:
   - Any suspicious mass or lesion by either core biopsy or fine-needle aspiration (FNA). Core

Differential Diagnosis

DISEASE	CLINICAL PRESENTATION	INVESTIGATIONS	MANAGEMENT
Breast cancer	• Breast lump • Skin changes • Nipple inversion • Blood-stained nipple discharge • Non-cyclic breast pain	• Triple assessment (i.e. clinical assessment, imaging and biopsy. See additional information)	• Surgery • Chemotherapy • Radiotherapy • Hormonal therapy
Fibroadenoma	• Discrete, firm, non-tender and highly mobile breast lump	• Triple assessment	• Reassurance • Excision if lump > 4 cm or age >40 years old
Breast cyst	• Smooth, discrete lump • May be painful	• Triple assessment	• Aspiration for simple cyst • Excision biopsy if clinically or radiologically suspicious
Mastitis	• Redness • Swelling • Warmth • Fever • Flu-like symptoms • Tender lump if blocked duct	• Not usually required	• Antibiotics • Drainage if abscess present
Breast abscess	• Hot and painful swelling • Usually occurs in lactating breast, following mastitis	• Triple assessment	• Aspiration under ultrasound guidance or • Surgical incision and drainage
Fat necrosis	• History of trauma	• Triple assessment	• Reassurance • Lump often disappears spontaneously
Galactocoele	• Subareolar mass • Milky nipple discharge	• Triple assessment	• Aspiration or • Excision

Table 1.11   Signs and symptoms of breast cancer

New lump	A new lump or thickening in the breast and/or armpit area
Nipple change	A newly inverted or retracted nipple
Skin change	A change in the skin of the breast, areola or nipple such as colour, dimpling, puckering or reddening
Shape change	A change in the breast shape or size
Nipple discharge	A discharge from the nipple that occurs without squeezing

biopsy provides full histology, therefore allows differentiation between carcinoma in situ and invasive breast cancer

Present Your Findings

Mrs Patterson is a 45-year-old woman who noticed a lump in her left breast 2 weeks ago. The lump is not painful, but she has noticed some changes to the skin overlying the lump. She has not noticed any nipple discharge or nipple changes. She feels otherwise generally well in herself. Mrs Patterson has a family history of breast cancer, with both her mother and maternal grandmother affected by breast cancer.

I feel that this may be a case of breast cancer, with differentials being fibroadenoma and breast cyst.

I would like to refer Mrs Patterson to the breast clinic for urgent further assessment, including history and examination, imaging and a biopsy of the breast lump.

❓ QUESTIONS AND ANSWERS FOR CANDIDATE

What are the broad treatment options used for breast cancer?

• Surgery
• Endocrine therapy; for example, tamoxifen, aromatase inhibitors and trastuzumab
• Radiotherapy
• Chemotherapy

What is the meaning and clinical relevance of oestrogen receptor (ER) and human epidermal growth factor receptor 2 (HER2) status?

• 60–70% of breast cancers express ER. The growth of these cancers can be controlled by hormonal therapies; for example, the ER antagonist tamoxifen and aromatase inhibitors, such as anastrozole or letrozole
• 25–30% of breast cancers overexpress HER2. Trastuzumab (Herceptin) is a monoclonal antibody directed against HER2 and can be given to patients with HER2-positive breast cancer

What are the differential diagnoses for nipple discharge and when should you refer urgently to breast clinic?

• Physiological; for example, pregnancy
• Duct ectasia
• Breast cancer
• Intraductal papilloma

You should refer urgently if there is unilateral, spontaneous bloody discharge.

 A Case to Learn From

A 42-year-old woman presented to her primary care doctor after finding a lump in her right breast on self-examination. The lump was non-tender and there were no other breast or nipple changes. Her primary care doctor could also palpate a lump on examination and made an urgent referral for the patient to breast clinic where a ductal carcinoma was confirmed. The patient underwent a wide local excision and adjuvant chemotherapy and made an excellent recovery. This case highlights the importance of promoting self-examination to pick up any worrying signs at an early stage and maximise chances of survival. Without regular self-examination and early detection of her breast lump, given that she was completely asymptomatic, this patient may not have had such a positive outcome.

 Top Tip

Remember that men can get breast cancer too! However, it is rare, with only 1 in 1000 men being diagnosed with breast cancer. Male breast cancer contributes to less than 1% of all breast cancer.

STATION 1.22: URINARY INCONTINENCE

SCENARIO

You are a junior doctor in primary care and have been asked to see Mrs Sanchez, a 54-year-old woman, who has presented with a 3-month history of urinary incontinence. She is afraid to leave the house in case she needs the toilet and it is starting to significantly affect her quality of life. Please take a history from Mrs Sanchez, present your findings and formulate an appropriate management plan.

 Cardinal Symptoms

Dysuria
Haematuria
Prolapse
Focal neurology

HISTORY OF PRESENTING COMPLAINT

URINARY INCONTINENCE

- Frequency: Daytime frequency, nocturia
- Volume: Amount of urine passed
- Type of incontinence: Determine if predominantly stress, urge or mixed incontinence:
  - Stress incontinence: Involuntary passage of small volumes of urine associated with increased intra-abdominal pressure, commonly when coughing, sneezing, laughing or exercising

- Urge incontinence: Overwhelming desire to void, little warning and patient may not reach toilet in time
- Dysuria: Establish if there is pain when micturating and since when
- Prolapse symptoms: Dragging sensation, sensation of a lump
- Fluid intake: Noting caffeine specifically
- Physical ability: Patient's level of mobility and accessibility of toilets

ASSOCIATED SYMPTOMS

Other symptoms to enquire about include:
- Haematuria and if so, establish how often and where in the stream the blood appears
- Faecal incontinence

PAST MEDICAL AND SURGICAL HISTORY

In this scenario, it is also important to enquire about:
- Recurrent urinary tract infections
- Diabetes mellitus: Can cause polyuria
- Neurological conditions
- Chronic cough
- Constipation
- Functional problems; for example, poor mobility, inaccessibility to toilets, cognitive deficit, behavioural problems
- Previous gynaecological surgeries

MEDICATION HISTORY

Enquire about prescribed medications (including any recent changes) and over-the-counter medications. Allergies should be included, with the specific reaction noted. In this scenario it is also important to note:
- Diuretics: Increased production of urine
- Anticholinergics, tricyclic antidepressants, antihistamines: Decrease bladder contractility. Anticholinergics may also lead to urinary retention and subsequent overflow
- Sedatives: Muscle relaxant

SOCIAL HISTORY

Social history includes enquiring about occupation, residence, lifestyle (diet, exercise, smoking, alcohol, substance abuse) and recent travel. Additionally in this scenario, consider:
- Smoking: Document pack years, calculated as the number of packs per day multiplied by the number of years smoked
- Alcohol and illicit drug use: Document units of alcohol consumed per week

- Mobility: Incontinence may be due to inability to get to the toilet secondary to poor mobility

FAMILY HISTORY

Ask about any significant family history, including:
- History of neurological conditions
- Malignancy

SYSTEMS REVIEW

On systems review, particularly pertinent questions to the above case may include questions regarding:
- Pregnancies: Number of pregnancies, type of deliveries, weight of babies and complications; for example, third-degree tears
- Cauda equina syndrome: Back pain, leg weakness, saddle anaesthesia
- LUTS: Urgency, frequency, hesitancy, dribbling, incontinence
- Diabetes: Polyuria and polydipsia, weight loss, increased thirst

Risk Factors for Stress Incontinence

- Increased age
- Previous vaginal delivery
- Obesity
- Previous pelvic surgery; for example, hysterectomy
- Chronic coughing; for example, secondary to COPD

ADDITIONAL INFORMATION

URODYNAMIC TESTING

Urodynamics is an investigation that assesses how the bladder and urethra are functioning. They are pivotal in diagnosing the cause and nature of a patient's incontinence. Specific tests that can be performed as part of urodynamics include:
- Postvoid residual volume: Whether the patient can empty their bladder completely
- Uroflowmetry: The speed at which the patient can empty their bladder and the rate of voiding
- Multichannel cystometry: Measuring the pressure in the rectum and bladder during bladder filling and voiding

Present Your Findings

Mrs Sanchez is a 54-year-old woman who has presented with a 3-month history of urinary incontinence. She describes frequent, involuntary passage of small amounts of urine throughout the day on coughing, exercising and laughing. She denies the presence of dysuria or haematuria and there are no symptoms suggestive of urge incontinence. She has had three children who were all born by vaginal delivery. Mrs Sanchez's quality of life appears to be significantly impacted by her urinary incontinence as she is often afraid to leave the house.

Mrs Sanchez is describing stress incontinence, which is likely secondary to weakness of the pelvic floor muscles.

I would like to examine Mrs Sanchez fully and perform a urine dip to rule out infection and glycosuria. I would advise lifestyle interventions; for example, caffeine reduction and regular pelvic floor exercises in the first instance, and refer to gynaecology for specialist input if required.

Differential Diagnosis

DISEASE	CLINICAL PRESENTATION	INVESTIGATIONS	MANAGEMENT
Urinary tract infection	• Urinary frequency • Dysuria • Suprapubic pain • Fever	• Urine dip • Urine MC&S	• Antibiotics
Overactive bladder syndrome	• Urge incontinence • Frequency • Overwhelming desire to void	• Urine dip • Urine MC&S	• Bladder training • Oxybutynin
Prolapse	• Dragging sensation • Sensation of a lump • Stress incontinence	• Speculum examination • Urine dip • Urine MC&S	• Lifestyle measures; for example, weight loss • Pelvic floor exercises • Vaginal pessary • Surgery
Atrophic vaginitis	• Postmenopausal • Vaginal dryness • Vaginal irritation	• May not be required	• Topical oestrogen
Cauda equina syndrome	• Leg weakness • Leg pain (often bilateral) • Bladder and/or bowel dysfunction • Saddle anaesthesia	• MRI spine	• High-dose steroids • MRI • Neurosurgery or radiotherapy

❓ QUESTIONS AND ANSWERS FOR CANDIDATE

What are the management options for stress incontinence?
- Conservative:
  - Weight loss
  - Pelvic floor exercises
  - Caffeine reduction
  - Vaginal pessaries
- Medical:
  - Duloxetine: Can help to increase urethral muscle tone
- Surgical:
  - Tension-free vaginal tape
  - Colposuspension
  - Sling procedure
  - Urethral bulking

What are the management options for urge incontinence?
- Conservative:
  - Caffeine reduction
  - Reduction in evening fluid intake
  - Bladder training
- Medical:
  - Antimuscarinic anticholinergics: For example, oxybutynin, tolterodine
- Surgical:
  - Sacral nerve stimulation
  - Injection of bladder wall with botulinum toxin
  - Augmentation cystoplasty
  - Urinary diversion

Name three potential complications of incontinence.
- Increased risk of institutionalisation
- Social isolation
- Depression
- Skin irritation

 A Case to Learn From

I saw a 75-year-old woman in primary care who was brought in by her daughter due to urinary incontinence. The patient's daughter was very concerned about her mother's symptoms and worried about the underlying cause. A detailed history revealed that the patient had significant osteoarthritis and used a walking stick around the house. She spent the majority of her time in the sitting room and the toilet was quite some distance away. A few simple changes allowed the patient easier access to the toilet and her incontinence improved. Always try to get a complete overview of the patient's circumstances in order to provide the best care.

 Top Tip

Some patients have a mixed pattern of stress and urge incontinence. Manage the patient initially according to the dominant symptom type.

STATION 1.23: UROLOGY: HAEMATURIA

SCENARIO

You are a junior doctor in the ED and have been asked to see Brian Stevens, a 55-year-old man, who presented with a 24-h history of frank, painless haematuria. He is otherwise fit and well with no significant medical history. Please take a history from Mr Stevens, present your findings and formulate an appropriate management plan.

 Cardinal Symptoms

Fever
Pain
Macroscopic or microscopic haematuria
Blood clots
Weight loss

HISTORY OF PRESENTING COMPLAINT

HAEMATURIA

- Onset: Any recent trauma or surgical procedures undertaken
- Duration: How long have symptoms been going on?
- Colour of urine: Bright red, brown, pink
- Clots: Frequency and size
- Pain: With haematuria or in general
- Timing of blood: At the beginning, during or end of stream of urine
- Exacerbating or precipitating factors: For example, exercise, trauma

ASSOCIATED SYMPTOMS

Other symptoms to enquire about include:
- Fever
- Weight loss
- Back pain
- Anorexia
- Malaise
- Lethargy

PAST MEDICAL AND SURGICAL HISTORY

In this scenario, it is also important to enquire about:
- Urinary tract infections
- Recent catheterisation
- Coagulopathy
- Malignancy
- Renal stones
- Prostate disease
- Rheumatological disease
- Respiratory disease

MEDICATION HISTORY

Enquire about prescribed medications (including any recent changes) and over-the-counter medications. Allergies should be included, with the specific reaction noted. In this scenario it is also important to note:
- Anticoagulants: Increase bleeding risk
- Nephrotoxic drugs: For example, NSAIDs, gentamicin, can damage the kidneys
- Cyclophosphamide: Can cause haematuria
- Rifampicin: Can discolour urine

SOCIAL HISTORY

Social history includes enquiring about occupation, residence, lifestyle (diet, exercise, smoking, alcohol, substance abuse) and recent travel. Additionally in this scenario, consider:

- Smoking: Document pack years, calculated as the number of packs per day multiplied by the number of years smoked
- Alcohol and illicit drug use: Document units of alcohol consumed per week
- Exercise: Strenuous exercise may cause transient haematuria
- Diet: Urine discoloration from beetroot ingestion
- Occupation: Work in dye, rubber and textile industries is associated with increased risk of bladder cancer
- Recent travel abroad: Fresh-water swimming is associated with a risk of urinary schistosomiasis

FAMILY HISTORY

Ask about any significant family history, including:

- Renal disease; for example, polycystic kidney disease
- Coagulopathy
- Malignancy

SYSTEMS REVIEW

On systems review, particularly pertinent questions to the above case may include questions regarding:

- Genitourinary: Dysuria, urgency, suprapubic pain, loin pain, incontinence, poor stream, dribbling, hesitance, menstruation
- Other: Rash, arthralgia, myalgia, recent upper respiratory tract infection, cough, haemoptysis, breathlessness, associated symptoms of anaemia

Risk Factors for Bladder Cancer

- Smoking
- Chemical or occupational exposure; for example to dyes, textiles, rubbers, paints, etc.
- Chronic bladder inflammation
- Previous cancer treatment near the bladder; for example, radiotherapy to the bowels
- Previous chemotherapy treatment
- Type 2 diabetes

ADDITIONAL INFORMATION

NICE GUIDELINES FOR URGENT UROLOGY REFERRAL OF A PATIENT WITH HAEMATURIA

- Age ≥ 45 years old and:
  - Unexplained visible haematuria without urinary tract infection

Differential Diagnosis

DISEASE	CLINICAL PRESENTATION	INVESTIGATIONS	MANAGEMENT
Urinary tract infection	• Urinary frequency • Dysuria • Suprapubic pain • Fever	• Urine dip • Urine MC&S	• Antibiotics
Renal stone	• Colicky loin to groin pain • Nausea and vomiting • Macroscopic or microscopic haematuria	• FBCs • U&Es • CRP • Clotting profile • Calcium • Phosphate • Uric acid • Urine dip • Urine MC&S • CT KUB	• Analgesia • Antiemetics • Antibiotics if infection • Most stones less than 5 mm pass spontaneously • Extracorporeal shock-wave lithotripsy or percutaneous nephrolithotomy for larger stones
Renal cancer	• Macroscopic or microscopic haematuria • Flank pain • Palpable flank mass • Weight loss	• FBCs • U&Es • LFTs • Clotting profile • Urine dip • Renal tract USS • CT abdomen	• Surgery • Chemotherapy • Targeted therapies • Palliative radiotherapy
Bladder cancer	• Frank, painless haematuria	• FBCs • U&Es • LFTs • Clotting profile • Urine dip • Cystoscopy	• Transurethral resection of bladder tumour (TURBT) • Radical surgery, radical radiotherapy, chemotherapy for advanced bladder cancer

Continued

Differential Diagnosis—cont'd

DISEASE	CLINICAL PRESENTATION	INVESTIGATIONS	MANAGEMENT
Glomerulonephritis	• Haematuria • Proteinuria • Nephritic or nephrotic syndrome • Chronic kidney disease	• FBCs • U&Es • CRP • ESR • Clotting profile • Immunoglobulins • Serum electrophoresis • Complement autoantibodies • Urine dip • Urine MC&S • Renal tract USS • Renal biopsy	• Management depends on cause of glomerulonephritis; for example, immunosuppressants
Prostate cancer	• Obstructive and/or irritative symptoms • Prostatism • Haematuria • Urinary retention	• Digital rectal examination • Prostate-specific antigen • Transrectal USS • Prostatic biopsy • MRI prostate and pelvis	• Watchful waiting • Radical prostatectomy • Radiotherapy • Hormone treatment • Chemotherapy

• Visible haematuria persisting or recurring after treatment of urinary tract infection
• Age ≥ 60 years old with unexplained microscopic haematuria
• Consider non-urgent referral if ≥ 60 years old and recurrent or persistent unexplained urinary tract infection

CAUSES OF HAEMATURIA

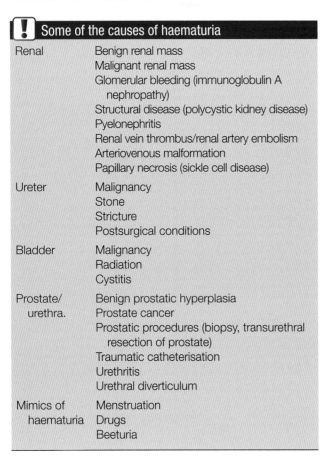

! Some of the causes of haematuria

Renal	Benign renal mass Malignant renal mass Glomerular bleeding (immunoglobulin A nephropathy) Structural disease (polycystic kidney disease) Pyelonephritis Renal vein thrombus/renal artery embolism Arteriovenous malformation Papillary necrosis (sickle cell disease)
Ureter	Malignancy Stone Stricture Postsurgical conditions
Bladder	Malignancy Radiation Cystitis
Prostate/urethra.	Benign prostatic hyperplasia Prostate cancer Prostatic procedures (biopsy, transurethral resection of prostate) Traumatic catheterisation Urethritis Urethral diverticulum
Mimics of haematuria	Menstruation Drugs Beeturia

🔍 Present Your Findings

Mr Stevens is a 55-year-old man who presented to the ED with a 24-h history of painless frank haematuria. He has not passed any clots. There is no history of trauma and no obvious precipitating factors. He denies any symptoms of infection. He is generally fit and well and is a smoker with a 30-year pack history.

My differential diagnosis would include a urological malignancy, benign prostatic disease or urinary tract infection. I would like to perform a full physical examination and ask for bloods, a urine dip and urinalysis initially. I would have a low threshold for investigating for malignancy with urine cytology, cystoscopy and CT KUB.

❓ QUESTIONS AND ANSWERS FOR CANDIDATE

Name three risk factors for renal stones.
• Infection
• Dehydration
• Metabolic disease; for example, hypercalcaemia/hypercalciuria, hyperoxaluria, hyperuricaemia, cystinuria
• Drugs; for example, diuretics, allopurinol, steroids, acetazolamide, calcium or vitamin D supplements

What are the different types of renal stones?
• Calcium oxalate
• Calcium phosphate
• Staghorn or triple phosphate
• Urate
• Cystine

What are the common causative organisms in urinary tract infections?
• *E. coli* (most common)
• *Proteus*
• *Pseudomonas*
• Streptococci
• Staphylococci

A Case to Learn From

As a junior doctor on a night shift, I was asked to review a patient on the ward who had been admitted with frank haematuria. The patient was now reporting lower abdominal pain and difficulty passing urine. I realised that this patient had acute urinary retention; therefore I passed a Foley catheter, but this did not drain. I therefore discussed the case with my senior on-call who explained that a known complication of haematuria with clots is clot retention, where large clots can obstruct the urethra and the management of this involved passing a three-way catheter with subsequent bladder irrigation, which allowed the clots to drain.

 Top Tip

If you find haematuria in a female patient, always remember to ask about her menstrual cycle and whether she is currently menstruating. If so, this could be the cause of finding blood in the urine and therefore a urine dip should be rechecked at a later date.

2 Examinations

Content Outline

Performing examinations is a fundamental part of clinical practice, no matter what specialty you enter. As a clinician, you are expected to examine patients appropriately and provide them with the dignity and respect that they deserve. You must know what you are trying to find out from the examination, so that you do not miss out on important information, and also that you do not carry out any unnecessary steps.

Carrying out an examination is much more than running through the steps of a sequence. You need to be aware of what is normal, in order for you to pick up on the abnormalities. Clinical signs can give you a lot of information and aid diagnosis, from general inspection through to carrying out special tests. The more you do the examinations, the sooner it will come naturally to you, as though by second nature, and you will come across as being more confident.

Study Action Plan

- Familiarise yourself with the steps of the examination first, in a systematic approach. Once you know the sequence, then get into the routine of carrying out the steps on friends, family or even a pillow!
- Once you begin clinical placements, try to examine real patients as much as you can. They give you a much more realistic reaction than when you are practising on friends or peers, and you may pick up on clinical signs as well

STATION 2.1: CARDIOVASCULAR

SCENARIO

You are a junior doctor in the emergency department (ED) and have been asked to see Mrs Smith, a 60-year-old woman, who has presented with shortness of breath and a new murmur. Please perform a relevant cardiovascular examination on Mrs Smith and present your findings.

PREPARATION

- WIPER:
  - *Wash* your hands
  - *Introduce* yourself
  - Ask about *pain*
  - Appropriately *expose*
  - *Reposition*
- Explain the examination to the patient and your reasons for performing it
- Gain verbal consent
- Give the patient privacy to expose themselves as required
- Start with the patient in a comfortable position (usually sitting in a chair or bed)
- Offer a chaperone

GENERAL INSPECTION

- Environment: Vomit bowls, medications, electrocardiogram (ECG) leads
- Patient: Pain or agitation, obesity, obvious swellings

EXAMINATION OF THE ARMS

- Signs of infective endocarditis: Look for clubbing (Fig. 2.1) and splinter haemorrhages. Turn the hand around and feel for Osler's nodes in the pulps of the fingers and look for Janeway lesions on the palms
- Capillary refill time (CRT): Push down on the finger pulp for 5 s. This should cause a loss of colour in the pulp of the thumb. Upon release, the time taken for the pulp to return to its normal colour is known as the CRT (Fig. 2.2)
- Radial pulses: Feel both simultaneously. Comment on whether they are regular or irregular, and whether there is a radio-radio delay between the two radial pulses (Fig. 2.3)

- Collapsing pulse: Ask the patient if they have any shoulder pain before lifting the arm (with the forearm above the head) (Fig. 2.4)
- Brachial or carotid pulses: Feel for the volume and character of the pulse. Think about whether the pulse is slow-rising (feature of aortic stenosis) or collapsing (feature of aortic regurgitation) (Fig. 2.3)
- BP: Assess for a narrow pulse pressure (feature of aortic stenosis) and a wide pulse pressure (feature of aortic regurgitation)
- Temperature: Feel for the patient's temperature peripherally

EXAMINATION OF THE FACE

- Hypercholesterolaemia: Look for xanthelasma or corneal arcus (Fig. 2.5)
- Central cyanosis: Look into the mouth
- Pallor: Look into the eyes
- Fundoscopy: Look for features of hypertensive and/or diabetic retinopathy and Roth spots (features of infective endocarditis)

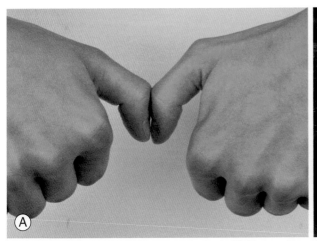
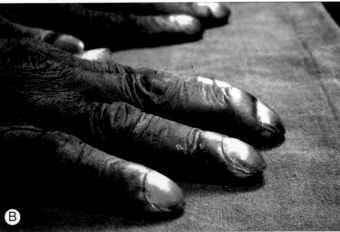

Fig. 2.1 (A) Assessing for clubbing: Look for a diamond formed between thumbnails. (B) Clubbed fingers with increased convexity of nail fold and loss of angle between nail bed/fold.

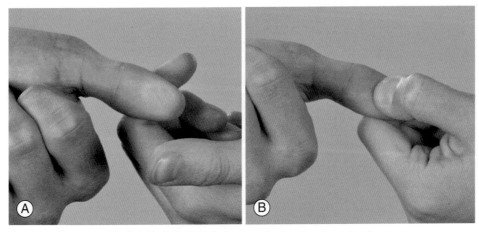

Fig. 2.2 (A, B) CRT: Note the loss of colour in pulp of thumb.

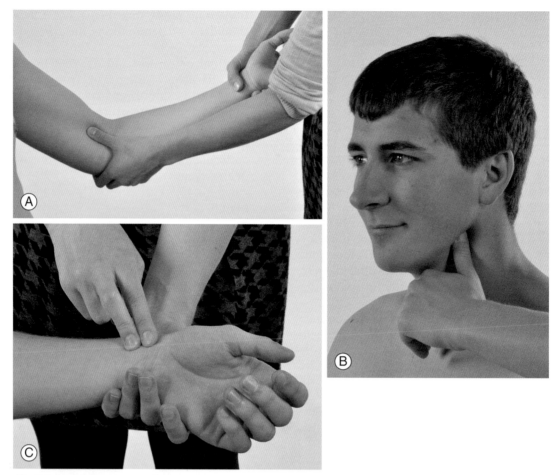

Fig. 2.3 Feeling for pulses: (A) Brachial (medial to bicep tendon), (B) carotid (between sternocleidomastoid and angle of mandible) and (C) radial (between radial styloid and tendon of flexor carpi radialis).

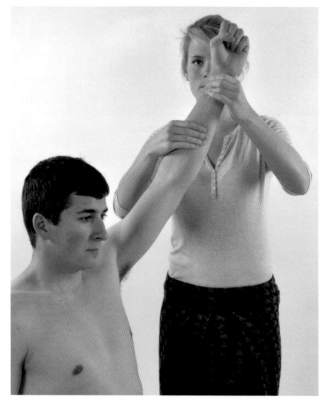

Fig. 2.4 Feeling for a collapsing pulse: Both by feeling the character of the pulse with one hand and feeling for pulsations in the anterior forearm muscles with the other hand.

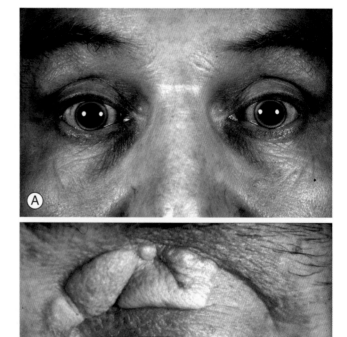

Fig. 2.5 (A) Corneal arcus and (B) xanthelasma.

EXAMINATION OF THE CHEST

INSPECTION

Look for:

- Devices: For example, pacemaker or implantable cardioverter defibrillator (ICD) (Fig. 2.6)
- Scars: Median sternotomy, lateral thoracotomy, pacemaker, mitral valvotomy, chest drains

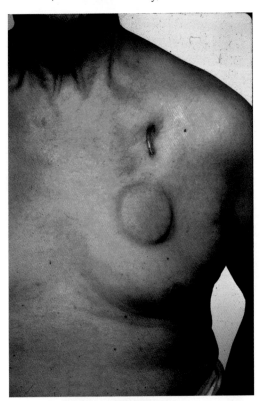

Fig. 2.6 Pacemaker or ICD.

- Chest wall deformities: For example, pectus excavatum ('funnel chest') or pectus carinatum ('pigeon chest') (Fig. 2.7)
- Visible pulsations: Also known as precordial impulses
- Blood vessel grafts: Look also at the legs and wrists
- Jugular venous pressure (JVP):
  - Look for pulsation behind the sternocleidomastoid muscle
  - Positioning is very important. Sit the patient at 45° if possible and ask them to relax
  - Ask them to turn their head slightly away from the side of the neck that you are inspecting
  - Look for the JVP
  - If the JVP is not seen, assess the hepatojugular reflux by placing the hand inferior to the liver edge and pressing gently to accentuate the JVP. Ask about abdominal pain first!

PALPATION

Feel for:

- Apex beat: Usually located in midclavicular line, fifth intercostal space
- Parasternal heaves: Feel for right ventricular heaves (under the nipple) and left ventricular heaves (left of the sternum)
- Thrills: Over the mitral, tricuspid, pulmonary and aortic areas

AUSCULTATION (FIG. 2.8)

- Auscultate all four areas of the precordium
- Check for radiation to both the carotids and axillae
- Ask the patient to roll on to the left side. Auscultate the mitral area to listen for mitral stenosis

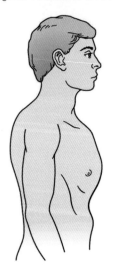

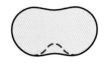

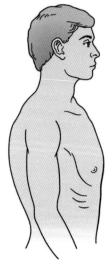

PECTUS CARINATUM

PECTUS EXCAVATUM

BARREL CHEST

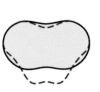

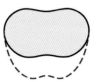

Fig. 2.7 Chest wall deformities: Pectus carinatum ('pigeon's chest') (left) and pectus excavatum ('funnel chest') (right).

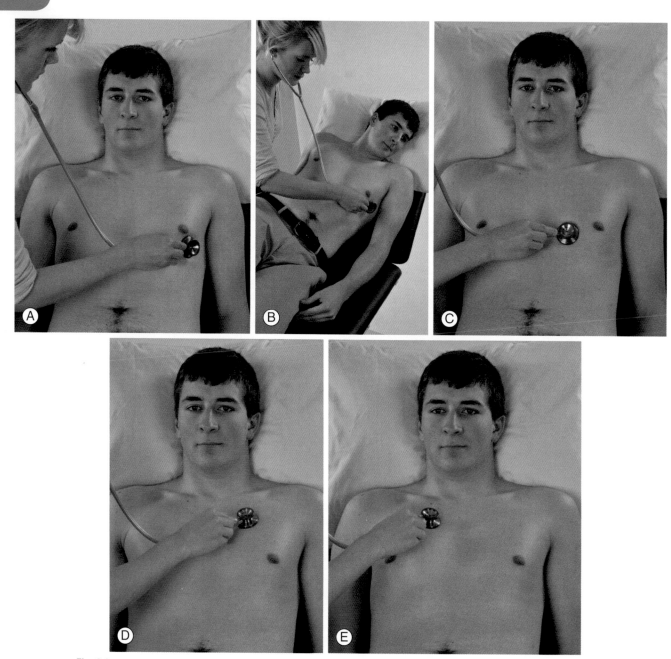

Fig. 2.8 (A–E) Auscultation: Start at the apex. Listen in the mitral area with the diaphragm, with the bell and then with patient rolled on to his left (for mitral stenosis). Listen in the tricuspid, pulmonary and aortic areas. Always simultaneously feel for a central pulse; for example, carotid, to time heart sounds and murmurs.

- Ask the patient to sit up, breathe in, breathe out and then hold their breath. Listen at the lower left sternal edge for aortic regurgitation (Fig. 2.9)
- Think about the heart sounds (including presence of S3 and S4) as well as any murmurs
- Listen at the lung bases for heart failure (Fig. 2.10)

EXAMINATION OF THE ABDOMEN AND LEGS

- Right heart failure: Assess for hepatomegaly, ascites, peripheral oedema
- Scars: Look for saphenous vein grafts

FINISHING

- Offer to:
  - Perform an ECG
  - Dipstick the urine
  - Perform a respiratory and peripheral arterial examination
- Thank the patient
- Check that they're comfortable and offer to help reposition them
- Wash your hands
- Leave the patient in privacy to get dressed

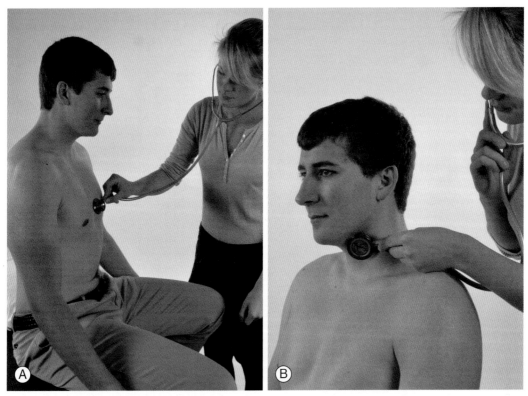

Fig. 2.9 Auscultation: Listening for (A) aortic murmur and (B) for radiation into the neck.

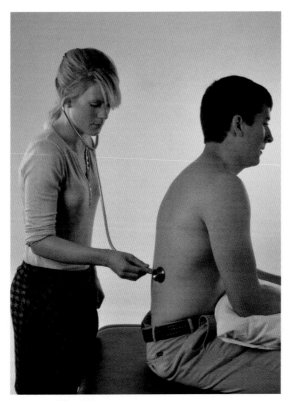

Fig. 2.10 Auscultation of the lung base.

⚠ Systolic murmurs: Comparison of aortic stenosis and mitral regurgitation

	AORTIC STENOSIS	MITRAL REGURGITATION
Aetiology	Valvular: • Most common • Congenital bicuspid valve, most common cause in 40–60-year-olds • Senile calcification, seen in over-60s • Inflammatory valvulitis; for example, rheumatic fever Subvalvular: • Fibromuscular ring • Hypertrophic cardiomyopathy Supravalvular: • Williams syndrome	Annulus: • Senile calcification Mitral valve leaflets: • Mitral valve prolapse syndrome • Connective tissue disorders • Infective endocarditis Chordae tendinae: • Connective tissue disorders • Infective endocarditis Papillary muscles: • Post myocardial infarction
Symptoms	• Asymptomatic • Breathlessness (due to left ventricular failure) • Angina (due to increased myocardial work) • Dizziness and syncope on exertion • Systemic emboli: Retinal or cerebral • Sudden death	Acute (non-compensated): • Pulmonary oedema with severe dyspnoea. Chronic (partially compensated): • Fatigue • Dyspnoea (on exertion)
Pulse	• Low volume • Slow rising • Faint • Pulsus alterans (in severe cases)	May have: • Atrial fibrillation (AF) • Atrial flutter
Blood pressure (BP)	• Low BP • Narrowed pulse pressure	• Not typically affected unless in heart failure
Precordium	• Systolic thrill in the aortic area (leaning forward and on expiration) • Heaving (rarely displaced) apex	• Systolic thrill in the mitral area • Laterally and downwardly displaced thrusting apex (due to dilated left ventricles) • Raised JVP • Pulmonary hypertension
Heart sounds	• Ejection systolic murmur (left sternal edge, on expiration, leaning forward, crescendo, decrescendo, radiating to carotid) • Ejection click, if the valve is mobile and bicuspid • Soft A2, may be inaudible if the valve is calcified • S4 heard	• Pansystolic murmur (apex, on expiration, blowing, patient leaning back at 45°, radiating to the back or axilla) • Soft S1 • S3 heard • Loud P2, if pulmonary hypertension develops • Mid-systolic click, if there is mitral prolapse
ECG	• Left ventricular hypertrophy • Left axis deviation • First-degree heart block (extension of calcification across the atrioventricular (AV) node)	• Left ventricular hypertrophy • AF may be present • P mitrale, if there is significant atrial dilatation
Chest X-ray (CXR)	• Calcified valve • Left ventricular hypertrophy	• Calcified valve • Left ventricular dilatation • Left atrial dilatation
Echocardiogram	• Unicuspid or bicuspid valve • Calcified valve • Increased blood flow velocity across the aortic valve (seen on Doppler scan)	• Left atrial dilatation • Left ventricular dilatation • Mitral valve prolapse • Infective vegetation • Pulmonary hypertension
Complications	• Arrhythmias • Myocardial infarction • Heart failure • Infective endocarditis • Emboli, from endocarditis or calcification	• Arrhythmias • Heart failure • Pulmonary hypertension • Infective endocarditis

❗ Diastolic murmurs: Comparison of aortic regurgitation and mitral stenosis

	AORTIC REGURGITATION	MITRAL STENOSIS
Aetiology	Valvular disease: • Infective endocarditis • Connective tissue disorders Aortic root disease: • Aortic dissection • Connective tissue disorders • Syphilis Mixed stenosis and/or regurgitation: • Rheumatic fever • Rheumatoid arthritis	• Rheumatic heart disease (almost all) • Congenital
Symptoms	• Similar presentation to aortic stenosis • Angina and syncope are less common • Breathlessness. • Generally well tolerated unless acute	• Breathlessness (due to pulmonary hypertension) • Fatigue • Haemoptysis • Systemic emboli • Chronic bronchitis (due to oedematous bronchial mucosa) • Chest pain • Palpitations • Enlarged atria and subsequent compression of the recurrent laryngeal nerve, oesophagus or left main bronchus
Pulse	• Collapsing ('water-hammer') pulse • Throbbing peripheral pulses	• Small volume • Atrial arrhythmia (AF is more common than mitral regurgitation)
BP	• Wide pulse pressure	• Not typically affected unless in heart failure
Precordium	• Diastolic thrill in the aortic area • Diffuse, displaced, forceful apex	• Diastolic thrill in the mitral area • Tapping apex • Raised JVP (due to right heart failure) • Parasternal heave (due to right ventricular hypertrophy)
Heart sounds	• Early diastolic murmur (left lower sternal edge, high-pitched, on expiration, leaning forward) • May be an ejection systolic 'flow' murmur due to volume overload • Soft A2	• Mid-diastolic murmur (apex, rumbling, on expiration, radiating to the axilla) • Opening snap • Loud P2 • Split S2
ECG	• Left ventricular dilatation (due to volume overload) • P mitrale, if there is significant atrial dilatation	• Right ventricular hypertrophy • AF
CXR	• Possible widened mediastinum (in aortic dissection) • Left ventricular dilatation	• Left atrial dilatation with or without (±) right heart dilatation • Pulmonary hypertension • Pulmonary oedema
Echocardiogram	• Dilated aortic root • Dilated left ventricle with vigorous contractions	• Mitral valve calcification • Left atrial dilatation • Pulmonary hypertension • Right ventricular hypertrophy, dilatation and failure
Complications	• Arrhythmias • Heart failure • Infective endocarditis	• Arrhythmias • Pulmonary hypertension • Right heart failure • Infective endocarditis

Present Your Findings

Mrs Smith is a 60-year-old woman presenting with short-ness of breath and a new heart murmur. She is comfortable at rest, on 2 L of oxygen. There are no stigmata of infective endocarditis. Her pulse is regular at a rate of 60 beats per min (bpm), slow rising and of normal volume. Pulse pressure is normal. On auscultation, she has an ejection systolic mur-mur in the aortic area, radiating to both of her carotid pulses. S1 is normal with a quiet S2. There are no additional heart sounds and there is no evidence of heart failure.

I feel the most likely diagnosis is aortic stenosis.

To complete my examination, I would like to perform a respiratory examination and look at the bedside ECG monitoring. I would like to take bloods, including: Full blood count (FBCs), urea and electrolytes (U&Es) and liver function tests (LFTs). I would request a CXR, ECG and an echocardiogram.

? QUESTIONS AND ANSWERS FOR CANDIDATE

How does the JVP differ from the carotid pulse?

Use the acronym MOPHAIR:

- *Multi-waveform*: For each cardiac cycle, there are two JVP 'waves' ('a' wave and 'v' wave), compared to one carotid wave
- *Occludable*: Lightly pressing on the internal jugular vein will occlude the JVP, but will not occlude the carotid pulse
- *Positional* variation: The JVP falls on sitting up
- *Hepatojugular* reflux: The JVP rises with light pressure on the liver
- Fills from *above*: After the JVP has been occluded (since this is the direction of blood flow)
- *Impalpable*: A pulse cannot be felt in the JVP
- *Respiratory* changes: The JVP falls on inspiration

What are the causes of AF?

Cardiac:

- Heart failure
- Ischaemic heart disease (IHD)
- Atrial dilatation
- Cardiac surgery
- Hypertension

Non-cardiac:

- Infection
- Hyperthyroidism
- Alcohol
- Pulmonary embolism (PE)

How would you grade a cardiac murmur?

- See Table 2.1

 A Case to Learn From

I saw a patient with a heart murmur in an exam. I was getting very confused, because it radiated to the neck and therefore seemed to be an ejection systolic murmur. However, it also ra-diated into the axilla and therefore seemed pansystolic in char-acter. In the end I just said there was a systolic murmur and that it could be either of the above. It turned out the patient had both! From this I took the lesson that you should be confi-dent in describing what you hear even if it doesn't seem likely.

 Table 2.1   Grading scale of cardiac murmurs

GRADE OF MURMUR	AUDIBILITY	THRILL
1	Barely audible	No
2	Audible after a few seconds of auscultation	No
3	Immediately audible – moderate intensity	No
4	Loud intensity	Yes
5	Very loud (may be heard with the stethoscope slightly off thoracic wall)	Yes
6	Loudest (may be heard with the stethoscope entirely off thoracic wall)	Yes

Top Tip

When introduced to a patient with a murmur, most students will only listen to the murmur on one occasion. I found that, providing the patient was happy, going back and listening to the murmur a second or third time really helped consolidate my pattern recognition skills.

STATION 2.2: RESPIRATORY

SCENARIO

You are a junior doctor in general medicine and have been asked to see Mrs Fredrickson, a 76-year-old wom-an, who has presented with severe difficulty in breath-ing and a cough. Please perform a relevant respiratory examination on Mrs Fredrickson and present your findings.

PREPARATION

- WIPER:
  - *Wash* your hands
  - *Introduce* yourself
  - Ask about *pain*
  - Appropriately *expose*
  - *Reposition*
- Explain the examination to the patient and your rea-sons for performing it
- Gain verbal consent
- Give the patient privacy to expose themselves to above the waist (cover the breasts with a blanket)
- Start in a comfortable position (usually at 45°)
- Offer a chaperone

GENERAL INSPECTION

- Environment: Use of oxygen (O_2) mask or nasal can-nula, inhalers, nebulisers, spacers, peak flow meter, sputum pot or a chest drain

• Patient: Pain or agitation, evidence of weight loss, drowsiness, cushingoid appearance, scars from drains or surgery, nature of breathing ± additional sounds (see Additional Information, below)

EXAMINATION OF THE HANDS

• Fingers: Clubbing, peripheral cyanosis
• Tremor: There may be a fine tremor caused by excessive use of beta-agonists or theophylline bronchodilators
• Tar staining: From cigarette smoking
• Pulse: Check the rate, rhythm and volume at the wrist. Chronic carbon dioxide (CO_2) retainers have warm peripheries and large-volume pulses since CO_2 is a vasodilator
• CO_2 retention flap or flapping tremor: Test by asking the patient to lift the arms until in front of them, cock the wrists back and hold for 30 s (Fig. 2.11)

EXAMINATION OF THE EYES

• Anaemia: Look for conjunctival pallor
• Horner's syndrome: Interruption in the sympathetic chain in the neck or brainstem, commonly due to a lung cancer at the apex of the lung invading the sympathetic chain (Fig. 2.12)

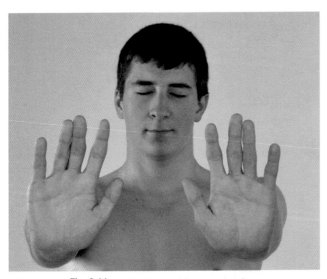

Fig. 2.11 Assessing for CO_2 retention flap.

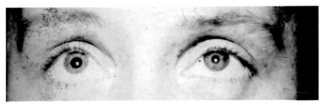

Fig. 2.12 Horner's syndrome: Note the ptosis and pupil constriction on left, which is associated with apical lung tumours.

EXAMINATION OF THE MOUTH

• Central cyanosis: Check at the lips and tongue
• Oral thrush: Check the mouth. It can be secondary to steroids

EXAMINATION OF THE NECK

ELEVATED JVP

• Causes include: Cor pulmonale, elevated intrathoracic pressures (for example, acute severe asthma or tension pneumothorax) and superior vena cava (SVC) obstruction

TRACHEAL POSITION

• Insert the tip of your finger into the suprasternal notch and press gently into the trachea
• Check that your fingertip fits easily into both sides and that the trachea is central
• Warn patients that this might feel uncomfortable
• Interpret findings (Table 2.2)

LYMPH NODES

• Palpate the neck from behind the patient (see Station 2.16: Neck Lump Examination) and the axillary lymph nodes whilst taking the weight of the arm with your non-palpating hand (Fig. 2.13)
• If a node is palpable, then describe its nature:
  • Is it rubbery (feature of Hodgkin's disease)?
  • Is it tender (feature of tonsillitis)?
  • Is it matted together (feature of tuberculosis (TB) and metastatic disease)?

EXAMINATION OF THE CHEST

INSPECTION

Look for:
• Chest wall deformities: See Table 2.3
• Lesions in the chest wall: Possible metastatic tumour nodules and neurofibromas
• Scars: From thoracic surgery; for example, lateral thoracotomy, chest drain
• Dilated superficial veins: Consider SVC obstruction. Note that elevation of the JVP does not vary with breathing (unlike with heart failure) since there is a fixed obstruction
• Asymmetry: Between the two axillae
Patterns you might see:
• Generalised indrawing of intercostal muscles: Implying that the patient cannot achieve adequate ventilation by normal inspiratory efforts. This is

Table 2.2 Interpretation of the tracheal position

'TRACHEA DEVIATED TOWARDS' PATHOLOGY	'TRACHEA DEVIATED AWAY' PATHOLOGY
Lobar collapse Pneumonectomy	Large pleural effusion Tension pneumothorax

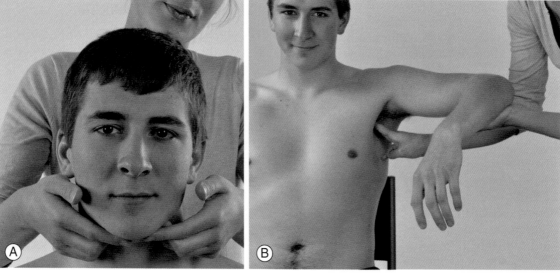

Fig. 2.13 Feeling for lymph nodes in the neck (A) and in the axilla (B).

〰 Table **2.3** Chest wall shape			
BARREL CHEST	**PECTUS EXCAVATUM**	**THORACIC KYPHOSCOLIOSIS**	**PECTUS CARINATUM**
• Increased anteroposterior (AP) diameter compared to the lateral diameter • Typically associated with lung hyperinflation or kyphoscoliosis	• Also known as 'funnel chest' • Depressed sternum (usually benign) • May be associated with pulmonary hypertension	• Excessive AP and lateral curvature of the spine • May be idiopathic or secondary to childhood poliomyelitis or spinal TB • Causes decreased ventilatory capacity and increased work of breathing	• Also known as 'pigeon chest' • Prominent sternum • May be an indicator of chronic respiratory disease in childhood

seen in patients with gross hyperinflation secondary to emphysema or asthma
- Local indrawing of a portion of the chest wall ('flail chest'): Usually seen in trauma patients who have sustained double fractures of a series of ribs or the sternum
- Purse-lipped exhalation: This prevents bronchial wall collapse and minimises work done in breathing. This is seen in patients with severe airway narrowing

PALPATION

Feel for:
- Local abnormalities: Seen on inspection
- Apex beat: If it is impalpable, consider diagnosis such as emphysema, obesity, dextrocardia and a large pleural effusion
- Chest expansion:
  - Assess upper, middle and lower zones (Fig. 2.14)
  - Place the fingertips firmly in the midaxillary line and pull the hands to towards the centre of the chest, maintaining this pressure to tighten

any loose skin. The thumbs should meet in the middle and remain off the patient. Ask the patient to take a deep breath. In a healthy individual the ribs move up and out; this can be seen by the outward, upward movement of your thumbs
- Any change is difficult to detect if it is bilateral
- Unilateral causes of reduced expansion include: Pneumothorax, pleural effusion, pneumonia and collapse

PERCUSSION

- Start at the supraclavicular fossae and work down
- All movement should come from your wrist joint and your middle finger should remain partially flexed
- Strike the middle phalanx of the middle finger of one hand with the distal phalanx of the middle finger of the other hand. The other fingers are not touching the chest
- Compare the note at equivalent positions on both sides (Fig. 2.15)

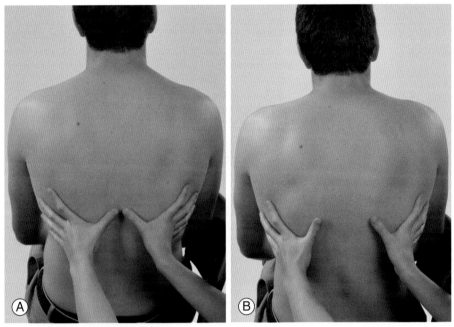

Fig. 2.14 Assessing for chest expansion by asking the patient to breathe out (A) and in (B).

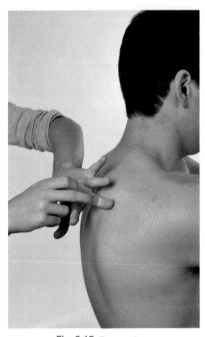

Fig. 2.15 Percussion.

Table 2.4	Interpreting percussion notes	
	RESONANT	**HYPERRESONANT**
Physiology	Normal	Large air-filled space; for example, in markedly emphysematous lung, pneumothorax
Character	Dull	Stony dull
Differential diagnoses	The lung is separated from the chest wall; for example, by pleural fluid, pleural thickening or pulmonary consolidation/ collapse	Characteristic of a large pleural effusion

- Map out any area of altered resonance by going from the normal to the abnormal area and interpret (Table 2.4)

AUSCULTATION

- Listen with the patient relaxed and breathing normally through an open mouth
- Auscultate the anterior chest wall, alternating between each side of the chest wall (to compare like with like), starting above the clavicle and finishing below the 11th rib

- Do not forget the lateral chest wall before auscultating the posterior chest wall
- In each area, assess the quality and amplitude of breath sounds whilst noting any added sounds (Table 2.5)
- Additional sounds include:
  - Crackles: Non-musical sounds with a crackling quality, due to a loss of stability of peripheral airways, which collapse on expiration. The high pressures of inspiration cause the abrupt reopening of alveoli and small bronchi, which produces the characteristic crackling noise, associated with infection, fluid and fibrosis
  - Wheeze: Musical-quality sound caused by continuous oscillation of opposing airway walls, implying narrowing of the small airways

Table 2.5 Types of breath sounds

	VESICULAR BREATHING	DIMINISHED VESICULAR BREATHING	BRONCHIAL BREATHING
Causes	Normal	Occurs if there is a thick chest wall; for example, pleural thickening, or if there is a reason for conduction of sound to the chest wall to be reduced; for example, emphysema or simply shallow breathing	Associated with pneumonic consolidation, which produces a uniform conducting medium. Also present at the border between the lung and a pleural effusion (due to an underlying compressed lung)
Character	Said to have a rustling quality. The sound should increase steadily during inspiration and then quickly fade during the first third of expiration	Similar in character to normal vesicular breathing, but quieter	Breath sounds are loud and blowing. Similar pitch and length of inspiration and expiration. Unlike normal vesicular breath sounds, there is an audible gap between inspiration and expiration

Typically present at the end of expiration as airways are normally narrow on expiration. If present on inspiration (when the airways are normally dilated), it implies severe airway narrowing, although in extremely severe airway obstruction, wheeze may be absent due to severely reduced airflow. Monophonic wheeze may be caused by an obstructing lesion, classically a tumour. Polyphonic wheeze is associated with more diffuse airway disease; for example, asthma

- Pleural rub: Creaking sound, produced by the movement of the visceral over the parietal pleura, when both sides have been roughened by fibrinous exudates or acute inflammation. Sounds like crunching snow or the creaking of leather. Typically, it is not audible on shallow breathing, but becomes clear on deep breathing. Causes include: Pneumonia, pleural effusion and PE

- Whispering pectoriloquy: This is performed by asking the patient to whisper '99' whilst auscultating the chest for vocal resonance (Fig. 2.16). Usually sounds of this volume are not heard, but in the setting of consolidation an increased transmission of sound occurs and thus louder 'whispering pectoriloquy' in the affected area. This is a useful way of differentiating pleural effusion (where there is reduced transmission of sound) from consolidation. Tactile vocal fremitus in principle assesses the same thing, but transmission of sound is felt rather than auscultated

EXAMINATION OF THE BACK

Repeat all of the steps mentioned above on the back, including: Inspection, palpation, percussion and auscultation. Note that when inspecting the back, the patient's arms should be folded across the chest at the front to ensure that the scapulae are opened up.

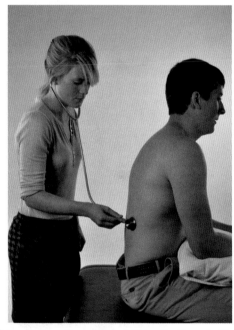

Fig. 2.16 Auscultation of lower zones, whilst asking the patient to say '99'.

FINISHING

- Offer to:
  - Check a peak flow
  - Examine a sputum sample
  - Dipstick the urine
- Thank the patient
- Check that they're comfortable and offer to help reposition them
- Wash your hands
- Leave the patient in privacy to get dressed

NATURE OF BREATHING

- Hyperventilation: Multiple causes, including anxiety, metabolic acidosis (Kussmaul respirations), toxins and head injury
- Hypoventilation: Indicating ventilatory failure
- Work of breathing: Signs of increased work of breathing include: Nasal flaring, tracheal tug, intercostal

recession, lip pursing and use of accessory muscles (sternocleidomastoid, pectoralis and platysma)
- Additional sounds: For example, cough, wheeze or stridor

CAUSES OF INTERSTITIAL LUNG DISEASE

- Idiopathic (cryptogenic) extrinsic allergic alveolitis:
  - Pigeon fancier's lung
  - Farmer's lung sarcoidosis
- Autoimmune:
  - Rheumatoid arthritis
  - Systemic sclerosis
  - Ankylosing spondylitis
- Occupational:
  - Asbestosis
  - Pneumoconiosis
  - Silicosis
- Drugs:
  - Methotrexate
  - Amiodarone
  - Nitrofurantoin
- Familial

CAUSES OF CLUBBING

- Carcinoma of bronchus
- Chronic suppurative lung disease; for example, cystic fibrosis (CF), empyema, bronchiectasis, lung abscess
- Fibrosing alveolitis
- Cyanotic heart disease
- Infective endocarditis
- Liver cirrhosis
- Idiopathic
- Inflammatory bowel disease (IBD)
- Familial

Present Your Findings

Mrs Fredrickson is a 76-year-old woman presenting with difficulty in breathing and a cough. She has breathlessness at rest, with pursed lips, use of accessory muscles and an audible wheeze. There is a green sputum pot at the bedside, with inhalers visible. Her chest is dull to percuss in the left base, with fine crackles, dullness to percuss and increased whispering pectoriloquy. I feel the most likely diagnosis is an infective exacerbation of chronic obstructive pulmonary disease (COPD). Differential diagnoses include: Asthma, heart failure and lung fibrosis.

To complete my examination, I would like to take a peak flow, inspect a sputum sample and dipstick the urine. I would like to start broad-spectrum antibiotics, take bloods including: FBCs, U&Es and C-reactive protein (CRP). I would also request a CXR.

❓ QUESTIONS AND ANSWERS FOR CANDIDATE

Name three causes of inspiratory crackles.
- Early inspiration: Small-airway disease; for example, bronchiolitis
- Mid-inspiration: Pulmonary oedema

- Late inspiration: Interstitial lung disease, COPD, pneumonia
- Inspiration and expiration: Bronchiectasis

Name three common causes of a wheeze.
- Asthma
- COPD
- Anaphylaxis
- Foreign-body inhalation
- Heart failure (cardiac wheeze)

How do you differentiate pleural effusion and consolidation on examination?
- Pleural effusion is 'stony dull' rather than dull
- Pleural effusion has reduced vocal resonance and/or tactile fremitus, whereas in consolidation it is increased

 A Case to Learn From

I clerked a patient with what clinically seemed like an atypical pneumonia. When I examined her lower limbs, she had reduced power throughout. I was concerned about Guillain–Barré syndrome (associated with mycoplasma pneumonia). When the consultant examined her, she initially had reduced power. However, the consultant just asked her to try harder and power was suddenly 5/5! Patient compliance is essential for accurate examination.

 Top Tip

It can be hard to assess for hypoventilation clinically. Many COPD patients with hypercapnia can look like they are hyperventilating even when they have alveolar hypoventilation.

STATION 2.3: ABDOMINAL

SCENARIO

You are a junior doctor in general surgery and have been asked to see Miss Payne, a 45-year-old woman, who has presented with severe abdominal pain and vomiting. Please perform a relevant abdominal examination on Miss Payne and present your findings.

PREPARATION

- WIPER:
  - *Wash* your hands
  - *Introduce* yourself
  - Ask about *pain*
  - Appropriately *expose*
  - *Reposition*
- Explain the examination to the patient and your reasons for performing it
- Gain verbal consent
- Give the patient privacy to expose themselves as required. When appropriate, expose from the xiphisternum to the pubic symphysis (PS)

- Provide a sheet to cover the patient's lower abdomen/pelvis
- Start in a comfortable position (with the patient sitting up at 45° and then lying flat)
- Offer a chaperone

GENERAL INSPECTION

- Environment: Vomit bowls, medications, abdominal drains, catheter bags
- Patient: Pain or agitation, muscle wasting (chronic diseases), abdominal distension, scars, nutritional status (large body habitus, cachexia), spider naevi, gynaecomastia, bruising, tattoos and peripheral oedema (signs of possible liver disease)

EXAMINATION OF THE HANDS

- Nails: Leukonychia ('white nails'; for example, secondary to low albumin), koilonychia ('spoon-shaped nails'; for example, secondary to iron deficiency), clubbing (Fig. 2.17)
- Palms: Palmar erythema (feature of chronic liver disease, hyperthyroidism), Dupuytren's contracture (feature of chronic liver disease)
- Liver flap: Ask the patient to cock both wrists up and hold that position for 30 s. Hand flapping is a positive sign of hepatic encephalopathy
- Pulse: Especially if you suspect a gastrointestinal bleed
- BP: Offer to measure the BP

EXAMINATION OF THE FACE, NECK AND CHEST

- Eyes: Ask the patient to lift their upper eyelid while looking down at the floor and note any jaundice or anaemia. Also look for Kayser–Fleischer rings (feature of Wilson's disease) and xanthelasma (feature of hypercholesterolaemia)

- Mouth: Gingivitis (feature of malnutrition), ulcers (feature of IBD), hydration, perioral pigmentation (feature of Peutz–Jeghers syndrome) and hepatic fetor ('bad breath')
- Lymph nodes: Ask the patient to sit forward and palpate their neck nodes. Troissier's sign is a palpable Virchow's node (in the left supraclavicular fossa), associated with gastrointestinal (GI) malignancy. While they're sitting forward, inspect the back for spider naevi and additional scars
- Chest: Hair loss (feature of chronic liver disease), gynaecomastia (feature of chronic liver disease, steroids), spider naevi often in the distribution of the SVC (feature of chronic liver disease and pregnancy). It is abnormal for men to have more than six, and for women to have more than four spider naevi

EXAMINATION OF THE ABDOMEN

- Reposition the patient by lying them flat with their hands by their side
- Think of the abdomen as being split into nine quadrants (Fig. 2.18) and visualise the organs underneath each one

INSPECTION

Look for:
- Shape: Generalised distension (think about the 'Five Fs': Fat, faeces, flatus, fluid, fetus), localised distension (mass, organomegaly), cachexia (feature of chronic disease, cancer, malnutrition)
- Scars: Anteriorly, posteriorly and in the flanks (Fig. 2.19). Look closely for laparoscopic scars and drain scars. Look under the skin folds in those with a large body habitus

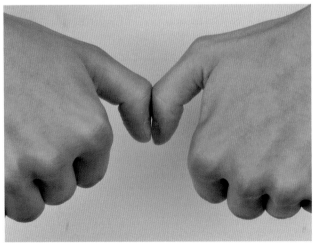

Fig. 2.17 Inspecting for clubbing: Look for a diamond formed between thumbnails.

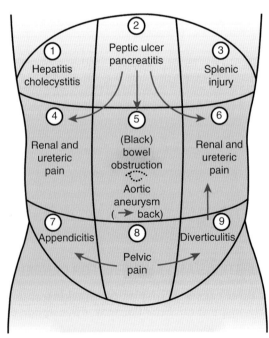

Fig. 2.18 The nine quadrants of the abdomen.

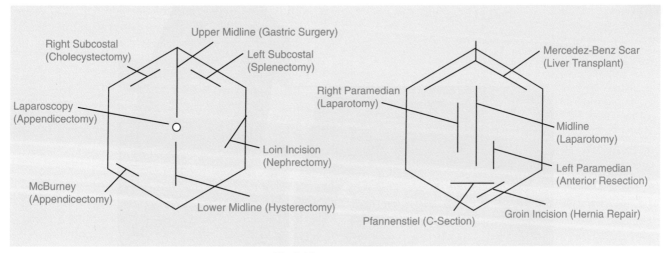

Fig. 2.19 Abdominal scars.

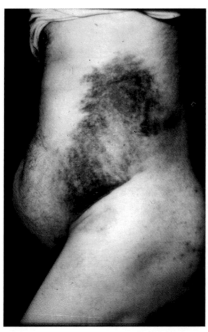

Fig. 2.20 Grey Turner's sign: Retroperitoneal bleeding associated with pancreatitis and ruptured AAA.

- Skin: Jaundice (feature of liver disease), Grey Turner's and/or Cullen's sign (retroperitoneal bruising associated with pancreatitis and/or ruptured abdominal aortic aneurysm (AAA)) (Fig. 2.20)
- Veins: Dilated abdominal wall veins, also known as 'caput medusae' (feature of portal hypertension) (Fig. 2.21)
- Cough: Ask the patient to blow out their tummy and cough. Pain may suggest peritoneal irritation. You can also see if hernias pop out

SUPERFICIAL PALPATION

- Kneel down to the level of the patient and look at the patient's face while palpating for signs of any pain

- Palpate the nine regions with one hand, looking out for tenderness and guarding
  - Voluntary guarding: Conscious anticipation of pain. The patient tenses their abdominal muscles to protect from pain prior to palpation. Avoided with distraction
  - Involuntary guarding: Innate reflex of the abdominal muscles to contract to protect from pain when palpated. Sign of peritonism and still present despite distraction

DEEP PALPATION

Repeat the process with superficial palpation, but this time, using both hands to palpate deeper. Again, assess for tenderness, guarding and any masses. Palpate five organs (Fig. 2.22):

- Liver: Begin in right iliac fossa, palpate with radial side of the index finger. Ask the patient to breathe in deeply and palpate on inspiration, feeling for the liver edge as it descends inferiorly. Keep moving your hand upwards until the liver is palpated. Measure the liver edge in fingerbreadths from the rib cage, commenting on surface, tenderness, pulsatility and any masses
- Spleen: Begin in the right iliac fossa, palpating with the fingertips. Keep moving up towards the left hypochondrium until you feel the spleen edge. Remember that you won't feel the spleen unless it's at least three times its normal size!
- Kidneys: Place one hand under the costal margin and the other in the right upper quadrant on the same side. Try to 'catch' the kidney between your hands as you press down
- Bladder: Distended bladder in the suprapubic region
- Abdominal aorta: Place each hand either side of the midline above the umbilicus. Feel for an expansile and pulsatile mass (features of AAA)

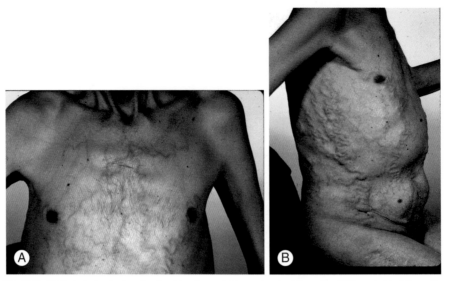

Fig. 2.21 Dilated abdominal wall veins (due to portal hypertension) from front (A) and side (B) profile.

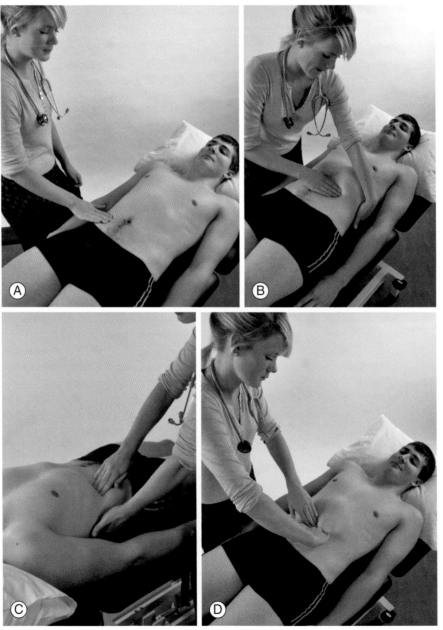

Fig. 2.22 (A–D) Deep palpation: Liver (starting in right iliac fossa), left kidney, right kidney and the aorta.

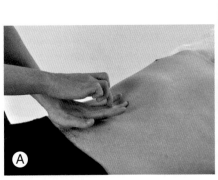
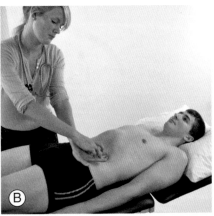
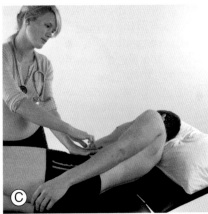

Fig. 2.23 Shifting dullness: Percuss the abdomen from the midline (A) to the periphery until dullness is noted (B). Keep your finger at this point and then ask the patient to roll towards you (C). Percuss again after 30 s and check if the percussion note is now resonant (positive test).

PERCUSSION

You may find it easier to percuss for each organ immediately after palpating for it instead of palpating every organ in order, and then percussing each one in the same order.

- Liver: Percuss from above and below the liver. Dullness will help determine the size of the liver. For the upper margin, percuss down from the chest. For the lower margin, percuss up from the right iliac fossa
- Spleen: Start in the right iliac fossa and move up towards the left hypochondrium
- Bladder: Consider percussing for the bladder in the suprapubic region
- Shifting dullness: This is a sign of ascites (Fig. 2.23)
- Fluid thrill: This is another sign of ascites (Fig. 2.24)

AUSCULTATION

Listen for:

- Bowel sounds: Listen over the ileocaecal valve for 30 s (Fig. 2.25). Bowel sounds may be present (normal), absent (for example, in paralytic ileus) or high-pitched and/or 'tinkling' (for example, in obstruction)
- Aortic bruits: Listen just above the umbilicus with the bell of the stethoscope
- Renal bruits: Listen 2 cm on either side of the umbilicus, with the bell of the stethoscope
- Liver bruits: If there is hepatomegaly, listen over the liver for a bruit (feature of hepatoma, acute alcoholic hepatitis, transjugular intrahepatic portosystemic stent shunt)

FINISHING

- Offer to:
  - Examine the external genitalia and hernial orifices
  - Look for peripheral oedema (sign of liver failure or nephrotic syndrome)

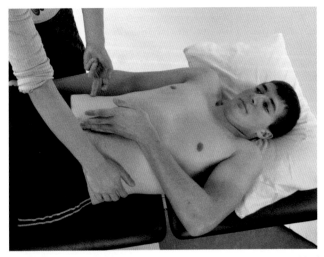

Fig. 2.24 Fluid thrill: Flick the skin on one side of the abdomen and feel for a 'thrill' on the other side with your hand. Place the patient's hand in the midline to stop transmission through the skin (since you only want to measure transmission through any fluid).

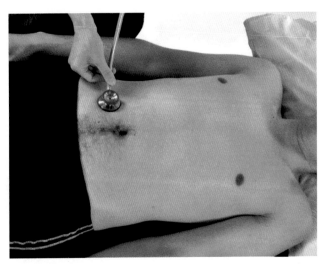

Fig. 2.25 Auscultating over the ileocaecal valve for bowel sounds.

- Perform a digital rectal examination (DRE)
- Dipstick the urine
- Thank the patient
- Check that they're comfortable and offer to help reposition them
- Wash your hands
- Leave the patient in privacy to get dressed

ADDITIONAL SIGNS TO ELICIT

- Rovsing's sign (feature of appendicitis): Tenderness in the right iliac fossa while palpating in the left iliac fossa
- Murphy's sign (feature of cholecystitis): Palpate over the site of the gallbladder, just under where the transpyloric plane crosses the costal margin. Ask the patient to inhale. Arrest of inspiration on palpation is positive

! Differentiating between a kidney and a spleen	
KIDNEY	**SPLEEN**
Moves inferiorly when enlarged	Moves to right iliac fossa when enlarged
Ballotable	Not ballotable
No notch	Has a notch
Does not move with respiration	Moves with respiration
Can get above it	Cannot get above it

CAUSES OF HEPATOMEGALY

- Cancer (primary hepatocellular carcinoma or secondary)
- Leukaemia
- Lymphoma
- Non-alcoholic fatty liver disease (NAFLD)
- Hepatitis
- Right heart failure

CAUSES OF SPLENOMEGALY

MASSIVE

- Chronic myeloid leukaemia (CML)
- Myelofibrosis
- Kala-azar (a parasitic disease)

MODERATE

- Lymphoma
- Chronic lymphocytic leukaemia (CLL)
- Malaria

MILD

- Epstein–Barr virus (EBV)
- Hepatitis
- Portal hypertension

- Felty's syndrome (a disorder characterised by the combination of rheumatoid arthritis, splenomegaly and neutropenia)

 Present Your Findings

Miss Payne is a 45-year-old woman presenting with abdominal pain, distension and vomiting, which is bilious as seen by bedside. Her abdomen is non-peritonitic, but distended with generalised tenderness. Her abdomen was tympanic with no shifting dullness. Bowel sounds were high-pitched. She has a scar in the right iliac fossa consistent with previous open appendicectomy.

I feel the most likely diagnosis is small-bowel obstruction, possibly secondary to adhesions. Differential diagnoses include: Large-bowel obstruction, pancreatitis and gastroenteritis.

To complete my examination, I would like to examine the hernial orifices, perform a DRE, inspect a stool sample and dipstick the urine. I would make her nil by mouth (NBM), insert a nasogastric (NG) tube on free drainage and start intravenous (IV) fluids. I would like to take bloods including: FBCs, U&Es, LFTs, amylase, coagulation, lactate and CRP. I would request a urinary beta-human chorionic gonadotrophin (β-hCG) test and organise an erect CXR and abdominal X-ray (AXR).

❓ QUESTIONS AND ANSWERS FOR CANDIDATE

Name three common causes of small-bowel obstruction.
- Adhesions postsurgery
- Hernias; for example, inguinal, femoral, incisional
- Malignancy
- Strictures; for example, Crohn's, radiation, ischaemic

How would you manage a patient with small-bowel obstruction?
- Assess the patient using an ABCDE approach
- 'Drip and suck' – NG tube insertion on free drainage and IV fluid hydration, with careful fluid balance
- Further imaging and surgery may be necessary in more severe cases

Name three causes of ascites.
- Hypoalbuminaemia: Cirrhosis (commonest), protein malnutrition or malabsorption, nephrotic syndrome
- Portal hypertension: Chronic liver disease
- Inflammation: Metastatic carcinoma, pelvic carcinoma (ovary), infection; for example, peritoneal TB

 A Case to Learn From

I was asked to examine a patient who was having an endoscopy for persistent anaemia. I noticed that they had spider naevi on the back of their right hand. On further examination, this patient had other signs of chronic liver disease, including gynaecomastia, axillary hair loss and a distended abdomen. Clinical signs like spider naevi can present in uncommon positions!

Top Tip

Don't forget that loud cardiac murmurs may be heard (and mistaken) as bruits over the liver.

STATION 2.4: HERNIA

SCENARIO

You are a junior doctor in the ED and have been asked to see Mr Jarral, a 91-year-old man, who has presented with abdominal pain and distension. He has also been vomiting and has noticed a lump in the groin. Please perform a relevant hernia examination on Mr Jarral and present your findings.

PREPARATION

- WIPER:
  - *Wash* your hands
  - *Introduce* yourself
  - Ask about *pain*
  - Appropriately *expose*
  - *Reposition*
- Explain the examination to the patient and your reasons for performing it
- Gain verbal consent
- Give the patient privacy to expose themselves as required, from the umbilicus down to the knees
- Start in a comfortable position (usually standing)
- Ensure that a chaperone is present

GENERAL INSPECTION

- Environment: Vomit bowls, hernia belts, medications
- Patient: Pain or agitation, large body habitus

EXAMINATION OF THE HERNIAL ORIFICES

INSPECTION

Look for:
- Masses: Compare both sides
- Scars: Previous surgery
- Skin: Note any erythema
- Accentuation: Pay particular attention to the inguinal, femoral and scrotal regions and ask the patient to cough to accentuate any hernia

PALPATION

- Gently feel the hernia, assessing for tenderness and observing the patient's face for discomfort
- Ask for a cough, feeling over the mass for a palpable cough impulse
- Define the local anatomy, highlighting each bony prominence in turn with a finger placement (this will help you appreciate the course of the inguinal ligament):
  - Pubic tubercle (PT): Hernias above and medial to your finger are likely to be inguinal,

whereas those below and lateral are more likely femoral
  - Anterior superior iliac spine (ASIS): Thus allowing you to find the midpoint between the ASIS and the PT, which is the midpoint of the inguinal ligament (the site of the deep inguinal ring)
  - Note that the 'mid-inguinal point' is different, as this is halfway between the ASIS and the PS
- Ask the patient if their hernia ever 'goes back in'. First ask the patient to reduce it on their own and if they cannot, attempt to do it yourself. The patient ideally should be supine in the Trendelenburg position (with the feet higher than the head) when you are trying to reduce an inguinal hernia
- Once reduced, keep fingers held over the site of reduction
- Then apply firm pressure with two fingers over the midpoint of the inguinal ligament whilst still pressing on the site of reduction
- Release the fingers from the site of reduction whilst keeping other fingers on the midpoint of the inguinal ligament
- Ask the patient to cough once more
- For an inguinal hernia, this will allow you to differentiate a direct from an indirect hernia:
  - If it is an indirect hernia, it is controlled and does not reappear
  - If it is a direct hernia, it is uncontrolled and does reappear
  - Note that the only definitive way to differentiate between the two is intraoperatively
- Standing up should make the hernia pop out again

AUSCULTATION

- Listen over the hernia for bowel sounds, particularly in large hernias

FINISHING

- Offer to:
  - Examine the contralateral side for hernias, the external genitalia, abdomen and rectum
- Thank the patient
- Check that they're comfortable and offer to help reposition them
- Wash your hands
- Leave the patient in privacy to get dressed

ANATOMY OF THE INGUINAL REGION (FIG. 2.26)

The Inguinal Canal

The communicating passage running obliquely from the deep ring to the superficial ring is known as the inguinal canal.

The four walls can be remembered as follows:
- Posterior: Transversalis fascia and conjoint tendon (medially)
- Anterior: External oblique
- Inferior: Inguinal ligament
- Superior: Conjoint tendon (of the internal oblique and the transversus muscles)

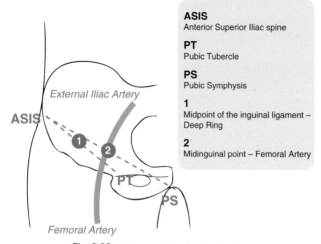

ASIS
Anterior Superior Iliac spine

PT
Pubic Tubercle

PS
Pubic Symphysis

1
Midpoint of the inguinal ligament –
Deep Ring

2
Midinguinal point – Femoral Artery

Fig. 2.26 Anatomy of the inguinal region.

In men, the inguinal canal conveys the spermatic cord and in women the round ligament. It also contains the ilioinguinal nerve, the genital branch of the genitofemoral nerve and lymphatics.

Midpoint of the Inguinal Ligament

This is the site of the deep inguinal ring, found halfway along the inguinal ligament. It is demarcated by an imaginary dashed line from the ASIS to the PT.

Mid-Inguinal Point

This is the site of the femoral artery, found halfway along the imaginary dashed line (Fig. 2.26), drawn from the ASIS to the PS.

Hesselbach's Triangle

This is the defined anatomical region within which hernias are direct. The borders are:
- Inferiorly: Inguinal ligament
- Superiorly: Inferior epigastric blood vessels
- Medially: Rectus abdominis

TYPES OF HERNIA

A description of different types of hernia is given in Table 2.6.

Present Your Findings

Mr Jarral is a 91-year-old man who has presented with abdominal pain and distension. He is comfortable at rest. He has a distended abdomen, with a visible lump over the right inguinal region. There are no associated skin changes. The lump is tender, reducible and controlled with pressure over the deep ring. Bowel sounds are present over the lump.

This is consistent with a diagnosis of a right-sided indirect inguinal hernia, although the question of being direct or indirect can only be confirmed during surgery.

To complete my examination, I would like to perform a full abdominal examination, examine the external genitalia and perform a DRE. I would like to refer him to the general surgeons for consideration of surgery or conservative management.

Table 2.6 Hernia types

TYPES OF HERNIA	DESCRIPTION
Inguinal	A protrusion of a viscus (commonly bowel) through the inguinal canal
Femoral	A protrusion of a viscus (commonly bowel) through the femoral canal
Incisional	A protrusion of a viscus (commonly bowel) through an acquired defect, which is iatrogenic (previous surgery) or from injury (knife wounds)
Richter's	Also known as a partial enterocele, this is a hernia involving only one side of the bowel wall
Amyand's	An inguinal hernia that contains the appendix
Spigelian	A hernia protruding through the spigelian fascia (aponeurosis of transversus abdominis muscle, which fills the space between the edge of the rectus and the muscle belly of the transversus). The fascia is widest (and therefore weakest) just below the level of the umbilicus, but Spigelian hernias can occur anywhere along this line
Littre's	A hernia involving Meckel's diverticulum

? QUESTIONS AND ANSWERS FOR CANDIDATE

What is the definition of a hernia?
- A protrusion of a viscus (or part of a viscus) through a defect in the wall of its containing cavity and into an anatomically abnormal position

What is the difference between an indirect and a direct inguinal hernia?
- Indirect inguinal hernia (80%): Viscus passes through the deep ring into the inguinal canal (therefore it is controlled by pressure over deep ring)
- Direct inguinal hernia (20%): Viscus passes through a defect in the abdominal wall, sometimes bulging into the inguinal canal

Name three complications of a hernia.
- Irreducible hernia: Cannot be reduced, but does not necessarily cause bowel obstruction or vascular compromise
- Obstructed hernia: Intestine within the hernia sac is obstructed
- Strangulated hernia: Irreducible hernia which results in vascular compromise and infarction of the obstructed bowel

---

 A Case to Learn From

I saw a child who was complaining of abdominal pain. The child hadn't noticed a lump and neither had his parents. However, it was clear on examination, and it turned out that he had a hernia that was intermittently obstructing. When it was surgically corrected, the symptoms improved. Always look for a hernia in any gastrointestinal examination!

Examine the patient both standing and lying. Start with whichever is convenient. Expose the scrotum in a male (other lumps may be there to trick you!) and check the other side while you're there.

Auscultation may be useful for a large hernia, but I don't think it is necessary. Contents are either bowel or omentum (rarely other small things; for example, appendix, ovary or bladder).

STATION 2.5: TESTICULAR

SCENARIO

You are a junior doctor in general surgery and have been asked to see Mr Smith, a 20-year-old man, who has presented with a swelling of his right testicle. Please perform a relevant testicular examination on Mr Smith and present your findings.

PREPARATION

- WIPER:
  - *Wash* your hands
  - *Introduce* yourself
  - Ask about *pain*
  - Appropriately *expose*
  - *Reposition*
- Explain the examination to the patient and your reasons for performing it
- Gain verbal consent
- Give the patient privacy to expose themselves as required and provide a sheet to cover the patient's genitalia
- Start in a comfortable position (standing)
- Ensure that a chaperone is present

GENERAL INSPECTION

- Environment: Vomit bowls, medications, urine sample
- Patient: Pain or agitation, gynaecomastia (Fig. 2.27), secondary sexual characteristics

EXAMINATION OF THE SCROTUM

INSPECTION

- Look at the front and back
- Note the size and shape of each scrotum
- Comment on:
  - Asymmetry
  - Lumps
  - Ulcers
  - Swellings

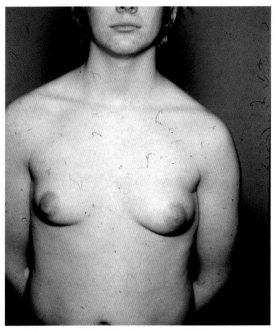

Fig. 2.27 Gynaecomastia.

- Rashes
- Scrotal oedema
- Scars; for example, from previous hernia surgery or exploration of the scrotum
- Distribution of pubic hair

Note that the left testicle is often lower than the right.

EXAMINATION OF THE PENIS

INSPECTION

- Comment on:
  - Asymmetry
  - Lumps
  - Ulcers
  - Discharge
  - Position of the urethral meatus

EXAMINATION OF THE TESTES

PALPATION

- Ask the patient if he is in any pain
- Warm your hands and put on gloves
- Ask the patient to stand up
- Examine the 'normal' side first
- Check if both testicles are present or if one may be undescended
- Note the size and symmetry of the testicles. If one is larger, note whether it is the whole testis or a discrete mass. If it is the latter, and you cannot get above the mass, consider a hernia (see Station 2.4: 'Hernia Examination). If it is the latter and you can get above the mass, then it is a scrotal mass (Tables 2.7 and 2.8). Ask the following four questions:
  1. Is it separate from, or part of, the testis?
  2. Is it cystic or solid?

⌁ Table **2.7**	Description of scrotal masses	
CONSISTENCY	**TESTICULAR**	**SEPARATE FROM TESTES**
Solid	If tender: Likely orchitis or testicular torsion If non-tender: Likely tumour or granuloma	If tender: Likely epididymitis
Cystic	If non-tender: Likely hydrocele	If non-tender: Likely epididymal cyst, hydrocele of the spermatic cord, varicocele or spermatocele

3. Is it tender or non-tender?
4. Does it transilluminate?
- Offer to transilluminate any masses that are present

FINISHING

- Offer to:
  - Feel the epididymis head, body and tail
  - Feel the spermatic cord using two fingers, tracing it from the testes to the inguinal region
  - Feel the inguinal lymph nodes for scrotal pathology. Note that testicular infection and malignancy tend to spread to the paraaortic nodes, not the inguinal nodes
  - Examine the abdomen and hernia
  - Dipstick the urine
  - Perform additional tests, including the cremasteric reflex and Phren's test
  - Provide the patient with information on how to self-examine, so that he can identify problems on his own
- Thank the patient
- Check that he is comfortable and offer to help reposition him
- Remove your gloves and wash your hands
- Leave the patient in privacy to get dressed

! Types of scrotal tumours

	TERATOMA	**SEMINOMA**	**LYMPHOMA**
Definition	• A germ cell tumour, with tissue components not normally found at that site	• Germ cell tumour • Histological diagnosis of 'pure seminomatous elements' (large round cells with vascular nuclei) and normal alpha-fetoprotein blood levels	• A solid tumour of the lymphoid cells
Age	• Mainly affects 20–30-year-olds	• Mainly affects 30–40-year-olds	• Mainly affects the elderly
Relative incidence	• 40–50%	• 40–50%	• 0–10%
Management	• Chemotherapy • Surgery	• Radiotherapy • Chemotherapy • Surgery	• Surgery • Chemotherapy • Radiotherapy
Prognosis	• Intermediate prognosis	• Highly curable if detected early	• Poorest prognosis; around 50% have systemic disease at presentation

CAUSES OF AN IMPALPABLE TESTIS

- Undescended testis
- Retracted testis; for example, due to cold hands
- Previous orchidectomy

CAUSES OF A SMALL TESTICLE

- Hypogonadism
- Cold temperature, causing muscle contraction

CAUSES OF A LARGE TESTICLE

- Hydrocele
- Varicocele
- Tumour

🔍 Present Your Findings

Mr Smith is a 20-year-old man presenting with right-sided testicular swelling.

The swelling is a smooth, well-circumscribed lump, measuring 4 × 6 cm, on the anterior aspect of the right testicle. It is soft, transilluminates and is non-tender. The left testicle is normal and examination of the rest of the external genitalia is unremarkable.

I feel the most likely diagnosis is a right-sided hydrocele.

To complete my examination, I would like to perform an abdominal examination, examine the hernia orifices and do a urine dipstick. I would request a testicular ultrasound and refer to urology.

Table 2.8	Differential diagnoses of scrotal masses
CONDITION	**INFORMATION**
Orchitis and epididymitis	• In young adults and adolescents, consider sexually transmitted infections (STIs), TB and mumps • In the elderly, consider *Escherichia coli* (*E. coli*) infection
Spermatocele	• Smooth, soft, well circumscribed • Typically arises from the head of the epididymis (superior aspect of testicle) • The fluid usually contains sperm
Cyst of the epididymis	• Smooth, soft, well circumscribed • Well above the testis and separate from it • Contains clear straw-coloured fluid • Transilluminates • If it is multilocular, it gives a 'Chinese lantern' appearance
Hydrocele	• A fluid collection, covering the anterior and lateral aspects of the testis • Soft, non-tender fullness • Transilluminates
Varicocele	• Dilated venous plexus along spermatic cord, like a 'bag of worms', found on examination when the patient is standing and reduces when lying flat • More common in the left than the right due to anatomical factors; for example, the lack of antireflux valves at the juncture of the left testicular vein and the left renal vein
Haematocele	• Haemorrhage into the tunica vaginalis usually secondary to trauma • Presents with pain, tenderness and rapid refilling of the sac on examination • Poor or absent transillumination because it is generally a solid clot
Torsed epididymal appendix	• Exquisite tenderness localised to the upper pole of the testis • Appears as a black dot on transillumination

❓ QUESTIONS AND ANSWERS FOR CANDIDATE

How would you explain to a patient how to self-examine in future?

• Examine whilst in the bath or shower (as heat softens the skin, making it easier to feel the testicles)
• Feel for lumps on the skin
• Feel for swellings inside the scrotum
• Examine each testicle separately and then compare both testicles. Note that it can be normal to have one that is larger and lower

• Use both hands and roll the testicle between the thumb and forefinger
• If there are any abnormalities or concerns, seek medical advice

What investigations would you do next in a patient with a suspected hydrocele and how would you manage this patient?

• Carry out ultrasound to assess for any underlying masses and fluid collection
• Hydrocele may only require conservative management
• Fluid may be aspirated, but to ensure no further recurrence, surgery is required

What histological features would differentiate a teratoma from other tumours?

• A teratoma is a germ cell tumour, with tissue components not normally found at that site; for example, teeth

 A Case to Learn From

We once saw a child with a very painful testicle. The skin was red and we suspected infection. However, in any acutely painful testicle (especially in children), consider testicular torsion, even if there is another diagnosis being considered more likely. In these circumstances, it would be a clinical diagnosis and you do *not* need an ultrasound for confirmation before commencing treatment. Testicular torsion is the most important differential in acute testicular pain and cannot be missed! It is a urological emergency and requires urgent surgical intervention.

Top Tip

Always examine the 'normal' side as well. There may be an asymptomatic lump that could be treated before it becomes a problem.

STATION 2.6: STOMA

SCENARIO

You are a junior doctor in general surgery and have been asked to see Mrs Pouch, a 40-year-old woman, in clinic, for a routine postoperative follow-up. She has a stoma bag in situ. Please perform a relevant stoma examination on Mrs Pouch and present your findings.

PREPARATION

• WIPER:
    • *Wash* your hands
    • *Introduce* yourself

- Ask about *pain*
- Appropriately *expose*
- *Reposition*
- Explain the examination to the patient and your reasons for performing it
- Gain verbal consent
- Give the patient privacy to expose themselves as required and provide a sheet to cover the patient's lower abdomen and pelvis
- Start in a comfortable position (usually with the patient lying down)
- Offer a chaperone

GENERAL INSPECTION

- Environment: Vomit bowls, medications
- Patient: Pain or agitation, stoma bag

EXAMINATION OF THE STOMA

- A stoma is an artificial (deliberate) connection between a hollow viscus and the skin surface
- Inspect the area around the stoma for signs of infection, fistula or skin excoriation
- Describing a stoma is best done in a systematic manner:
  - Site: Describe in relation to the nine quadrants of the abdomen
  - Bag: Contents may include: Nothing, solid stool (colostomy), liquid stool (ileostomy) or urine (urostomy) (Fig. 2.28)
  - Surface: Either flush with the skin (minimally raised/less protuberant) or with a protruding spout
  - Openings: Single-lumen (end) or double-lumen (loop)
  - Skin: Note the health of the mucosa (colour) and surrounding skin

EXAMINATION OF THE ABDOMEN

INSPECTION

- Especially scars that can give vital clues as to the operative history

PALPATION

- Palpation is not normally expected
- Be gentle and enquire about pain

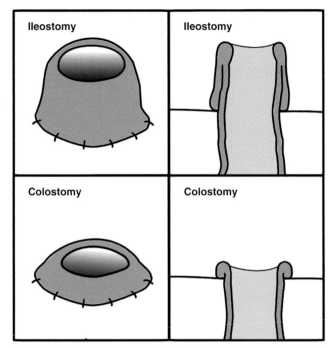

Fig. 2.28 Ileostomy vs. colostomy.

- Be cautious while removing the bag to avoid leakage
- With gloves and lubricant on the index finger, insert it into the opening to assess:
  - Stenosis: Feel for narrowing of the opening conduit
  - End type: Confirm the number of openings as they are not always easy to visualise

FINISHING

- Offer to:
  - Assess for parastomal and incisional hernias by asking the patient to cough
  - Place a new ostomy appliance at the site or the patient may prefer to do this for themselves
  - Perform an abdominal examination, including an assessment for the presence of an anus
- Thank the patient
- Check that they're comfortable and offer to help reposition them
- Remove your gloves and wash your hands
- Leave the patient in privacy to get dressed

! Types of stoma bags

	ILEOSTOMY	COLOSTOMY	UROSTOMY
Surgical procedure	• Panproctocolectomy; for example, in ulcerative colitis • Anterior resection; for example, in colorectal cancer	• Abdominoperoneal resection, i.e. with no anus; for example, in colorectal cancer • Hartmann's procedure, i.e. with the anus present; for example, in colorectal cancer	• Total cystectomy; for example, in bladder cancer
Site	• Right lower quadrant	• Left lower quadrant	• Usually right-sided, but can vary
Bag contents	• Liquid stool	• Semiformed stool	• Urine
Surface opening	• Raised from the skin in a spout	• Flush with the skin or minimally raised	• Usually as a spout, like an ileostomy

Present Your Findings

Mrs Pouch is a 40-year-old woman attending a routine outpatient appointment. She is comfortable at rest and has a stoma located in the lower right quadrant of her abdomen. The stoma appears healthy, with liquid stool, and a single lumen which is raised from the skin. There is a midline laparotomy scar and no evidence of incisional or parastomal hernia.

I feel the most likely diagnosis is an end ileostomy, which is healthy.

To complete my examination, I would like to perform a full abdominal examination, including assessing for an anus. Routine follow-up would continue with the stoma care community team.

? QUESTIONS AND ANSWERS FOR CANDIDATE

Name three potential complications that might occur post stoma creation.
• Immediate: Haemorrhage
• Early: Ischaemia, adhesions, diarrhoea
• Late: Skin excoriation, parastomal hernia, stenosis, fistulas, psychosexual complications, nutritional deficiency, prolapse

What two procedures might result in someone having a colostomy and how might you tell the difference on examination?
• Abdominoperoneal resection (no anus)
• Hartmann's procedure (with the anus present)

What is the difference between a loop colostomy and an end colostomy?
• Loop colostomy: A loop of colon is pulled out into the abdomen and then opened up and stitched to skin
• End colostomy: One end of the colon is pulled through a hole in the abdomen and stitched to the skin

A Case to Learn From

At medical school, we were all given colostomies to wear for a week: In the shower, in the swimming pool, in intimate settings. It proved a useful learning opportunity for appreciating the psychological impact of having a stoma, particularly when a patient first starts to use one. Always be aware of this and enquire when appropriate.

Top Tip

It's often nicer to ask the patient to replace their own ostomy device if you have taken it off, so ask them what they'd prefer, particularly if they are looking very well, as they often do in an exam!

STATION 2.7: RECTAL

SCENARIO

You are a junior doctor in general surgery and have been asked to perform a DRE on Mr Wilson, a 69-year-old man, who has presented with vomiting, abdominal pain and reduced bowel movements. Treat and address the model as you would a real patient and perform a DRE, stating your positive and negative findings. He has already consented to the procedure.

PREPARATION

• WIPER:
  • *Wash* your hands
  • *Introduce* yourself
  • Ask about *pain*
  • Appropriately *expose*
  • *Reposition*
• Explain the examination to the patient and your reasons for performing it

- Gain verbal consent
- Give the patient privacy to expose themselves as required and only remove the underwear when necessary. Provide a sheet to cover the patient's lower body
- Place an incontinence sheet between the patient's buttocks and the bed. This ensures that no faecal staining of the bed occurs during the examination
- Start in a comfortable position (usually with the patient lying in bed, then when appropriate, position the patient in the left lateral position, with knees drawn to the chest [Fig. 2.29])
- Ensure that a chaperone is present

GENERAL INSPECTION

- Environment: Vomit bowls, stool charts
- Patient: Pain or agitation

INSPECTION

- Gently separate the buttocks with your left hand.
- Inspect the anus and perianal area, looking for:
  - Fissures
  - Skin tags
  - Erythema
  - Sinuses or fistulae
  - Pilonidal sinuses
  - Haemorrhoids

PROCEDURE

- Lubricate your right index finger
- Separate the buttocks with your left hand and gently apply pressure with the pulp of the finger to enter the anus. This will overcome the sphincter tone
- Warn the patient when you are going to insert your finger
- Insert your finger through the anus, aiming towards the umbilicus
- Palpate the anterior, right lateral, posterior and left lateral walls in turn

- Note any pain that may be elicited
- Comment on:
  - Size
  - Surface
  - Consistency of the prostate gland (in males)
  - Presence of any other masses or stool in rectum
- Test the anal tone by asking the patient to squeeze his buttocks or bear down on your finger
- Withdraw your finger
- Inspect your finger for faeces, blood, mucus or melaena
- Offer the patient some paper towel to clean themselves. The patient may require assistance if they are unable to do this independently

FINISHING

- Offer to:
  - Perform an abdominal examination
  - Inspect a stool sample
  - Dipstick the urine
- Thank the patient
- Check that they're comfortable and offer to help reposition them
- Remove your gloves and wash your hands
- Leave the patient in privacy to get dressed

! Signs and symptoms of different colorectal tumours based on the general location		
RIGHT-SIDED TUMOUR	**LEFT-SIDED TUMOUR**	**RECTAL TUMOUR**
• Often painful • Palpable abdominal mass • Weight loss • Anaemia	• Change in bowel habit • Palpable mass • Pain is a less frequent feature • May have blood and/or mucus per rectally	• Change in bowel habit • Blood and/or mucus per rectally • Rarely associated with pain

🔍 Present Your Findings

Mr Wilson is a 69-year-old man presenting with vomiting, abdominal pain and reduced bowel movements. With his consent, I performed a rectal examination on him. On inspection, there was evidence of a fistula in the 9 o'clock position, with tenderness of the rectum on palpation and soft stool with blood and/or mucus mixed in with it.

I feel the most likely diagnosis is IBD, although I would also consider malignancy in this age group.

To complete my examination, I would like to perform a full abdominal examination, inspect a stool sample and dipstick the urine. I would make him NBM and start IV fluids. I would like to perform an AXR and take bloods, including: FBCs, U&Es, LFTs, amylase, coagulation, lactate, erythrocyte sedimentation rate (ESR) and CRP.

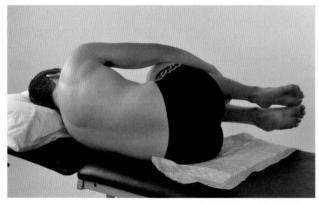

Fig. 2.29 Positioning of patient for a rectal examination. Only remove underwear when needed.

❓ QUESTIONS AND ANSWERS FOR CANDIDATE

Name three common causes of rectal bleeding.
- Haemorrhoids
- Anal fissures
- Colon polyps
- Colorectal cancer
- IBD
- Crohn's disease
- Ulcerative colitis
- Intestinal infections
- Diverticular disease
- Angiodysplasia
- Perfuse bleeding from the upper GI tract; for example, oesophageal varices, gastritis, gastric carcinoma

If blood was found on examination, what features might suggest malignancy as a more likely explanation?
- Older age
- Unexplained weight loss
- Altered bowel habit
- Abdominal pain
- Fatigue
- Family history and/or personal history of colorectal cancer

How would you manage a large rectal bleed?
- Activate major haemorrhage protocol
- Urgent bloods, including: Cross-match, FBC, U&Es, LFTs, bone profile and blood gas
- Two large-bore IV access and fluid or blood as a bolus
- Urgent surgical review

 A Case to Learn From

When I was in theatre as a student, a consultant asked us to perform a rectal examination for our learning on a patient who was asleep. Four of us did it, appreciating the malignancy of the prostate. However, we retrospectively found out that the patient had not been consented and it had been assumed and done while the patient was anaesthetised. Never assume consent, and if unsure, always check the consent form yourself.

 Top Tip

Take your time doing the rectal examination. If you're not sure about your findings, it's much better for the patient that you take a little longer than having to perform the procedure again.

STATION 2.8: CRANIAL NERVES

SCENARIO

You are a junior doctor in general medicine and have been asked to see Mr Wade, a 48-year-old man, who has presented with a droopy eyelid. Please perform a relevant cranial nerve (CN) examination on Mr Wade and present your findings.

PREPARATION

- WIPER:
  - *Wash* your hands
  - *Introduce* yourself
  - Ask about *pain*
  - Appropriately *expose*
  - *Reposition*
- Explain the examination to the patient and your reasons for performing it
- Gain verbal consent
- Give the patient privacy to expose themselves as required
- Start in a comfortable position (usually with the patient sat down)
- Offer a chaperone

GENERAL INSPECTION

- Environment: Vomit bowls, medications, walking aids
- Patient: Pain or agitation, ptosis (CN III). eye position (CN III, IV, VI), pupil symmetry (CN II, III), facial symmetry (CN VII), sternocleidomastoid and trapezius bulk (CN XI), speech (CN V, VII, IX, X, XII), skin lesions (for example, neurofibromatosis [Fig. 2.30])

EXAMINATION OF THE EYE

INSPECTION

- Ptosis: Drooping of the upper eyelid (feature of Horner's syndrome, third-nerve palsy, congenital abnormality, senile ptosis, myasthenia gravis [Fig. 2.31])
- Exophthalmos: Anterior bulging of the eyeball (feature of Graves' disease or secondary to a retro-orbital mass)
- Enophthalmos: Eyeball recession within the orbit (could be congenital, traumatic causes or secondary to Horner's syndrome)

EXAMINATION OF THE OLFACTORY NERVE (CN I)

- Ask about any changes in sense of smell or taste of food
- CN I could be tested formally by covering each nostril and testing with a battery of standardised smells; for example, peppermint

EXAMINATION OF THE OPTIC NERVE (CN II)

- Ask regarding glasses or contact lens use
- Visual acuity: Test one eye at a time with a Snellen chart or, as a simple bedside screen, get the patient to read something

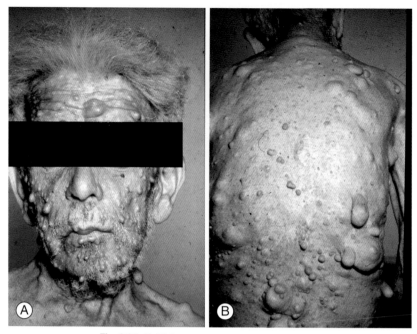

Fig. 2.30 (A, B) Skin lesions of neurofibromatosis.

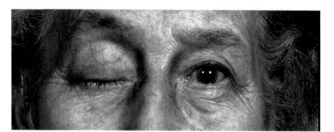

Fig. 2.31 Right-eye ptosis.

- Visual fields: Sit opposite the patient and ask them to look straight ahead. Test the four quadrants of both eyes separately, by moving a finger into the visual field from outside it, then see if there is evidence of neglect by testing both eyes simultaneously (Fig. 2.32)
- Blind spot: Test for blind spots using a red hat pin
- Offer to perform fundoscopy

EXAMINATION OF THE OCULOMOTOR, TROCHLEAR AND ABDUCENS NERVES (CN III, IV, VI)

- Eye movements: Ask the patient, while keeping their head still, to follow the movements of your finger in all directions (pursuit movements). Ask about double vision and look for nystagmus (Fig. 2.33)
- Accommodation reflex: Ask the patient to look to a distant point; for example, a curtain, then at something closer; for example, your pen torch (Fig. 2.34)
- Pupillary light reflexes: Test for both direct and consensual light reflexes and look for a relative afferent pupillary defect (RAPD). For both reflexes above, the sensory limb is dependent on CN II and the motor limb on CN III

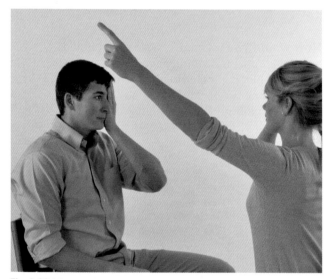

Fig. 2.32 Visual field assessment: Ensure that you cover your eye that is directly opposite the one that isn't being tested (i.e. cover your right eye when testing the patient's left eye).

EXAMINATION OF THE TRIGEMINAL NERVE (CN V)

- Feel the contraction of masseter and temporalis muscles under your fingers whilst the patient clenches his jaw (Fig. 2.35)
- Ask the patient to open his jaw against your resistance
- Test facial sensation by first, demonstrating the sensation centrally; for example, at the sternum. Then test light touch to the corresponding areas for ophthalmic, maxillary and mandibular branches on both sides of the patient's face whilst his eyes are closed (Fig. 2.36)

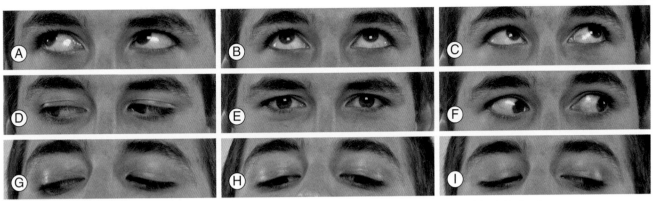

Fig. 2.33 (A–I) Assessing ocular movements (CN III, IV, VI) by asking the patient to look in eight directions.

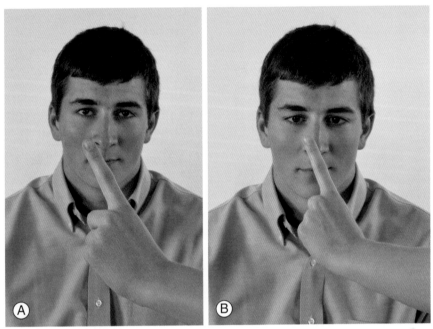

Fig. 2.34 Testing accommodation by asking the patient to focus on your finger (A) and then to focus on an object in the distance (B). Look for convergence of the eyes and constriction of the pupils.

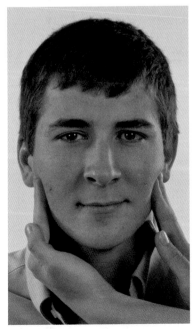

Fig. 2.35 Masseter palpation.

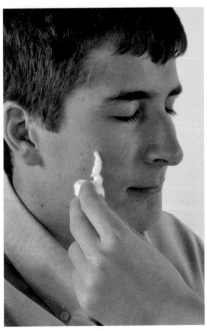

Fig. 2.36 Sensation in the maxillary division of the trigeminal nerve. Note the patient's eyes are shut to prevent cheating!

- Offer to assess pain and temperature sensation in the same areas
- Offer to assess corneal reflex using cotton wool (Fig. 2.37) and jaw jerk reflex by striking the chin while the mouth is open (Fig. 2.38)

EXAMINATION OF THE FACIAL NERVE (CN VII)

- Test in order of branches (Fig. 2.39):
  - Temporal: Raising the eyebrows
  - Zygomatic: Scrunching the eyes
  - Buccal: Blowing out the cheeks
  - Mandibular: Showing teeth or whistling
  - Cervical: Sticking the chin forward
- Ask the patient to relax between tests
- Fig. 2.40 demonstrates a patient with facial nerve palsy

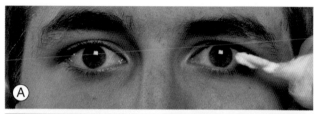
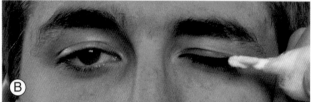

Fig. 2.37 (A, B) Corneal reflex test: Blink in response to stimulation of the cornea with a cotton-wool wisp is normal.

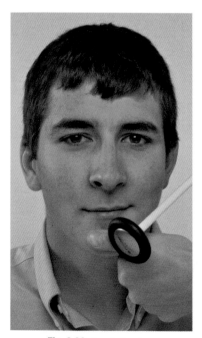

Fig. 2.38 Jaw jerk reflex.

EXAMINATION OF THE VESTIBULOCOCHLEAR NERVE (CN VIII)

- Sit to the side of your patient and remember to start with the unaffected side first
- With one hand, obscure the entrance to the contralateral ear canal and rub gently. Do this by pushing the tragus into the canal. This will muffle this ear and ensure that you are only testing one ear at a time. With the other hand, cover the patient's eyes so that they cannot lip read (Fig. 2.41)
- Ensure that you are at full arm's length
- Whisper a combination of a number and a letter; for example, 'N4', and ask the patient to repeat what you are saying. Get increasingly louder until they can hear you
- Perform Rinne's and Weber's tests (see Station 2.23: Ear Examination)
- Offer to assess balance

EXAMINATION OF THE GLOSSOPHARYNGEAL AND VAGUS NERVES (CN IX AND X)

- Ask the patient to (Fig. 2.42):
  - Cough
  - Swallow water
  - Open their mouth and say 'ahh' (while you look for uvular deviation)
- Offer to test the gag reflex by sticking a tongue depressor gently into the back of the throat

EXAMINATION OF THE ACCESSORY (SPINAL ROOT) NERVE (CN XI)

- Ask the patient to (Fig. 2.43):
  - Shrug their shoulders against resistance
  - Put their chin on to their left shoulder and then on to their right shoulder. Ask the patient to do both of these against resistance

EXAMINATION OF THE HYPOGLOSSAL NERVE (CN XII)

- Inspect the patient's mouth while open, looking for fasciculations (Fig. 2.44A)
- Ask the patient to stick out their tongue and inspect it for wasting and deviation (Fig. 2.44B)
- Ask the patient to push their tongue into their cheek and resist the movement by pushing on to their tongue from the outside of the cheek (Fig. 2.44C)

FINISHING

- Offer to:
  - Perform a full neurological examination, including: Cerebellar, upper- and lower-limb examination
  - Assess sweating on both sides of the face
  - Perform vibration and temperature testing

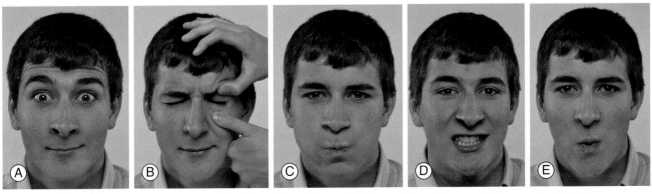

Fig. 2.39 Facial nerve testing: (A) Raising the eyebrows (temporal); (B) scrunching up the eye, with the examiner trying to open them (zygomatic); (C) blowing out the cheeks (buccal); (D) showing teeth; or (E) whistling (mandibular).

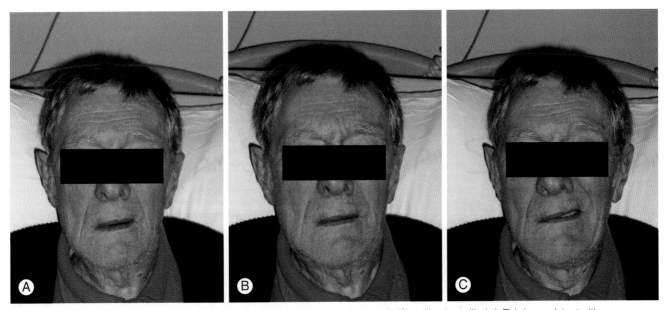

Fig. 2.40 Facial nerve palsy: (A) Baseline; (B) raising eyebrows (temporal); (C) smiling (mandibular). This is consistent with a lower motor neurone lesion since there is no forehead sparing.

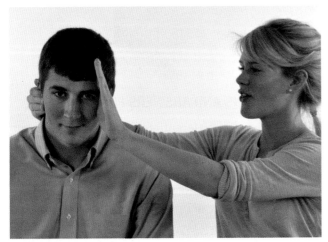

Fig. 2.41 Whisper test, while obscuring the patient's eyes to avoid any lip reading.

- Perform a fundoscopy
- Perform a cognitive assessment, including speech
- Thank the patient
- Check that they're comfortable and offer to help reposition them
- Wash your hands
- Leave the patient in privacy to get dressed

❗ Interpretation of visual fields	
VISUAL FIELD LOSS	**VISUAL PATHWAY DEFECT**
Total blindness in one eye	Complete lesion of the optic nerve
Bitemporal hemianopia	Optic chiasma lesion
Homonymous hemianopia	Contralateral hemisphere lesion
Homonymous quadrantanopia	Optic radiation lesion

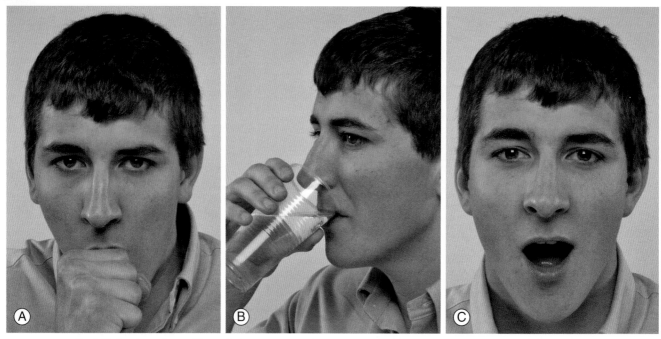

Fig. 2.42 Ask the patient to (A) cough, (B) swallow and (C) say 'ahh' so that you can look in the mouth for uvular deviation.

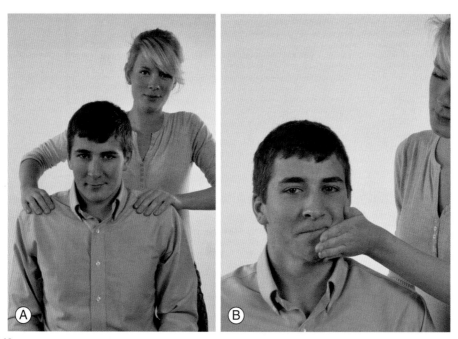

Fig. 2.43 (A) Shoulder shrug (against resistance) and (B) putting the chin on to the left shoulder (against resistance).

Present Your Findings

Mr Wade is a 48-year-old man presenting with a droopy eyelid. He has a left-sided miosis, enophthalmos and a partial ptosis. There was a slow direct pupillary response to light on the left side compared with the right. There were no other significant abnormalities.

I feel the most likely diagnosis is Horner's syndrome.

To complete my examination, I would like to do a full neurological assessment, including cerebellar and peripheral nerve testing, perform fundoscopy, assess sweating on both sides of the face and do a cognitive assessment. I would like to take bloods, including: FBCs, U&Es, LFTs, bone profile, thyroid function test (TFTs), ESR and CRP. I would also request a CXR in case this is related to a Pancoast's tumour.

QUESTIONS AND ANSWERS FOR CANDIDATE

How would you differentiate an upper motor neurone VII cranial nerve lesion from a lower motor neurone lesion?
- The muscles of the forehead have bilateral cortical representation. Therefore, in an upper motor neurone lesion; for example, a cerebral infarct, there is sparing of the forehead. The patient would still be able to raise their eyebrows equally on both sides

What are the classic features of Horner's syndrome?
- Miosis with notable asymmetry in pupil size
- Droopy eyelid

- Anhidrosis (reduced sweating)
- Sunken appearance to the eyes
- Delayed pupil dilatation in dim light

What features might be associated with a middle cerebral artery stroke?

- Primarily face and upper-limb areas of motor cortex (and sensory)
- Spatial perception is abnormal if the stroke is in the non-dominant hemisphere
- Language centres are abnormal if the stroke is in the dominant hemisphere
- Homonymous hemianopia
- Deviation of the head and eyes towards the side of the lesion

 A Case to Learn From

I examined a patient once who I thought had perfectly normal sensation in their face. However, the examination was repeated by my senior, who identified a clear sensory loss pattern in the V3 branch of the trigeminal nerve. The difference? He took the time to touch gently and made moving from one dermatome to another very irregular so that the patient couldn't second guess when sensation was about to be tested. Don't rush when testing sensations!

 Top Tip

It is actually much more reliable to look for fasciculations when the tongue is resting in the mouth than when it is protruded.

STATION 2.9: PERIPHERAL NERVES (UPPER LIMB)

SCENARIO

You are a junior doctor in the ED and have been asked to see Mr Reilly, a 64-year-old man, who has recently had a fall and fractured his humerus. He is now struggling to perform everyday tasks with his right hand.

Please perform a relevant neurological examination on Mr Reilly's upper limbs and present your findings.

PREPARATION

- WIPER:
  - *Wash* your hands
  - *Introduce* yourself
  - Ask about *pain*
  - Appropriately *expose*
  - *Reposition*
- Explain the examination to the patient and your reasons for performing it
- Gain verbal consent
- Give the patient privacy to expose themselves as required
- Start in a comfortable position (usually sitting or standing)
- Offer a chaperone

GENERAL INSPECTION

- Environment: Walking aids, wheelchairs, arm support
- Patient: Pain or agitation. A good acronym to use for patient inspection is SWIFT:
  - *Scars*
  - *Wasting* of muscles
  - *Involuntary* movements
  - *Fasciculations*
  - *Tremor*

PRONATOR DRIFT

Ask the patient to hold his arms out in supination (palms facing the ceiling) and close his eyes. If you see pronator drift (palm(s) turning involuntarily to face the floor), think upper motor neurone lesion (Fig. 2.45).

ASSESSMENT OF TONE:

- Ensure that the patient is relaxed

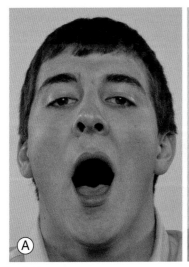 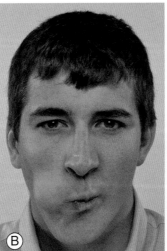 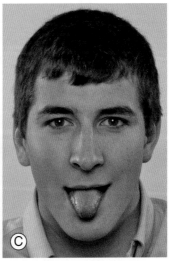

Fig. 2.44 (A) Inspecting the inside of the mouth, (B) Pushing the tongue on to the inside of the cheek and (C) Sticking the tongue out.

- Hold the patient's hand in a handshake position, then use your other hand to support their elbow, taking the weight of their arm (Fig. 2.46)
- Ask if the patient has any pain
- Move the patient's arm for them, ensuring that they are relaxed and don't resist any movements
- Test tone by:
  - Elbow flexion
  - Supination; Slowly, then feel for a supinator 'catch'
  - Wrist circumduction: Feel for cogwheeling

ASSESSMENT OF POWER

- Give clear instructions and demonstrate the movements in advance if needed (Fig. 2.47)
- Always compare both sides
- Be consistent in your testing style. Dynamic testing is asking the patient to perform a movement, i.e. 'push me away', 'pull me towards you'. Static testing is asking the patient to resist a movement, i.e. 'bend your elbow, now don't let me straighten it.'
- Perform the actions described:
  - Shoulder abduction
  - Elbow flexion
  - Elbow extension

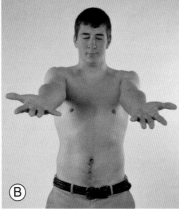
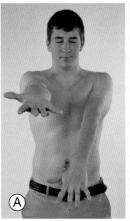

Ⓐ Ⓑ

Fig. 2.45 (A, B) Pronator drift.

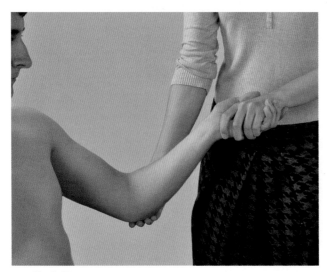

Fig. 2.46 Taking the weight off the arm for tone assessment.

- Wrist flexion
- Wrist extension
- Grip strength
- Finger abduction
- Thumb abduction
- Rate the power on the Medical Research Council (MRC) scale (Table 2.9)
- When scoring power at each joint, the following standardised scale is used by clinicians:

ASSESSMENT OF REFLEXES

- Biceps reflex (C5): Strike the bicep tendon in the antecubital fossa. Note flexion of the elbow
- Brachioradialis reflex (C6): Strike the brachioradialis tendon roughly 5–7 cm above the wrist. Note supination of the wrist
- Triceps reflex (C7): This can be difficult to elicit. Ensure that you take the weight of the arm as you strike the tricep tendon at the elbow (Fig. 2.48)

  Reinforce reflexes as necessary; for example, by asking the patient to clench his teeth. Reflexes are best obtained when the patient is relaxed. Biceps and brachioradialis are best elicited when the arms are positioned in the lap. Triceps are best elicited when the elbow is bent at 90°. With one hand supporting the wrist, strike the triceps tendon just above the olecranon.

ASSESSMENT OF COORDINATION

See Station 2.11: Cerebellar Examination but as minimum, perform finger–nose testing and assess for dysdiadochokinesia.

ASSESSMENT OF SENSATION

A number of factors limit reliable testing of sensation. These include the challenge of getting the patient to keep their eyes shut, the difficulty in applying the same amount of pressure each time you touch the patient and the presence of calloused skin.

Different modalities test different tracts. Normally light touch, proprioception and pain suffice, but vibration and temperature (Fig. 2.49) can also be tested. Do all of these with the patient's eyes shut.

SENSATION TESTING

- Provide a reference stimulus by touching the sternum first
- Test by dabbing (rather than stroking) in each dermatome whilst the patient's eyes are closed (Fig. 2.50)
- Regularly ask if one side is any different from the other
- To ensure that you're covering all dermatomes and the major nerves, test the following areas:
  - Upper, lateral aspect of the arm (axillary nerve (C5)), also known as the 'regimental patch'
  - Outer forearm (lateral cutaneous nerve of forearm [C6])
  - Middle finger (median nerve [C7])

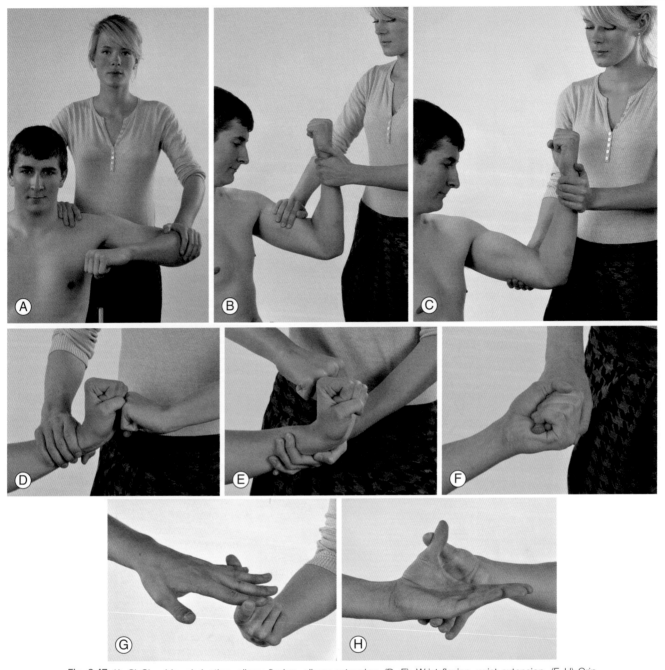

Fig. 2.47 (A–C) Shoulder abduction, elbow flexion, elbow extension. (D, E): Wrist flexion, wrist extension. (F–H) Grip strength, finger abduction, thumb abduction. Note that, in each assessment, the joint being tested is isolated, using the other hand if necessary. This ensures that the test is specific for the joint in question.

- First dorsal web space (radial nerve [C7])
- Little finger (ulnar nerve [C8])
- Medial aspect of the antecubital fossa (medial cutaneous nerve of forearm [T1])
- Repeat for pain, using a Neurotip
- Test proprioception starting with a small-amplitude movement in the most distal joint (Fig. 2.51)
- Test vibration sense (Fig. 2.52)

FINISHING

- Offer to:
  - Perform a full neurological examination, including: Cerebellar, cranial nerve and lower-limb examination

- Perform a vascular exam of the upper arm
- Test temperature and vibration sensation
- Assess function; for example, asking the patient to do up a button
- Perform fundoscopy
- Perform a cognitive assessment, including speech
- Perform a DRE if there any concerns regarding cauda equina syndrome
- Thank the patient
- Check that they're comfortable and offer to help reposition them
- Wash your hands
- Leave the patient in privacy to get dressed

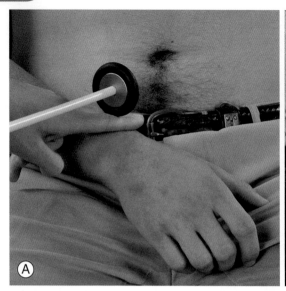
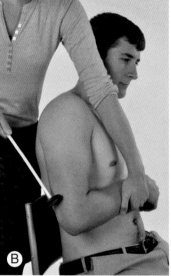
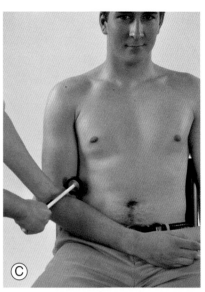

Fig. 2.48 Testing of the tricep (A), bicep (B) and brachioradialis (C) reflexes.

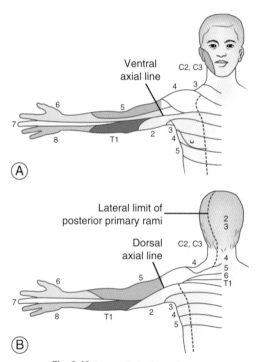

Fig. 2.49 Upper-limb dermatomes.

! Differentiating between upper and lower motor neurone lesions

	UPPER MOTOR NEURONE	LOWER MOTOR NEURONE
Inspection	• Pronator drift	• Muscle wasting and fasciculation
Tone	• Increased • May be reduced in severe acute upper motor neurone lesions in the initial stages	• Decreased or normal
Power	• Not often useful in the differentiation between upper and lower motor neurone lesions	• Not often useful in the differentiation between upper and lower motor neurone lesions
Tendon reflexes	• Brisk or increased reflexes • May be reduced in severe acute upper motor neurone lesions in the initial stages	• Presence of clonus • Decreased or absent
Plantar	• Upgoing	• Downgoing

Table 2.9   MRC power scale

0 – No movement
1 – Flicker of movement
2 – Isogravitational movements only
3 – Able to move against gravity
4 – Able to move against resistance but not fully
5 – Full power
One of the problems with this scale is that 4 encompasses such a wide range of power that its utility can be limited. Also, testing movements specifically against and with gravity is difficult to do properly.

🔍 Present Your Findings

Mr Reilly is a 64-year-old man who has presented following a fractured humerus. On examination, he is comfortable at rest. He has 0/5 power of wrist and finger extension on the right side. There is reduced sensation in the first dorsal web space on the right hand. There is loss of the brachioradialis reflex on the right side, despite reinforcement. There are no other abnormalities.

Given the sparing of triceps power and reflex, I feel the most likely diagnosis is a right radial nerve palsy secondary to humeral fracture.

I would like to examine the cranial nerves and lower limbs, perform a vascular assessment of the upper limb and examine for fractures elsewhere. I would like to refer to physiotherapy and optimise analgesia.

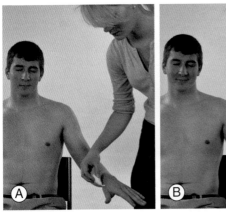

Fig. 2.50 (A, B) Assessing light touch and pain. Ensure that the patient's eyes are shut.

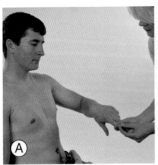

Fig. 2.51 (A, B) Testing proprioception: Ensure that you hold the finger from the sides to avoid excessive sensory stimulation. Ensure that the patient's eyes are shut.

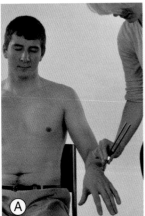

Fig. 2.52 (A, B) Testing vibration sense: Place the tuning fork on a bony prominence and ask the patient when they feel the vibration stop. Ensure that the patient's eyes are shut.

❓ QUESTIONS AND ANSWERS FOR CANDIDATE

What muscles in the hand are supplied by the median nerve?
- 'LOAF' muscles:
  - *Lumbricals* (first and second)
  - Thenar eminence (*opponens* pollicis, *abductor* pollicis brevis, *flexor* pollicis brevis)

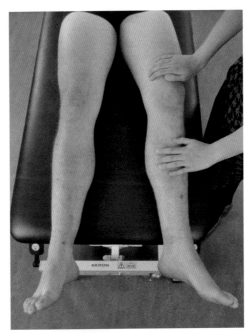

Fig. 2.53 Assessing for tone.

What is the sensory distribution of the ulnar nerve?
- Medial forearm
- Medial wrist
- Medial one and a half digits

If you are unable to elicit a reflex in the arm, how might you reinforce it?
- Ask the patient to clench his teeth

🗨 A Case to Learn From

I once reviewed a patient who had been in a car accident. There was a concern that he had injured his radial nerve due to a humerus injury. On initial examination, his power seemed reduced and we were not able to assess sensation well because there was so much pain. However, after giving adequate analgesia and after the patient had become more relaxed, he reported normal sensation and power was 5/5. Patient compliance is important, as is documenting why a patient can't achieve a movement, be that pain, stiffness or non-compliance.

💡 Top Tip

Don't think too much about what your findings mean when you are doing the exam. It is more important to describe your findings accurately than to interpret them accurately. Go through a checklist of what you are going to test, how you are going to test it and then think about interpretation afterwards.

STATION 2.10: PERIPHERAL NERVES (LOWER LIMB)

SCENARIO

You are a junior doctor in a neurology clinic and have been asked to see Mr Romberg, a 64-year-old man,

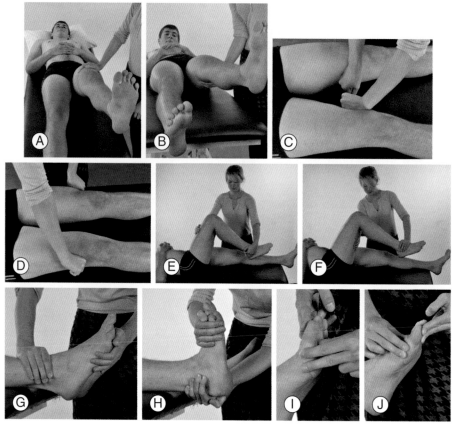

Fig. 2.54 (A–J) Actions to assess for power in the lower limbs. Hip flexion (A), extension (B), adduction (C), and abduction (D). Knee flexion (E) and extension (F). Ankle plantar flexion (G) and extension (H). Hallux/toe extension (I) and flexion (J).

who has long-standing diabetes mellitus. He is concerned that he is continually injuring his feet without realising it. Please perform a relevant neurological examination of Mr Romberg's lower limbs and present your findings.

PREPARATION

- WIPER:
  - *Wash* your hands
  - *Introduce* yourself
  - Ask about *pain*
  - Appropriately *expose*
  - *Reposition*
- Explain the examination to the patient and your reasons for performing it
- Gain verbal consent
- Give the patient privacy to expose themselves as required
- Start in a comfortable position (standing, then when appropriate, have him lie flat while exposing the legs)
- Offer a chaperone

GENERAL INSPECTION

- Environment: Walking aids, wheelchairs, shoes (especially tailor-made orthoses), glasses

- Patient: Pain or agitation. A good acronym to use for patient inspection is SWIFT:
  - *Scars*
  - *Wasting* of muscles
  - *Involuntary* movements
  - *Fasciculations*
  - *Tremor*

GAIT

- If possible, get the patient up and see how they can manage to walk from one end of the room to the other. Observe the whole body, look for signs of pain and observe how they turn. This can be done at the beginning or the end of the examination.
- Gaits to look for include:
  - Festinant: Parkinson's disease
  - Antalgic: For example, due to osteoarthritis of hip
  - Scissoring: Cerebral palsy
  - Ataxic: Cerebellar dysfunction
  - Marche à petits pas: Diffuse cerebrovascular disease
  - Footslapping: Sensory polyneuropathy
- Consider additional examinations whilst the patient is standing; for example, tandem walk and Romberg's test as appropriate (see Station 2.11: Cerebellar Examination)

ASSESSMENT OF TONE

- Ask the patient to lie flat on their back
- Ensure that the patient is relaxed and that the limbs are floppy
- Roll the patient's legs from side to side, looking at the feet for resistance (Fig. 2.53)
- Abruptly lift the knee and note the movement of the lower leg. In hypertonia, the ankle will come off the examination couch, even if the patient is relaxed
- Passively flex and extend the knee joint

ASSESSMENT OF POWER

- Give clear instructions and demonstrate the movements in advance if needed (Fig. 2.54)
- Always compare both sides
  Be consistent in your testing style. *Dynamic* testing is asking the patient to perform a movement, i.e.
- push me away,
- pull me towards you

Static testing is asking the patient to resist a movement, i.e.
- bend your elbow, now don't let me straighten it
- Rate the power on the MRC scale
- While performing the actions, note the nerve roots listed in Table 2.10

ASSESSMENT OF REFLEXES

- Knee tendon reflex (L3/4): Strike the ligamentum patellae. When eliciting a knee reflex, look for contraction of the quadriceps muscle (Fig. 2.55)
- Ankle tendon reflex (S1/2): Obtaining ankle reflexes can be difficult. The foot should be pulled up with one hand into dorsiflexion, before striking the Achilles with the tendon hammer. Another method is to get the patient to kneel on a chair, with ankles dangling off the side
  Reinforce if reflexes are absent by asking the patient, just before striking the tendon, to clench their teeth or to flex their fingers, interlock them and then pull them

Table 2.10	Nerve roots in the leg		
MOVEMENT	**MUSCLE**	**NERVE**	**ROOT**
Hip flexion	Iliopsoas	Lumbar sacral plexus	L1, L2
Hip extension	Gluteus maximus	Inferior gluteal	L5, S1
Knee flexion	Hamstring	Sciatic	L5, S1
Knee extension	Quadriceps	Femoral	L3, L4
Ankle plantar flexion	Gastrocnemius	Posterior tibial	S1
Ankle dorsiflexion	Tibialis anterior	Deep peroneal	L4, L5
Hallux or toe extension	Extensor hallucis longus	Deep peroneal	L5

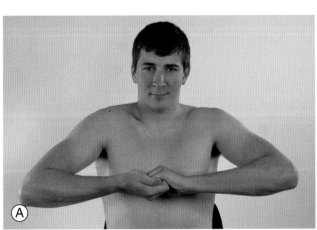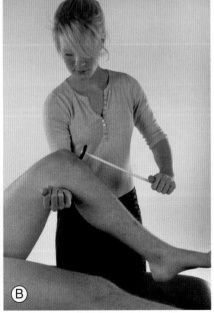

Fig. 2.55 Reinforcement with the Jendrassik manoeuvre (A) and knee reflex (B).

as hard as they can in opposite directions (Jendrassik manoeuvre) (Fig. 2.55A).

ADDITIONAL REFLEXES

- Plantar reflex: Use the blunt end of an object; for example, the reverse end of a pen, to run up the lateral aspect of the sole of an unsocked foot. A normal response is for the big toe to flex downwards. In an abnormal response, the big toe extends and the other toes splay out (Fig. 2.56)
- Ankle clonus: Rapidly flex the foot into dorsiflexion. Clonus is when the foot subsequently beats, rapidly moving from flexion to extension. More than five beats is abnormal (Fig. 2.57)

ASSESSMENT OF CO-ORDINATION

- In the supine position, ask the patient to run their left heel from the right knee down along the shin of their right leg. Ask them then to make an arc in the air with their heel and repeat the previous movement. This should then all be repeated with opposite legs (Fig. 2.58)
- An abnormal response is if this cannot be completed smoothly; for example, they can't roll their heel along their shin or they cannot land easily on their leg after the arc

ASSESSMENT OF SENSATION

- Provide a reference stimulus by touching the sternum first
- Test by dabbing (rather than stroking) in each dermatome whilst the patient's eyes are closed

- Regularly ask if one side is any different from the other
- To ensure that you're covering all dermatomes and the major nerves, test the following areas:
  - Upper outer thigh (lateral cutaneous nerve of thigh [L2])
  - Inner aspect of thigh (femoral nerve [L3])
  - Medial lower leg (saphenous nerve [L4])
  - Upper outer aspect of lower leg (common peroneal nerve [L5])
  - Dorsal surface, medial aspect of big toe (superficial peroneal nerve [L5])
  - Heel of foot (tibial nerve [S1])
  - Posterior aspect of knee (sciatic nerve [S2])
- Repeat for pain using a Neurotip (Fig. 2.59)
- Test proprioception, starting with a small amplitude movement in the most distal joint (Fig. 2.60)
- Test vibration sense (Fig. 2.61)
- If spinal cord pathology is suspected; for example, demyelinating lesion from multiple sclerosis, then it's important to assess the sensory level at which sensation changes (decreases, increases or alters) when moving in a caudal to cranial direction. If abnormalities are present, consider temperature testing (using hot/cold; for example, a glass tube filled with warm water and cold tuning fork), vibration testing (Fig. 2.61) and cerebellar function testing

FINISHING

- Offer to:
  - Perform a full neurological examination, including: Cerebellar, cranial nerve and lower-limb examination
  - Perform a vascular exam of the upper arm

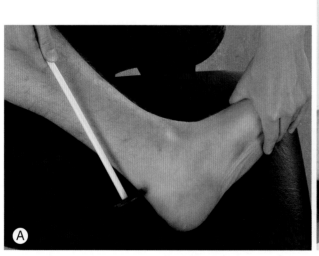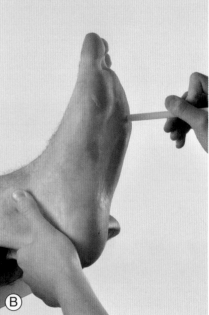

Fig. 2.56 Ankle reflex (A) and plantar reflex (B).

- Test temperature and vibration sensation
- Assess function; for example, asking the patient to do up a button
- Perform fundoscopy
- Perform a cognitive assessment, including speech
- Perform a DRE if there are any concerns regarding cauda equina syndrome
- Thank the patient
- Check that they're comfortable and offer to help reposition them
- Wash your hands
- Leave the patient in privacy to get dressed

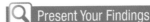 **Present Your Findings**

Mr Romberg is a 64-year-old man who presented with increasing foot injuries. On examination, he is overweight and walks with the aid of one stick. He has a foot-slapping gait and a positive Romberg's test. He has decreased sensation to light touch and pain up to the ankle, in a stocking distribution. Motor examination is unremarkable. Mr Romberg has a bilateral symmetrical sensory neuropathy.

Given the stocking distribution of sensory loss, I feel the most likely diagnosis is diabetic polyneuropathy.

I would like to examine the upper limbs and cranial nerves, check the fundi, dipstick the urine and check the other organ systems for complications of diabetes. I would like to perform blood tests, including: FBCs, U&Es, LFTs, B_{12} and folate, TFTs, blood glucose and HbA_{1c}.

!	**Causes of peripheral neuropathy**
Genetic	• Charcot–Marie–Tooth disease • Friedreich's ataxia
Metabolic	• Diabetes mellitus • Chronic renal failure • Porphyria • Amyloidosis • Liver failure
Toxic	• Alcoholism • Drugs; for example, vincristine, phenytoin • Heavy metals
Inflammatory	• Guillain–Barré syndrome • Systemic lupus erythematosus (SLE)
Nutritional	• Vitamin B_{12} deficiency

? **QUESTIONS AND ANSWERS FOR CANDIDATE**

Name three common causes of footdrop.
- Common peroneal nerve palsy
- Sciatic nerve palsy
- Motor neurone disease (MND)
- L4/5 route lesion
- Stroke

What type of gait might be seen in a post-hemiplegic stroke?
- Hemiplegic gait, with circumduction

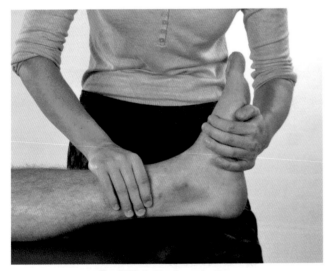

Fig. 2.57 Ankle clonus testing.

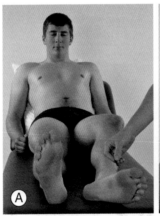 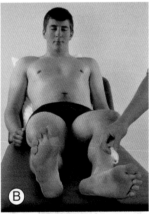

Fig. 2.59 Assessing light touch (A) and pain (B). Ensure that the patient's eyes are shut.

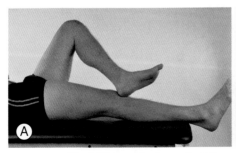 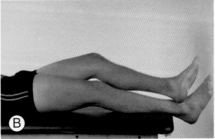 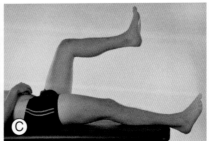

Fig. 2.58 Coordination testing: The ankle should be placed on the knee (A), rolled down the shin (B), lifted back up to the knee in an arc (C) and the cycle repeated.

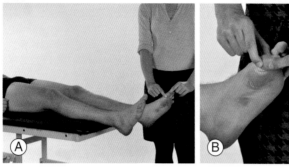

Fig. 2.60 (A, B) Proprioception: Ensure that you hold the toe from the sides to avoid excessive sensory stimulation. Ensure that the patient's eyes are shut.

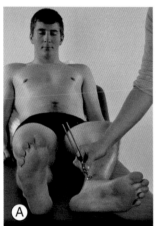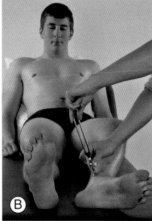

Fig. 2.61 (A, B) Vibration sense: Place the tuning fork on a bony prominence and ask the patient when they feel the vibration stop. Ensure that the patient's eyes are shut.

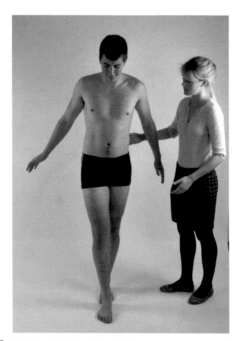

Fig. 2.62 Tandem walking. Ensure that you remain close to the patient, to support them in case they become unstable.

- The affected leg will be dragged in a semicircle due to weakness of the distal muscles and hypertonia

What is Brown-Séquard syndrome?
- Lateral disruption to only one side of the spinal cord
- Ipsilateral loss of light touch, proprioception and vibration
- Contralateral loss of pain and temperature
- Fibres of the spinothalamic tract cross early on entry to the spinal cord, whereas the dorsal columns do not decussate until they ascend to the medulla
- Causes include:
  - Trauma
  - Pressure effects of vertebral metastases
  - Cervical spondylosis
  - Transverse myelitis
  - Multiple sclerosis

A Case to Learn From

Mrs J was a 60-year-old woman who presented with a 1-day history of left-sided weakness, affecting her leg more than her arm. She was a smoker, with a strong family history of stroke. On examination, her left leg was hypotonic with no power. She had decreased reflexes of the ankle and knee on the left side compared with the right and was unable to walk unassisted. A computed tomography (CT) head was ordered, although I was confused given the classic lower motor neurone signs. However, it confirmed an anterior cerebral artery territory stroke. I learnt from this case that upper motor neurone lesions (in the early stages) may present with typical lower motor neurone signs.

Top Tip

If you don't get a tendon reflex, it is more likely to be down to poor technique or lack of patient compliance than the reflex not being there. Ensure the patient is fully relaxed before striking the tendon, and practise as much as you can on well people before the exam.

Top Tip

Be aware of patients who have neurological signs that don't fit with any obvious neurological pattern. In these cases, it is worth repeating the exam, but if they persist, it may be non-organic disease.

STATION 2.11: CEREBELLAR

SCENARIO

You are a junior doctor in general medicine, and have been asked to see Mr Gordon, a 75-year-old male, who has presented with persistent falling. He also finds that when reaching for objects, he keeps missing them. Please perform a relevant cerebellar examination on Mr Gordon and then present your findings.

PREPARATION

- WIPER:
  - *Wash* your hands
  - *Introduce* yourself
  - Ask about *pain*
  - Appropriately *expose*
  - *Reposition*
- Explain the examination to the patient and your reasons for performing it
- Gain verbal consent
- Give the patient privacy to expose themselves as required
- Start in a comfortable position (usually sitting)
- Offer a chaperone

GENERAL INSPECTION

- Environment: Walking aids, wheelchairs, shoes (especially tailor-made orthoses), glasses
- Patient: Pain or agitation, dishevelled appearance (may suggest alcohol excess), signs of chronic liver disease (for example, palmar erythema, spider naevi)

GAIT

- Ask the patient to walk up and down the room. Look for a broad-based gait with irregular stride rhythm or length and instability
- To pick up more subtle ataxic gait, ask the patient to tandem walk, i.e. walking by placing one foot in front of the other as if on a tightrope (Fig. 2.62)

EXAMINATION OF THE EYES

- Slow-pursuit movements: Hold up a pen and ask the patient to follow its movement with their eyes, keeping their head still. Move it horizontally and vertically, as for ocular muscle examination, in all directions. Hold their gaze at lateral and vertical positions to try and elicit nystagmus
- Rapid eye movements: Make a fist with one hand and an open palm with the other. Rapidly shout 'fist' and 'palm', while asking the patient to look at the respective hand in response. Look for square-wave jerks (SWJ) and saccadic intrusions (SI). A saccade is a fast eye movement (Fig. 2.63)
  - SWJs are inappropriate saccades that take the eye away from its focus. There is then a pause, followed by a corrective saccade back to the original target
  - SIs are similar, but not necessarily followed by a return movement. They may be associated with cerebellar disease

EXAMINATION OF SPEECH

- Slurring of speech: Ask the patient to say 'British constitution', 'West Register Street' and 'baby hippopotamus'

- Staccato speech: Ask the patient how to make a cup of tea

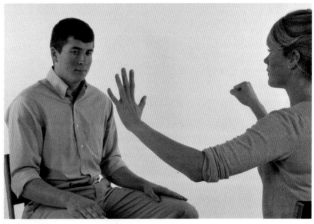

Fig. 2.63 Rapid eye movement testing: The patient alternates between looking at the fist and palm on the examiner's command.

EXAMINATION OF THE UPPER LIMBS

- Cerebellar rebound: With the patient's arms held out in front of him, press his arm downwards and let go, with him resisting. When you let go, he should try to restore his arms to the original position. Look for overshoot
- Finger–nose test: Ask the patient to bring his index finger out to touch your finger, which should be positioned at roughly arm's length away from him. Then ask him to touch his nose and repeat from your finger to his nose as quickly and accurately as he can. Look for intention tremor and poor coordination (Fig. 2.64)
- Dysdiadochokinesis: Ask the patient to slap his hand with the palm of his other hand, then to slap it with the other side of his hand (dorsal) and repeat, lifting his hand up in between, and as fast as he can. Look for poor coordination

FINISHING

- Offer to:
  - Perform a full neurological examination, including peripheral and cranial nerve examination
  - Perform fundoscopy
  - Perform a cognitive assessment, including speech
  - Perform a urine dipstick
- Thank the patient
- Check that they're comfortable and offer to help reposition them
- Wash your hands
- Leave the patient in privacy to get dressed

DANISHH MNEMONIC

DANISHH is a useful mnemonic to remember the important sections of a cerebellar examination:
- *Dysdiadochokinesia*
- *Ataxia*
- *Nystagmus*

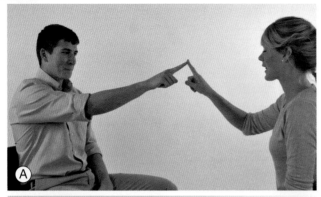

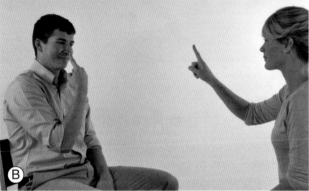

Fig. 2.64 (A, B) Finger–nose testing. Ensure that the patient is at full arm's length when touching your finger.

- *Intention* tremor
- *Slurred,* staccato speech
- *Hypotonia*
- *Heel*–shin test

🔍 Present Your Findings

Mr Gordon is a 75-year-old male who has presented with persistent falling. On examination, Mr Gordon has an ataxic gait. On testing ocular pursuit movements, nystagmus was elicited at mid-lateral gaze and he demonstrated ocular dysmetria on testing fast saccadic eye movements. He has slurred speech, intention tremor and past-pointing. I also note that he has stigmata of chronic liver disease.

I feel the most likely diagnosis is cerebellar dysfunction, perhaps secondary to ethanol excess.

I would like to do a full neurological examination, take an alcohol history and complete an abdominal examination. I would like to take bloods, including: FBCs, U&Es, LFTs, TFTs, B$_{12}$, folate, CRP, ESR and blood glucose and also consider a magnetic resonance imaging (MRI) brain scan.

❓ QUESTIONS AND ANSWERS FOR CANDIDATE

What is nystagmus?
- Nystagmus is rhythmical, involuntary, oscillatory movement of the eye that can be elicited when the eyes look horizontally or vertically
- This can be a normal variant at extremes of horizontal gaze

- If it occurs at less than 30° from the midline, it is pathological

Name three causes of cerebellar syndrome.
- Alcohol
- Drugs; for example, phenytoin
- Multiple sclerosis
- Hereditary ataxias; for example, Friedreich's ataxia
- Tumours of the posterior fossa
- Metastatic disease; for example, lung or breast primary tumour
- Infection; for example, varicella zoster and legionella

What is the imaging modality of choice for looking at the cerebellum?
- MRI

🗨 A Case to Learn From

We saw a man with increasing levels of clumsiness reported by his wife, but he was adamant that there wasn't a problem. Although he walked slowly, there wasn't anything obvious neurologically wrong with him. It was only after we asked him to tandem walk that he became very unstable. An MRI scan revealed a cerebellar tumour. Always remember to assess the gait, as it can reveal a lot!

💡 Top Tip

The evaluation of cerebellar signs is rather dependent on a prior motor and sensory examination. Some features of cerebellar disease such as incoordination can indeed be an expression of proprioceptive loss or weakness.

STATION 2.12: PARKINSON'S DISEASE

SCENARIO

You are a junior doctor in neurology outpatients and have been asked to see Mr Smith, a 62-year-old man, who has been referred by his primary care physician with signs of parkinsonism. Please perform a relevant examination on Mr Smith and present your findings.

PREPARATION

- WIPER:
  - *Wash* your hands
  - *Introduce* yourself
  - Ask about *pain*
  - Appropriately *expose*
  - *Reposition*
- Explain the examination to the patient and your reasons for performing it
- Gain verbal consent
- Give the patient privacy to expose themselves as required
- Start in a comfortable position (usually sitting)
- Offer a chaperone

GENERAL INSPECTION

- Environment: Walking aids, wheelchairs, shoes (especially tailor-made orthoses), glasses
- Patient: Pain or agitation, hypomimia (reduced degree of facial expression), hypophonia (soft speech), drooling, resting tremor of hands and/or feet

TREMOR

- Ask the patient to close his eyes and slowly count backwards from 20 (this should elicit and accentuate any tremor)
- See if any other tremor is evident. Ask the patient to hold his arms straight out with the palms facing the floor (postural)
- Perform the finger–nose test to look for intention tremor due to cerebellar disease
- Note that the finger–nose test should dampen a Parkinson's disease tremor, but accentuate a benign essential tremor
- A Parkinson's disease tremor is normally markedly asymmetrical. Remember that up to a third of patients with idiopathic Parkinson's disease will not have a tremor

BRADYKINESIA

- Using one hand first, ask the patient to move his fingers towards his thumbs as though closing a duck's beak, then open and close the imaginary beak. Ask him to repeat this as quickly and as accurately as he can
- Ask him to mimic playing the piano with both hands as fast as possible in mid-air
- Look for bradykinetic fade in both of the above movements (Fig. 2.65)

MICROGRAPHIA

- Ask the patient to write a sentence; for example, 'Little red riding hood'
- Ask the patient to repeat it about five times
- Look for abnormally small writing

RIGIDITY

- Passively circumduct a wrist and then flex and/or extend at the elbow (Fig. 2.66)
- Repeat on the other side
- Feel for lead pipe rigidity (rigidity throughout movement) and cogwheeling (ratchety stiffness of limb through passive movement)

GAIT AND POSTURAL INSTABILITY

PULL TEST (FIG. 2.67)

- With the patient still standing, warn him that you need to test his tendency to fall backwards

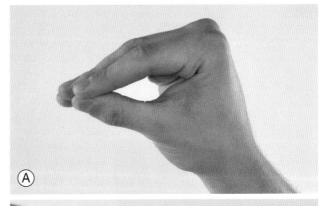
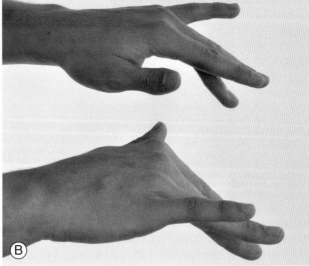

Fig. 2.65 Testing for bradykinesia. (A) Duck beak movements and (B) piano-playing movements.

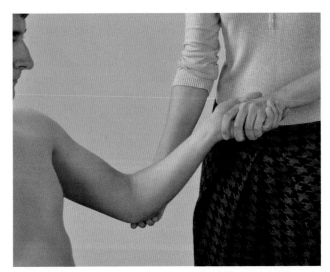

Fig. 2.66 Taking the weight off arm for tone assessment.

(retropulsion) and will need to pull him back, but you will be behind to support him
- Then, with both hands on each of the patient's shoulders, pull him back sharply

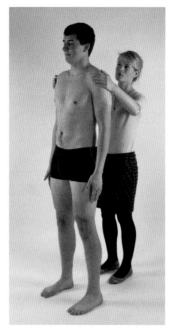

Fig. 2.67 Pull test: Patient sharply pulled back from the shoulders.

- Ask the patient to walk normally from one side of the room to the other, and then to turn around and come back
- Look for gait ignition failure, festinance, reduced arm swing, stooped posture and en bloc turning
- In idiopathic Parkinson's disease, postural instability is a late sign to develop. Therefore, if this was present early or at onset, an alternative diagnosis should be sought

PARKINSON-PLUS SYNDROMES

The Parkinson-plus syndromes are all neurodegenerative disorders, in which parkinsonian features occur alongside other symptoms and signs.
- Examine eye movements; for example, look for vertical downward ophthalmoplegia (feature of progressive supranuclear palsy (PSP))
- Measure the erect and supine BP (multiple system atrophy (MSA))

FINISHING

- Offer to:
  - Perform a full neurological examination, including: Cerebellar, peripheral and cranial nerve examination
  - Perform fundoscopy
  - Perform a cognitive assessment including speech
  - Dipstick the urine
- Thank the patient
- Check that they're comfortable and offer to help reposition them
- Wash your hands
- Leave the patient in privacy to get dressed

! Key terms relating to Parkinson's disease and parkinsonism

TERM	DESCRIPTION
Bradykinetic fading	Performed movements get progressively slower
Cogwheeling	Intermittent, regular elicitation of resistance on passive movement of a limb, due to co-occurrence of tremor and rigidity
Festinant gait	Involuntary acceleration of rate of steps
Gait ignition failure	Difficulty initiating walking
Lead pipe rigidity	Increased tone throughout range of passive movement
Micrographia	Small, spidery handwriting
Retropulsion	The tendency to step backwards involuntarily if pulled from behind

🔍 Present Your Findings

Mr Smith is a 62-year-old man who has presented with signs of parkinsonism. He has a unilateral, pill-rolling, resting tremor of his right hand, dampened by movement. He has bradykinesia of his right side and has marked micrographia. He has bilateral rigidity with noticeable cogwheel rigidity at the right wrist. He walks with the aid of one stick and has a stooped, festinant gait. There is no evidence of Parkinson-plus syndromes.

I feel the most likely diagnosis is Parkinson's disease.

I would like to do a full neurological examination, including cerebellar, peripheral and cranial nerve examination, perform fundoscopy and do a cognitive assessment, including speech. I would consider commencing Mr Smith on medication; for example, levodopa.

❓ QUESTIONS AND ANSWERS FOR CANDIDATE

Name three differential diagnoses of Parkinson's disease.
- Vascular Parkinson's disease
- Dementia with Lewy bodies
- Anti-dopaminergic drugs; for example, phenothiazines, metoclopramide
- Parkinson-plus syndromes
- Wilson's disease
- Dementia pugilistica

Name three examples of Parkinson's plus syndromes.
- PSP: Vertical gaze dysfunction, frequent falling
- MSA: Urogenital problems, i.e. incontinence and/or erectile dysfunction, and/or orthostatic hypotension. Cerebellar, as opposed to parkinsonian, features may occur
- Lewy body dementia: Cognitive impairments, visual hallucinations, paranoia and inability to focus or concentrate

Name three medications available to treat Parkinson's disease.
- Levodopa
- Dopamine agonists
- Monoamine oxidase-B inhibitors

 A Case to Learn From

I was walking around the ward and suddenly bumped into a patient. He had Parkinson's disease and even with the most minimal impact, he crashed to the floor. I felt awful, but the learning point I got out of it was the degree of postural instability people with Parkinson's might have and that they can 'topple like a falling tree'!

 Top Tip

Don't assume that in Parkinson's disease the tremor will be bilateral.

STATION 2.13: PERIPHERAL VASCULAR

SCENARIO

You are a junior doctor in vascular surgery and have been asked to see Mr O'Neil, a 60-year-old man, who has developed pain in his right leg on walking and at rest. Please perform a relevant vascular examination of Mr O'Neil and present your findings.

PREPARATION

- WIPER:
  - *Wash* your hands
  - *Introduce* yourself
  - Ask about *pain*
  - Appropriately *expose*
  - *Reposition*
- Explain the examination to the patient and your reasons for performing it
- Gain verbal consent
- Give the patient privacy to expose themselves as required
- Start in a comfortable position (usually lying on the bed)
- Offer a chaperone

GENERAL INSPECTION

- Environment: Walking aids, medications
- Patient: Pain or agitation, tar stains, corneal arcus (Fig. 2.68), xanthelasmata and/or xanthoma, previous surgical scars

EXAMINATION OF THE LEGS

INSPECTION

- Look between the toes

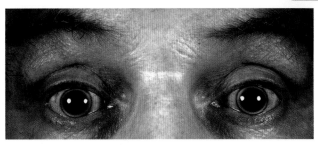

Fig. 2.68 Corneal arcus.

- Examine the heels and under any dressings
- Note the muscle bulk, particularly looking for asymmetry and swelling
- Note any nail changes
- Inspect the skin, noting:
  - Colour (pale, blue, dusky red or black (ischaemic), brown)
  - Ulcers (Table 2.11) or breaks:
    Site: Arterial ulcers generally appear on pressure areas; for example, the malleoli, fifth metatarsal base, metatarsal heads, toes and heel. Venous ulcers usually appear in the gaiter region of the lower leg (80% medial, 20% lateral) (Fig. 2.69).
    Shape, depth and edges: Arterial ulcers are small, regularly shaped, deep and with a 'punched-out' appearance and a sloughy or necrotic base. Venous ulcers are shallow, irregularly shaped, large with a green sloughy appearance over a pink and granulating base.
  - Scars
  - Hair loss
  - Thickening of the skin
  - Dry skin
- Varicose veins and signs of chronic venous disease

PALPATE

- Temperature: Cool if the vascular supply is compromised
- CRT: Under 2s is normal after pressing the nail bed for 5 s (Fig. 2.70)
- Oedema
- Sensation
- Tender: Squeeze the calf gently; it will be tender in acute limb ischaemia

PULSES

- Femoral:
  - Situated at the mid-inguinal point midway between the anterior superior iliac spine and the PS. Remember the acronym NAVAL, from lateral to medial: *nerve, artery, vein and lymphatics*
  - Press firmly down and towards the patient's head in the groin crease. Use two or three fingers

Table **2.11**   Ulcer characteristics

	VENOUS	ARTERIAL	NEUROPATHIC
Site	• Gaiter area (around the medial malleolus and calf)	• Distal extremities and pressure areas (heel and under the metatarsal heads)	• Pressure areas (heel and under the metatarsal heads)
Pain	• Painful or painless	• Painful	• Painless
Edge and base	• Sloping edges with a red granulation base (sometimes white)	• Punched-out edges with no red granulation base • The base can be slough or infective	• Punched-out and clean edges
Skin changes	• Haemosiderin deposits • Venous eczema • Lipodermatosclerosis	• Trophic changes; for example, hair loss and thin skin • Cold	• Often normal surrounding skin
Other	• Varicose veins	• Absent distal pulses	• Sensory loss

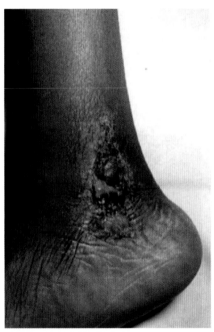

Fig. 2.69 Venous ulcer. (Source: Tibbs, D.J., 2013. Varicose veins and related disorders. Butterworth-Heinemann.)

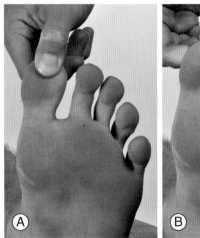 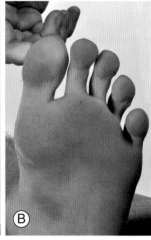

Fig. 2.70 (A, B) Capillary refill.

- Popliteal:
  - This is notoriously difficult to palpate, even though it is quite large and strong
  - Flex the patient's knee to 30° but don't let the patient bend it themselves
  - Place your thumbs on the patella, place your other fingers in the popliteal fossa and try to sandwich the popliteal pulse between your fingers and the back of the tibia
  - If the popliteal pulse is very easy to feel, this should alert you to a possible aneurysm (Fig. 2.71)
- Posterior tibial:
  - This is best palpated posterior to the medial malleolus
  - Place your fingers on the artery and push it up against the bony medial malleolus to feel its pulse (Fig. 2.72)
- Dorsalis pedis:
  - Draw an imaginary horizontal line between the malleoli
  - Drop a perpendicular line down from this to meet the first interspace (between the big toe and second toe). The dorsalis pedis is palpated one-third of the way down this perpendicular line from the malleoli (Fig. 2.73)
- If any pulses are absent, use a handheld Doppler

AUSCULTATE

- Femoral bruits
- Buerger's test:
  - Raise the limb slowly (up to an angle of 45°), flexing at the hip joint
  - Once the limb appears pale, note the angle. This is known as Buerger's angle. The poorer the arterial supply to the lower limb, the smaller the angle will be. If the limb does not appear pale, wait 2 min further when you reach 45°. The limb should not turn pale in a healthy individual
  - After this, ask the patient to sit with their legs hanging off the side of the bed
  - Normally, the legs will turn a pink colour. An abnormal result is signified by 'sunset rubor' (dusky

red colour). This is reactive hyperaemia, due to arteriole dilatation to remove toxic metabolites
- Note that this can be painful for patients, so be gentle and remember to ask if they are experiencing any pain (Fig. 2.74)

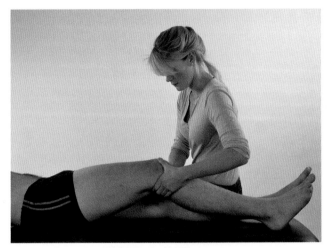

Fig. 2.71 Popliteal pulse.

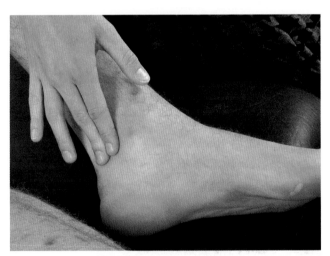

Fig. 2.72 Posterior tibial pulse.

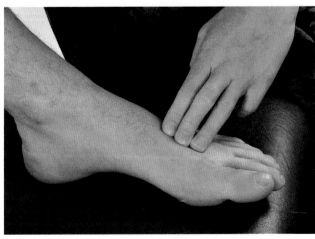

Fig. 2.73 Dorsalis pedis.

EXAMINATION OF THE ABDOMEN

- Rule out an AAA by inspecting for any obvious palpations in the abdomen and palpating for a pulsatile mass
- Auscultate the aorta and renal arteries for vascular bruits, which are suggestive of turbulent blood flow which may indicate arterial disease

FINISHING

- Offer to:
  - Perform a full cardiovascular examination
  - Palpate for an abdominal aneurysm (Fig. 2.75)
  - Perform fundoscopy
  - Measure ankle brachial pressure index (ABPI)
  - Dipstick the urine

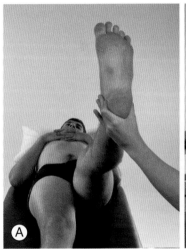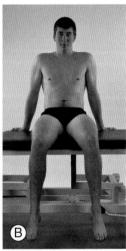

Fig. 2.74 Buerger's test: (A) Raise the limb; (B) patient sitting on the edge of the bed with legs hanging off the end.

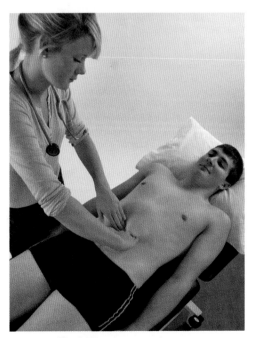

Fig. 2.75 Palpating for an AAA.

- Assess functional ability in a corridor walking test
- Thank the patient
- Check that they're comfortable and offer to help reposition them
- Wash your hands
- Leave the patient in privacy to get dressed

FURTHER INVESTIGATIONS

- Angiography, spiral CT or MRI
- Doppler or duplex assessment

 Present Your Findings

Mr O'Neil is a 60-year-old man who presented with right-leg pain on walking and at rest. He has tar-stained fingers and corneal arcus. His right leg is thin, pale and cool up to the knee. There is evidence of hair loss. CRT is 3 s peripherally. The right femoral pulse is palpable, but no pulses distal to this are present. Power is normal, but there is reduced sensation at the toes. There is a small, painful necrotic-looking ulcer at the tip of the big toe on his right foot. It is of regular shape, 0.5 cm deep and has a punched-out appearance of an arterial ulcer. Buerger's angle is 30°, with sunset rubor seen. Examination of the left leg was unremarkable.

I feel the most likely diagnosis is critical limb ischaemia.

To complete my examination, I would like to measure an ABPI, check distal pulses with a Doppler and perform a full cardiovascular examination. I would refer urgently to vascular surgery, with consideration of urgent imaging of the lower-limb vasculature.

❓ QUESTIONS AND ANSWERS FOR CANDIDATE

Name three signs of an acutely ischaemic limb.
Soft signs (which tend to come first):
- Pulseless
- Pallor
- Perishingly cold
  Hard signs:
- Pain
- Paraesthesia
- Paralysis

How do you measure ABPI?
- Take the systolic BP in the legs using a Doppler probe over dorsalis pedis/posterior tibial arteries
- Divide it by the systolic pressure in the arms

Give three examples of cardiovascular risk factors for peripheral arterial disease.
  Non-modifiable:
- Older age
- Male gender
- Family history
  Modifiable:
- Smoking
- Alcohol
- Poor diet
- Sedentary lifestyle
- Raised body mass index (BMI)
- Raised cholesterol
- Obesity

 A Case to Learn From

A patient with known AF developed an embolic stroke. Whilst an inpatient, he then developed an acutely ischaemic left arm. This was initially missed, because the upper-limb sensation loss was felt to be due to the stroke. However, a more careful examination revealed signs of acute ischaemia, with loss of sensation as well as pain, pallor, reduced radial pulse and a cold limb. The patient required urgent vascular intervention. Patients with AF can develop multiple emboli in close succession and possible signs of an ischaemic limb need to be thoroughly evaluated.

💡 **Top Tip**

Make sure that you appreciate the difference between intermittent claudication (calf pain on walking, limb not at risk) and critical limb ischaemia (rest pain, ulceration or gangrene, limb at risk).

STATION 2.14: VARICOSE VEIN

SCENARIO

You are a junior doctor in vascular clinic and have been asked to see Mr Wilson, a 45-year-old man, who is known to suffer from varicose veins. Please perform a relevant vascular examination on Mr Wilson and present your findings.

PREPARATION

- WIPER:
  - *Wash* your hands
  - *Introduce* yourself
  - Ask about *pain*
  - Appropriately *expose*
  - *Reposition*
- Explain the examination to the patient and your reasons for performing it
- Gain verbal consent
- Give the patient privacy to expose themselves as required
- Start in a comfortable position (usually sitting)
- Offer a chaperone

GENERAL INSPECTION

- Environment: Compression stockings, wound dressings, bandages in close proximity or on the patient
- Patient: Pain or agitation

EXAMINATION OF THE LEGS

INSPECTION

Varicose veins follow the path of the two major veins:

- Long saphenous: Ascends in front of the medial malleolus and runs along the medial side of the leg, going behind the medial condyles and along the medial side of the thigh, passing through the fossa ovalis and ending in the femoral vein at the saphenofemoral junction (SFJ)
- Short saphenous: Ascends behind the lateral malleolus and runs laterally, crossing to the middle at the lower part of the popliteal fossa and ending in the popliteal vein, between the heads of the gastrocnemius. Also gives off a branch that joins the long saphenous vein
- There may also be thin, thready, superficial varicosities

Signs of chronic venous disease:

- Lipodermatosclerosis: Indurated areas of brown/red/orange thickened skin caused by fibrosis of subcutaneous fat (need to palpate for this)
- Saphena varix: A dilatation at the top of the long saphenous vein due to valvular incompetence. Can reach the size of a golf ball or larger
- Venous eczema: Caused by leakage of irritant venous contents on to the skin surface
- Venous/malleolar flare: Spider-like venous tortuosities around the malleoli
- Skin pigmentation: Haemosiderin deposition
- Atrophie blanche: White scar tissue with 'dotted' capillaries
- Oedema
- Inverted champagne bottle appearance: Narrow around the ankle, due to chronic venous insufficiency leading to fibrosis
- Venous ulcers

PALPATION

- Temperature and tenderness: Heat and tenderness of superficial thrombophlebitis
- Lipodermatosclerosis: Scarring and contraction of the subcutaneous fat. May only be appreciated by gentle palpation. Compare the consistency of the subcutaneous fat on one leg with that on the other leg
- Phlebitis: Along the veins
- SFJ incompetence: Get the patient to cough whilst feeling at the SFJ (4 cm below the femoral vein). Reflux will manifest as a forced expansion and/or palpable thrill. Follow the vein up along its path
- Saphenopopliteal junction (SPJ) incompetence: Check for a cough impulse whilst feeling behind the knee
- Pitting oedema

PERCUSSION:

- Tap test: Tap the vein above (proximally) whilst feeling below, with a finger held on to the more distal portion of the vein. This allows for assessment of valvular incompetence

TRENDELENBURG TEST

- To assess for SFJ incompetence (Fig. 2.76):
  - With the patient lying flat on a couch, lift the leg up to drain the veins
  - Tie the tourniquet initially at the SFJ high in the thigh
  - Ask the patient to stand. The aim is to see if you can stop the veins re-engorging when the leg is lowered again
  - If the varicosities refill once the leg is lowered, with the tourniquet at the SFJ, then any distal perforators are incompetent
- The 'modified' test involves subsequently attaching the tourniquet distally, at varying distances along the leg, to identify the location of the incompetent perforators
- Other sets of perforators include:
  - Hunterian perforator (mid-thigh)
  - Dodd perforator (approximately one handbreadth above the knee)
  - Boyd perforator (approximately one handbreadth below the knee)
  - Cockett perforators (5, 10 and 15 cm above the ankle)

FINISHING

- Offer to:
  - Perform venous duplex ultrasound, to assess site of venous incompetence and patency of deep veins

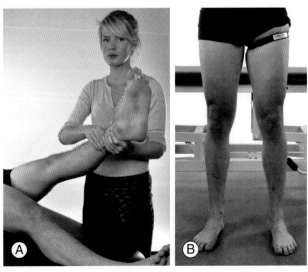

Fig. 2.76 Trendelenburg test: Lifting the leg up, and 'milking' the veins (A) and then after applying a tourniquet at the SFJ and asking patient to stand (B).

- Thank the patient
- Check that they're comfortable and offer to help re-position them
- Wash your hands
- Leave the patient in privacy to get dressed

CAUSES OF VARICOSE VEINS

Varicose veins are normal veins dilated under increased venous pressure.

In healthy veins one-way valves direct venous blood flow upward and inward, from capillaries to superficial veins to deep veins to the heart.

Varicose veins are most commonly due to valve incompetence, but may also be due to:

- High pressure in the superficial veins; for example, dialysis shunts or spontaneous arteriovenous malformations
- Hereditary vein wall weakness
- Outflow obstruction; for example, intravascular thrombosis or external compression
- Pregnancy

Present Your Findings

Mr Wilson is a 45-year-old man presenting with varicose veins. He has dilated superficial veins on the medial side of both legs, extending to above the knee joint. He has bilateral ulcers in the gaiter region, with 'sloping' edges and granulation tissue. There is also evidence of venous eczema, haemosiderosis, lipodermatosclerosis and atrophie blanche on both legs. There is no temperature difference, tenderness or oedema evident. A cough impulse is palpable at both SFJs.

I feel the most likely diagnosis is long saphenous varicose veins with chronic venous disease.

To complete my examination, I would like to perform venous duplex ultrasound and an abdominal examination to identify any masses. I would then explore the impact of the varicose veins on Mr Wilson and discuss conservation and operative management options with him.

❓ QUESTIONS AND ANSWERS FOR CANDIDATE

What are the management options of varicose veins?
Conservative:

- Lifestyle changes: Weight loss, exercise
- Education: Keep the leg elevated, skin care, prevent injury
- Graded compression stockings: Usually class 2 (< 30 mmHg) or class 3 (< 40 mmHg)
- Care: Regular debridement and cleaning or dressing of ulcers

Surgical:

- For more severe cases; for example, phlebitis, ulcers, bleeding, eczema
- Ligation and vein stripping
- Sclerotherapy
- Endovenous procedures; for example, radiofrequency or laser ablation of the long or short saphenous veins

How can you tell the difference between short and long saphenous varicose veins?

- It is more likely to be long saphenous if it goes above the knee and if it is medial

What is an important contraindication to using compression stockings?

- Cannot be used with concomitant arterial pathology or this will lead to ischaemia
- Requires ABPI before use

🗨 A Case to Learn From

I once saw a patient who had varicose veins but who had presented with an unrelated problem. I started talking to her about management options and she looked shocked. The varicose veins were mild and really didn't trouble her. In the early stages, varicose veins aren't anything to worry about and it is the patient's choice whether they require intervention.

💡 Top Tip

Remember that as good as clinical testing is for venous incompetence, Doppler will always be better, so ensure that you mention this at the end of your examination.

STATION 2.15: ULCER

SCENARIO

You are a junior doctor in vascular surgery and have been asked to see Mr Simpson, a 67-year-old man with diabetes, whose wife has noticed an ulcer under his foot. Please examine Mr Simpson's foot ulcer and present your findings.

PREPARATION

- WIPER:
  - *Wash* your hands
  - *Introduce* yourself
  - Ask about *pain*
  - Appropriately *expose*
  - *Reposition*
- Explain the examination to the patient and your reasons for performing it
- Gain verbal consent
- Give the patient privacy to expose themselves as required
- Start in a comfortable position (usually sitting)
- Offer a chaperone

GENERAL INSPECTION

- Environment: Compression stockings, wound dressings, bandages in close proximity or on the patient

- Patient: Pain or agitation, signs of cardiovascular risk factors; for example, xanethalasma/xanthoma, raised BMI, signs of thyroid disease

GENERAL INSPECTION

- Remember to look from all aspects, including between the toes and the soles of the feet
- Comment on:
  - Site: Use anatomical terms and centimetres from the nearest bony prominence
  - Size: Measure or estimate the width of the ulcer
  - Shape: Describe the shape
  - Skin: Surrounding skin can suggest the underlying pathology
  - Scars: From previous ulcers (atrophie blanche), skin grafts or other surgery like stripping
  - Base: Granulation tissue (red), slough (dead), pus, bone or tendon
  - Edge: Punched-out (arterial or neuropathic), sloping (venous or healing), undetermined margins overhanging the ulcer (infection or pressure sores)
  - Depth: Shallow or deep. Estimate in millimetres if possible
  - Colour: Red, white, necrotic

PALPATION

- Ask the patient if they are in any pain prior to palpation
- Comment on:
  - Tenderness: Look at the patient's face
  - Temperature: Feel the surrounding skin with the back of your hand
  - Lymph nodes: Local drainage
  - Local tissue: Assess the neurovascular status of the limb for suggestive pathology

FINISHING

- Offer to:
  - Perform a vascular examination, assessing the pulses and looking for signs of chronic venous insufficiency
  - Measure ABPI
  - Perform a peripheral nerve examination of the legs
  - Check blood glucose
  - Perform a urine dipstick
- Thank the patient
- Check that they're comfortable and offer to help reposition them
- Remove your gloves and wash your hands

DEFINITION OF AN ULCER

An ulcer is a break in the normal continuity of an epithelial or endothelial surface. This is a descriptive process much like that of a lump, which can yield spot diagnoses.

Features of Chronic Venous Insufficiency

- Oedema
- Hyperpigmentation
- Venous dermatitis
- Chronic cellulitis
- Cutaneous infarction (atrophie blanche)
- Ulceration

🔍 Present Your Findings

Mr Simpson is a 67-year-old male presenting with a foot ulcer. The ulcer is round, 5 × 3 cm, located above his left medial malleolus. There are varicose veins in the long saphenous distribution with skin changes, namely haemosiderin deposition, eczema and lipodermatosclerosis. The base of the ulcer has red granulation tissue and is shallow, with sloping edges and an irregular margin. The skin is warm to touch and non-tender and distal pulses are present.

I feel the most likely diagnosis is venous ulceration.

To complete the examination, I would like to perform a full vascular examination, including a Doppler ultrasound and measuring ABPI. I would also like to perform a peripheral nerve examination, check blood sugar as well as glycated haemoglobin (HbA_{1c}) levels and dipstick the urine. I would also discuss both conservative and surgical management of the venous disease with the patient.

❓ QUESTIONS AND ANSWERS FOR CANDIDATE

Name three causes of ulcers.
Arterial (large-vessel):
- Atherosclerosis
Arterial (small-vessel):
- Diabetes mellitus
- Vasculitides
- Rheumatoid arthritis
Neuropathic (peripheral neuropathy):
- Idiopathic
- Diabetes mellitus
- Alcohol
- Vitamin deficiency
Venous (venous stasis):
- Varicose veins
- Deep-vein thrombosis (DVT)
- Immobility of the limb

What investigation options are available for further ulcer assessment?
- This will be guided by the pathology suggested from your clinical evaluation
- Investigations include:
  - Punch biopsy: To assess histological change
  - Portable 8-MHz Doppler ultrasound probe: To assess venous flow (reflux indicated by a second audible 'whoosh') and arterial pulses (stenosis indicated by typical waveform)
  - Colour duplex: To define venous adequacy; for example, incompetent perforator veins, and to

visualise the blood flow within arteries; for example, popliteal stenosis
- Arteriography: To assess branch flow within lower-limb arteries

What are some of the conservative measures to treat a venous ulcer?
- Four-layer bandaging, which heals 70% of ulcers in 3 months
- Keep the limb elevated and protected from injury
- Regular cleaning and removal of slough to encourage granulation tissue
- Once healed, commence on class II compression stockings after checking that ABPI is ≥0.8

 A Case to Learn From

We had a patient come on to the ward with an ST elevation myocardial infarction (STEMI). They were taken to the cath lab, had their vessel opened up and were ready to go home. It was only when a medical student examined them that an arterial ulcer was discovered on their feet. Often patients would not think to talk about, or notice, an ulcer, so in those with risk factors for arterial disease, it is important to double check.

 Top Tip

Always look at the feet for yourself when inspecting ulcers, including pulling the toes apart to look between them.

STATION 2.16: NECK LUMP

SCENARIO

You are a primary care physician and have been asked to see Mr Gardner, a 60-year-old man, who has presented with a neck lump. Please perform a relevant examination on Mr Gardner and present your findings.

PREPARATION

- WIPER:
  - *Wash* your hands
  - *Introduce* yourself
  - Ask about *pain*
  - Appropriately *expose*
  - *Reposition*
- Explain the examination to the patient and your reasons for performing it
- Gain verbal consent
- Give the patient privacy to expose themselves as required
- Start in a comfortable position (sitting)
- Offer a chaperone

GENERAL INSPECTION

- Patient: Pain or agitation, low or high BMI, hoarse voice, dyspnoea or stridor, exophthalmos, inappropriately dressed for current weather

EXAMINATION OF THE NECK

INSPECTION:

- Inspect the neck, looking at it from eye level
- Look for masses in the front, sides or back of the neck by walking around the patient
- Describe the mass as you would any lump:
  - Site: In relation to anatomical sites
  - Size: Approximate width and length in centimetres
  - Shape: Round, oval, irregular
  - Colour: Erythematous, skin-coloured or otherwise
  - Edge: Smooth or irregular
  - Skin: Scars suggesting previous surgery; for example, thyroid or carotid incisions
- Ask the patient to:
  - Open their mouth and protrude their tongue. You may identify a thyroglossal cyst, which moves upwards with this action
  - Take a mouthful of water and swallow as you are inspecting. You may identify movement, which suggests a thyroid mass
- Repeat both of the above while gently palpating from behind, as neck lumps may be difficult to identify on inspection alone
- Take the time to appreciate the patient as a whole; for example, noticing features suggestive of thyroid disease. The age of the patient can point towards likely pathology; for example:
  - Childhood congenital lesions; for example, branchial cysts
  - Adolescent lymphadenopathy from infective causes such as glandular fever
  - Older neoplastic disease

PALPATION

- Approach the patient from behind and gently place the pads of your fingers on each side of the neck
- Ensure that the patient is warned and, as always, observe for signs of discomfort or tenderness
- Show the examiner, in a thorough and practised routine, the sequential palpation of the anatomical triangles of the neck, including: The parotid region, submandibular region and lymph node (Fig. 2.77)
- Example sequence:
  - Palpate the submandibular area with your left hand on the patient's left side and your right hand on the patient's right side
  - Move your hands progressively inward, to meet over the submental area

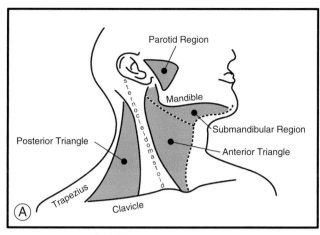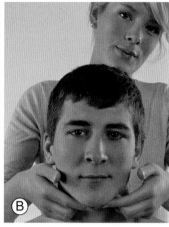

Fig. 2.77 Feeling for neck lymph nodes: Anatomy (A) and technique (B).

- Palpate down the midline to the thyroid
- Do the thyroid examination with swallowing and then with tongue protrusion (whilst still palpating)
- Then move up both anterior borders of the sternocleidomastoid, with each hand at the mastoid process, following the posterior border of the sternocleidomastoid to the supraclavicular fossa
- Palpate this and finish by following the trapezius to the occiput
- Once a lump is found, identify the remaining descriptive qualities:
  - Tenderness: Look at the patient's face (looking around from behind) and ask if pressing causes any pain
  - Temperature: Feel the surrounding skin
  - Consistency: Smooth, irregular, cystic or solid
  - Mobility: Mobile with the skin or attached to deeper underlying tissue
  - Pulsatility: Relating to vascular masses
  - Bruit: Relating to vascular masses
  - Transillumination: Cystic or solid

FINISHING

- Offer to:
  - Look in the mouth, as well as palpate the floor of mouth
  - Examine the nose and ears
  - If a parotid mass is obvious, then it would be appropriate to continue to examine the face and scalp, including the facial nerve
  - Perform further investigations; for example, ultrasound, routine bloods (including TFTs and inflammatory markers), fine-needle aspiration, CT/MRI and early ears, nose and throat (ENT) review if you suspect malignancy
- Thank the patient
- Check that they're comfortable and offer to help reposition them
- Wash your hands

- Leave the patient in privacy to get dressed

🔍 **Present Your Findings**

Mr Gardner is a 60-year-old male who has presented with a neck lump. The lump is in the right anterior triangle of the neck. It measures 2 × 1 cm. It is firm, has a smooth surface, is well circumscribed, non-tender to palpation and is mobile over deep tissue. There is a central punctum. There is no pulsation or transillumination. There is no associated lymphadenopathy.

I feel the most likely diagnosis is a sebaceous cyst.

To complete my examination, I would like to look in the mouth, as well as palpate the floor of the mouth and examine the nose and ears. I would like to order an ultrasound of the lump to confirm the diagnosis and then discuss with Mr Gardner the management options of conservative, drainage or surgical removal.

❓ **QUESTIONS AND ANSWERS FOR CANDIDATE**

Name three possible causes of parotid swelling.
- Infection; for example, viral, bacterial
- Autoimmune; for example, Sjögren's syndrome
- Malnutrition
- Alcohol abuse
- Malignancy; for example, pleomorphic adenoma
- Drugs

What are the borders of the anterior triangle of the neck?
- Midline: Sternocleidomastoid
- Inferior: Mandible

If you found a neck lump in a patient with suspected thyroid disease, what other features might you look for?
- Hypothyroid: Weight gain, dry skin, pallor, hair loss, peripheral oedema, hyporeflexia, pretibial myxoedema
- Hyperthyroid: Tachycardia or AF, hypertension, warm or moist skin, lid lag, hand tremor, weight loss, muscle weakness

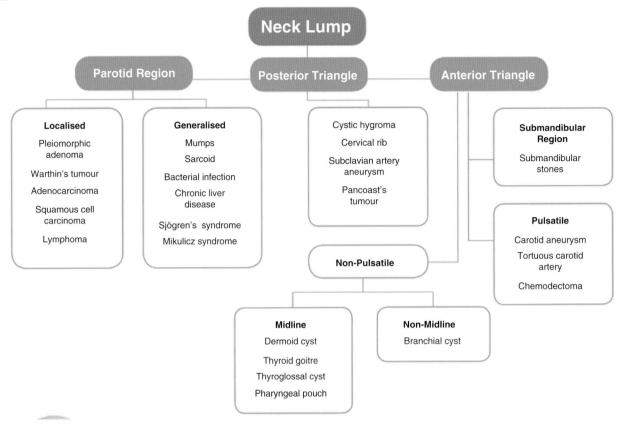

Fig. 2.78 Causes of neck lump.

 A Case to Learn From

In an OSCE examination a student began describing a large lump in the patient's neck on inspection. The patient looked a little horrified and afterwards the examiner exclaimed, 'she's got a lovely neck!' There was no mass there. If you're not sure whether someone has a lump in the neck, make sure you palpate it before telling the examiner about it!

 Top Tip

Submandibular stones are seldom palpable from the outside. One would need to palpate the floor of mouth to detect them.

STATION 2.17: THYROID

SCENARIO

You are a junior doctor in general medicine and have been asked to see Mr Hashimoto, a 50-year-old man, who has presented with weight loss and profound diarrhoea. He has also developed a lump in his neck. Please perform a relevant thyroid examination on Mr Hashimoto and present your findings.

PREPARATION

- WIPER:
  - *Wash* your hands

- *Introduce* yourself
- Ask about *pain*
- Appropriately *expose*
- *Reposition*
- Explain the examination to the patient and your reasons for performing it
- Gain verbal consent
- Give the patient privacy to expose themselves as required
- Start in a comfortable position (usually sitting)
- Offer a chaperone

GENERAL INSPECTION

- Environment: Mobility aids (due to proximal myopathy in hyperthyroidism)
- Patient: Pain or agitation, hair, skin, behaviour, build, clothing

EXAMINATION OF THE HANDS:

- Thyroid acropachy: Clubbing, soft-tissue swelling and periosteal new bone formation
- Onycholysis: Loosening or separation of the fingernail from the bed
- Sweating
- Palmar erythema: Redness of the palms can be associated with hyperthyroid states

- Fine tremor
- Arrhythmias: Assess the rate and rhythm of the patient's radial pulse. Bradycardia can be associated with hypothyroidism, whereas tachycardia and AF can be associated with hyperthyroidism

EXAMINATION OF THE EYES

- Chemosis: Oedema of the conjunctiva
- Periorbital oedema
- Erythema
- Assess for:
  - Exophthalmos: Protrusion of the eye anteriorly, associated with Graves' disease. Look from the side and look down on the eyes from behind the patient (Fig. 2.79)
  - Ophthalmoplegia: Examine CN III, IV and VI
  - Lid lag: Ask the patient to follow your finger with their eyes as you sharply drop your finger from eye level downwards (Fig. 2.80)

EXAMINATION OF THE NECK

INSPECTION

- Inspect the neck from front and side, looking for:
  - Scars
  - Hyperaemia
  - Swelling
  - Distended neck veins

Note that the normal thyroid gland should not be visible on general inspection. If you can visualise it, then it is abnormal.

PALPATION

- Palpate the neck from behind, assessing for:
  - Masses (Fig. 2.81): Site, size, shape, surface, consistency, edge, mobility, fluctuance, transillumination, bruits (Fig. 2.82), relationship to skin and deep structures
  - Lymph nodes: Submental, submandibular, down anterior chain, supraclavicular, posterior chain,

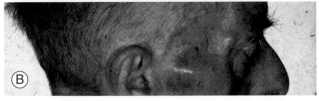

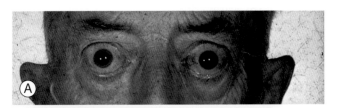

Fig. 2.79 Thyrotoxicosis: (A) Note that the entire white of the eye can be seen outlining the iris, due to lid retraction and exophthalmos. (B) Note the protruding eyeballs visible from side view.

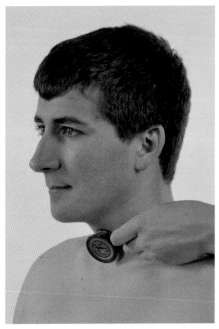

Fig. 2.81 Auscultation for a thyroid bruit.

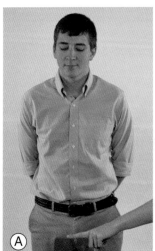

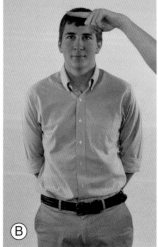

Fig. 2.80 (A, B) Assessing for lid lag (delay in movement of the eyelid as the eye moves downward).

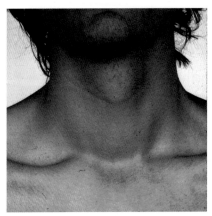

Fig. 2.82 Visible neck lump consistent with a goitre.

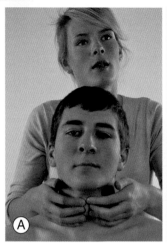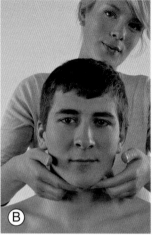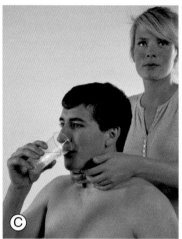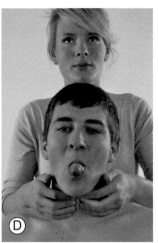

Fig. 2.83 (A, B) Palpating lymph nodes, (C) Sipping water and (D) Sticking tongue out.

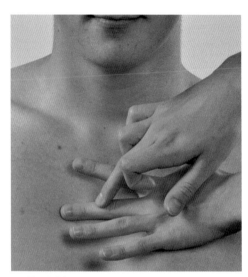

Fig. 2.84 Percussion for a retrosternal goitre.

parotid and mastoid areas and occipital nodes (Fig. 2.83A, B)
- Temperature
- Palpate the trachea from front:
  - Warn the patient that they might experience discomfort
  - Check for deviation, which can be caused by a large goitre

While you are inspecting and palpating, ask the patient to:
- Sip water, hold it in the mouth and then swallow on your command (Fig. 2.83C)
- Stick out their tongue (a thyroglossal cyst will move) (Fig. 2.83D)

EXAMINATION OF THE CHEST

- Percuss for extension of retrosternal goitre (Fig. 2.84)

FINISHING

- Offer to:
  - Perform a cardiovascular examination

- Examine reflexes
- Examine the legs for pretibial myxoedema
- Assess for proximal myopathy
- Check BP
- Perform a urine dipstick
- Thank the patient
- Check that they're comfortable and offer to help reposition them
- Wash your hands
- Leave the patient in privacy to get dressed

! Differential by type of lump

TYPE OF LUMP	DIFFERENTIAL DIAGNOSES
Smooth or diffuse	• Hashimoto's disease • Graves' disease • Iodine deficiency
Solitary nodule	• Cyst • Colloid nodule • Adenoma • Carcinoma • Dominant nodule multinodular goitre
Multiple nodules	• Multiple cyst • Multinodular goitre

🔍 Present Your Findings

Mr Hashimoto is a 50-year-old man who has presented with weight loss, profound diarrhoea and a neck lump. On examination, he is a very thin man who appears anxious with a fine bilateral hand tremor and an irregularly irregular pulse. He has marked exophthalmos, lid lag and failure of upward gaze. He has a 2 × 2 cm neck lump which does not move on tongue protrusion, but does elevate on swallowing. This lump is non-tender, has a well-circumscribed, smooth border and is firm in consistency.

I feel the most likely diagnosis is hyperthyroidism, most likely Graves' disease.

To complete my examination, I would like to measure the BP, dipstick the urine and perform an ECG. I would like to take bloods, including: FBCs, U&Es, LFTs, bone profile, blood glucose and TFTs.

QUESTIONS AND ANSWERS FOR CANDIDATE

Name three indications for surgery in Graves' disease.
- Failure of medical treatment
- Intolerance of medication
- Large goitre
- Poor compliance with medication
- Patient choice

Name three complications of a thyroidectomy.
- Bleeding thyroid crisis (fast AF, pulmonary oedema)
- Hypoparathyroidism
- Hypocalcaemia
- Damage to the recurrent laryngeal nerve
- Recurrent hyperthyroidism
- Late hypothyroidism

What is the most sensitive test for optic nerve compression?
- Loss of colour vision

A Case to Learn From

We saw a patient in AF, who unusually cardioverted with a simple Valsalva manoeuvre. They had their baseline bloods checked, including electrolytes, but no TFTs. Although there were no signs now suggesting any element of thyroid disease, we added them on, and low and behold, it was a new diagnosis of hyperthyroidism. Conditions like hyperthyroidism can present with one symptom, so have a low threshold for testing for it.

Top Tip

Movement of a thyroglossal cyst on tongue protrusion is almost impossible to detect on inspection. It is essential to palpate whilst doing this manoeuvre.

STATION 2.18: CUSHING'S SYNDROME

SCENARIO

You are a junior doctor in general medicine and have been asked to see, Mrs Kain, a 30-year-old woman, who has presented with feelings of low mood, weight gain and amenorrhoea for 3 months. Please perform a relevant examination of Mrs Kain's endocrine system and present your findings.

PREPARATION

- WIPER:
  - *Wash* your hands
  - *Introduce* yourself
  - Ask about *pain*
  - Appropriately *expose*
  - *Reposition*
- Explain the examination to the patient and your reasons for performing it

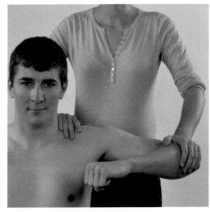

Fig. 2.85 Testing for proximal myopathy.

- Gain verbal consent
- Give the patient privacy to expose themselves as required
- Start in a comfortable position (usually sitting)
- Offer a chaperone

GENERAL INSPECTION

- Environment: Medications, particularly glucocorticoids
- Patient: Pain or agitation, hair, skin, behaviour, build, obvious truncal obesity, moon facies, dorso-cervical fat pad

EXAMINATION OF THE UPPER LIMBS

- Bruising: Particularly on the back of the hands and forearms
- Wounds: Minor injuries are more likely to persist due to poor healing
- Trunk-to-limb ratio: The centripetal adiposity associated with Cushing's syndrome results in relatively thin arms with a large trunk ('orange on a matchstick' appearance)
- Muscle strength: Check for proximal myopathy. Ask the patient to raise both arms out like chicken wings and assess for power by saying 'keep your arms up' while you push down on the patient's arms. Check each arm individually, not both arms simultaneously (Fig. 2.85)
- Skin fold thickness: Pinch the skin and gently lift it. Thin skin is associated with Cushing's syndrome (Fig. 2.86)
- BP: May be elevated

EXAMINATION OF THE FACE

- Facial 'mooning': Look at the patient head on. With 'mooning', the cheeks may obscure the junction of the ear with the side of the face
- Acne
- Plethoric cheeks

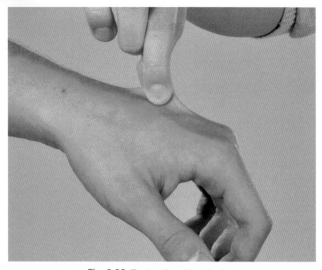

Fig. 2.86 Testing for skin thinning.

- Hirsutism
- Hair thinning
- Cataracts

EXAMINATION OF THE NECK

- Inspect and palpate the supraclavicular fossae for 'fat pads'

EXAMINATION OF THE BACK

- Inspect and palpate the back for interscapular fat pads ('buffalo hump') and thoracic kyphosis
- Comment on stature and any clinical evidence of osteoporosis, scoliosis or loss of distance between lower ribs and the top of the pelvis due to crush fractures of lumbar vertebrae

EXAMINATION OF THE CHEST

- Inspect for breathlessness and auscultate for wheeze (due to respiratory illness, for which long-term oral steroids may cause a cushingoid appearance)
- In males, examine for gynaecomastia by looking and palpating (if applicable) for breast tissue

EXAMINATION OF THE ABDOMEN

- Inspect for:
  - Centripetal adiposity
  - Scars of adrenalectomy
  - Purple striae on the abdomen (Fig. 2.87)

EXAMINATION OF THE LOWER LIMBS

- Trunk-to-limb ratio (as with the upper limbs)
- Proximal myopathy: Ask the patient to cross the arms over the chest and then to stand from sitting (Fig. 2.88)

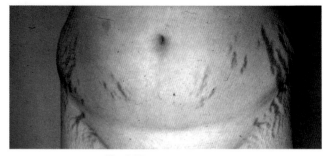

Fig. 2.87 Abdominal striae.

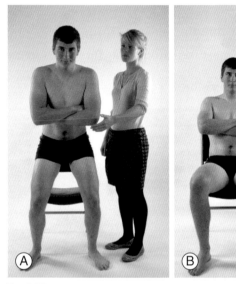

Fig. 2.88 (A, B) Testing for proximal myopathy. Ensure that you are close to the patient as they stand, in case they fall.

- Thin skin
- Bruising
- Leg ulcers
- Oedema

FINISHING

- Offer to:
  - Perform a cardiovascular examination
  - Check the BP
  - Dipstick the urine
- Thank the patient
- Check that they're comfortable and offer to help re-position them
- Wash your hands
- Leave the patient in privacy to get dressed

COMPLICATIONS OF CUSHING'S SYNDROME

- Cardiovascular disease; for example, stroke, myocardial infarction, peripheral vascular disease
- Thromboembolic events; for example, DVT or PE
- Type 2 diabetes
- Hypertension
- Hypercholesterolaemia

- Osteoporosis or fractures
- Infections
- Depression

 Present Your Findings

Mrs Kain is a 30-year-old woman presenting with low mood, weight gain and amenorrhoea. On examination, she has centripetal obesity, dorsal fat pads, multiple bruising to the forearms and thin skin. Her face is plethoric and she has acne. She has a proximal myopathy with 3/5 power for hip flexion and 3/5 power for shoulder abduction.

I feel the most likely diagnosis is Cushing's syndrome.

To complete my examination, I would like to measure her BP and perform a urinalysis. I would like to check a random cortisol level, as well as FBCs, U&Es, LFTs, bone profile and a blood glucose.

❓ QUESTIONS AND ANSWERS FOR CANDIDATE

Name three clinical features from your examination that have the best predictive value in supporting a diagnosis of Cushing's syndrome (rather than obesity or depression).
- Hypertension
- Myopathy
- Bruising

Name three complications of transsphenoidal hypophysectomy (treatment for pituitary adenoma).
- Cerebrospinal fluid rhinorrhoea
- Diabetes insipidus
- Hypopituitarism
- Visual field disturbance (though only with very poor surgical technique)
- Persistence of disease
- Recurrence of disease

Name three causes of Cushing's syndrome.
Exogenous steroids:
- For diseases such as rheumatoid arthritis, asthma and IBD
Endogenous steroids:
- Pituitary adenoma (Cushing's disease)
- Pituitary microadenoma producing excess adrenocorticotropic hormone (ACTH), which increases cortisol production by adrenal glands
- Adrenal adenoma or carcinoma ectopically secretes cortisol, which in turn reduces ACTH levels

 A Case to Learn From

We saw a patient with a new diagnosis of Cushing's syndrome. It was picked up by a surgeon during a preoperative assessment for a hernia and it was not based on concerns from the referring doctor or the patient, but purely by eyeballing the patient. If you see a patient with centripetal obesity, then have a low threshold for sending a cortisol level, even if they don't have any other symptoms.

 Top Tip

Remember that there is a patient in front of you when you are presenting! Don't use phrases like 'buffalo hump'; say interscapular fat pad instead.

STATION 2.19: ACROMEGALY

SCENARIO

You are a junior doctor in general medicine and have been asked to see Mr Black, a 34-year-old man, who has noticed that his hands and feet have swollen up over the last few months. His wedding ring no longer fits his finger and his shoe size has increased. He also reports increased sweating. Please perform a relevant examination on Mr Black's endocrine system and present your findings.

PREPARATION

- WIPER:
  - *Wash* your hands
  - *Introduce* yourself
  - Ask about *pain*
  - Appropriately *expose*
  - *Reposition*
- Explain the examination to the patient and your reasons for performing it
- Gain verbal consent
- Give the patient privacy to expose themselves as required
- Start in a comfortable position (usually sitting)
- Offer a chaperone

GENERAL INSPECTION

- Environment: Medications
- Patient: Pain or agitation, hair, skin, behaviour, build and height, limb and digit lengths

EXAMINATION OF THE HANDS

INSPECTION

- Look at the shape and size of the hands. 'Spade-like', enlarged hands are common in acromegaly. If you are unsure, compare them with your own hands

PALPATION

- Ask the patient to stick their palms out in front of them and gently feel them:
  - The skin may feel moist and rubber-like. The palms may be boggy. This is due to increased sweating and oiliness. This is an important sign of *active* disease

- In thick skin, check skin fold thickness by gently pinching the skin on the back of the hand and comparing it with your own (Fig. 2.89)
- Assess for evidence of carpal tunnel syndrome
- Check the sensation in the median nerve distribution (lateral palm)
- Perform Phalen's and Tinel's test (see 'Hand and Wrist Examination') (Fig. 2.90)
- Feel the radial pulse (Fig. 2.91). Tachycardia is associated with a high-output cardiac state

EXAMINATION OF THE ARMS

- Axillary hair loss: Hypopituitarism may be associated with acromegaly
- Proximal myopathy: Ask the patient to raise both arms like chicken wings (after demonstrating the manoeuvre yourself). Check for power by saying 'don't let me push down' whilst pushing down on the patient's arms. Check each arm individually, not both arms simultaneously
- Measure BP: It is often increased

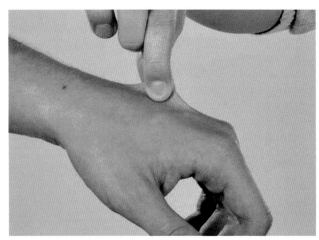

Fig. 2.89 Assessing for skin thinning.

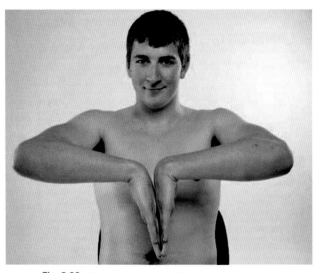

Fig. 2.90 Phalen's test for medial nerve compression.

EXAMINATION OF THE FACE

Look for (Fig. 2.92):
- Prominent supraorbital ridges
- Prognathism
- Protrusion of the lower jaw/underbite
- Large nose, ears and lips
- Coarse facial appearance

Ask the patient to:
- Stick out their tongue: It may be large (Fig. 2.93)
- Show you their gums: Look for an increased space between the teeth (diastema) (Fig. 2.94)
- Repeat a simple phrase: They may have a husky voice

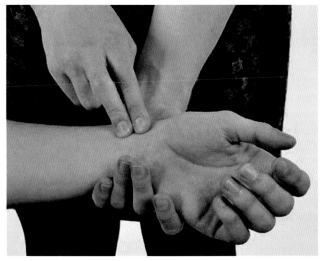

Fig. 2.91 Radial pulse.

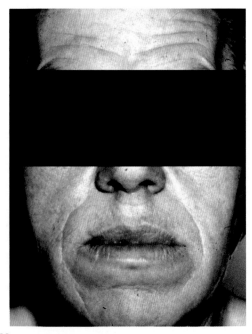

Fig. 2.92 Acromegaly features. Note the prominent supraorbital ridges, protrusion of lower jaw and coarse facial appearance.

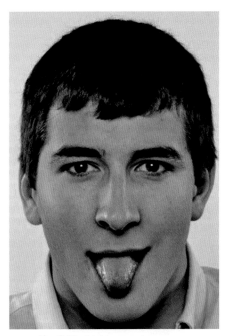

Fig. 2.93 Sticking out the tongue.

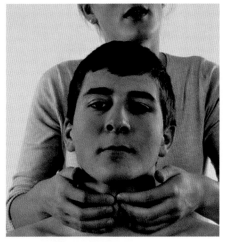

Fig. 2.95 Feeling for goitre.

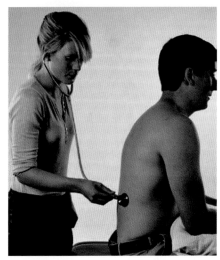

Fig. 2.96 Auscultating the lung bases.

EXAMINATION OF THE CHEST

- Apex beat: Cardiomegaly
- Auscultate the precordium: Third heart sound
- Auscultate the lung bases: Left heart failure (Fig. 2.96)

EXAMINATION OF THE ABDOMEN

- Hepatomegaly: Sign of right heart failure

EXAMINATION OF THE LOWER LIMBS

- Proximal myopathy: Assess for weakness in the legs by asking the patient to get up from a sitting position without using their arms (Fig. 2.97)
- Oedema: Heart failure
- Enlarged feet
- Increased heel pad thickness

FINISHING

- Offer to:
  - Perform a cardiovascular examination

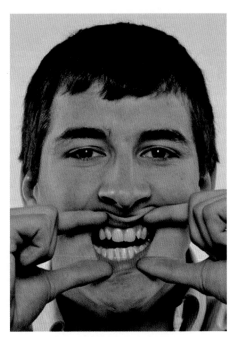

Fig. 2.94 Showing gums.

- Move their eyes following your finger: Assessing visual fields (see 'Eye Examination'). Optic chiasm compression may lead to a bitemporal hemianopia

EXAMINATION OF THE NECK

- Check JVP: Heart failure secondary to hypertension, cardiomyopathy or both
- Goitre: Approximately 10% of patients with acromegaly have a goitre (Fig. 2.95)

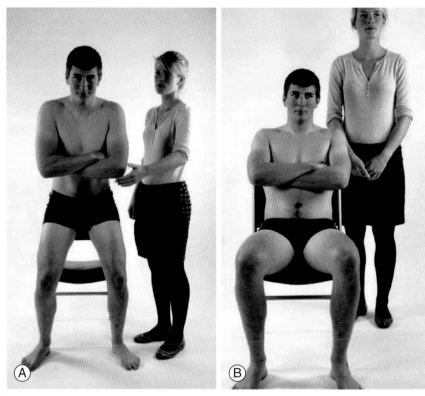

Fig. 2.97 Testing for proximal myopathy. Ensure that you are close to the patient as they stand, in case they fall.

- Check the BP
  - Review old photos (to look for physical changes)
  - Dipstick the urine
- Thank the patient
- Check that they're comfortable and offer to help reposition them
- Wash your hands
- Leave the patient in privacy to get dressed

CAUSES OF ACROMEGALY

- Pituitary tumours: Most commonly benign adenoma
- Non-pituitary tumours: Less common; for example, lung cancer, which may secrete growth hormone or growth hormone-releasing hormone

Q Present Your Findings

Mr Black is a 34-year-old man who has presented with hand and foot swelling over the last few months. On examination, he has thick, moist skin, with 'bogginess' in both palms. He has prominent supraorbital ridges with relatively large nose, lips and tongue. There was evidence of reduced sensation in the distribution of the media nerve bilaterally, with paraesthesia elicited during Tinel's test.

I feel the most likely diagnosis is acromegaly associated with carpal tunnel syndrome.

To complete my examination, I would like to measure his BP, examine the visual fields, review old photos and perform a urinalysis. I would like to check growth hormone/insulin-like growth factor 1 (IGF-1) levels, as well as taking bloods, including: FBCs, U&Es, LFTs, bone profile and a blood glucose.

? QUESTIONS AND ANSWERS FOR CANDIDATE

How would you confirm the diagnosis of acromegaly?
- Measure growth hormone levels during an oral glucose tolerance test
- In acromegaly, the growth hormone level is not suppressed after consuming the carbohydrate load
- There may even be a paradoxical rise in growth hormone levels

What treatment options are there for acromegaly?
- Medical:
  - Somatostatin analogues, for example, octreotide, can cause tumour shrinkage and are often given preoperatively to increase the chances of surgical cure
  - Dopamine agonists
  - Growth hormone receptor antagonists
- Surgery:
  - Transsphenoidal surgery to debulk the tumour
- Radiotherapy

Name three complications of acromegaly.
- Diabetes
- Hypertension
- Cardiomyopathy
- Carpal tunnel syndrome
- Osteoarthritis
- Proximal muscle weakness
- Sleep apnoea
- Visual loss (bitemporal hemianopia)
- Colon cancer

A Case to Learn From

We once saw a patient who was adamant that their appearance had changed, but they didn't look particularly unusual. It was only when we looked at old photos that it became clear that their features had dramatically changed and became a lot coarser. The pictures were our clue to acromegaly. Old photos are key to allowing patients' subjective report of changes to be converted to objective evidence of change.

 Top Tip

Don't get acromegaly confused with gigantism. Once the growth plates have fused in childhood, excess growth hormone won't lead to excess height, although it will still lead to bony changes.

STATION 2.20: BREAST

SCENARIO

You are a junior doctor in breast surgery and have been asked to see Ms Dodd, a 25-year-old woman, who has noticed a breast lump. Please perform a relevant breast examination on Ms Dodd and present your findings.

PREPARATION

- WIPER:
  - *Wash* your hands
  - *Introduce* yourself
  - Ask about *pain*
  - Appropriately *expose*
  - *Reposition*
- Explain the examination to the patient and your reasons for performing it
- If the presenting complaint is unilateral, then enquire about its location so you can examine the asymptomatic breast first
- Gain verbal consent
- Give the patient privacy to expose herself as required. Provide a sheet to cover the patient's chest and ensure she is undressed from the waist up
- Start in a comfortable position (with the patient usually sitting in a chair or bed)
- Ensure that a chaperone is present

GENERAL INSPECTION

- Patient: Pain or agitation

EXAMINATION OF THE BREASTS

INSPECTION

- Check in five positions:
  - At rest
  - Raising both arms above the head

- Sitting and pushing the body up off the bed with both hands
- Putting hands on hips and pushing inwards
- With the patient leaning forward, observe the breasts for muscle tethering of breast lump
- Observe for:
  - Asymmetry: For example, in size or appearance
  - Swelling or masses
  - Skin changes: For example, scaling of the nipple and areola associated with Paget's disease of the breast, peau d'orange, dimpling of the skin associated with inflammatory breast cancer, erythema, skin puckering associated with malignancy, invasion of the suspensory ligaments of the breast
  - Nipple changes: For example, nipple inversion, which can be normal or associated with breast cancer, abscess, mammary duct ectasia, nipple discharge, which can be physiological but is sometimes associated with mastitis or breast cancer

PALPATION

- Put on a pair of gloves
- Ask the patient to lie back to 45° and relax her head on the pillow while placing the arm on the same side of the breast to be examined behind her head.
- Start with the unaffected breast
- Palpate four quadrants in turn (with the flat of the fingers, not the palm)
- Feel the area underneath nipple and areola
- Feel for the axillary breast tail tissue
- Feel the axilla while supporting the arm
- Repeat on the other breast
- For any lump, describe:
  - Size
  - Location
  - Shape
  - Colour
  - Tenderness
  - Temperature
  - Consistency: Soft/firm/hard
  - Surface: Smooth/irregular
  - Borders: Well defined/ill defined
  - Tethering/Mobility
  - Overlying skin changed
- Ask the patient to attempt to produce discharge, if present, by squeezing the nipple between the index finger and the thumb

FINISHING

- Offer to:
  - Check supraclavicular lymph nodes from behind
  - Check for hepatomegaly and lymphoedema
  - Palpate for bony tenderness
  - Auscultate lung bases
- Thank the patient

- Check that they're comfortable and offer to help reposition them
- Remove your gloves and wash your hands
- Leave the patient in privacy to get dressed

⚠ Non-malignant causes of breast lumps

COMMON	RARE
• Fibroadenoma	• Galactocele
• Fibrocystic change	• Lipoma
• Sebaceous cyst	• Fat necrosis
• Acute mastitis or abscess (if in association with breastfeeding or smoking)	• Gynaecomastia

🔍 Present Your Findings

Ms Dodd is a 25-year-old woman presenting with a new breast lump. It is a 2 × 2 cm, mobile, well-circumscribed lump at the 6 o' clock position of her left breast. The lump is soft, mobile, non-tender and has no associated skin changes. There is no axillary or cervical lymphadenopathy.

I feel the most likely diagnosis is a benign fibroadenoma.

To complete my examination, I would like to auscultate the lung bases, examine for hepatomegaly and lymphadenopathy, and palpate for bony tenderness. I would like to refer Ms Dodd to a one-stop breast clinic for triple assessment.

❓ QUESTIONS AND ANSWERS FOR CANDIDATE

What is the most common breast malignancy?
- Invasive ductal carcinoma

What is tamoxifen?
- Selective oestrogen receptor modulator (SERM)
- Used in oestrogen receptor-positive breast cancer

What does triple assessment involve?
- Triple assessment for early detection of breast cancer involves:
  - History and examination: Clinically
  - Imaging: Mammography or ultrasound
  - Histology: Core biopsy and/or fine-needle aspiration (FNA)

A Case to Learn From

I examined a patient once and was convinced she had a benign fibroadenoma. She was well with a small, mobile, non-tender lump. I discussed the case with my consultant, wanting to send the patient home, but he insisted we still had her checked out in the triple assessment clinic, especially given that she had a few sinister factors in the history. It turned out that she had a malignancy and this was only picked up on imaging and biopsy. Have a low threshold for referral for any new breast lump!

Top Tip

Breast examination is one case where you don't just offer a chaperone, you bring one in routinely. It can be important for both the patient and the doctor.

STATION 2.21: DERMATOLOGICAL

SCENARIO

You are a junior doctor in primary care and have been asked to see Mrs Barton, a 45-year-old woman, who has presented with a rash on her scalp and elbows. Please perform a relevant dermatological examination on Mrs Barton and present your findings.

PREPARATION

- WIPER:
  - *Wash* your hands
  - *Introduce* yourself
  - Ask about *pain*
  - Appropriately *expose*
  - *Reposition*
- Explain the examination to the patient and your reasons for performing it
- Gain verbal consent
- Give the patient privacy to expose themselves as required
- Start in a comfortable position (usually sitting in a chair or bed)
- Offer a chaperone

GENERAL INSPECTION

- Patient: Pain or agitation, signs of systemic disease; for example, unwell in meningococcal sepsis, swollen joints in psoriatic arthritis

EXAMINATION OF INDIVIDUAL LESIONS

APPEARANCE

- Pustule: Lesion containing pus
- Erosion: Loss of epidermis
- Ulcer: Loss of epidermis and dermis
- Weal: Circumscribed, elevated area of dermal oedema
- Macule: Flat, circumscribed area of skin discoloration
- Papule: Circumscribed raised lesion < 5 mm in diameter at the widest point
- Nodule: Circumscribed raised lesion > 10 mm in diameter at the widest point
- Plaque: Circumscribed, disc-shaped, elevated lesion
  - Small < 2 cm
  - Large > 2 cm

Note that when differentiating a nodule and plaque, there is inconsistency in describing lesions between 5 and 10 mm.

- Vesicle: Lesion < 5 mm in diameter at the widest point, containing fluid
- Bulla: Lesion greater than 10 mm in diameter at the widest point, containing fluid (Fig. 2.98)
  Note that when differentiating a vesicle and bulla, there is inconsistency in describing lesions between 5 and 10 mm.

SITE

- Psoriasis: Knees, elbows, scalp and lower back
- Eczema: Flexures
- Acne: Face and upper trunk
- Basal cell carcinoma (BCC): Head and neck
- Herpes zoster infection: Nerve distribution (Fig. 2.99)
- Contact dermatitis (Fig. 2.100)

SHAPE

- Round
- Oval (Fig. 2.101)
- Annular
- Linear
- Irregular

SURFACE

- Smooth vs. rough
- Crust or scale (lift to see what is underneath)
- Keratin horn
- Excoriation, maceration, lichenification

ADDITIONAL FEATURES

- Size
- Colour (and blanching)
- Outline can be well demarcated vs. ill defined (Fig. 2.102)
- It is important to appropriately classify burns, and this may involve removing blisters to review the skin surface underneath

SPECIAL TECHNIQUES

- Scraping a psoriatic plaque for capillary bleeding
- Nikolsky's sign in some blistering diseases; for example, toxic epidermal necrolysis or pemphigus vulgaris (rubbing of the skin results in exfoliation of the epidermis)

FINISHING

- Offer to:
  - Examine the nails in psoriasis
  - Examine the fingers and wrists in scabies
  - Examine the toe webs in fungal infection
  - Examine the mouth in lichen planu
- Thank the patient
- Check that they're comfortable and offer to help reposition them
- Wash your hands
- Leave the patient in privacy to get dressed

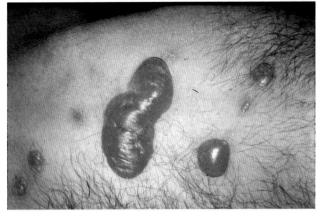

Fig. 2.98 A bulla.

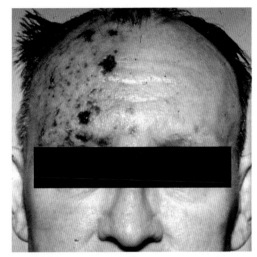

Fig. 2.99 Herpes zoster infection. Note that it is confined to the ophthalmic division of the trigeminal nerve.

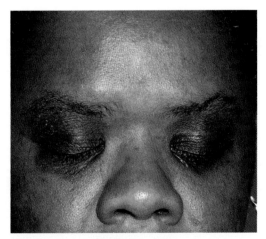

Fig. 2.100 Allergic contact dermatitis – patient wore gold earings and was likely touching eyelid after touching ear rings. (Source: Shiland, B.J., 2018. Mastering Healthcare Terminology. Elsevier.)

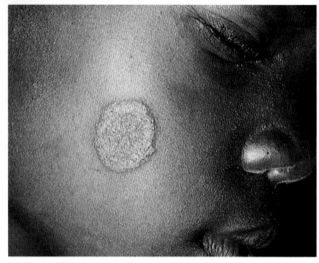

Fig. 2.101 Tinea corporis. (From Hurwitz S: *Clinical pediatric dermatology: a textbook of skin disorders of childhood and adolescence*, ed 5, 2016, Elsevier.)

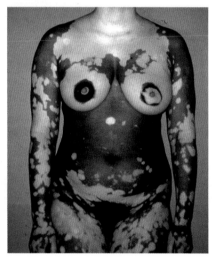

Fig. 2.102 Vitiligo. (Source: Micheletti, R.G., Elston, D., McMahon, P.J., & James, W.D. (2023). *Andrews' Diseases of the Skin Clinical Atlas*. Elsevier Inc.)

⚠ Types of skin changes in psoriasis

SKIN CHANGES IN PSORIASIS	DESCRIPTION
Chronic plaque	• Salmon pink • Well demarcated • Silvery/white scaling • Located over extensor surfaces, scalp, behind ears, naval, natal clefts • May develop on scars (Koebner phenomenon)
Guttate	• Raindrop lesions • Small, red scaly plaques • Located at the trunk, upper arms and thighs
Inverse or flexural	• Shiny and smooth • May be a crack in the skin crease • Red
Pustular	• Dry, red and tender skin • Very quick onset • Associated with systemic symptoms; for example, fever and dehydration
Erythrodermic	• Usually occur on a background of worsening or unstable psoriasis • Erythroderma • May be precipitated by infection, alcohol, medications; for example, antimalarials and lithium

🔍 Present Your Findings

Mrs Barton is a 45-year-old woman presenting with a rash on her elbow and scalp. These are pink, well-demarcated plaques with a white-silver scaling. She has plaques on the extensor surfaces of both elbows, her scalp, and behind her ears. There is further plaque overlying an abdominal scar from a previous caesarean section. Her fingernails show pitting, ridging and onycholysis.

I feel the most likely diagnosis is psoriasis with secondary nail changes.

To complete my examination, I would like to examine her joints for evidence of psoriatic arthropathy. Treatment options may include emollients, vitamin D analogues, tar, dithranol and narrow-band ultraviolet B therapy.

❓ QUESTIONS AND ANSWERS FOR CANDIDATE

Name three nail changes that you might see with psoriasis.
- Pitting
- Ridging
- Discoloration
- Subungal hyperkeratosis
- Onycholysis

What pattern of joint involvement might you see in psoriasis?
- There are five different patterns of joint involvement:
  - Distal interphalangeal (DIP) joint swelling
  - Rheumatoid arthritis pattern of symmetrical small-joint swelling
  - Monoarthritis
  - Ankylosing spondylitis or sacroiliitis
  - Arthritis mutilans

Describe the aetiology of psoriasis.
- A family history is present in 35% of patients
- A child with one affected parent has approximately 25% probability of being affected, approximately 60% if both parents are affected
- Risk factors (precipitating factors):
  - Koebner phenomenon: Trauma, including surgical scars
  - Infection; for example, streptococcal sore throat may precipitate guttate psoriasis

- Drugs; for example, β-blockers, lithium, non-steroidal anti-inflammatory drugs (NSAIDs) and antimalarial medications can worsen or precipitate psoriasis
- Sunlight exposure, although beneficial, aggravates psoriasis in 10% of cases
- Psychological stress may worsen psoriasis
- Alcohol

 A Case to Learn From

We had a patient who had been labelled with osteoarthritis for years. They were then examined in an OSCE examination. It was the first time someone looked behind the ears properly. Psoriatic plaques were noted and their diagnosis was changed to psoriatic arthritis. Always be thorough in your assessment, particularly in an exam.

 Top Tip

Despite people saying corticosteroids are not widely used for psoriasis, experiences are that they are. It is, of course, possible you can get rebound or go pustular from them, but this is often more of a problem with systemic steroids.

STATION 2.22: HAEMATOLOGICAL

SCENARIO

You are a junior doctor in haematology and have been asked to see, Mrs Hodgkins, a 44-year-old woman, who has been feeling 'under the weather' for the last few weeks. She has lost considerable weight, bruises more easily than before and has recently been sweating profusely. Please perform a relevant haematological examination on Mrs Hodgkins and present your findings.

PREPARATION

- WIPER:
  - *Wash* your hands
  - *Introduce* yourself
  - Ask about *pain*
  - Appropriately *expose*
  - *Reposition*
- Explain the examination to the patient and your reasons for performing it
- Gain verbal consent
- Give the patient privacy to expose themselves as required
- Start in a comfortable position (usually with the patient sitting)
- Offer a chaperone

GENERAL INSPECTION

- Patient: Pain or agitation

INSPECTION

- Look for:
  - Muscle wasting (chronic diseases)
  - Nutritional status (cachexia)
  - Spider naevi
  - Gynaecomastia
  - Bruising
  - Tattoos
  - Peripheral oedema (signs of possible liver disease)
  - Colour: Pallor (anaemia), plethora (polycythaemia), jaundice, purpura or bruising (thrombocytopenia, reduced clotting factors)

EXAMINATION OF THE HANDS

- Pulse: Rate, rhythm, volume (may have sinus tachycardia with anaemia) (Fig. 2.103)
- Skin crease pallor: Anaemia
- Telangiectasia: Hepatic dysfunction
- Koilonychia: Iron deficiency anaemia
- CRT: Should be under 2 s
- Temperature: Pyrexial or apyrexial

EXAMINATION OF THE FACE

- Tongue: Colour, smoothness (atrophic glossitis and/or a fissured appearance is associated with vitamin B_{12} deficiency)
- Lips: Angular stomatitis (Fig. 2.104), telangiectasia
- Gum: Hypertrophy (associated with leukaemia) or bleeding (Fig. 2.105)
- Buccal mucosa: Petechiae
- Tonsils: Enlarged tonsils could imply infection or a palatal or pharyngeal lymphoma
- Conjunctivae: Pallor, jaundice
- Fundi: Haemorrhage, signs of hyperviscosity; for example, engorged veins, papilloedema (secondary to polycythaemia)

EXAMINATION OF LYMPH NODES

- Location:
  - Neck: Submental, submandibular, deep cervical, preauricular, postauricular, occipital, supraclavicular, infraclavicular
  - Other: Epitrochlear, axillary, inguinal, femoral (Fig. 2.106)

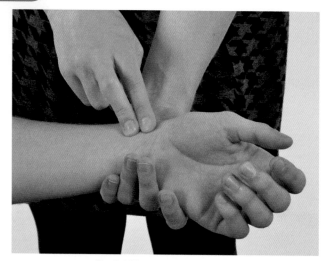

Fig. 2.103 Assessing the pulse.

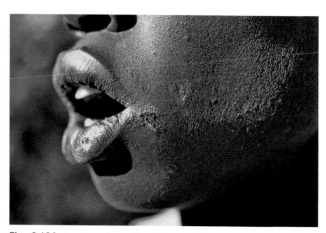

Fig. 2.104 Angular stomatitis. (Source: Nabarro, L., Morris-Jones, S. and Moore, D., 2018. Peters' Atlas of Tropical Medicine and Parasitology. Elsevier.)

Comment on:
- Size
- Consistency (Fig. 2.107):
  - Hard: Like pressing your forehead. Malignancy (lymphoma less likely)
  - Rubbery: Like pressing the end of your nose. Malignancy (especially lymphoma)
  - Soft: Like pressing your lips. Most likely associated with infection
- Tenderness

EXAMINATION OF THE ABDOMEN

- Examine the abdomen as per Station 2.3: Abdominal Examination
- Assess for hepatomegaly and splenomegaly. Hepatosplenomegaly suggests lymphoproliferative or myeloproliferative disease. Hepatomegaly is smooth and/or non-tender in haematological disease and common causes include lymphoma and leukaemia
- Palpate the inguinal lymph nodes

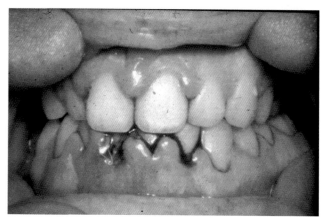

Fig. 2.105 Bleeding gums.

EXAMINATION OF THE LEGS

- Peripheral circulation and any associated gangrene (toes)
- Oedema (from lymphatic obstruction)

FINISHING

- Offer to:
  - Perform an abdominal examination
  - Examine the joints
  - Dipstick the urine
- Thank the patient
- Check that they're comfortable and offer to help reposition them
- Remove your gloves and wash your hands
- Leave the patient in privacy to get dressed

! Causes of splenomegaly by size

MODERATE (3–5 FINGER BREADTHS)	MASSIVE (> 5 FINGER BREADTHS)
• Lymphoma	• CML
• Chronic leukaemia	• Myelofibrosis

🔍 Present Your Findings

Mrs Hodgkins is a 44-year-old woman presenting with lethargy, weight loss, bruising and sweating over the last few weeks. On examination, she is comfortable at rest. She is underweight, sweating and has a temperature of 38°C. She has moderate hepatosplenomegaly. There is also evidence of bilateral leg oedema with palpable inguinal and axillary lymph nodes, which are smooth and non-tender.

I feel the most likely diagnosis is lymphoma. Differential diagnoses include infection and autoimmune disease.

To complete my examination, I would like to perform an abdominal examination, examine the joints, dipstick the urine and request a CXR. I would like to take bloods, including: FBCs, U&Es, LFTs, bone profile, amylase, coagulation, lactate, ESR and CRP.

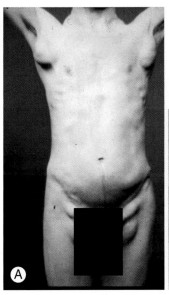
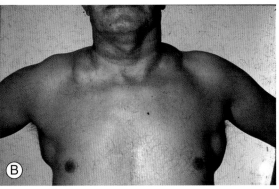
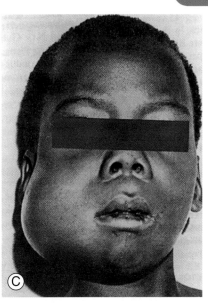

Fig. 2.106 Lymphadenopathy visible on inspection: Axillary and groin (A); axillary and neck (B), face (C). (Source: (C) Cook, G.C., & Zumla, A. (2009). *Manson's tropical diseases*. Elsevier.)

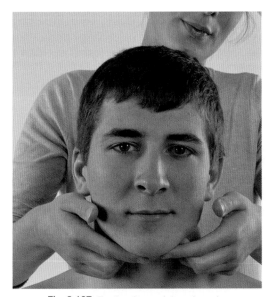

Fig. 2.107 Feeling for neck lymph node.

❓ QUESTIONS AND ANSWERS FOR CANDIDATE

How do you differentiate between an enlarged spleen and a kidney?
- A spleen has a notch, is dull to percuss, moves down with inspiration and you cannot get between it and the ribs

- A kidney has no notch, is resonant to percuss, does not move with inspiration and you can get your fingers over it
- Ultrasound will give confirmation

What might you see with haemarthrosis?
- Haemarthrosis is bleeding into the joints
- It can cause deformity, swelling, tenderness and restricted joint movement
- It is often associated with infection, but can also be associated with congenital bleeding disorders; for example, haemophilia A and B

Name three causes of microcytic anaemia.
- Iron deficiency
- Thalassaemia
- Sideroblastic anaemia
- Lead toxicity

🐘 A Case to Learn From

We saw a patient with mild neutropenia and didn't think too much of it, as it was in the context of a child who was otherwise well. It just happened to be the case that the sibling came into hospital for an infection and was also well, but with low neutrophils. We referred the family to haematology and they and their mother received a new diagnosis of congenital neutropenia. In familial conditions where patients are relatively well, it may be the case that multiple members have lived undiagnosed, despite having clues on their blood test results.

Top Tip

When examining the axillary lymph node, take the weight of the arm and get the patient to relax fully. This will make palpation easier and will make it more comfortable for the patient.

STATION 2.23: EAR

SCENARIO

You are a junior doctor in primary care and have been asked to see, Mrs Mason, an 82-year-old woman, who has presented with worsening hearing. Please perform a relevant hearing examination on Mrs Mason and present your findings.

PREPARATION

- WIPER:
  - *Wash* your hands
  - *Introduce* yourself
  - Ask about *pain*
  - Appropriately *expose*
  - *Reposition*
- Explain the examination to the patient and your reasons for performing it
- Gain verbal consent
- Give the patient privacy to expose themselves as required
- Start in a comfortable position (usually sitting)
- Offer a chaperone

GENERAL INSPECTION

- Environment: Guide dog, walking aids
- Patient: Pain or agitation, hearing aids

EXAMINATION OF THE EXTERNAL EAR

- Inspect the preauricular area for an endaural incision scar (suggests previous ear surgery) (Fig. 2.108)
- Inspect the pinna and comment on any lesions seen
- Inspect the postauricular area for a postauricular incision scar (suggests previous surgery to the ear, i.e. you may find a mastoid cavity)
- Palpate the postauricular area (evidence of cochlear implant (the bone-anchored hearing aid (BAHA) abutment of a cochlear implant may be palpable here) and the mastoid area for tenderness (mastoiditis)

EXAMINATION OF THE AUDITORY MEATUS AND TYMPANIC MEMBRANE

- Select the appropriate-sized speculum. There are two types:

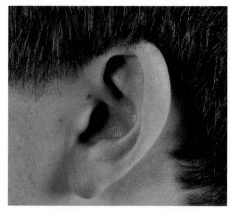

Fig. 2.108 External ear inspection.

- 4 mm: Safer (less likelihood of damaging the ear canal and drum) and greater visibility
- 3 mm: Paediatrics or for a small ear canal
- Turn the light source to full brightness and test that it is bright enough
- Grip the otoscope like a pencil. For the right ear use the right hand and for the left ear use the left hand
- Hold the otoscope by placing your little finger on the patient's zygoma. This acts as an anchor, preventing damage to the inner ear if sudden movement of the patient's head occurs
- Elevate the pinna upwards and backwards with your free hand. You may also need the patient to tilt their head away from you
- Put the speculum on the back of the tragus, under direct vision, and then slowly insert the speculum whilst looking through the earpiece
- Comment on the ear canal (wax, signs of infection) and the tympanic membrane. A healthy drum is translucent and pinky-grey (Fig. 2.109). If it is abnormal, describe the location and nature of the pathology according to whether it is in the pars flaccida or pars tensa. If it is in the pars tensa, describe what quadrant it is in (for example, anteroinferior, posterosuperior). In general, the tympanic membrane is a circle with a 1-cm diameter. Try to describe the size of any perforation

EXAMINATION OF HEARING

WHISPER TEST

- This is a crude bedside method of establishing hearing levels (Fig. 2.110)
- Sit to the side of your patient; remember to start with the good side first
- With one hand, obscure the entrance to the contralateral ear canal and rub gently (do this by pushing the tragus into the canal). This will muffle this ear and ensure that you are only testing one ear at a time

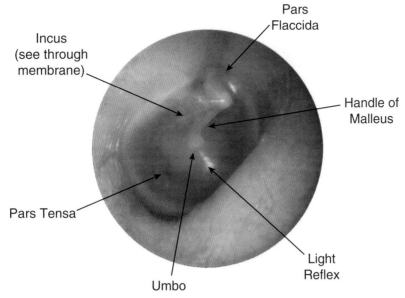

Fig. 2.109 Anatomy of the ear.

- With the other hand, cover the patient's eyes so that they cannot lip read
- Ensure that you are at full arm's length
- Whisper a combination of a number and a letter; for example, 'N4', and ask the patient to repeat what you are saying. Get increasingly louder until they can hear you

RINNE'S TUNING FORK TEST

- Tap a 512-Hz tuning fork on your elbow (not on a piece of furniture). Check that you have made the tuning fork ring by placing it next to your own ear first
- Place it in the following two positions and ask where the patient hears it loudest:
  - Position 1: On the mastoid process
  - Position 2: In front of the ear
- When holding the tuning fork on a bony process, always support the other side of the head with your free hand
- When holding the tuning fork in front of the ear, make sure that the two prongs are upright, pointing toward the ceiling and in line with the ear canal's entrance
- To interpret the results:
  - Rinne's positive: Normal hearing or sensorineural deafness. Air conduction is greater than bone conduction (louder in front of ear than on mastoid process)
  - Rinne's negative: Conductive deafness. Bone conduction is greater than air conduction (louder on mastoid process than in front of ear)

WEBER'S TUNING FORK TEST

- Tap the tuning fork as before and place the base on the vertex of the head or forehead. Support the patient's head with your other hand

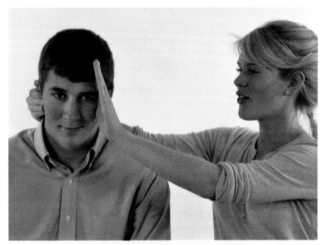

Fig. 2.110 Whisper test.

- Ask the patient whether they hear the sound loudest on the left, right or in the middle:
  - Normal (or symmetrical loss): Sound heard in the midline, equally in both ears
  - Sensorineural deafness: Sound loudest in the less-affected ear
  - Conductive deafness: Sound loudest in affected ear

FINISHING

- Offer to:
  - Examine the facial nerve
  - Request a pure-tone audiogram and tympanogram
- Thank the patient
- Check that they're comfortable and offer to help reposition them
- Wash your hands

⚠ Common ear pathology and presentation of associated otoscopy findings

IMAGE	DESCRIPTION

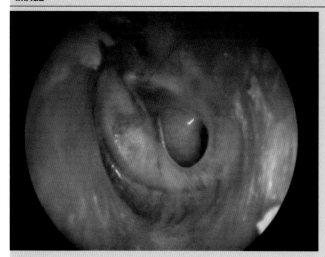

Fig. 2.111 Perforation.

This image demonstrates a 10% central perforation in the posterior inferior quadrant, but an otherwise normal ear drum. It would be reasonable to perform a puretone audiogram and a tympanogram.

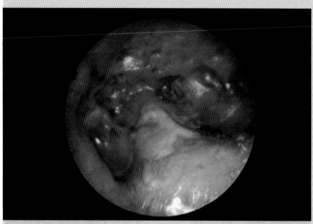

Fig. 2.112 Mastoid cavity.

This image demonstrates an obvious cavity in the superoposterior aspect of the ear canal that is consistent with a mastoid cavity, perhaps indicating previous surgery for a cholesteatoma. The tympanic membrane is intact with a positive light reflex. Conductive hearing loss can occur due to ossicular erosion with cholesteatomas; therefore it would be reasonable to perform a pure-tone audiogram

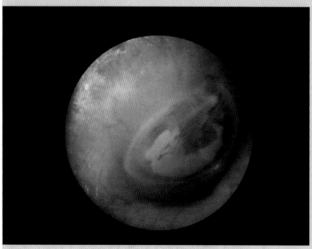

Fig. 2.113 Tympanoslcerosis.

This image demonstrates an opacification of the tympanic membrane consistent with tympanosclerosis. It would be reasonable to perform a tympanogram in order to see if there is reduced motility of the drum and a pure tone audiogram to see if there is any associated conductive hearing loss

Present Your Findings

Mrs Mason is an 85-year-old woman presenting with worsening hearing. On examination of the external ear, there are no pinnal lesions or deformities, no mastoid tenderness and no evidence of previous ear surgery. She wears no hearing aids or implant devices. On examination of the external auditory meatus and tympanic membrane, she has bilateral dry ears with no mastoid cavities. Her right tympanic membrane looks healthy and normal, but her left tympanic membrane has a 10% central perforation in the posterior inferior quadrant. This ear was Rinne's negative, suggesting conductive hearing loss. There was no lateralisation on Weber's test. Whispering test was normal in both ears.

I feel the most likely diagnosis is conductive hearing loss secondary to perforation.

To complete my examination, I would like to perform a pure-tone audiogram and a tympanogram.

❓ QUESTIONS AND ANSWERS FOR CANDIDATE

Name three common causes of a perforated eardrum.
- Acute otitis media
- Complication of grommet insertion
- Barotrauma

What pattern of hearing loss might you get with otosclerosis in the right ear?
- Fusion of stapes, therefore conductive hearing loss

- Rinne's negative (right ear)
- Rinne's positive (left ear)
- Weber's lateralising to left

When would you treat otitis media with antibiotics?
- Most cases do not require antibiotics because they are viral
- Consider in those who are less than 2 years old with bilateral infection, those with otorrhoea, those with prolonged infection and those who are very unwell or who have complications

 A Case to Learn From

Once I was doing a hearing assessment on a child. Initial results convinced me they had a sensorineural deafness pattern, but there were no reports of hearing problems previously. I continued with the assessment, waited for the child to be a bit more relaxed and repeated the exam. Auditory assessment was subsequently normal. Remember that compliance is key to getting accurate results, especially from a paediatric patient!

💡 Top Tip

Remember that anyone can move while you are examining them, particularly children. Don't forget to put your finger on the patient's zygoma so that if they move you still have control over the otoscope.

3 Orthopaedic Examinations

Content Outline

Before dealing with individual joints, here are some general principles that are applicable to all orthopaedic examinations:

1. Do not cause the patient additional pain.
2. Expose the joint and surrounding structures adequately.
3. Always examine the 'normal' limb, comparing it with the 'abnormal' limb.
4. Always assess the joint above and below the 'abnormal' one.
5. Assess active before passive movements.
6. Use standard terminology when describing deformities and movements.

A good way to prepare before starting any examination is:

- Introduce yourself and wash your hands
- Confirm patient identity
- Explain the examination to the patient and reasons for performing it
- Gain verbal consent
- Expose both left and right joint. Patients can wear shorts or use a sheet to cover themselves to maintain dignity
- Offer a chaperone if appropriate
- Ask if the patient has current pain and if so, where, in order to ensure that you do not exacerbate pain

Study Action Plan

- Start by familiarising yourself with the routine for each examination. This can be done on friends or even dolls/teddy bears!
- Once you are confident with the steps, then practise on real patients with clinical signs
- It is useful to be familiar with the normal range of movement for each joint so you can identify abnormal movements more easily
- When practising in groups, talk through what you are doing to help consolidate the steps, remembering: Look, feel, move, special tests and distal neurovascular integrity

STATION 3.1: CERVICAL SPINE

SCENARIO

You are a junior doctor working in orthopaedics and have been asked to see Leanne Jamieson, a 68-year-old woman, who has been referred by her primary care physician with a stiff and painful neck. She is also complaining of headaches in the back of her head. Please examine Mrs Jamieson's cervical spine and then present your findings.

PREPARATION

- WIPER:
  - *Wash* your hands
  - *Introduce* yourself
  - Ask about *pain*
  - Appropriately *expose*
  - *Reposition*
- Explain the examination to the patient and your reasons for performing it
- Gain verbal consent
- Give the patient privacy to expose themselves as required
- Start in a comfortable position (usually sitting in a chair or bed)
- Offer a chaperone

The following is designed for an examination in a patient who does not have a suspected unstable cervical spine.

LOOK

- Important to note whether changes are symmetrical or asymmetrical
- Ask the patients to remove enough clothing to expose the neck and upper thorax
- Inspect from front, side and back, looking for:
  - General inspection: Posture or position of the neck
  - Muscle: Spasm or muscle wasting

- Scars: For example, longitudinal midline posterior scars or transverse scars adjacent to the midline anteriorly are indicative of previous surgery
- Skin changes: Including any lumps
- Loss of normal lordosis: Commonly due to muscle spasm (best seen from the side)

FEEL

Ensure to ask patients if they have pain and clarify the location.
- Spinous processes: Palpate along the midline for tenderness starting from the occiput and moving downwards. The C-spine from C2 downwards is palpable. C7 and T1 spinous processes are the largest
- Facet joints: Move your fingers 2.5 cm lateral to the spinous processes to palpate facet joints for tenderness. The facet joints between C5 and C6 are those that are most often involved in osteoarthritis and may be painful on palpation
- Muscles: Palpate the paraspinal and trapezius muscles for tenderness
- Supraclavicular: Palpate for a cervical rib. Overdevelopment of the seventh cervical vertebra can affect the subclavian artery and the first thoracic nerve
- Crepitus: Spread your hands on each side of the neck and ask the patient to flex and extend the spine

MOVE

Do not move in trauma where the cervical spine is suspected (Fig. 3.1). Assess with the patient sitting in a chair.

FLEXION
- The patient should be able to touch chin to chest
- Normal is 80°
- Chin–chest distance can be measured

EXTENSION
- Make sure that the patient is seated
- The plane of the nose and forehead should normally be nearly horizontal
- Normal is 50°

ROTATION
- The chin normally falls just short of the plane of the shoulders
- Normal is 80°

LATERAL FLEXION
- The patient should nearly be able to touch the ear on to the shoulder
- Normal is 45°
Passive movements can be assessed very gently if there are reduced active movements.

SPECIAL TESTS

LHERMITTE'S TEST
- Electric shock-like sensations in the spine or limbs on neck flexion
- Can be caused by multiple sclerosis, myelopathy from cervical spondylosis, vitamin B_{12} deficiency or whiplash injury

HOFFMAN'S TEST
- There is a positive Hoffman's sign when the middle fingernail gets flicked downwards and you observe adduction and flexion of the thumb of the same hand
- It can be caused by multiple sclerosis or spinal cord compression (cervical myelopathy)

GAIT
- Gait should also be assessed as gait disturbance and ataxia can be seen in patients with cervical spondylotic myelopathy See Station 3.9: Gait, arms, legs and spine (GALS)

NEUROVASCULAR ASSESSMENT (FIG. 3.2 AND TABLE 3.1)

Examine the limbs, paying particular attention to:
- Lower motor neurone signs in the upper limbs; for example, hypotonia, wasting, fasciculations, hyporeflexia

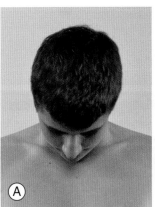 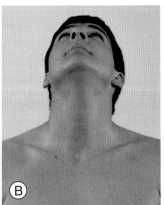 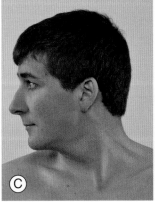 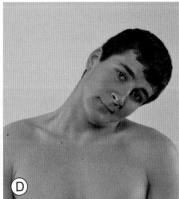

Fig. 3.1 Neck movements: (A) flexion; (B) extension; (C) rotation; and (D) lateral flexion.

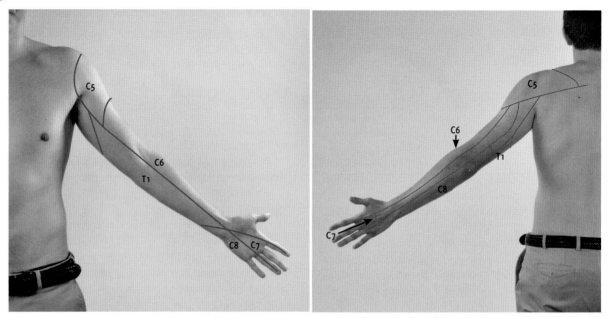

Fig. 3.2 (A, B) Upper-limb dermatomes.

Table 3.1   **Nerve roots and the respective dermatome, myotome and reflex**

NERVE ROOT	DERMATOME	MYOTOME	REFLEX
C5	• Over the deltoid	• Shoulder abduction	• Biceps • Supinator
C6	• Thumb • Radial aspect of the forearm (dorsal and palmar)	• Elbow flexion (also C5)	• Biceps • Triceps • Supinator
C7	• Palmar and dorsal surface of middle finger	• Elbow extension (also C8)	• Triceps
C8	• Palmar aspect of the little finger • Ulnar aspect of the forearm • Dorsal surface of the little finger	• Finger flexion	• Nil

- Upper motor neurone signs in the lower limbs; for example, hypertonia, weakness, upgoing plantar reflex, hyperreflexia
- Perform a per rectum (PR) examination to assess the anal tone, palpate and percuss for an enlarged bladder and examine for saddle anaesthesia if concerned over cord compression

CERVICAL RIB AND THORACIC OUTLET SYNDROME

- Inspect the hands: May be perishingly cold, discoloured and atrophic
- Palpate the radial pulse and then apply traction to the arm for several seconds: Reduction of radial pulsation after this manoeuvre suggests the presence of a cervical rib (Fig. 3.3)

FINISHING

- Offer to:
  - Examine the shoulder, as shoulder pain can be referred to the neck
- Thank the patient

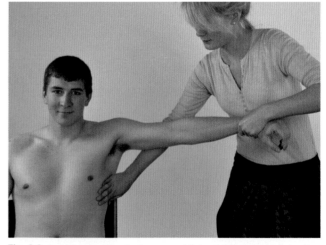

Fig. 3.3 Applying traction to the arm whilst palpating the radial pulse, to assess for a cervical rib.

- Check they're comfortable and offer to help reposition them
- Wash your hands
- Leave the patient in privacy to get dressed

CERVICAL SPINE PATHOLOGIES

⚠ Common cervical spine pathology

CATEGORY	DIAGNOSIS	PRESENTATION
Bone	Fracture	• History of trauma or strain • Tenderness • Pain may radiate to the arms • May also have associated head or long-bone injury

	Cervical rib	• Can cause thoracic outlet syndrome
		  • Neurogenic: Neck pain, numbness in fingers
		  • Vascular: Cold hands, weak pulse

Joint	Rheumatoid arthritis	• Neck pain • Limited range of movement • Occiput headache • May have signs of brachial plexus root compression in the upper limbs
Disc	Acute intervertebral disc prolapse	• History of strain • Sudden onset of pain • May have a wry neck on inspection • Stiffness • May have paraesthesia in the arms
	Chronic disc degeneration (cervical spondylosis) and osteoarthritis	• Gradual onset of pain and stiffness • Stiffness worse in the morning • Pain may worsen with activity • Pain may radiate to the shoulders • Limited range of movement
Soft tissue	Whiplash	• History of trauma • Gradual development of neck pain • Nausea, dizziness, headache • Paraesthesia • Spasms • Reduced range of movement • May not be symptomatic until 6–12 h after the event
	Acute torticollis	• Rotated and flexed neck due to spasm of sternocleidomastoid muscle • History of repetitive mode of activity or unusual posture or position

TRAUMA

- In trauma situations with possible cervical spine injury, it is important to follow the ABCDE approach:
  - *Assess* airway, then stabilise the cervical spine
  - *Breathing*
  - *Circulation*
  - *Disability*
  - *Exposure*, using log roll
- The cervical spine should not be moved or examined thoroughly until it has been cleared as safe to do so by a senior clinician

Present Your Findings

Mrs Jamieson is a 68-year-old woman who presented with neck pain and stiffness. She has also been suffering from occiput headaches. A thorough history revealed that she has rheumatoid arthritis of the hands and knees; a walking stick was noted. On cervical spine examination, crepitus was felt during movement. It was also noted that range of movement was limited both actively and passively. On neurovascular examination, hyperreflexia of both upper limbs was noted.

This is suggestive of an upper motor neurone problem. This may be as a result of the effect of rheumatoid arthritis on the cervical spine, with differentials being chronic disc degeneration. To complete my examination, I would like to examine the shoulders, perform X-rays of the cervical spine and request magnetic resonance imaging (MRI) to assess for spinal cord compression.

A Case to Learn From

A patient saw their primary care physician after sustaining whiplash following a minor car accident. They had tried to manage the pain at home and were wearing a neck collar that they already had in their house. The doctor explained that it was important to keep their neck mobile and that a neck collar should not be worn in this instance. If there is no plausible mechanism of cervical spine fracture, then a neck collar is unlikely to be needed.

❓ QUESTIONS AND ANSWERS FOR CANDIDATE

What X-rays would you request in a suspected cervical spine fracture?
- Anteroposterior (AP) and lateral X-rays of the cervical spine (C1–T1) and a peg view

How would you manage whiplash?
- Keep the neck mobile
- Simple analgesia
- Ice packs
- Physiotherapy if chronic

How would you manage a patient with a possible unstable cervical spine fracture?
- In-line triple mobilisation – collars, blocks and tape
- Analgesia
- AP and lateral X-rays of the cervical spine (C1–T1) and a peg view
- Discussion with neurosurgeons and/or orthopaedics, depending on the results of X-ray
- Further imaging may be required; for example, computed tomography (CT) or MRI

 Top Tip

Examination of the spine is most easily carried out standing behind a seated patient.

 Top Tip

Assess for posterior midline tenderness before assessing movements, to avoid aggravating an unstable cervical spine injury.

STATION 3.2: THORACOLUMBAR SPINE

SCENARIO

You are a junior doctor working in orthopaedics, and have been asked to see Simon MacPherson, an 85-year-old man, who has recently developed back pain. He is known to have prostate cancer. Please examine his thoracolumbar spine and present your findings.

PREPARATION

- WIPER:
  - *Wash* your hands
  - *Introduce* yourself
  - Ask about *pain*
  - Appropriately *expose*
  - *Reposition*
- Explain the examination to the patient and your reasons for performing it
- Gain verbal consent
- Give the patient privacy to expose themselves as required
- Start in a comfortable position (usually sitting in a chair or bed)
- Offer a chaperone

LOOK

Important to note whether:
- Changes are symmetrical or asymmetrical

Ask the patient to remove his clothing so that the entire back can be inspected.
- Inspect from front, side and back, looking for:
  - General inspection: Walking aids, frailty
  - Gait: By asking the patient to walk to the door and back

Difficulty with tip-toe walking indicates S1 weakness
Difficulty with heel walking indicates L5 weakness
  - Asymmetry: Shoulder asymmetry or pelvic tilt
  - Muscle: Spasms or wasting
  - Scars: Previous surgery
  - Skin changes: For example, café au lait spots may suggest neurofibromatosis. Fat pad or hairy patch may suggest spina bifida
  - Scapula: Winged scapula may suggest long thoracic nerve injury
- Check whether the shoulders, hips, knees and ankles are parallel
- Assess both the thoracic and lumbar curvatures:
  - Increased thoracic kyphosis is a feature of osteoporosis, advanced ankylosing spondylitis and Scheuermann's kyphosis
  - Flattening or reversal of lumbar lordosis is a common finding in prolapsed intervertebral disc, osteoarthritis of the spine, infections of the vertebral bodies and ankylosing spondylitis
  - Look for lateral curvature: May be a sign of scoliosis
- Ask the patient to stand with their back against the wall. The heels, pelvis, shoulders and occiput should all be able to touch the wall simultaneously (Fig. 3.4). In patients with ankylosing spondylitis or increased thoracic kyphosis this may be difficult or impossible

FEEL

Ensure to ask patients if they have pain and clarify the location. With the patient standing, palpate the:
- Spinous processes from T1 to the sacrum
- Sacroiliac joints for tenderness
- Paraspinal musculature

PERCUSSION

- Lightly percuss the spine, starting at the top of the neck, going down to the sacrum
- Significant pain is associated with infection, malignancy and fractures

MOVE

Flexion, extension and lateral flexion are movements of the lumbar spine. Rotation occurs in the thoracic spine.

FLEXION

- Ask the patient to touch their toes while keeping their legs straight
- Normal is 90°

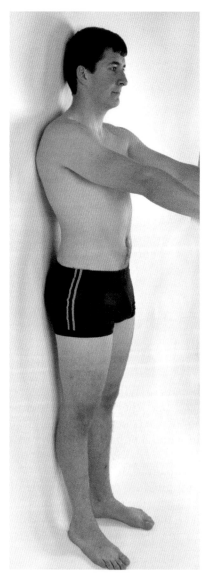

Fig. 3.4 Assessing the curvature of the spine. Note the position of the heels, pelvis, shoulders and occiput.

- Watch closely for curvature of the spine, smoothness of movement and any restriction, remembering that hip flexion can compensate for a stiff lumbar spine
- Measure flexion through the modified Schober method (Fig. 3.5)
- Locate the dimples of Venus, which overlie the sacroiliac joints
- Using a tape measure mark 10 cm above the dimples of Venus with a pen (point A), and 5 cm below (point B)
- Anchor the top of the tape with a finger at point B and ask the patient to flex forward as far as possible
- The distance between point A and point B increases with lumbar flexion. Measure the change in this distance with the above manoeuvre
- This is normally 6–7 cm. Anything < 5 cm is suggestive of spinal pathology

EXTENSION (FIG. 3.6A)

- Ask the patient to arch their back, assisting them by steadying the pelvis
- Normal is 30°

LATERAL FLEXION (FIG. 3.6B)

- Ensure that the legs are straight
- Ask the patient to slide their hands down the side of each leg in turn – the left hand down the left leg and the right hand down the right leg
- Normal is 25°

ROTATION (FIG. 3.6C)

- With the patient seated, ask them to twist their shoulders around to each side
- Rotation is measured between the plane of shoulders and the pelvis
- Normal is 40°

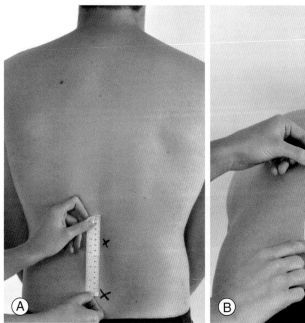
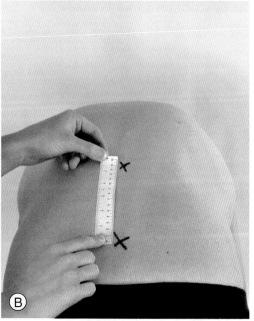

Fig. 3.5 (A, B) Modified Schober method for assessing flexion.

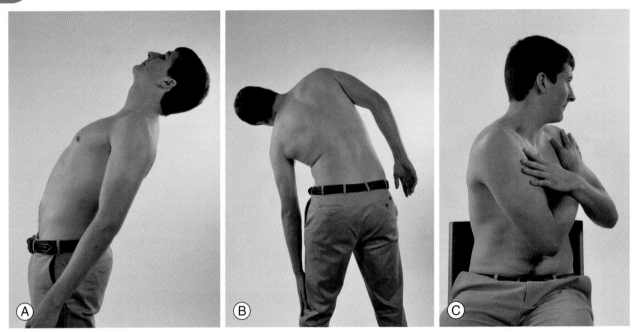

Fig. 3.6 Assessing (A) extension, (B) lateral flexion and (C) rotation.

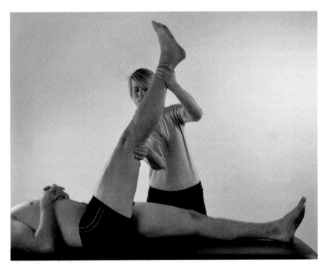

Fig. 3.7 Straight-leg raise with the angle to measure demonstrated.

SPECIAL TESTS

STRAIGHT-LEG RAISE

- Assesses L4, L5, S1 nerve roots, thus L4/5, L5/S1 and S1/S2 disc spaces (Fig. 3.7)
- With the patient lying on his back, maximally flex his hip whilst keeping the leg straight
- The test is positive if the patient experiences pain going down the entire lower limb, past the knee. Frequently there will be pain and tightness that affect the posterior thigh only; this is not a positive test
- Measure the angle between the bed and the leg
- Normal is 80–90° hip flexion

TIBIAL STRETCH TEST

- Assesses L4–S3 nerve roots (Fig. 3.8)

- With the patient lying supine, passively flex the knee to 90° and then flex the hip to 90°, before extending the knee, keeping the hip flexed to 90°
- Apply pressure over both hamstring tendons in the one leg
- Observe for pain
- Then apply pressure over the middle of the popliteal fossa, where the tibial nerve runs
- Pain when the nerve is pressed, but not when the hamstring tendons are pressed, is a positive finding

FEMORAL STRETCH TEST

- Assesses L2–L4 nerve roots (Fig. 3.9)
- With the patient lying on their front, flex the knee to 90° and maximally extend the hip
- Pain in the back or radiating down the anterior thigh is a positive result

NEUROVASCULAR ASSESSMENT

- Neurological assessment of the lower limbs assesses dermatomes (Fig. 3.10), myotomes and reflexes
- PR examination assesses the anal tone and for saddle anaesthesia
- See Table 3.2 for more information

FINISHING

- Offer to:
  - Examine the hips, shoulders and cervical spine.
- Thank the patient
- Check they're comfortable and offer to help reposition them
- Wash your hands
- Leave the patient in privacy to get dressed

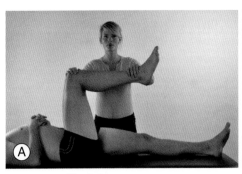
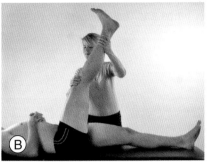
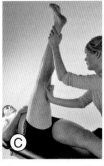
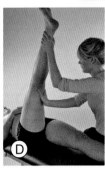

Fig. 3.8 Tibial stretch test: (A) flexing the knee and hip; (B) straightening the knee; (C) pressure over the hamstring tendons; and (D) pressure over the tibial nerve.

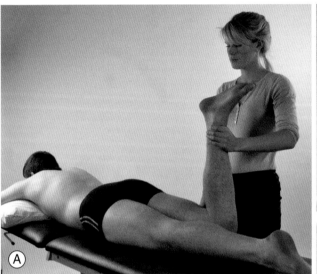
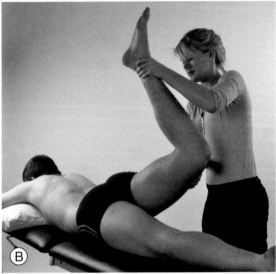

Fig. 3.9 (A, B) Femoral stretch test.

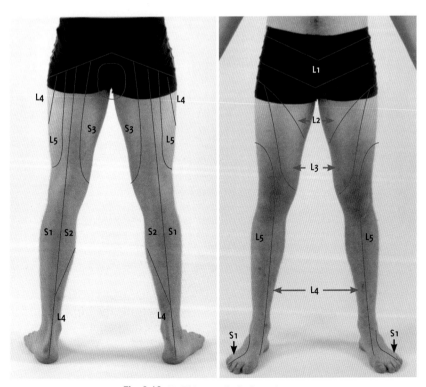

Fig. 3.10 (A, B) Lower-limb dermatomes.

⎯⋏⎯ Table **3.2**   **Nerve roots in the lower limbs and their respective dermatome, myotome and reflex**

NERVE ROOT	DERMATOME	MYOTOME	REFLEX
L2	Medial upper thigh	Hip flexion	Nil
L3	Medial lower thigh	Knee extension	Knee
L4	Medial calf	Ankle dorsiflexion	Knee
L5	First dorsal web space, lateral calf and dorsum of the foot	Great toe dorsiflexion	Nil
S1	Lateral sole of the foot and posterolateral calf	Plantar flexion	Ankle

❗ Common thoracolumbar spine diagnoses

CATEGORY	DIAGNOSIS	PRESENTATION

Traumatic	Fracture	• Major trauma
		• Pathological fracture: > 70-year-olds
		  • Extensive use of steroids
		  • Pain following minor fall, coughing or heavy lifting
		  • Vertebral tenderness on examination

Idiopathic	Mechanical back pain	• Back pain, which may radiate to the buttocks • Pain worse on movement • May have had episodes of back pain in the past, which has settled • No neurological, bladder or bowel symptoms
Degenerative	Degenerative disc disease	• Chronic and acute presentations • Lower-back pain, which may radiate to the buttocks • Restricted range of movement
	Cauda equina syndrome	• Severe back pain • Lower motor neurone weakness • Flaccid tone in lower limbs • Loss of reflexes in lower limbs bilaterally • Absent plantars • Perianal or saddle anaesthesia • Decreased anal tone • Bladder, bowel or sexual dysfunction
Inflammatory	Ankylosing spondyloarthritis	• Back pain and stiffness worse in the morning • Improves with movement • Young males typically affected • Extra-articular symptoms: Anterior uveitis, psoriasis, inflammatory bowel disease (IBD)
Infection	Discitis	• Pain may be severe and worse with activity • May be of insidious onset • Pain may wake the patient up at night • May have neurological signs
Neoplastic	Metastatic spinal cord compression	• Severe back pain • Upper motor neurone weakness • Bilateral weakness in flexors • Increased tone in lower limbs • Brisk reflexes in lower limbs bilaterally • Upgoing plantars • ± Sensory disturbances
	Spondylolisthesis (vertebral body slipped over another)	• Back pain and stiffness • May have tingling sensation or numbness down the legs • Difficulty walking • Tight hamstrings • Kyphosis

Present Your Findings

Mr MacPherson is an 85-year-old man who has presented with back pain. On examination, this man has tenderness over his lumbar spinal and paraspinal muscles to palpation and percussion. He has a decreased range of hip flexion and extension bilaterally. Straight-leg test was positive at 65° flexion. Neurologically, he has hypoaesthesia over the L4–S1 dermatomes and flaccid weakness of ankle and toe dorsiflexion and plantar flexion bilaterally. Both ankle reflexes are absent. In addition, he has perianal hypoaesthesia on PR examination with reduced anal tone.

These findings are consistent with a diagnosis of metastatic spinal cord compression, most likely secondary to prostatic cancer bone metastasis. This is a medical emergency. To complete my examination, I would like to request an urgent MRI, commence steroid therapy and consider for further neurosurgical and/or oncological intervention.

❓ QUESTIONS AND ANSWERS FOR CANDIDATE

How is metastatic spinal cord compression managed?
- Analgesia
- Oral dexamethasone
- Urgent MRI spine
- Early discussion with neurosurgery and oncology, with the possibility of neurosurgical decompression or palliative radiotherapy

Give three red flags for neoplastic involvement of spine.
- Age < 20 or > 50 years old
- History of malignancy
- Pain waking the patient at night
- Pain not improved by rest
- Pain not relieved by conservative management
- Pain in the thoracic region
- Systemic symptoms; for example, fever, weight loss and night sweats

What tumours are more likely to metastasise to bone?
- Prostate
- Breast
- Kidney
- Thyroid
- Lung

Note: Use the mnemonic: 'lead kettle' to remember these: Pb is lead on the periodic table.

 A Case to Learn From

I once saw a patient with ankylosing spondylitis for a review. His back symptoms were stable and settled. It was only on systems review that the patient revealed that he had eye pain and photophobia which were causing him trouble when looking at screens at work. The patient was urgently referred to ophthalmology to treat the anterior uveitis. Always remember to perform a systems review as patients may not always provide you with this information themselves.

 Top Tip

Remember the clinical patterns associated with upper motor neurone and lower motor neurone lesions – this is an easy question to ask in an exam!

 Top Tip

Patients with chronic back pain may have a discoloration of the skin, erythema ab igne, related to hot water bottle use.

STATION 3.3: SHOULDER

SCENARIO

You are a junior doctor working in orthopaedics and have been asked to see Stephen O'Humeral, a 50-year-old non-binary person complaining of pain in and around his right shoulder. The pain is worse when trying to reach into his kitchen cupboards, and he has now been referred in by his primary care physician. Please examine Mr O'Humeral and present your findings.

PREPARATION

- WIPER:
  - *Wash* your hands
  - *Introduce* yourself
  - Ask about *pain*
  - Appropriately *expose*
  - *Reposition*
- Explain the examination to the patient and your reasons for performing it
- Gain verbal consent
- Give the patient privacy to expose themselves as required
- Start in a comfortable position (usually sitting in a chair or bed)
- Offer a chaperone

LOOK

Important to note whether:
- Changes are symmetrical or asymmetrical
  Ask the patients to remove enough clothing to expose the shoulder and joints above and below:
- Inspect both shoulders from front, side and back, starting with the normal shoulder, looking for:
  - General inspection: Check for deformity, swelling, scars and asymmetry
  - Muscle bulk: Assess the deltoid, pectoralis, supraspinatus and infraspinatus muscles, looking for muscle wasting
  - Scapula: Look at the scapula for winging, which would suggest long thoracic nerve palsy

FEEL

Ensure to ask patients if they have pain and clarify the location.

- Ask the patient to tell you if palpation causes pain
- Feel the temperature of the clavicle, acromioclavicular joint, scapular spine and biceps tendon, comparing both sides
- Palpate each of the following, assessing for tenderness, bony abnormalities, for example, osteophytes, swelling and deformity:
  - Sternoclavicular joint
  - Clavicle
  - Acromion
  - Coracoid
  - Scapular spine
  - Biceps tendon
- Extend the shoulder, bringing the supraspinous tendon anterior to the acromion, allowing it to be palpated
- Palpate the surrounding muscles, subacromial space and greater tuberosity, assessing for tenderness

MOVE

First, screen cervical spine movements by asking the patient to:

- Nod head back and forth
- Look left then right
- Try to touch ear to each shoulder

Assess shoulder function by asking the patient to:

- Put their hands behind their head (Fig. 3.11)
- Put their hands to the mouth
- Reach high up on the back (Fig. 3.12A)
- Reach their hands to the lower back
- Perform circular 'stirring' movements with each upper limb (Fig. 3.12B)
- Determine the range of active, then passive, movements

FLEXION (FIG. 3.13A)

- Normal is 0–180°

EXTENSION (FIG. 3.13B)

- Normal is 0–60°

ABDUCTION

- Whilst palpating the inferior pole of the scapula with your hand, assess the proportion of movement occurring at the glenohumeral joint versus the amount coming from the scapula rotating
- Normal is 0–150° (Fig. 3.14)

EXTERNAL ROTATION

- Ask the patient to flex their elbow to 90°, holding it to the side of their body, with the fist pointed forward. Then ask them to rotate their arm outwards (Fig. 3.15)

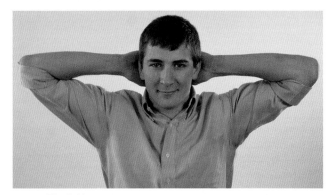

Fig. 3.11 Assessing function: Hands behind the head.

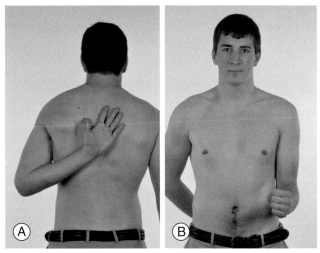

Fig. 3.12 Assessing function: (A) Reaching up the back and (B) making 'stirring' movements.

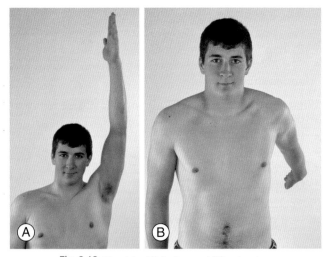

Fig. 3.13 Shoulder (A) flexion and (B) extension.

- Normal is 0–90°
- External rotation is restricted in frozen shoulder

INTERNAL ROTATION

- Ask the patient to rotate their arm across their back and then walk their thumb up their vertebrae
- Record the highest vertebra that the thumb can touch

- Normal is the mid thoracic level (Fig. 3.15C)
- Assess movements passively, feeling for crepitus with one hand over the shoulder joint

SPECIAL TESTS

IMPINGEMENT SYNDROME

Assesses for a painful arc:
- Passively abduct the shoulder
- Once it is fully abducted, release and ask the patient to adduct it slowly
- Pain between 60 and 120° implies a painful arc
- Pain during this manoeuvre is almost pathognomonic of supraspinatous tendonitis

SCARF TEST

Assesses for acromioclavicular joint pathology:

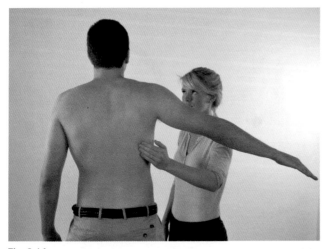

Fig. 3.14 Abduction, with the examiner palpating the lower pole of the scapula.

- Ask the patient to flex their shoulder and elbow to 90° and then place the hand on the opposite shoulder
- Apply a posteriorly directed force over the flexed elbow
- Pain indicates acromioclavicular joint pathology

ROTATOR CUFF

- Each of the four muscles forming the rotator cuff needs to be assessed (Fig. 3.16)
- In the following tests, positive findings are:
  - Loss of power, which suggests a tear
  - Pain, which suggests tendonitis

Supraspinatous:
- Assess the first 15° of shoulder abduction against resistance
- Jobe's test is shoulder abduction against resistance with the thumb pointing down to the floor

Infraspinatous and teres minor:
- Assess external rotation against resistance, elbows flexed to 90° and arms adducted
- This test is more specific if the shoulder is flexed to 30° before externally rotating it, as this diminishes the contribution of the deltoid

Gerber's lift-off test
- Assesses the function of subscapularis
- Test internal rotation against resistance by asking the patient to lift their hands off their back whilst you try to keep them there

BICIPITAL TENDONITIS

- Supinate the forearm and then flex the shoulder against resistance
- Similar to the rotator cuff muscles:
  - Loss of power suggests a tear
  - Pain suggests tendonitis (Fig. 3.17)

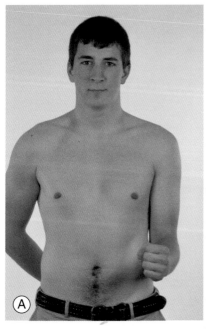
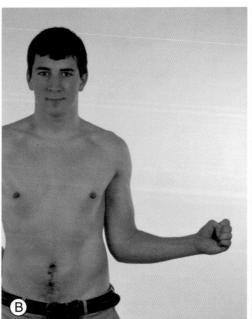
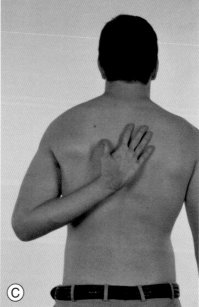

Fig. 3.15 (A, B) External rotation and (C) internal rotation.

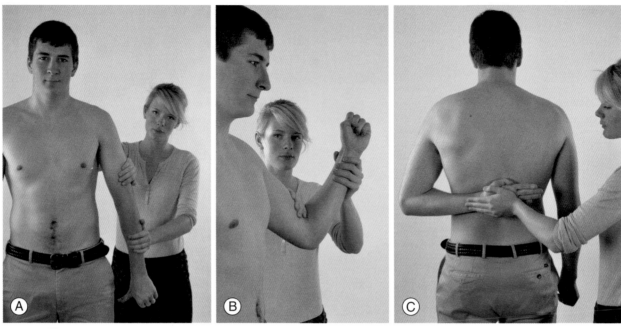

Fig. 3.16 Assessing the rotator cuff: (A) Supraspinatous – Jobe's test; (B) infraspinatous and teres minor; and (C) subscapularis.

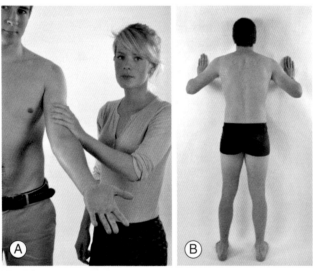

Fig. 3.17 (A) Assessing for bicipital tendonitis; (B) testing for a 'winged scapula' by asking the patient to push against a wall and observing for abnormal protrusion of the scapulae.

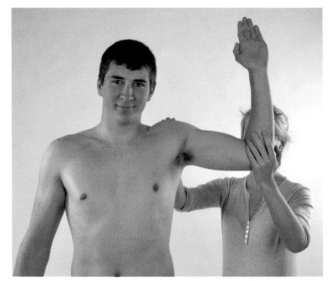

Fig. 3.18 The shoulder apprehension test.

WINGED SCAPULA (3.17B)

- Assesses for long thoracic nerve injury
- Ask the patient to push forcefully against a wall with the palms of both hands, whilst standing facing the wall
- Look at their back for a 'winged scapula', where the scapula protrudes from the back in an abnormal way
- This suggests damage to the long thoracic nerve supplying the serratus anterior

SHOULDER APPREHENSION TEST (FIG. 3.18)

- Stand behind the patient and ask them to abduct their shoulder to 90°, flex their elbow to 90° and externally rotate so that the fingers are pointing towards the ceiling
- Put one of your hands over their shoulder and with your other hand, hold their elbow
- Push forward on their shoulder and pull back on the elbow
- Apprehension to this manoeuvre is a positive test, suggesting previous dislocation

NEUROVASCULAR ASSESSMENT

- Assess sensation at the regimental badge area (the skin covering the inferior region of the deltoid muscle). This is supplied by the axillary nerve

- In anterior shoulder dislocation, the axillary nerve may be compressed, leading to abnormal sensation
- Assess dermatomes and myotomes (C5–T1) (Station 3.1: Cervical spine)
- Palpate the radial pulse. If not present, palpate the brachial pulse
- Check capillary refill time and ensure that the hand is warm and well perfused

FINISHING

- Offer to:
  - Examine the neck (specifically cervical spine) and elbow
- Thank the patient
- Check they're comfortable and offer to help reposition them
- Wash your hands
- Leave the patient in privacy to get dressed

⚠️ Common diagnosis from shoulder examination

DIAGNOSIS	PRESENTATION
Impingement syndrome	• Usually middle-aged • Good range of passive movement • Pain worse on overhead movements • Painful arc test positive (60–120°)
Rotator cuff tear	• Often elderly, occasionally younger patients from trauma • Painless limited range of movement • Special tests positive depending on location of tear
Frozen shoulder (adhesive capsulitis)	• Usually middle-aged • May have history of diabetes or thyroid disease • Sudden-onset pain and stiffness • Limited external rotation strongly suggestive
Calcific tendonitis	• Usually middle-aged • May have diabetes • Sudden-onset shoulder pain • Pain may increase at night • Limited range of movement
Glenohumeral osteoarthritis	• Usually elderly • Limits external rotation
Shoulder dislocation	• Usually younger patients, sometimes elderly from falls • Asymmetrical and displaced on inspection • Anterior dislocations are more common • Posterior dislocations are unusual and usually with a history of seizures or electrocution • Pain • Limited range of movement

AXILLARY NERVE INJURY

Signs of an axillary nerve injury include:
- Pain to deltoid and anterior shoulder of the affected side
- Loss of movement in the shoulder area of the affected side
- Loss or reduction in sensation in the regimental badge region of the affected side
- Weakness to the deltoid or teres minor muscles; for example, difficulty with abduction and external rotation

🔍 Present Your Findings

Mr O'Humeral is a 50-year-old non-binary person who presented with right-shoulder pain and difficulties reaching overhead. On examination, their right shoulder is tender over the acromion. There are no signs of infection in the joint. Active abduction is difficult for the patient to initiate due to pain, but there is a full range of movement for passive abduction. In addition, there is a painful arc between 70 and 120°. The other movements at the shoulder are normal, including the other rotator muscles. The left shoulder is normal, as is examination of the elbow and neck.

These findings are in keeping with a diagnosis of chronic tendonitis, also known as impingement syndrome. To complete my examination I would like to test the neurovascular status of the arm, provide adequate analgesia and refer to physiotherapy.

❓ QUESTIONS AND ANSWERS FOR CANDIDATE

What are the names of some special tests for assessing rotator cuff tear, the muscle they test and the muscle action?
- Jobe's test, supraspinatous, abduction
- Resisted external rotation, infraspinatous and teres minor, external rotation
- Gerber's lift-off test, subscapularis, internal rotation

What are the three phases of frozen shoulder recovery?
- Freezing phase (3 months)
- Frozen phase (6 months)
- Thawing phase (12 months)

What investigation would be useful if suspecting a rotator cuff tear?
- MRI

A Case to Learn From

A patient with shoulder pain was being cared for in primary care. The patient had chronic shoulder pain and was managed conservatively with simple analgesia, rest and physiotherapy. The pain that the patient reported was worsening and began to impact on their quality of life. Following referral to secondary care, the patient was diagnosed with cervical spine disease. It is always vital to examine the joints above and below the joint with the presenting complaint.

> **Top Tip**
>
> When a patient comes in with shoulder dislocation, it is important to consider that anterior shoulder dislocations can affect the axillary nerve. The dislocation of the shoulder or the reduction manoeuvre for it can cause traction injuries to the axillary nerve. Therefore, it is important to document the status of the axillary nerve before and after manipulation.

STATION 3.4: ELBOW

SCENARIO

You are a junior doctor in orthopaedics and have been asked to see William Murray, a 35-year-old painter and decorator who has presented with right-elbow pain and reduced grip strength in the right hand. The pain has developed gradually over the last year and now his elbow is causing him difficulty at work. He has been referred in by his primary care physician. Please examine Mr Murray and present your findings.

PREPARATION

- WIPER:
  - *Wash* your hands
  - *Introduce* yourself
  - Ask about *pain*
  - Appropriately *expose*
  - *Reposition*
- Explain the examination to the patient and your reasons for performing it
- Gain verbal consent
- Give the patient privacy to expose themselves as required
- Start in a comfortable position (usually sitting in a chair or bed)
- Offer a chaperone

LOOK

Important to note whether:
- Changes are symmetrical or asymmetrical

Ensure that the patient is standing in the anatomical position. Ask the patient to remove enough clothing to expose the elbow and joints above and below.
- Inspect from the front, back, medial and lateral sides of the elbow, looking for:
  - General inspection: Asymmetry, scars
  - Carrying angle: 5–15° of cubitus valgus is normal to stop the arm hitting the hip whilst walking. Cubitus varus, forearm towards body, suggests previous paediatric supracondylar fracture. Cubitus valgus suggests non-union of previous fracture (Fig. 3.19)
  - Deformities: Fixed flexion deformity

- Skin changes: Rheumatoid nodules, psoriatic plaques
- Signs of inflammation: Olecranon bursitis may present as erythema and swelling of elbow
- Muscle wasting: Biceps and triceps

FEEL

Ensure to ask patients if they have pain and clarify the location.
- Assess the temperature of the elbow using the back of your hand. Do not forget to check the front and back of the elbow
- Palpate:
  - Olecranon process
  - Medial and lateral epicondyle
  - Radial head
- Palpate the distal biceps tendon:
  - Ask the patient to flex the elbow to 90°
  - Palpate over the anterior crease in the elbow using three fingers to feel a tensed tendon

MOVE

- Determine the range of active, then passive, movements

ELBOW FLEXION

- Normal is 0–150°

ELBOW EXTENSION

- Normal is 0°

PRONATION

- Normal is 70°
- Ask the patient to push their elbows into their sides, and flex the elbow to 90°

SUPINATION

- Normal is 90°

Additionally, do not forget to feel the elbow joint for crepitus with one hand, whilst actively assessing range of movement with the other.

SPECIAL TESTS

FUNCTION

Assess function by asking the patient to:
- Raise their hands to the mouth: Eating
- Reach their hands to the buttocks: Toileting

COZEN'S TEST

- Tests for lateral epicondylitis or tennis elbow (Fig. 3.20)
- Tests active wrist extension against resistance
- Palpate the lateral epicondyle

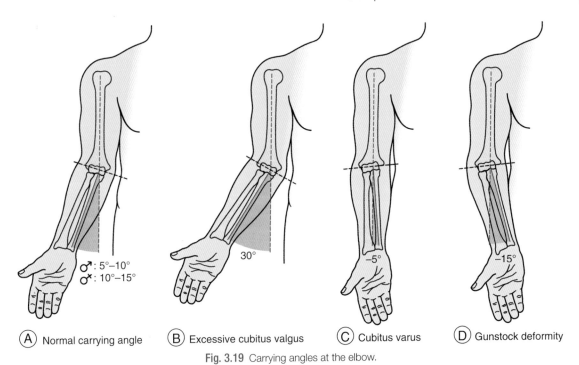

(A) Normal carrying angle   ♂: 5°–10° ♀: 10°–15°

(B) Excessive cubitus valgus   30°

(C) Cubitus varus   −5°

(D) Gunstock deformity   −15°

Fig. 3.19 Carrying angles at the elbow.

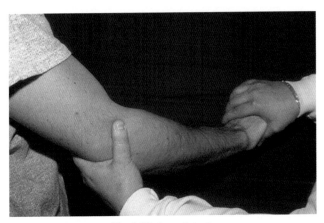

Fig. 3.20 Cozen's test.

- Ask the patient to clench their hand into a fist and extend their wrist
- Push down gently on the extended wrist, whilst asking the patient to continue extending wrist
- Positive finding would be if the test reproduces pain

GOLFER'S ELBOW TEST

- Tests for medial epicondylitis or golfer's elbow (Fig. 3.21)
- Tests active wrist flexion against resistance
- Ensure that the patient's elbow is flexed at 90° and feel the medial epicondyle with one hand
- Ask the patient to make a fist and flex their wrist
- Gently try to extend the wrist with your other hand, asking the patient to continue flexing, opposing the resistance
- Positive finding is manoeuvre reproducing pain

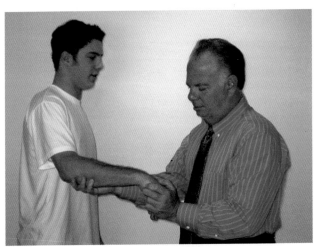

Fig. 3.21 Golfer's elbow test.

NEUROVASCULAR ASSESSMENT

- Perform a full peripheral nerve examination on the upper limbs
- Perform a vascular assessment of the upper limbs

FINISHING

- Offer to:
  - Examine the shoulder and wrist
- Thank the patient
- Check they're comfortable and offer to help reposition them
- Wash your hands
- Leave the patient in privacy to get dressed

! Common diagnoses from elbow examination

DIAGNOSIS	PRESENTATION	EXAMINATION FINDINGS
Elbow osteoarthritis	• Painful joint • Morning stiffness • Exacerbated by exercise • Limited range of movement impeding daily activities • 'Locking' may be felt by the patient	• Limited range of movement • Crepitus may be felt • If long-standing disease, then may have ulnar nerve signs (see cubital tunnel syndrome)
Lateral epicondylitis: 'Tennis elbow'	• Pain and burning on lateral elbow • Pain may radiate down extensors • Develops over time • Caused by repetitive supination and pronation in extension. The patient may have hobby/work that involves this movement; for example, backhand swings during tennis	• Cozen's test positive • Weak grip strength
Medial epicondylitis: 'Golfer's elbow'	• Pain and burning on medial elbow • Develops over time • Caused by repetitive wrist flexion and pronation. The patient may have hobby/work that involves this movement	• Golfer's test positive
Ulnar nerve entrapment: 'Cubital tunnel syndrome'	• Numbness and tingling in the hands or fingers. The ulnar nerve supplies the little finger and half of the ring finger • Common provoking factors in the history include keeping the elbow bent for a long time and leaning on the elbow	• Weak grip strength • May have muscle wasting if long-standing disease
Elbow dislocation	• Usually following a fall on outstretched hand	• Presents with gross deformity • Pain • Limited range of movement

Present Your Findings

Mr Murray is a 35-year-old male who presented with elbow pain and reduced grip strength of the right arm. On examination, there was a small amount of tenderness of the lateral right epicondyle on palpation. Range of movement was normal. Cozen's test was positive.

This is consistent with a diagnosis of lateral epicondylitis (tennis elbow), with differentials being radial nerve syndrome (compression of the posterior interosseous nerve), cervical radiculopathy, elbow osteoarthritis and a fracture of the radius or olecranon.

To complete my examination, I would like to check the neurovascular status of the elbow, examine the shoulder and hand and order an ultrasound or MRI if there were doubts over the diagnosis. I would also ensure adequate analgesia and offer activity modification advice.

? QUESTIONS AND ANSWERS FOR CANDIDATE

What is the management of epicondylitis?
Conservative:
• Activity modification
• Analgesia
• Physiotherapy
• Orthosis
• Corticosteroid injection

Surgical:
• Surgical release

What is the terrible triad of the elbow?
An elbow fracture-dislocation pattern associated with high trauma:
• Posterior dislocation of elbow
• Radial head fracture

• Coronoid process fracture

What investigations may be of use for ulnar nerve entrapment?
To rule out pathology, the following investigations can be used:
• Ultrasound or MRI for bony mass or anatomical cause of entrapment
• X-ray of elbow if bony deformities suspected
• X-ray of cervical neck for cervical rib
• Blood tests to rule out anaemia, diabetes and hypothyroidism, which are all associated with peripheral neuropathy
• Nerve conduction studies to determine the function of nerve

A Case to Learn From

A patient presented to hospital with acute left lateral elbow pain. It was presumed lateral epicondylitis (tennis elbow) and initially there was no plan to image her elbow. She later disclosed to a nurse that she had slipped over a week ago and landed on her left side. Further imaging demonstrated a small avulsion fracture. Ensure you take a full history, including trauma. Patients may not disclose things that happened more than a few days previously as they may not feel it pertinent to their presenting complaint.

Top Tip

Examiners will appreciate you paying close attention to the inverted triangle on the posterior aspect of the elbow. This is formed by the medial and lateral epicondyles, and the olecranon. Palpation of this area with the elbow flexed and during pronation and supination is essential.

STATION 3.5: HAND AND WRIST

SCENARIO

You are a junior doctor in orthopaedics and have been asked to see Caitlyn King, a 45-year-old woman who has presented with pain and stiffness of the finger joints. This has been an ongoing problem for the past year and she has been referred in by her primary care physician. Please examine Mrs King and present your findings.

PREPARATION

- WIPER:
  - *Wash* your hands
  - *Introduce* yourself
  - Ask about *pain*
  - Appropriately *expose*
  - *Reposition*
- Explain the examination to the patient and your reasons for performing it
- Gain verbal consent
- Give the patient privacy to expose themselves as required
- Start in a comfortable position (usually sitting in a chair or bed)
- Offer a chaperone

LOOK

Important to note whether:
- Changes are symmetrical or asymmetrical
- Changes mainly involve the small joints in the hands or the wrists
- Ask the patient to remove enough clothing to expose the hands, wrists and elbows
- Inspect from front, side and back, looking for:
  - General inspection: Frailty, splints, muscle wasting, asymmetry
  - Cushingoid features: Long-term steroid use
  - Signs of systemic disease: Swelling, redness
  - Tremor: With the patient's hands outstretched
  - Ear: Tophi on ear (gout) (Fig. 3.22), skin changes behind the back of the ear (psoriasis, eczema)
- Inspect the elbows for:
  - Rheumatoid nodules
  - Psoriasis
  - Scars

With the patient's palms down (Fig. 3.23), look for:
- General inspection: Asymmetry and deformity
- Shortening: Psoriatic arthritis
- Swelling and erythema: Infection, gout
- Muscle: Wasting
- Skin: Scars, thinning and bruising of skin can indicate steroid use
- Wrists:
  - Radiocarpal subluxation: Rheumatoid arthritis

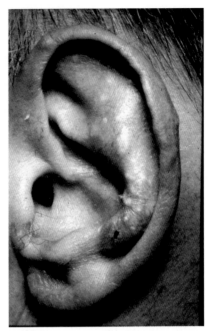

Fig. 3.22 Gouty tophi visible on general inspection.

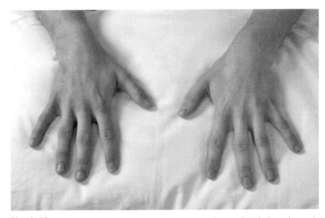

Fig. 3.23 Palms down: Using a pillow to rest the patient's hands on is often the most comfortable way to inspect them.

- Dorsum:
  - Wasting: Ulnar nerve palsy
- Metacarpophalangeal (MCP) joint:
  - Ulnar deviation and subluxation: Rheumatoid arthritis
- Fingers:
  - Swan neck deformity: Flexion at the MCP and distal interphalangeal (DIP) joints, extension at the proximal interphalangeal (PIP) joint
  - Boutonnière deformity: Extension at the MCP and DIP joints, flexion at the PIP joint
  - Z-shaped deformity of the thumb: Flexion at the MCP joint, hyperextension at the PIP joint
  - Mallet finger: Involuntary flexion of the distal phalanx of a finger
  - Nodes: Heberden's (found at the DIP joints) or Bouchard's (found at the PIP joints) nodes suggestive of osteoarthritis

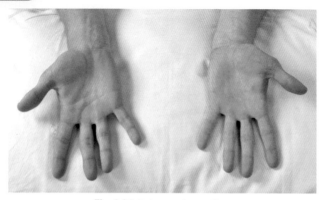

Fig. 3.24 Palms-up inspection.

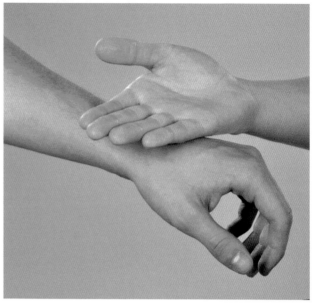

Fig. 3.25 Feeling the hands for the temperature.

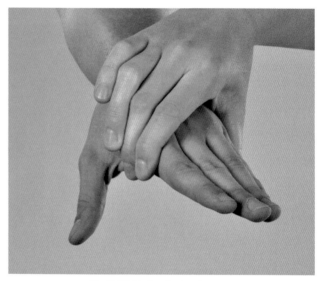

Fig. 3.26 Feeling for tenderness.

- Nails:
  - Psoriasis: Pitting, onycholysis
  - Nail fold infarcts
  With the patient's palms up (Fig. 3.24), look for:
- Problems turning the hand: Associated with radio-ulnar joint abnormality
- Wrists:
  - Scars from carpal tunnel release operation or surgery for rheumatoid arthritis
- Palms:
  - Palmar erythema
  - Muscle wasting: Involving either the thenar eminence, hypothenar eminence or both
If only thenar eminence: Suggests median nerve damage and possible carpal tunnel syndrome.
If only hypothenar eminence: Suggests ulnar nerve damage.
  - Scars: Dupuytren's contracture release surgery

FEEL

Ensure to ask patients if they have pain and clarify the location.
- With the patient's palms up:
  - Palpate radial pulses together and capillary artery refill time
  - Feel the temperature at both wrists and the MCP joints on both sides to compare
  - Feel for thickening of the palmar fascia and tendon nodules:
Dupuytren's contracture is fixed flexion contraction of hands, caused by thickening of the palmar aponeurosis.
  - Feel the bulk of the thenar and hypothenar eminences
- Ask the patient to turn their hands with the palms down:
  - Using the back of the hand, assess the temperature at the patient's forearm, wrists and MCP joints (Fig. 3.25)
  - Ask whether the patient is in pain and, importantly, looking at the patient's face, squeeze across a row of MCP joints, assessing for tenderness (Fig. 3.26)
- Bimanually palpate any MCP, PIP and DIP joints that are swollen or tender. This should be done by having your thumbs above and index finger below the joint (Fig. 3.27)
  - Any signs of active synovitis: The joint being warm, swollen, tender, rubbery
  - Are there any hard, bony swellings? Bouchard's nodes (at the PIP joints) and Heberden's nodes (at the DIP joints)
  - Bimanually palpate the wrist, ensuring to look at the patient's face for pain
  - Run your hand up the patient's arms to their elbows, looking for rheumatoid nodules or psoriatic plaques

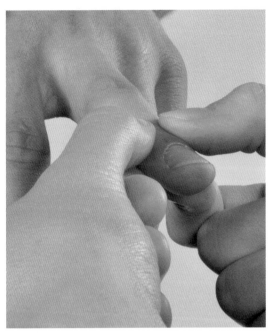

Fig. 3.27 Bimanually palpating the PIP joint.

MOVE

- Move actively before passively

EXTENSION

- Straighten fingers fully

FLEXION

- Make a fist

ABDUCTION AND ADDUCTION (FIG. 3.28)

- Abduct and adduct fingers
- Touch the tip of each finger with the thumb on the same hand (opposition)

WRIST EXTENSION AND FLEXION (FIG. 3.29)

- Make a prayer and reverse prayer sign
- Assess wrist extension and flexion passively

ULNAR DEVIATION OF THE WRIST

- To assess ulnar deviation, stabilise the forearm with one hand. Then, while grasping the metacarpals from the radial side with the other hand, apply traction in the ulnar direction
- Do the opposite for radial deviation. Ulnar deviation should be greater than radial

SUPINATION AND PRONATION

- This may also be done when asking the patient to turn their hands on inspection
- Repeat passively if there is limited range of movement, or pain, ensuring to look at the patient's face

SPECIAL TESTS

PHALEN'S TEST (FIG. 3.30)

- Hold the wrist in forced flexion, reverse prayer position, for 60 s

- Paraesthesia in the distribution of the median nerve suggests carpal tunnel syndrome

TINEL'S TEST (FIG. 3.31)

- Percuss over the carpal tunnel for 30 s
- Paraesthesia in the distribution of the median nerve is suggestive of carpal tunnel syndrome

FUNCTION (FIG. 3.32)

Ask the patient to:
- Grip two of your fingers: Power grip
- Pinch your finger: Pincer grip
- Pick up an object; for example, a coin: Precision grip
- Bring their hands to their mouth (eating)
- Put their hands behind their head (dressing)
- Put their hands over their spine (toileting)

NEUROVASCULAR ASSESSMENT

Assess sensation by ensuring that the patient's eyes are closed. Touch the following areas of both hands to compare, asking if they feel the same:
- Radial: First dorsal web space
- Median: Tip of index finger
- Ulnar: Dorsolateral surface of hand

Assess power, ensuring to compare both sides.
- Radial: You push against extended wrists of the patient
- Median: You try to break a grip of the patient's thumb and little finger pinched together
- Ulnar: The patient tries to abduct their fingers while you press them together

When assessing nerves, do so systematically. Carry out an inspection, then assess sensation, followed by motor function (Table 3.3).

The difference between the hand of benediction and the claw hand (Fig. 3.33) can be confusing. Remember:
- The hand of benediction only occurs when the patient tries to make a fist, whereas the claw hand occurs at rest
- There is flexion at the MCP joints of the ring and index fingers in the hand of benediction, whereas the MCP joints of these fingers are extended in the claw hand

FINISHING

- Offer to:
  - Examine the elbow
- Thank the patient
- Check they're comfortable and offer to help reposition them
- Wash your hands
- Leave the patient in privacy to get dressed

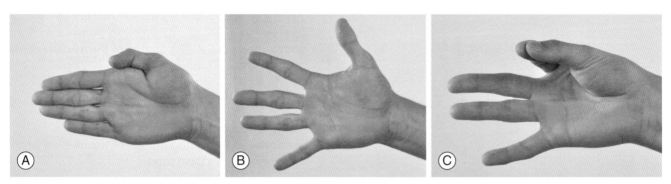

Fig. 3.28 Assessing active movement: (A) Adduction; (B) abduction; and (C) opposition.

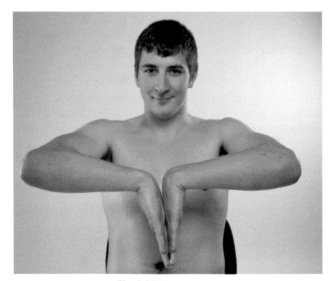
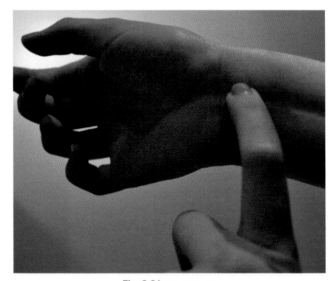

Fig. 3.29 Assessing active movement. Assess flexion with the reverse prayer sign (A) and wrist extension with the prayer sign (B).

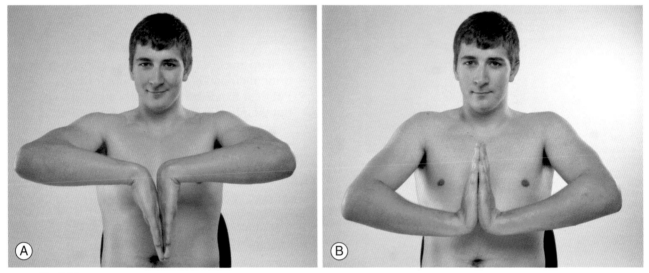

Fig. 3.30 Phalen's test.

Fig. 3.31 Tinel's test.

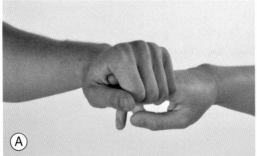
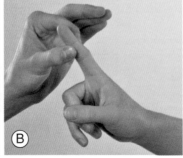
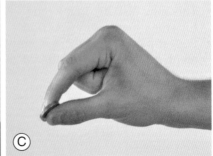

Fig. 3.32 Testing function: (A) Power grip; (B) pincer grip; and (C) precision grip.

! Common hand and wrist diagnoses and how to differentiate between them

	RHEUMATOID ARTHRITIS	OSTEOARTHRITIS	PSORIATIC ARTHRITIS
Typically affected joints	• MCP joints	• DIP, PIP, carpometacarpal (CMC) joint of the thumb	• DIP joints.
Palmar features	• Wasting of the thenar eminence • Palmar erythema • Z thumb deformity • Reduced range of movement • Boutonnière and swan neck deformities • Raised temperature	• Diffuse atrophy • Reduced range of movement • Normal temperature	• Reduced range of movement • Erythema
Dorsal features	• Wrist subluxation • Soft-tissue swelling • Wasting of intrinsic muscles (guttering)	• Squaring of the CMC joints • Bouchard's nodes (at the PIP joints) • Heberden's nodes (at the DIP joints) • Crepitus	• Nail changes • Dactylitis, 'sausage finger'
Radiological features	• Loss of joint space • Erosions • Periarticular osteoporosis • Deformity • Soft-tissue swelling	• Loss of joint space • Subchondral sclerosis • Bone cysts • Osteophytes	• Arthritis mutilans, 'telescoping' • Erosions, 'pencil-in-cup' deformity • Joint subluxation • Soft-tissue swelling, 'sausaging' • Bone proliferation, 'fuzzy'

ASSESSING TENDONS

Suspect a tendon injury if the patient is unable to perform any of the tests listed in Table 3.4.

Present Your Findings

Mrs King is a 45-year-old woman who presented with bilateral painful and stiff finger joints. On examination, the MCP joints were swollen with erythema bilaterally. Additionally, there was slight radiocarpal subluxation and ulnar deviation. Z thumb was also observed in the right hand. Range of movement was limited bilaterally, and function was also poor. Neurovascular status was intact.

This is consistent with a diagnosis of rheumatoid arthritis, with differentials being psoriatic arthritis, osteoarthritis and gout. To complete my examination I would like to examine the elbow, perform an X-ray, perform relevant blood tests and refer to rheumatology. I would also ensure adequate analgesia.

? QUESTIONS AND ANSWERS FOR CANDIDATE

What are the structures that run through the carpal tunnel?
• Four flexor digitorum profundus tendons
• Four flexor digitorum superficialis tendons
• Flexor pollicis longus tendon
• Median nerve

What is the motor function for each nerve?
• Median: Abducts thumb, flexes fingers
• Radial: Extends fingers and wrist

• Ulnar: Claws fourth and fifth finger, spreads second and third fingers, adducts thumb

Where at the hand would you test for sensation for each nerve?
• Radial: First dorsal web space
• Ulnar: Radial border of index finger
• Median: Ulnar border of fifth finger

A Case to Learn From

One time, a patient in her late 50s presented with swollen and stiff fingers. She was diagnosed with osteoarthritis. It wasn't until a few consultations later that the doctor noticed some nail pitting and small scaly, red patches developing on the patient's hand. Interestingly, some patients with psoriatic arthritis will develop arthritis before psoriasis, so it is important not to forget about psoriatic arthritis as a differential.

Top Tip

Remember to ask about hand dominance and any hobbies or occupations that require dexterity or a high level of function. Additionally, in the case of lacerations, examine the hand in the position it was when injured; for example, a clenched fist.

Top Tip

Patients with rheumatoid arthritis often have painful hands. Be sure not to cause the patient any harm during your examination. Ask the patient to turn their hands over themselves rather than doing it for them.

Table 3.3   Assessments of nerves

	RADIAL NERVE	MEDIAN NERVE	ULNAR NERVE
Muscle wasting	• None – no intrinsic muscles are supplied by the radial nerve	• Thenar eminence	• Small muscles of hand (except thenar eminence)
Sensation	• First dorsal web space	• Radial border of the index finger	• Ulnar border of the fifth finger
Motor supply	• Triceps brachii, anconeus, brachioradialis, extensor carpi radialis longus • Deep branch: Extensor carpi radialis brevis, supinator • Posterior interosseous: Extensor digitorum, extensor digiti minimi, extensor carpi ulnaris, extensor pollicis brevis, extensor pollicis longus, extensor indicis and abductor pollicis longus (Fig. 3.33)	• Supplies the 'LOAF' muscles of the hand (lateral two lumbricals, opponens pollicis, abductor pollicis brevis and flexor pollicis brevis) plus all of the flexors of the forearm (except flexor carpi ulnaris and the ulnar part of flexor digitorum profundus)	• Supplies all muscles of the hand except 'LOAF' plus flexor carpi ulnaris and the ulnar part of flexor digitorum profundus
Motor testing	• Ask the patient to extend their fingers against resistance, and then the wrist, with the arm flexed to 90° at the elbow and pronated (Fig. 3.34A) • Ask the patient to extend their thumb against resistance (Fig. 3.34B)	• Try to break a grip of the patient pressing their thumb tip into their index fingertip, making an OK sign • Abduct the thumb against resistance (Fig. 3.35)	• Assess finger adduction by asking the patient to hold a piece of card between their extended fourth and fifth fingers • Assess finger abduction by asking the patient to abduct their extended index finger against resistance • Froment's sign: Grip a piece of card between the adducted thumb and palm. A positive Froment's sign is when the interphalangeal joint flexes as the patient tries to compensate for a weak thumb adductor with flexor pollicis longus, which is innervated by the median nerve. A negative test shows no significant flexion of the PIP (Fig. 3.36)
Posture	• Wrist drop (Fig. 3.37)	• Hand of benediction: Proximal lesion of the median nerve results in the hand of benediction when the patient tries to make a fist • The patient is unable to flex the MCP, PIP or DIP joints of the index and middle fingers due to loss of innervation to the lateral two lumbricals. The ring and little finger can flex at these joints	• Claw hand • Occurs at rest • Loss of innervations of the medial two lumbricals results in extension at the MCP joints of the ring and little fingers due to unopposed action of the extensor digitorum • If the lesion is at the wrist, some flexion will be observed at the PIP and DIP joints because innervation of the medial half of flexor digitorum profundus is intact • If the lesion is at the elbow, the claw will be less marked due to paralysis of the medial half of the flexor digitorum profundus, with resultant loss of flexion at the PIP and DIP joints

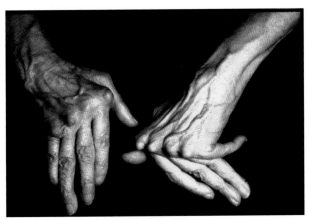

Fig. 3.33 Bilateral symmetrical arthropathy, showing ulnar deviation of the fingers, swelling of the MCP joints, guttering/muscle wasting (between extensor tendons over the metacarpals).

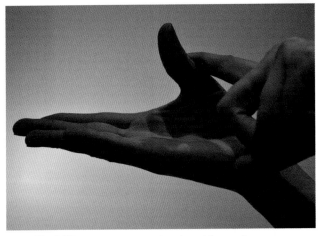

Fig. 3.35 Testing the motor function of the median nerve.

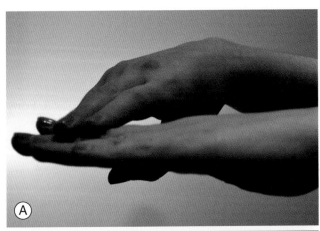

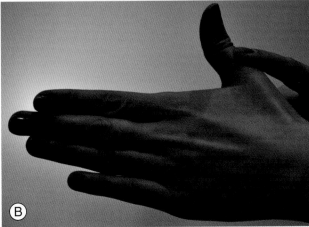

Fig. 3.34 (A, B) Testing the motor function of the radial nerve.

STATION 3.6: HIP

SCENARIO

You are a junior doctor working a busy shift in the emergency department (ED). Andrew Trendelenburg is an 82-year-old man who has fallen at home. His left lower limb looks shorter than his right and it also looks rotated. Please examine his hips and present your findings.

PREPARATION

- WIPER:
  - *Wash* your hands
  - *Introduce* yourself
  - Ask about *pain*
  - Appropriately *expose*
  - *Reposition*
- Explain the examination to the patient and your reasons for performing it
- Gain verbal consent
- Give the patient privacy to expose themselves as required
- Start in a comfortable position (usually sitting in a chair or bed)
- Offer a chaperone

LOOK

Important to note whether:
- Changes are symmetrical or asymmetrical

Ask the patient to remove enough clothing to expose both hips.
- Inspect from front, side and back, looking for:
  - General inspection: Age, frailty, body mass index (BMI), scars, redness, swelling, walking aids, comorbidities
  - Alignment: From all angles, ensure that the patient's shoulders are in line with the pelvis. Kyphosis at the back. Ensure that the pelvis is level, feeling for the iliac crests. If not, it can cause apparent leg shortening
  - Muscle wasting: Quadriceps and gluteus may be affected, suggestive of lack of use from osteoarthritis
  - Deformity: Fixed flexion deformity
  - Gait: Ask the patient to walk across the room whilst you assess for:
    - Antalgic gait: Limping, often an indication of osteoarthritis
    - Trendelenburg gait: The pelvis tilts away from the affected hip and the trunk tilts towards the

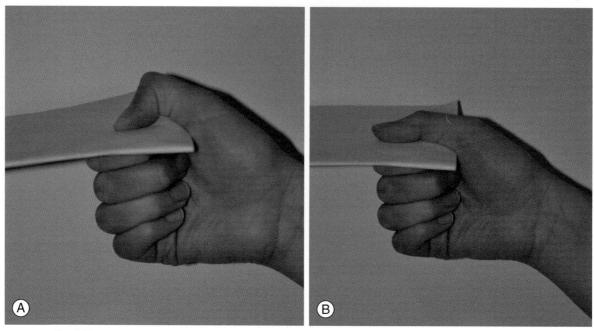

Fig. 3.36 Testing the motor function of the ulnar nerve. (A) Negative Froment's test; (B) positive Froment's test.

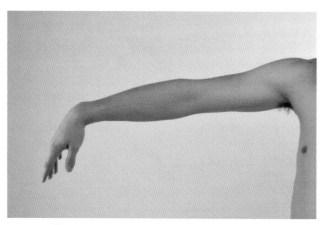

Fig. 3.37 Wrist drop due to a radial nerve lesion.

affected hip. Often there has been previous hip surgery or L5 radiculopathy
- Ask the patient to lie supine on the couch:
  - Look at the feet to identify any rotation of the lower limbs: Neck of femur fracture

FEEL

Ensure to ask patients if they have pain and clarify the location.
    With the patient supine on the couch:
- Temperature: It may be difficult to detect any changes, as the hip is a deep joint
- Palpate:
  - Greater trochanter: Hand's breadth below the iliac crest. Also, roll the leg from side to side with one hand, whilst the other hand palpates the greater trochanter. If pain is elicited, it suggests trochanteric bursitis

- Anterior superior iliac spine: Tenderness or bony abnormalities indicate osteoarthritis

MOVE

- Screen the lumbar spine by asking the patient to raise their leg straight off the couch as hip pain may come from the spine

ACTIVE HIP FLEXION

- Ask the patient to flex their knee to 90°, then flex their hip fully
- Normal is 120°

PASSIVE HIP FLEXION

- Take another 20° with one hand stabilising the pelvis

ROTATION

- With hip still flexed, test internal rotation by moving the foot laterally (normal 40°). Test external rotation by moving the foot medially
- Normal is 45° (Fig. 3.44)

ABDUCTION AND ADDUCTION

- Ask the patient to extend their leg; place one hand on the iliac crest of the opposite side of the pelvis to ensure that the pelvis is stabilised
- Using the other hand, abduct then adduct the hip
- Normal abduction is 45°
- Normal adduction is 30°

EXTENSION

- Ask the patient to roll on to their side (if possible) to assess extension (normal is 20°)

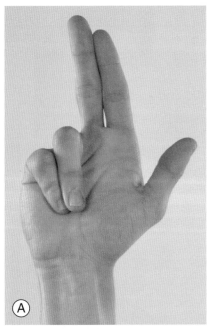
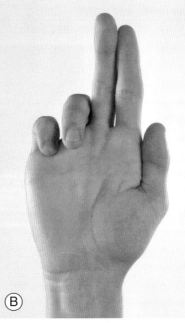
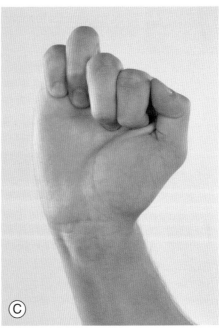

Fig. 3.38 From left to right: (A) The hand of benediction occurring when trying to make a fist. Note the fourth and fifth MCP joints are flexed. (B) The claw hand occurring at rest. Note the fourth and fifth MCP joints are extended. (C) The claw hand when trying to make a fist. Note the fourth and fifth MCP joints remain extended.

Table 3.4   Tests for various tendons in the hands and wrists

TENDON	ACTION	IMAGE OF THE ACTION
Flexor digitorum profundus	Ask the patient to flex their DIP joint whilst keeping the PIP, MCP and wrist joints extended	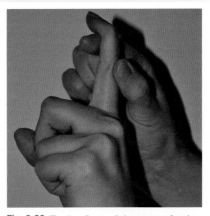 **Fig. 3.39** Testing flexor digitorum profundus.
Flexor digitorum superficialis	Hold the non-test fingers fully extended and ask the patient to flex the PIP joint you are examining	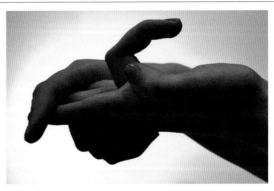 **Fig. 3.40** Testing flexor digitorum superficialis.

Continued

Table 3.4 Tests for various tendons in the hands and wrists—Cont'd

TENDON	ACTION	IMAGE OF THE ACTION
Extensor digitorum	Ask the patient to extend their fingers whilst their wrist is held in the neutral position	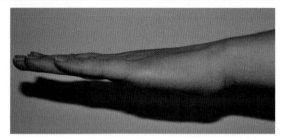 Fig. 3.41 Testing extensor digitorum.
Flexor and extensor pollicis longus	Ask the patient to flex and extend their interphalangeal joint of the thumb whilst holding the proximal phalanx of the thumb	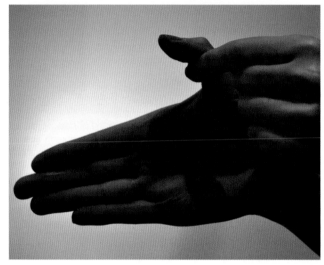 Fig. 3.42 Testing flexor and extensor pollicis longus
Extensor pollicis brevis	Ask the patient to extend their thumb like a hitch-hiker	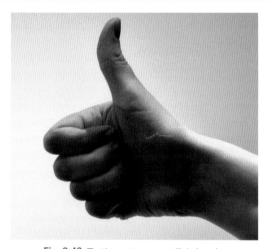 Fig. 3.43 Testing extensor pollicis brevis.

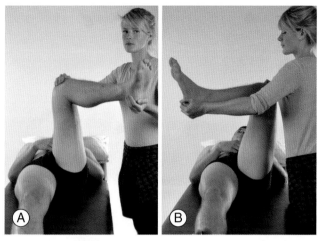

Fig. 3.44 (A) Internal rotation; (B) external rotation.

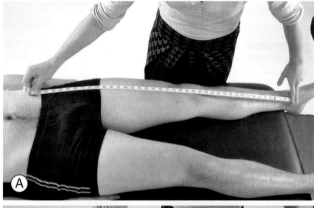

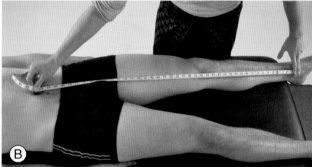

Fig. 3.45 (A) True leg length measurement; (B) apparent leg length measurement.

SPECIAL TESTS

LEG LENGTH DISPARITY (FIG. 3.45)

- True length: Measured from the anterior superior iliac spine to the medial malleolus on both legs
- Apparent length: Compare with the distance from the umbilicus to the medial malleolus
- If there is a true leg length discrepancy, ask the patient to flex their knees (if able) whilst keeping their heels together; this allows you to see whether the shortening is below or above the knee
- If the abnormality is above the knee, place your thumbs on the anterior superior iliac spines, and with your fingers, feel for the tops of the greater trochanters to assess whether the pathology is proximal to the trochanters

THOMAS TEST

- Tests for fixed flexion of the hip
- Place one hand under the lower back, to ensure that the resting lordosis is removed
- Fully flex the non-test hip with your other hand until the lumbar spine touches the fingers of the hand under the back
- Look at the opposite leg. If it is lifted off the couch as a result of this manoeuvre, there is a fixed flexion deformity in that hip
- A positive test implies a hip flexion contracture

TRENDELENBURG'S TEST (FIG. 3.46)

- With the patient standing, crouch in front of them and gently place one of your hands on each anterior superior iliac spine, so that you can monitor the movement of the pelvis
- Ask the patient to stand on each leg in turn
- Hold for about 30 s
- In a negative test, the pelvis remains level or the raised-leg side may rise
- In a positive test, the pelvis will dip on the raised-leg side, due to failure or weakness of the hip abductors on the opposite side, and the patient's body will move towards the supporting leg

NEUROVASCULAR ASSESSMENT

- Assess sensation along the dorsum and sole of the foot: Branches of the sciatic nerve
- Assess sensation of the anterior and medial thigh and medial calf: branches of the femoral nerve
- Palpate for the dorsalis pedis and posterior tibial arterial pulses

FINISHING

- Offer to:
  - Examine the other hip, spine and knees
- Thank the patient
- Check they're comfortable and offer to help reposition them
- Wash your hands
- Leave the patient in privacy to get dressed

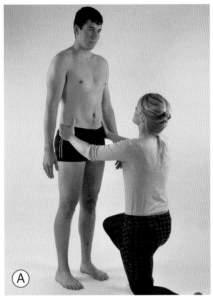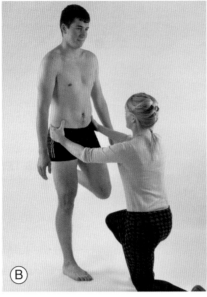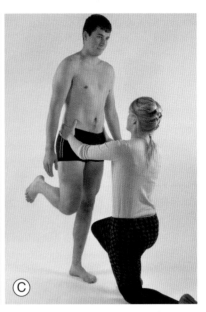

Fig. 3.46 (A–C) A negative Trendelenburg's test.

⚠ Common hip diagnoses in adults

DIAGNOSIS	HISTORY	EXAMINATION FINDINGS
Osteoarthritis	• Gradual onset of pain • Stiffness worse after activity • Pain exacerbated by activity • May affect everyday activities	• Antalgic gait • Tender on palpation • Limited range of movement • Crepitus
Trochanteric bursitis	• Lateral hip pain • Acute or insidious onset • Difficulty climbing stairs • Pain worse lying on affected side	• Pain on palpation of the trochanter • Pain exacerbated on internal and external rotation
Neck of femur fracture	• History of trauma • Anterior groin pain	• Inability to weight bear • Tenderness • Limited range of movement • Leg shortening and external rotation
Avascular necrosis	• Pain in the anterior groin that is exacerbated by weight bearing • Pain may gradually get worse • Pain may present at rest or night • History of hip fracture or dislocation, steroid use or alcoholism	• Antalgic gait • Tenderness on palpation • Restricted range of movement • A neurological finding may be present if a nerve is compressed due to necrosis of bone

⚠ Causes of true leg shortening

Pathology proximal to the greater trochanter	Pathology distal to the greater trochanter
Fractured neck of femur	Fractures
Post hip arthroplasty	Osteomyelitis
Hip dislocation	Septic arthritis
Arthritis	Epiphyseal injury
Slipped upper femoral epiphysis	Polio
Perthes' disease	Rare conditions; for example, hemihypertrophy

🔍 Present Your Findings

Mr Trendelenburg is an 82-year-old male who presented to the ED following a fall at home. On examination, he is in obvious discomfort. He has a shortened and externally rotated left lower limb. He is tender over the greater trochanter and is unable to move his left lower limb due to pain. The limb is distally neurovascularly intact. The right lower limb is normal.

This is consistent with a diagnosis of a fractured left neck of femur. To complete my examination I would like to ensure that the patient has adequate analgesia and request an AP pelvis and lateral left hip X-rays.

❓ QUESTIONS AND ANSWERS FOR CANDIDATE

What would a positive Trendelenburg test show?
- Pelvis dips on the raised-leg side
- Patient's upper body will move towards supporting the leg

What are the surgical options for a neck of femur fracture?

Depends on the type of fracture and level of functioning of the patient. Some general pointers are:
- Extracapsular: Generally dynamic hip screw
- Subtrochanteric: Generally intermedullary nail
- Intracapsular:
  - If undisplaced in young patients: Cannulated screws
  - If displaced or undisplaced in elderly patients: Hemiarthroplasty or total arthroplasty
  - In a young patient, reduction and cannulated screw fixation can also be considered for a displaced intracapsular fracture

Which nerve innervates the gluteus maximus?
- Inferior gluteal

 A Case to Learn From

I once saw a patient who had no pain at all, but he was just struggling to weight bear. No one really knew why and only after taking a full history did we discover that he has a history of rheumatoid arthritis, for which he was taking regular painkillers. A neck of femur fracture may present with no pain at all. It is important to ask if the patient takes any other pain relief medication for other conditions, or if they consume any other substances which may reduce pain; for example, alcohol.

 Top Tip

Remember to assess for leg length discrepancy and a fixed flexion deformity. Thomas' test is important but easy to get wrong under pressure!

 Top Tip

Use common sense when examining patients. If they are lying on a couch, assess gait at the end of the examination, whereas if they are standing or sitting, gait can be examined at the start, as can Trendelenburg's test.

STATION 3.7: KNEE

SCENARIO

You are a junior doctor on your orthopaedics rotation and you have been asked to see Sara Emerald, a 68-year-old woman, who has presented with chronic right-knee pain and reduced walking ability. She has been referred by her primary care physician to an orthopaedic clinic. Please examine Mrs Emerald and present your findings.

PREPARATION

- WIPER:
  - *Wash* your hands
  - *Introduce* yourself
  - Ask about *pain*
  - Appropriately *expose*
  - *Reposition*
- Explain the examination to the patient and your reasons for performing it
- Gain verbal consent
- Give the patient privacy to expose themselves as required
- Start in a comfortable position (usually sitting in a chair or bed)
- Offer a chaperone

LOOK

- Important to note whether changes are symmetrical or asymmetrical
- Ask the patient to remove enough clothing to expose the knees, and the joints above and below
- Inspect from front, side and back, looking for:
  - General inspection: Walking aids, wheelchair, nutritional status, scars, erythema, swelling, psoriasis
  - Alignment: Only truly assessed when standing and weight bearing, legs in genu valgus or in genu varus (Fig. 3.47)
  - Muscle wasting: quadriceps
  - Deformity: fixed flexion deformity
  - Length: shortening of leg
  - Gait:

  Antalgic gait: Pain
  Stiff-knee gait: Cerebral palsy
- Ask the patient to lie semisupine on the couch; meanwhile you inspect the knee for:
  - Open incision scars, laparoscopic scars
  - Obvious effusions
- Measure the thigh circumference 15 cm above the tibial tuberosity for wasting (Fig. 3.48)

FEEL

- Feel both knees with the back of your hands and comment on the temperature
- Flex the knee to 90°. Palpate knee structures in an orderly fashion using one finger at a time. Start furthest from the pain
- Feel the back of the knee for Baker's cyst
- Extend the knee and feel for effusion by performing the following; this may be assessed in several ways:
  - Look: For loss of dimples medial to the knee cap
  - Patellar tap: Larger effusions. Grip your left hand on the quadriceps muscles and slide down until you are above the patella. Hold your left hand there, emptying the suprapatellar pouch. With

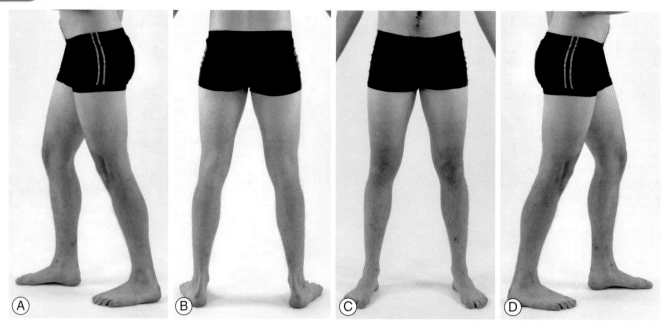

Fig. 3.47 Inspection of the knees with the patient standing to assess alignment.

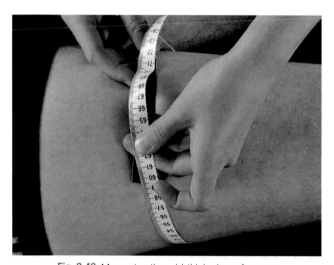

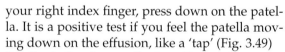
Fig. 3.48 Measuring the mid-thigh circumference.

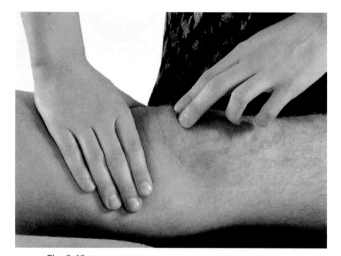
Fig. 3.49 Assessing for an effusion with the patellar tap.

your right index finger, press down on the patella. It is a positive test if you feel the patella moving down on the effusion, like a 'tap' (Fig. 3.49)

- Patellar ballot: Large effusions. Empty the suprapatellar pouch as above, holding your left hand above the knee. Press on the patella firmly with the thumb towards the femur. It is a positive test if you feel bulging under your left hand
- Sweep test (Fig. 3.50): Small effusions. Sweep distally to proximally along the medial side of the knee, which moves the synovial fluid. Then sweep along the lateral side of the knee but proximally to distally. It is a positive find if the fluid bulges on to the medial side

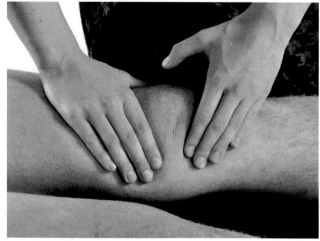
Fig. 3.50 Assessing for an effusion with the sweep test.

MOVE

- Screen the lumbar spine by performing a straight-leg test (station 3.2: Thoracolumbar spine)

- Screen the hip by asking the patient to flex the hip and with your hands, internally and externally

rotate the hip (station 3.6: Hip examination)
- Note whether the movement is painful or stiff and the location of this

KNEE FLEXION (FIG. 3.51)

- Ask the patient to move her heel as close to her bottom as possible
- Normal is about 140°

KNEE EXTENSION

- Ask the patient to straighten her leg out on to the couch (Fig 3.52A)
- Normal is that the patient should be able to get it flat on to the couch
- Inability to extend fully indicates an extensor lag: Disruption of the extensor mechanism or quadriceps weakness
- Passively flex then extend the knee with one hand over the knee, feeling for crepitus (Fig. 3.52B)
- Hyperextend the knees by raising both ankles off the couch (> 10° is hyperextended)

SPECIAL TESTS

PATELLAR APPREHENSION

- This tests for patellar dislocation (Fig. 3.53)
- Fully extend the knee and apply a lateral force to the patella whilst slowly flexing the knee
- It is a positive test if it is painful or there is resistance to flexion

ANTERIOR AND POSTERIOR DRAWER TESTS

- These test the anterior and posterior cruciate ligaments for laxity or rupture (Fig. 3.54)
- Flex the knee to 90° and sit on the patient's foot. Ensure to ask beforehand if they have pain in their foot
- Grab the tibia with both hands. Put your thumbs on the tibial tuberosity and wrap fingers around the back of the tibia
- Ask the patient to relax and check that the hamstrings are relaxed using your fingers
- From this position, move the tibia towards you
- It is a positive test if there is significant movement of it away from the femur: anterior cruciate ligament injury
- Now push the tibia away from you. Again, it is a positive test if there is significant movement of the tibia away from the femur and posterior sag: posterior cruciate ligament injury (Fig. 3.55)

LACHMAN'S TEST

- This test is more sensitive for anterior cruciate ligament injury (Fig. 3.56)
- Flex the knee to 20°
- Place one hand under the lower leg (behind the proximal tibia) and grasp the top of the femur with the other hand
- Attempt to glide surfaces forwards and backwards over each other
- There should be no gliding if the knee is stable
- It is a positive test if gliding occurs

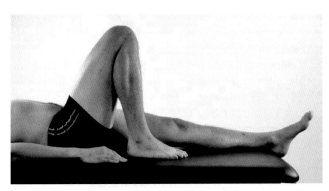

Fig. 3.51 Knee flexion.

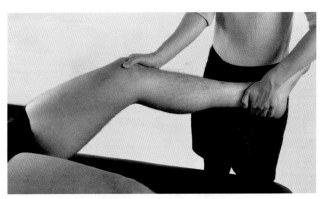

Fig. 3.53 Patellar apprehension test.

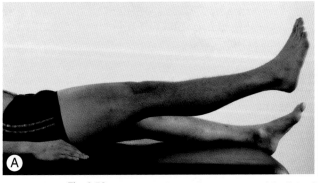
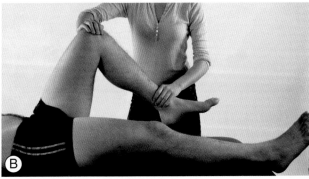

Fig. 3.52 Knee extension and assessment of the integrity of the extensor mechanism (A), feeling for crepitus (B).

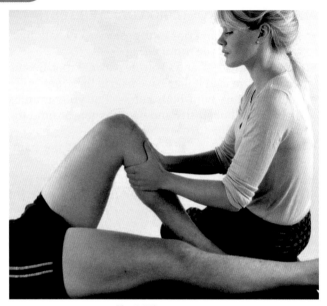

Fig. 3.54 Drawer test.

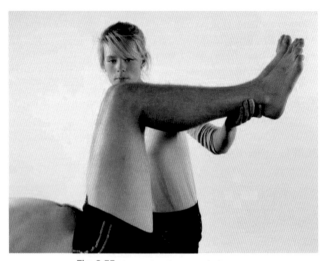

Fig. 3.55 Assessing for a posterior sag.

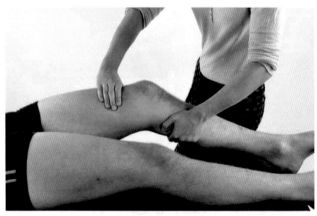

Fig. 3.56 Lachman's test.

MEDIAL AND LATERAL COLLATERAL LIGAMENT STRESS TESTS

- These test for laxity or rupture (Fig. 3.57)
- Extend the knee fully

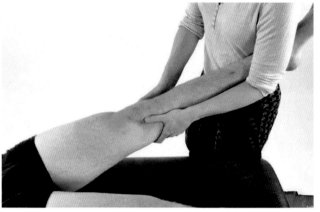

Fig. 3.57 Position for collateral stress tests.

- Place the distal tibia of the leg being tested between your elbow and side
- Place your right hand on the lateral knee and your left hand on the medial calf
- Apply valgus stress by pushing both hands: Suggests medial collateral ligament injury if there is extreme pain or obvious laxity
- Place your left hand on the medial knee and the right hand on the lateral calf
- Apply varus stress by pushing both hands: Suggests lateral collateral ligament injury if there is extreme pain or obvious laxity
- If this is stable, repeat with the knee flexed to 30° to assess if there is minor laxity

MCMURRAY'S TEST

- This tests for meniscal tear (Fig. 3.58)
- Flex the knee to 90°
- Place the fingers of one hand on the joint line
- Hold the calf with the other hand
- Externally rotate the foot whilst also abducting the hip. Flex and extend the knee (medial menisci)
- Internally rotate the foot whilst also adducting the hip. Flex and extend the knee (lateral menisci)
- It is positive if there is pain or clicking. Note that it can be extremely painful

NEUROVASCULAR ASSESSMENT

- Perform a full peripheral nerve examination on the lower limbs
- Perform a vascular assessment of the lower limbs, assessing the popliteal, tibial and dorsalis pedis pulses (Fig. 3.59)

FINISHING

- Offer to:
  - Examine the hips and ankles
- Thank the patient
- Check they're comfortable and offer to help reposition them
- Wash your hands
- Leave the patient in privacy to get dressed

! Common diagnoses from knee examinations

DIAGNOSIS	EXAMINATION FINDINGS
Knee osteoarthritis	• Fixed knee flexion • Joint line tenderness • Bony prominences • Small effusion • Limited range of movement
Rheumatoid arthritis	• Hot joint • Effusion • Joint line tenderness • Limited range of movement • May be symmetrical
Soft-tissue injury (ligamentous/ menisci)	• Antalgic gait • Effusion • Limited range of movement • Special tests may be positive
Septic arthritis	• Erythema • Hot joint • Large effusion • Sudden onset • Extremely painful joint line
Gout or pseudogout	• Erythema • Hot joint • Large effusion • Sudden onset • Extremely painful joint line
Psoriatic arthritis	• Psoriasis • Joint tenderness, especially tibial tuberosity where tendons attach (enthesitis) • Effusion • Limited range of movement • Extra-articular features: Eye changes
Reactive arthritis	• Sudden onset of effusion • Erythema • Joint line tenderness • Extra-articular features: Keratoderma blennorrhagica, oral ulcers, urethritis, eye changes

Present Your Findings

Mrs Emerald is a 68-year-old woman who presented with chronic right-knee pain and reduced walking ability. On examination, a walking stick was observed. The knees were in slight valgus. Tenderness was observed along the joint line of the right knee, particularly the lateral compartment. A small effusion was present and crepitus identified. Range of movement was limited. Active flexion reached 100°, and this was increased to 120° passively.

This is consistent with a diagnosis of osteoarthritis of the right knee, with differentials being rheumatoid arthritis or psoriatic arthritis. To complete my examination, I would like to check the neurovascular status of the limb, examine the hip and the ankle, calculate the BMI and perform a weight-bearing X-ray. I would also ensure adequate analgesia.

QUESTIONS AND ANSWERS FOR CANDIDATE

What are the four common findings of osteoarthritis on X-ray?
- Sclerosis
- Cysts
- Osteophytes
- Narrowing of joint space

What are some of the complications of knee replacement surgery?
- Peroneal nerve palsy
- Infection
- Pulmonary embolism

What investigation would be ordered if ligament rupture was suspected?
- MRI to look at soft tissue such as tendons and ligaments

A Case to Learn From

A patient came into the ED with a very red and swollen joint, on a background of gout. It had appeared suddenly. She was afebrile and had no preceding illnesses. The working diagnosis was gout and an aspiration was sent for analysis. When the results came back, they showed white cell count of 60,000 μL and over 75% polymorphonuclear leukocytes, consistent with septic arthritis. A red, hot, swollen, painful knee of sudden onset should be considered as septic arthritis until proven otherwise (even without an initial temperature). This is because such infection can cause irreversible destruction to the joint. Aspirates should be taken before commencing antibiotics and should be sent off for culture and histology.

Top Tip

Ask about timing of injury. Haemarthrosis develops rapidly, but a knee effusion usually takes several hours to become apparent.

Top Tip

Use only one finger/thumb at a time to palpate for tenderness. If you use both hands simultaneously and the patient complains of pain, you cannot be sure which site is the painful site and will have to inflict more discomfort to confirm the tender area.

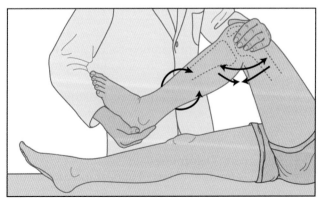

Fig. 3.58 McMurray's test.

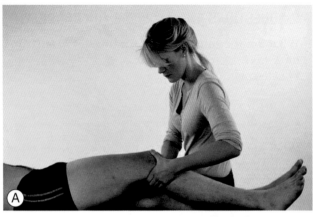
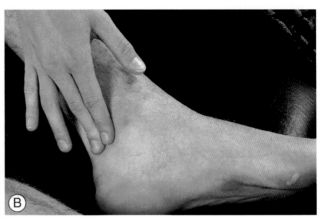

Fig. 3.59 (A) Popliteal pulse and (B) tibial pulse.

STATION 3.8: FOOT AND ANKLE

SCENARIO

You are a junior doctor working in the ED and have been asked to see John Weber, a 43-year-old male, who has presented with severe left ankle pain. He was playing football this morning and suddenly felt pain in his ankle whilst on the court. Please examine Mr Weber and present your findings.

PREPARATION

- WIPER:
  - *Wash* your hands
  - *Introduce* yourself
  - Ask about *pain*
  - Appropriately *expose*
  - *Reposition*
- Explain the examination to the patient and your reasons for performing it
- Gain verbal consent
- Give the patient privacy to expose themselves as required
- Start in a comfortable position (usually sitting in a chair or bed)
- Offer a chaperone

LOOK

Important to note:
- Whether changes are symmetrical or asymmetrical
Ask the patient to remove enough clothing to expose the feet, ankles and knees.
- Inspect from front, side and back, looking for:
  - General inspection: Walking aids (crutches, walking stick), frailty, BMI, signs of systemic illness
  - Alignment: Deformities
  - Achilles tendon: Unusual appearance; for example, swelling
  - Medial arches (Fig. 3.60):

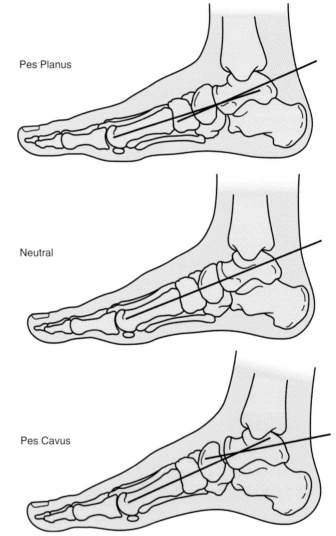

Fig. 3.60 Medial arch abnormalities (above); hindfoot inspection showing valgus and varus deformity (lower).

- Pes cavus: High arches, often Charcot–Marie–Tooth
- Pes planus: Flat feet, often congenital
- Patient's shoes: Abnormal sole patterns, comfort aids

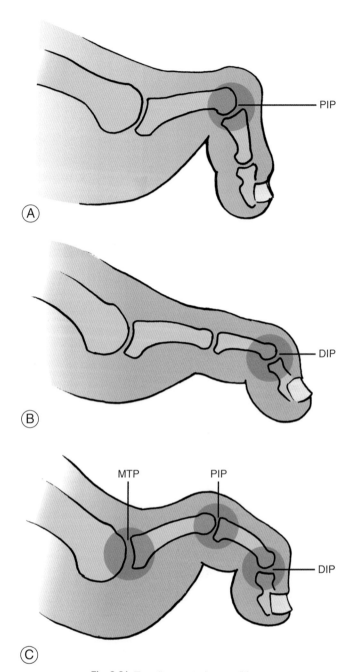

(A)

(B)

(C)

Fig. 3.61 Toe alignment abnormalities.

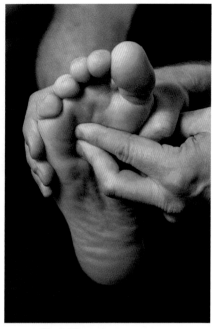

Fig. 3.62 Metatarsal squeeze.

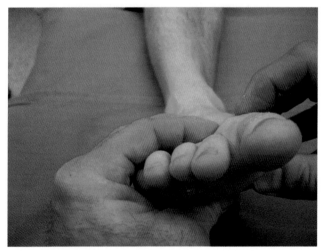

Fig. 3.63 Palpation of tarsal bones using a bimanual approach.

- Forefoot:
  - Nail changes or rashes: Psoriasis
  - Toe alignment: Claw toe, hammer toe, mallet toe (Fig. 3.61)
  - Intrinsic muscle wasting: Diabetes
  - Calluses
  - Ulcers
- Plantar surfaces:
  - Calluses: Ill-fitting footwear
  - Ulcers: Diabetes

FEEL

- Signs of systemic disease: Pain or swelling
- Pulses:

- Dorsalis pedis: Lateral to extensor hallux longus
- Posterior tibial
- Temperature: Using the back of your hand, feel for the temperature at the ankle joint and down the forefoot
- Squeeze along each individual toe
- Metatarsal squeeze (Fig. 3.62): Using one hand, grasp the patient's foot at the metatarsal heads and squeeze together
- Palpation:
  - Using a bimanual approach, hold the patient's foot and use both of your thumbs to palpate the tarsal (Fig. 3.63) and metatarsal bones
  - Palpate the medial malleolus, anterior ankle joint and lateral malleolus
  - Using your thumb and your second and third finger, palpate the subtalar joints (Fig. 3.64)

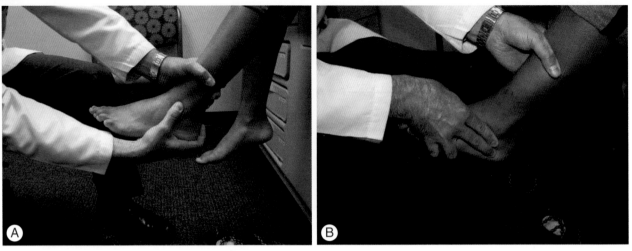

Fig. 3.64 Palpation of the subtalar joint.

- Using the palm of your hand and fingers, palpate the Achilles tendon, feeling for any thickness or tenderness

MOVE

- Ensure to steady the ankle with one hand, in order to avoid ankle movement interference

INVERSION AND EVERSION

- Place your hand at the lateral and then medial borders of the foot and ask the patient to try to touch your hand
- Normal range of movement is 30° for inversion and 20° for eversion

Move your hand down to grasp the midfoot with your hand to avoid ankle movement interference.

DORSIFLEXION AND PLANTAR FLEXION OF THE BIG TOE

- Ask the patient to point toes to the ceiling and to curl toes inwards
- Normal range of movement is 70° for dorsiflexion and 45° for plantar flexion
- Remove your hand from the foot

ANKLE DORSIFLEXION AND PLANTAR FLEXION

- Ask the patient to try to bring their foot towards them and press down like pressing on a car pedal, respectively
- Normal range of movement is 40° for dorsiflexion and 20° for plantar flexion
  Examine any joints with limited movement passively.

MIDTARSAL JOINT MOVEMENT

- Hold the ankle joint with one hand and the forefoot with the other hand. Apply a twisting motion (Fig. 3.65)

SUBTALAR JOINT MOVEMENT

- Hold the ankle joint with one hand and the heel with the other hand. Invert and evert the foot (Fig. 3.66)

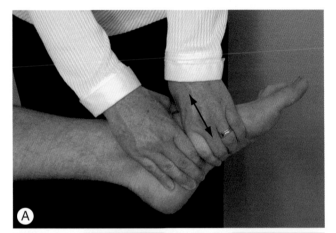

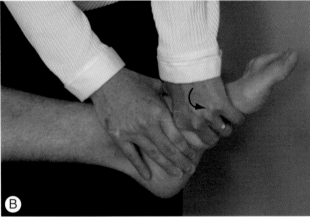

Fig. 3.65 Assessing midtarsal joint movement.

SPECIAL TESTS

GAIT ASSESSMENT

- Ask the patient to walk across the room, turn and walk back
- Look at the gait for:
  - Symmetry
  - Normal cycle of heel strike: May avoid if tender heel
  - Toe-off: May avoid pushing off toes if forefoot is tender

- High-stepping gait if foot drop

SIMMONDS'/THOMPSON'S TEST (FIG. 3.67)

- Ask the patient to lie face down on the couch, with feet hanging off of the bed
- With both hands, squeeze the calf muscle
- In a normal examination, the foot should plantar flex
- Test is positive if no movement occurs and indicates Achilles tendon tear or rupture

OTHER JOINTS

- Examine both knees and hips

NEUROVASCULAR ASSESSMENT

- Perform a full peripheral nerve examination on the lower limbs
- Perform a vascular assessment of the lower limbs

FINISHING

- Offer to:
  - Examine both knees and hips
- Thank the patient
- Check they're comfortable and offer to help reposition them
- Wash your hands
- Leave the patient in privacy to get dressed

[!] Common diagnoses from foot and ankle examination

AREA AFFECTED	CONDITION	EXPLANATION
Forefoot	• Hallux valgus	• Bunion: Medial deviation of the first metatarsal and lateral deviation of the hallux
	• Hallus rigidus	• Osteoarthritis of the big toe
	• Claw toe	• Hyperextension at the MCP joints and flexion at the interphalangeal joints
	• Hammer toe	• Extension at the MCP joints, flexion at the PIP joints and extension at the DIP joints
	• Mallet toe	• Hyperflexion at the DIP joints
	• Phalange fracture	• May be swollen • May be distal, middle or proximal phalangeal fracture
	• Gout	• Hot, swollen joint • Often the first metatarsophalangeal (MTP) joint
Midfoot	• Pes cavus	• High arches: Often neurological cause
	• Pes planus	• Flat arches: Commonly seen in adults
	• Metatarsal fracture	• Stress fracture of the fifth metatarsal is more common
Hindfoot	• Calcanovalgus	• Excessive dorsiflexion of the foot
	• Calcanovarus	• Dorsiflexed, adducted, and inverted foot
	• Calcaneous fracture	• Requires a high-energy mechanism
	• Talus fracture	• Requires a high-energy mechanism
	• Plantar fasciitis	• Common • May be painful or irritated on walking
Ankle	• Ankle ligamentous injury	• Common • Lateral ligaments more commonly affected, especially anterior talofibular ligament
	• Malleolus fracture	• Lateral more common than medial
	• Ankle osteoarthritis	• Osteoarthrits of the tibiotalar joint • Often have history of ankle fracture or tibial pilon fracture
	• Achilles tendon injury	• Sudden onset: Difficulty weight bearing

[Q] Present Your Findings

Mr Weber is a 43-year-old male who presented with sudden-onset severe left-ankle pain and reduced ability to weight bear. On examination, the left posterior ankle appears swollen and additionally is tender on palpation. Range of movement was limited, with decreased plantar flexion of the left ankle. Gait was also impaired, with an inability to weight bear fully on the ankle. Furthermore, Thompson's test was positive.

This is consistent with a diagnosis of an Achilles tendon tear or rupture, with differentials being gastrocnemius tear, posterior tibialis tendon injury and an ankle fracture. To complete my examination I would like to check the neurovascular status of the foot, examine the knee, calculate the BMI, perform an ultrasound scan and order a weight-bearing AP and lateral X-ray of the foot to exclude a fracture. I would also ensure adequate analgesia and refer to orthopaedics.

❓ QUESTIONS AND ANSWERS FOR CANDIDATE

What are the areas to test for nerve sensation in the foot?
- Deep peroneal nerve: First web space
- Superior peroneal nerve: Dorsum of foot
- Tibial nerve: Plantar foot

How do you manage hallux valgus (bunion)?
- Conservative: Shoe modification, orthroses, pads
- Surgical: Surgical correction, importantly for symptoms and not cosmetic

What would be the management steps for an ankle ligamentous injury?
- RICE:
  - Rest
  - Ice
  - Compression
  - Elevation
- Analgesia
- Physiotherapy

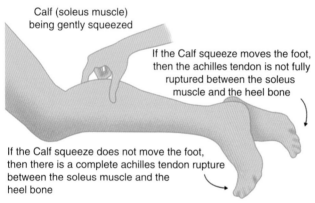

Calf (soleus muscle) being gently squeezed

If the Calf squeeze moves the foot, then the achilles tendon is not fully ruptured between the soleus muscle and the heel bone

If the Calf squeeze does not move the foot, then there is a complete achilles tendon rupture between the soleus muscle and the heel bone

Fig. 3.67 Simmonds' test.

📖 A Case to Learn From

A patient had come into the ED after jumping from the third floor of a building. He presented with pain in both feet and a bilateral calcaneal fracture was seen on radiograph. This was treated, but later, he started complaining of pain at his hips. It is important to remember that there may be other fractures if a patient presents with a high-energy trauma fracture. Often other radiographs and a CT are required to look for spine, pelvis and tibial plateau fractures, which may occur from a high-axial load on the skeleton.

💡 Top Tip

Beware of bruising to the plantar surface, which may indicate a bony injury such as a calcaneal fracture or Lisfranc injury – these ought not to be missed!

💡 Top Tip

Familiarise yourself with the sensory innervation of the foot and ankle. This is important clinically and a slick assessment will impress the examiners!

STATION 3.9: GAIT, ARMS, LEGS AND SPINE (GALS)

SCENARIO

You are a junior doctor working in rheumatology and are asked to see Caroline Lamb, a 45-year-old woman, who has been referred by her primary care physician due to increasingly stiff joints. Please perform a GALS screen on her and present your findings.

PREPARATION

- WIPER:
  - *Wash* your hands

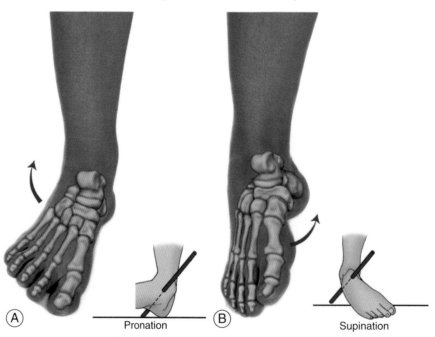

(A) Pronation   (B) Supination

Fig. 3.66 Assessing subtalar joint movements.

- *Introduce* yourself
- Ask about *pain*
- Appropriately *expose*
- *Reposition*
- Explain the examination to the patient and your reasons for performing it
- Gain verbal consent
- Give the patient privacy to expose themselves as required
- Start in a comfortable position (usually sitting in a chair or bed)
- Offer a chaperone

SCREENING QUESTIONS

Start by asking the patient the following questions:
- Is there any pain or stiffness in the muscles, joints or back?
- Can the patient dress herself completely without any difficulties?
- Can the patient walk up and down the stairs without difficulty?

GAIT

Assess the gait cycle by asking patient to walk a few steps, turn and walk back (Fig. 3.68). Look at the following:
- Symmetry
- Smoothness
- Ability to turn quickly

GENERAL INSPECTION

With the patient standing, conduct a general inspection and observe for the following:
- Front:
  - Shoulder bulk and symmetry
  - Elbow extension
  - Quadriceps bulk and symmetry
  - Feet: Forefoot abnormalities, midfoot deformities and foot arches
- Behind:
  - Shoulder muscle bulk and symmetry
  - Spinal alignment
  - Level iliac crests
  - Gluteal muscle bulk and symmetry
  - Popliteal swelling
  - Calf muscle bulk and symmetry
  - Hindfoot abnormalities
- Side:
  - Cervical lordosis
  - Thoracic kyphosis
  - Lumbar lordosis
  - Knee flexion or hyperextension

ARMS

- Ask the patient to put their hands behind their head (Fig. 3.69), which assesses:

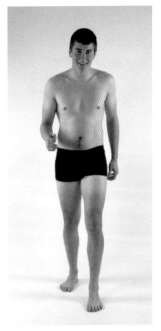

Fig. 3.68 Assessment of gait.

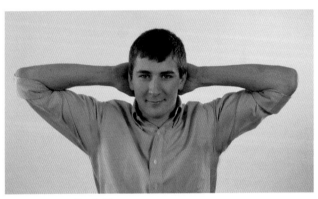

Fig. 3.69 Hands behind head position.

- Shoulder abduction
- External rotation
- Elbow flexion
- Ask the patient to hold their arms out, palms down and fingers outstretched. Observe the back of the hands and wrists for swelling and deformity
- Ask the patient to turn their hands over; look for muscle bulk and symmetry
- Ask the patient to make a fist
- Assess grip strength by asking the patient to squeeze your fingers (Fig. 3.70)
- Assess fine precision pinch by asking the patient to bring each finger in turn to meet the thumb
- Gently squeeze across MCP joints for tenderness, suggesting inflammation (Fig. 3.71). Be sure to tell the patient first and look at the patient's face for pain

LEGS

With the patient supine on the couch, examine their legs:
- Whilst feeling for crepitus, assess passive flexion and extension of both knees

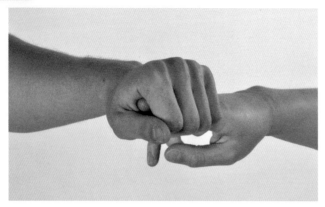
Fig. 3.70 Grip strength.

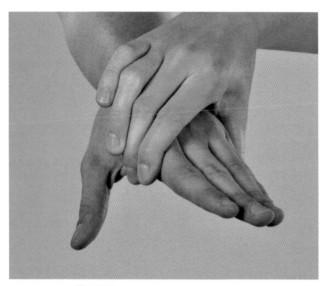
Fig. 3.71 Squeezing across MCP joints.

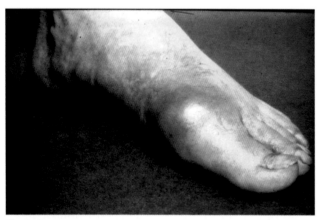
Fig. 3.72 Swelling of the first MTP joint in acute gout. This is likely to be tender.

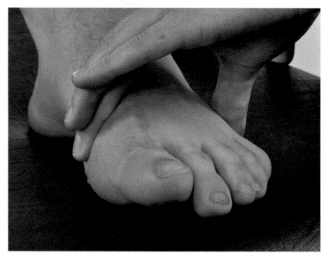
Fig. 3.73 Assessing for MTP tenderness.

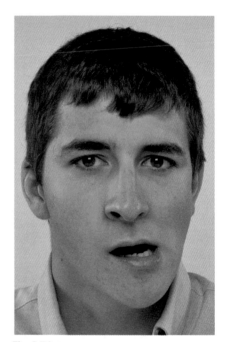
Fig. 3.74 Assessing temporomandibular joint.

- Perform a MTP squeeze, assessing for tenderness which suggests inflammation (Fig. 3.73). Ensure to warn the patient first and look at the patient's face for pain

SPINE

With the patient standing (this can be done at the start when assessing gait), examine the spine:
- Inspect the spine from behind for scoliosis
- Ask the patient to bring their ear to their shoulder on either side to assess lateral flexion
- Examine the temporomandibular joint by asking the patient to open their mouth and move the jaw from side to side (Fig. 3.74)
- Place your fingers on the patient's lumbar vertebrae and then ask the patient to bend and touch their

- With the patient's hips and knees flexed to 90°, hold the knee and ankle and internally rotate both hips
- Perform a patellar tap (Station 3.7: Knee examination)
- From the end of the couch, inspect the feet for calluses, swelling and deformity (Fig. 3.72)

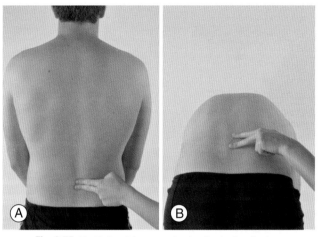

Fig. 3.75 (A, B) Crudely assessing lumbar spine flexion.

〰 Table **3.5**	An example of a GALS scoring table	
Pain?	Pain in both hands	
Problems walking?	No	
Problems dressing?	Difficulty buttoning and zipping	
	Appearance	Movement
Gait	√	√
Arms	X	X
Legs	√	√
Spine	√	√

toes to assess lumbar and hip flexion. Your fingers should move apart on flexion, and back together on extension. This is Schober's test (Fig. 3.75).

GALS SCORING TABLE

Note any abnormal finding; for example, swelling over the dorsum of both wrists and swan neck deformities in all fingers in both hands – possible rheumatoid arthritis (Table 3.5).

FINISHING

- Offer to:
  - Record findings on a GALS scoring table
  - Perform detailed examination of the joints with suspected abnormalities
- Thank the patient
- Check they're comfortable and offer to help reposition them
- Wash your hands
- Leave the patient in privacy to get dressed

Present Your Findings

Mrs Lamb is a 45-year-old woman who has presented with early-morning pain and stiffness, affecting the small joints of the hands. She is having difficulty with dextrous tasks, such as buttoning shirts. On examination, there is prominent deformity of the MCP joints with ulnar deviation of the fingers, and Z-shaped thumbs bilaterally. There is bilateral symmetrical joint swelling and tenderness affecting all MCP and MTP joints, with reduced range of movement in her hands. Her gait, lower-limb and spinal examinations are otherwise unremarkable.

This is consistent with a diagnosis of rheumatoid arthritis of the hands. To complete my examination I would like to perform blood tests to aid diagnosis, ensure adequate analgesia and ensure a senior rheumatology review.

❓ QUESTIONS AND ANSWERS FOR CANDIDATE

What are some of the clinical signs of osteoarthritis in the hands?
- Heberden's nodes at the DIP joints and Bouchard's nodes at the PIP joints
- Weak grip
- Tender metacarpal squeeze

What blood tests are useful for diagnosing rheumatoid arthritis?
- Anti-cyclic citrullinated peptide, rheumatoid factor, anti-citrullinated protein/peptide antibody
- Erythrocyte sedimentation rate/C-reactive protein
- Full blood count: May have normochromic normocytic anaemia or thrombocytosis

What does the Schober test examine?
- Thoracolumbar flexion
- Useful in examination for ankylosing spondylitis

A Case to Learn From

At the beginning of my training, I used to ask patients to squeeze my fingers to assess their grip strength, but I would assess one hand after the other. This led to me missing the sign that one of my patients had a weaker grip strength in one hand compared to the other, as I had no baseline to compare it with. Since then, I have been asking patients to squeeze my fingers with both hands at the same time, so that I can compare one side with the other.

Top Tip

Some children may respond better if playing 'Copy Cat'. Ask mum or dad to do the movements first or demonstrate the actions yourself.

Communication

Content Outline

Effective communication skills complement a doctor's knowledge and clinical skills, as well as helping to promote a positive patient interaction. Poor communication skills can lead to misunderstandings and loss of patient trust. It is important to communicate clearly, sensitively and succinctly. This chapter will give you a variety of scenarios to practise and develop this key skill.

Some relevant background knowledge of the topics will be provided in the stations of this chapter. There are also questions at the end of each scenario to test your knowledge. However, success in any communication skills OSCE relies on being able to sieve through this information, to identify what is most important to the patient in front of you, and perhaps to add information based on the specific circumstances presented.

A flexible generic framework can provide a useful structure to follow. Remember to spend time gauging who your patient is and their ideas, concerns and expectations. The same word might mean different things to two different patients. There is no spiel that can be memorised on 'cystic fibrosis counselling', only a framework to be adapted to the patient in front of you.

Study Action Plan

Unlike history taking or examination, it is difficult for medical students to practise communication skills on patients. However, the following may help:

- Observe communication skills in clinical scenarios and learn from them
- Develop your own framework to guide your communication. Some frameworks are suggested in the text. However, remember always to adapt to each patient
- Practise with friends, not only to assess each other at how you communicate facts, but also to confirm that you identify and appropriately address patient concerns

STATION 4.1: EXPLAINING HYPERTENSION

SCENARIO

You are a junior doctor in a primary care practice and have been asked to see Sonya Patel, a 47-year-old woman who has presented with persistently high readings of 156/98 mmHg on home blood pressure monitoring. Investigations for diabetes and underlying kidney disease have been negative. Please take a brief history of potential risk factors and explain Mrs Patel's diagnosis to her.

CORE CONCEPT

- The most common cause of hypertension is unknown (essential hypertension), but it can also be secondary to underlying renal disease and endocrine problems, including Cushing's disease and phaeochromocytoma
- Blood pressure may be raised in pregnancy or as a result of common medications; for example, the oral contraceptive pill, steroids and some antidepressants. It is vital to explore potential risk factors as this will change your management
- Hypertension is a common chronic condition that is often asymptomatic but can predispose to serious consequences, including strokes and heart attacks. This is important to explain to patients

Common Concerns

What do the numbers mean?	• Blood pressure readings are read out as one number 'over' another • The top number is the pressure in the arteries when the heart is contracting – it is the highest the blood pressure gets • The bottom number is the pressure in the arteries when the heart is relaxing – this is the lowest the blood pressure gets
What are the risks of having high blood pressure?	• High blood pressure can lead to a wide range of complications. It can affect your brain, leading to tissue damage, a stroke or dementia. It can affect your heart and its ability to pump blood round the body. It can also cause damage to your kidneys and your eyes
Do I have to take medication for life?	• In most cases, patients do not need to take medication and lifestyle changes can improve outcomes. However, if the blood pressure is high and sustained enough, antihypertensive medications may be needed for life. They can still be stopped or changed if the patient develops side effects or conditions which are contraindicated with their use

GATHERING INFORMATION AND COMMUNICATIONS

This case has two parts:
1. Taking a brief history to identify potential risk factors contributing to hypertension
2. Explaining the diagnosis

IDENTIFYING RISK FACTORS

Though patients with hypertension are mostly asymptomatic, it is important to ask for potential risk factors that contribute to hypertension.

LIFESTYLE

- Lack of physical activity and being overweight or obese
- Diet; in particular, high levels of salt in foods
- Excessive alcohol intake
- Stress

COMORBIDITIES

- Family history of hypertension
- Personal history of:
  - Diabetes
  - Kidney disease
  - Thyroid disease
  - High blood pressure in pregnancy

DRUG HISTORY

- Many medications can increase blood pressure as a side effect. For example:
  - Oral contraceptive pill
  - Steroids
  - Non-steroidal anti-inflammatory drugs (NSAIDs)
  - Certain selective serotonin-noradrenaline reuptake inhibitor (SSNRI) antidepressants; for example, venlafaxine

EXPLANATION OF THE DIAGNOSIS

When explaining a condition, it may be helpful to have the following structure (four Cs):
- Condition: What the condition is
- Complications: What it could lead to
- Causes: What could have led to this condition developing
- Combat: The treatment for this condition

WHAT AND WHY?

- Explanation of what high blood pressure is physiologically, in terms of forces on the artery walls
- What can happen to the heart if you have high blood pressure; for example, the heart pumping harder and getting bigger
- Hypertension can increase the risk of:
  - Strokes
  - Heart attacks
  - Kidney problems

AETIOLOGY

Explain the causes of hypertension:
- The majority of cases are essential hypertension, where the cause is unknown
- Hypertension can be due to an underlying problem; for example, diabetes, hormone imbalances, or kidney problems
- Lifestyle risk factors, including:
  - Lack of physical activity
  - Being overweight or obese
  - Having a lot of salt in the diet
  - Regularly drinking alcohol over the recommended limit

MANAGEMENT

- Conservatively, aim to maintain a healthy diet, increase the level of exercise and quit smoking
- Medically, certain tablets can help to reduce blood pressure. Discuss with the patient this option and how they feel about it

ADDITIONAL INFORMATION

WHITE-COAT HYPERTENSION

In some cases, patients' blood pressure is only elevated when it is being directly measured by a healthcare professional. This is known as 'white-coat hypertension'. In order to rule this out, the blood pressure may need to be checked multiple times, or patients can be sent home with a 24-h blood pressure monitor, which will check their blood pressure multiple times throughout the day.

ANTIHYPERTENSIVE MEDICATIONS

Table 4.1 gives a list of commonly used antihypertensives.

 Present Your Findings

Mrs Patel is a 47-year-old estate agent who is normally fit and well and does not take any regular medications. She reports a family history of hypertension. In terms of her lifestyle, she does not drink but admits that she does not exercise often.

Today I have explained that she has high blood pressure and have advised her to take up exercise and to maintain a healthy diet. I have also recommended starting her on ramipril, in order to help bring down her blood pressure. She will be reviewed again in 2 months' time to reassess her blood pressure following lifestyle changes and commencing ramipril.

? QUESTIONS AND ANSWERS FOR CANDIDATE

What should patients aim for their blood pressure to be?
- If under 80 years old, below 140/90 mmHg
- If above 80 years old, a blood pressure of below 150/90 mmHg is acceptable
- If the patient has a history of heart disease, diabetes, stroke or kidney disease, then the target should be <130/80 mmHg

What are the red-flag symptoms associated with phaeochromocytoma?
- Episodic headache
- Profuse sweating
- Palpitations
- Tremor associated with hypertension

What changes would you expect to find on fundoscopy in a patient with hypertensive retinopathy?
- Arteriovenous nicking
- Cotton-wool spots
- Retinal haemorrhages
- Optic disc swelling

 A Case to Learn From

A patient was newly diagnosed with hypertension and was to be started on ramipril. They were very keen to avoid medication so, after lifestyle modifications, were able to come off the antihypertensive. Not all medications are lifelong!

 Top Tip

Get into the role. Treat the actor as a real patient. You will be more natural and that's what we want from communication skills stations.

Table 4.1 Details on some antihypertensive medications

DRUG CLASS	EXAMPLES	SIDE EFFECTS	ADDITIONAL INFORMATION
Angiotensin-converting enzyme inhibitors (ACEi)	• Ramipril • Lisinopril	• Cough • Dizziness	• Regular monitoring of renal function and potassium levels is required
Angiotensin II receptor blockers (ARBs)	• Candesartan • Valsartan	• Hyperkalaemia • Headache • Dizziness	• Used as an alternative to ACEi if they cause a cough • Regular monitoring of renal function and potassium levels is required
Calcium channel blockers (CCBs)	• Amlodipine • Diltiazem	• Flushing • Headaches • Peripheral oedema	• Other CCBs apart from amlodipine and diltiazem interact with grapefruit juice, which can increase levels of the drug in the body, leading to a dangerous drop in blood pressure
Thiazide-like diuretics	• Indapamide • Bendroflumethiazide	• Constipation/diarrhoea • Dizziness • Electrolyte imbalance	• Regular monitoring of renal function and potassium levels is required

STATION 4.2: LIFESTYLE ADVICE POST MYOCARDIAL INFARCTION

SCENARIO

You are a junior doctor working on the cardiology ward and have been asked to speak to James Smith, a 55-year-old accountant, who was admitted with chest pain and underwent primary angioplasty for an ST elevation myocardial infarction (STEMI). He is now recovering well following his procedure and is about to be discharged from hospital. Please explore why he was at risk for developing heart disease and what lifestyle measures could be adopted to reduce his risk of another event.

CORE CONCEPT

Whilst there are non-modifiable risk factors that increase a patient's risk of having a heart attack, there are many that can be altered to prevent recurrence.

LIFESTYLE ADVICE

- *Weight*:
  - Aim to maintain a normal body mass index (BMI) of 20–25
  - If obese, advise weight loss (healthy diet and exercise)
- *Alcohol*:
  - Limit consumption or drink in moderation
  - The current recommendation is <14 units a week for both men and women
- *Fruit* and vegetables:
  - Eat five to eight portions a day
- *Fat*:
  - Maintain a well-balanced diet by reducing total fat intake
  - Offer dietician input and perhaps explore the possibility of cooking classes
- *Low* salt:
  - Reduce salt intake to less than 6 g/day (this helps to reduce blood pressure)
- *Exercise*:
  - Engage in regular aerobic physical exercise
  - Exercise ideally 30 min/day, ideally on most days of the week but for at least 3 days a week
- *Smoking*:
  - Reduce or quit smoking
  - You can discuss nicotine replacement therapy (NRT) and referral to a smoking cessation service

The above lifestyle advice can be remembered using the mnemonic WAFFLES.

All patients recovering from a heart attack should receive counselling about their recovery, which should include information regarding their new medications, lifestyle changes and follow-up care.

CARDIAC REHABILITATION

All patients who have had heart attacks should be followed up by a cardiac rehabilitation team and be encouraged to attend their sessions. The cardiac rehabilitation team is a multidisciplinary team consisting of cardiologists, physiotherapists, specialist nurses and dieticians who will support patients with their recovery. Programmes cover:
- Physical activity
- Education about lifestyle risk factors
- Relaxation
- Psychological support

Common Concerns

When can I drive again?	The Driver and Vehicle Licensing Agency (DVLA) states that if you hold a driving licence, then you do not have to inform the DVLA after a heart attack but you should stop driving for:
	• 1 week if you have had a heart attack and successful angioplasty
	• 4 weeks if you have had a heart attack and unsuccessful angioplasty
	• 4 weeks if you have had a heart attack but no angioplasty
	If you hold a bus, coach or lorry licence:
	• You must inform the DVLA and stop driving for 6 weeks
	• After 6 weeks, you must undergo a medical assessment with your primary care physician to see if you are fit to drive
When can I go back to work?	Patients may not be able to return to work for 6 weeks following a heart attack. When they do return, they may want to ask employers for a phased return, in order to support their recovery
What do I do if I get chest pain again?	The British Heart Foundation recommends:
	1. Stopping what you are doing
	2. Sitting down and resting
	3. Using glyceryl trinitrate (GTN) spray or tablet. The pain should recede after 5 min. Repeat GTN if the pain is still ongoing
	4. Call 999 immediately if the pain is not relieved by the second GTN dose

GATHERING INFORMATION AND COMMUNICATIONS

This case has two parts:
1. Clarifying the situation that led the patient to come into hospital
2. Providing post-discharge plans and advice

CLARIFYING THE SITUATION

Establish the patient's current level of understanding. You can do this by eliciting a short history.

Make sure to ask about:

- A brief history about the event itself, of particular note:
  - Presenting complaint
  - Any preceding symptoms of increasing chest pain
  - Whether the patient underwent stenting or managed with medications alone
- Non-modifiable risk factors; for example:
  - Previous heart attacks
  - Family history of cardiac problems
- Modifiable risk factors, including:
  - Diet, including: Salt, fat, fruit and vegetable intake
  - Exercise
  - Smoking
  - Alcohol intake
  - Conditions; for example: Dyslipidaemia, hypertension, obesity
  - Environmental stress

POST-DISCHARGE PLANS AND ADVICE

In reality, a patient may have multiple risk factors which need addressing, whilst the scenario may only ask you to address a particular issue.

POST-DISCHARGE

Cardiac rehabilitation programmes are an essential part of a patient's recovery and provide support through this process:

- For everyone who is recovering from a heart attack
- A number of different sessions with the cardiac rehabilitation team looking at different aspects of your life, including diet and exercise improvement, as well as psychological support

EXERCISE

- Exercise can reduce the risk of further heart problems by reducing blood pressure, controlling weight and reducing stress and anxiety
- During recovery, it is important gradually to increase the amount of exercise. The aim is eventually to do a total of at least 150 min of moderate activity per week:
  - Initially, start off by walking on the flat and gradually increase the workload
  - Avoid heavy lifting at the start but do household chores at your own comfort
- Cardiac rehabilitation classes can also help, as the physiotherapist can alter the exercise programme to suit the patient's needs

DIET

Emphasise the importance of maintaining a healthy balanced diet, as it can help to reduce the risk of further complications:

- Maintain a well-balanced diet by reducing total fat intake
- Try to keep within the recommended limits of alcohol per week, < 14 units in a week

CLOSING THE CONSULTATION

Making lifestyle changes can be difficult for a number of reasons:

- Patients may not know where to look for help
- They may be unaware of the benefits
- They may be embarrassed
  It may also help to set goals:
- Propose a short-term and achievable aim and offer material for the patient to take away and read
- Ensure follow-up is arranged if required

POST-MYOCARDIAL INFARCTION MEDICATIONS

Following a heart attack, patients will often be discharged with multiple new medications to familiarise themselves with. These medications are mostly related to modifying risk factors in order to prevent further heart attacks but some, for example, the GTN spray, are related to symptom relief. The medications can be more easily remembered using the acronym BRAGS (Table 4.2).

> **🔍 Present Your Findings**
>
> Mr Smith is a 55-year old ex-smoker who had a STEMI, treated with a coronary stent. He has a background history of hypertension and has a positive family history, as his father had a heart attack at the age of 50. He is an accountant who does not exercise at all and reports having 20 units of alcohol a week.
>
> Today I have advised him that in order to reduce the risk of another heart attack occurring, he should aim to increase his physical activity gradually. I have also informed him that the cardiac rehabilitation team will follow him up following discharge to support his recovery.

❓ QUESTIONS AND ANSWERS FOR CANDIDATE

Name three common differential diagnoses for acute chest pain:

- Acute coronary syndrome (ACS)
- Aortic dissection
- Pulmonary embolism
- Musculoskeletal causes
- Gastro-oesophageal reflux disease (GORD)

How would you differentiate between unstable angina (UA), non-ST elevation myocardial infarction (NSTEMI) and STEMI?

- Please see Table 4.3 for an overview on differentiating between these three conditions

Name three causes of raised troponin.
- Myocardial infarction
- Renal failure
- Sepsis
- Pulmonary embolism

 A Case to Learn From

A patient was readmitted to the ward with chest pain a few weeks after he had had stenting for a previous heart attack. Upon further questioning, it turned out that the patient had not been taking his dual antiplatelets and, as a result, the stent had become thrombosed, causing symptoms of another heart attack. This shows how important it is to counsel patients about secondary prevention methods before discharge.

 Top Tip

Following a heart attack, patients are often discharged with many new medications as well as being given lifestyle advice. It is important to counsel them not just on what to take, but also how long to take the medications as some medications, for example, clopidogrel, may be time-limited.

STATION 4.3: EXPLAINING STATINS

SCENARIO

You are a junior doctor working in a primary care practice and are asked to see Ken Adams, a 45-year-old man, who has undergone cardiovascular screening and, as a result, has been prescribed statins as

Table 4.2 The BRAGS acronym may help to remember which medications patients are started on following a heart attack

	MEDICATION	EXAMPLE	METHOD OF ACTION	KEY POINTS
B	Beta-blockers	• Bisoprolol	• Reduces heart rate and blood pressure	• Caution in those with asthma, as may promote bronchoconstriction
R	ACEi	• Ramipril • Lisinopril	• Reduces blood pressure	• Most common side effect is postural hypotension
A	Antiplatelets	• Aspirin • Clopidogrel • Ticagrelor • Prasugrel	• Antiplatelet activity reduces the risk of clots forming, therefore reducing the risk of further heart attacks	• Dual antiplatelets (aspirin plus one other) are started for those who have had stents and are usually taken for 1 year, then aspirin alone lifelong
G	GTN spray/sublingual tablets		• Coronary artery vasodilatation, therefore increasing the oxygen supply to the heart	• Can be used for symptomatic relief
S	Statins	• Atorvastatin • Simvastatin • Rosuvastatin	• Reduce cholesterol by inhibiting β-hydroxy β-methylglutaryl (HMG)-CoA reductase	• High doses are required for secondary prevention

Table 4.3 Differentiating between UA, STEMI and NSTEMI

ACS	ST CHANGES ON ELECTROCARDIOGRAM (ECG)	RISE IN CARDIAC ENZYMES
STEMIS	✔	✔
NSTEMI	✘	✔
UA	✘	✘

he has a 12% (moderate) risk of developing cardio-vascular disease (CVD) in the next 10 years. Please take a brief history covering his cardiovascular risk factors and then counsel him about statin use.

CORE CONCEPT

CARDIOVASCULAR RISK SCREENING

In order to identify who is at high risk of CVD, the following groups of patients are screened:

- Patients over 40 years old
- Patients of any age who have a strong family history of CVD or hypercholesterolaemia
  Screening involves:
- Checking for any history of risk factors, for example:
  - Smoking
  - Diet high in saturated fats and low in fruit, vegetable and fibre
  - High alcohol intake
  - Lack of physical activity
  - Obesity
- Checking cholesterol and glucose
- Blood pressure measurement
  A score is then calculated based on these factors to generate a risk score:
- >20%: High risk
- 10–20%: Moderate risk
- <10%: Low risk
  Patients who are considered to be at least moderate risk and those with pre-existing CVD, diabetes or chronic kidney disease are offered risk factor modification treatment, which includes statins.

STATINS

Statins reduce the risk of CVD by lowering the amount of cholesterol in the blood, therefore reducing fatty deposition in arterial walls and atheroma build-up. They are also associated with a number of side effects, including muscle pain. Recently, there has been a lot of negative press about statins and as a result, a number of patients are reluctant to take statins.

When counselling patients about medications, make sure to cover the following points:

- The reason why we are prescribing this drug
- What statins are and how they work
- When the patient needs to take the medication and the dosage
- The side effects and contraindications to be aware of
- What to do if side effects occur or a dose is missed

Common Concerns

What is the frequency of side effects?	• 5–10% of patients can have myalgia, which presents with muscle and tendon pain, stiffness, muscle weakness and cramping • Rhabdomyolysis is a very severe, but rare, complication of statins • The mean duration of statin treatment before developing side effects is 6 months, therefore symptoms that develop in those who have been on statins over many years are unlikely to be due to statins
What if I cannot tolerate statins?	• Dose reduction • Change to a different statin (possible as some statin are metabolised in a different ways)
Can I make any lifestyle changes?	• Stop smoking • Take regular exercise • Eat a healthy diet, avoiding foods high in saturated and *trans* fat; for example, red meat, processed foods and dairy products • Lose weight if overweight or obese

GATHERING INFORMATION AND COMMUNICATIONS

This case has two parts:
1. Taking a brief history to identify cardiovascular risk factors
2. Counselling the patient about statins

IDENTIFYING RISK FACTORS

Whilst assessing a patient's risk of developing CVD, it is important to cover the following points.

PAST MEDICAL HISTORY

- Hypertension
- Diabetes
- Chronic kidney disease
- Previous heart attacks and stroke

FAMILY HISTORY

- Any cardiovascular conditions
- Familial hypercholesterolaemia, including other inherited lipid conditions

LIFESTYLE

- Smoking
- Diet high in saturated fats and low in fruit, vegetable and fibre
- High alcohol intake
- Lack of physical activity
- Obesity

COUNSELLING ON STATIN USE

WHY?

Explain the risk of CVD in simple terms, making sure you relate it to the patient:
- Inform the patient what their risk of having a cardiovascular event in the next 10 years is
- Help the patient understand better by describing it as a likelihood in a group of 100 people
- Explain that, other than lifestyle interventions, patients are also offered statins to lower their risk

Explain the relationship between cholesterol and heart disease.
- Ensure that you provide any necessary context to the patient
- Explain that reducing blood cholesterol level will reduce the risk of future cardiovascular events, including heart attacks and strokes
- Explain that there are two types of cholesterol in the body. One type is high-density lipoprotein (HDL), which is beneficial at high levels. The other type is low-density lipoprotein (LDL), which is harmful at high levels
- Explain that high levels of the 'bad' cholesterol, LDL, can lead to fatty material building up in the artery walls. This can increase the likelihood of clots forming, which puts patients at risk of cardiovascular events

WHAT?

Explain how to lower cholesterol levels:
- Lifestyle interventions, including smoking cessation, increasing amount of exercise uptake and a balanced, healthy diet
- Explain that statins are medications that can lower blood cholesterol level and are offered to patients at a certain amount of risk

WHEN?

Explain when the drug is to be taken:
- The National Institute for Health and Care Excellence (NICE) recommends that patients prescribed statins for primary prevention should be started on 20 mg atorvastatin once a day. For those prescribed statins for secondary prevention, this should be increased to 80 mg atorvastatin
- Explain to the patient that statins are lifelong medications taken daily in the evening to reduce their cardiovascular risk

SIDE EFFECTS

If patients are aware of the common side effects, they may be more compliant with taking the medication. Some are listed below:
- Feeling sick (nausea)
- Feeling tired
- Headaches
- Indigestion and change in bowel habits
- Muscle aches and cramps
- Liver damage (monitored by blood tests)
- In very rare circumstances, statins can lead to rhabdomyolysis
- Statins can also interact with certain foods (for example, grapefruit) and some antibiotics, including clarithromycin. Advise the patient to make members of healthcare staff aware that they are on statins so that interactions can be minimised

WHAT IF?

- Try and answer any obvious questions you think the patient may have
- Advise the patient to inform their primary care doctor if they experience any side effects, so that appropriate blood tests can be organised if required
- Inform the patient that if they miss a dose, they should take it as soon as possible once they realise. However, if it has been 12 h since the missed dose, then wait until the next dose. Do not double up the dose the next day to make up for the missed dose

STATIN INDUCED MYOPATHY

This is a spectrum of disorders, which can range from:
- Asymptomatic increases in creatinine kinase
- Myalgia; for example, muscle and tendon pain, cramps, muscle weakness
- Myositis
- Rhabdomyolysis

LIFESTYLE METHODS OF REDUCING CHOLESTEROL

- Take regular exercise, as this can help to increase levels of HDL cholesterol
- Stop smoking
- Maintain a well-balanced diet by reducing total fat intake

MONITORING

- Before starting treatment, bloods should be taken for:
  - A full lipid profile
  - Liver function tests (LFTs)
- If a patient reports muscle pain, then stop the drug and check liver function and creatinine kinase
- Repeat LFTs:

- After 3 months of treatment and again after 1 year
- After any further dose increases

Present Your Findings

Mr Adams is a 45-year-old man with a background history of hypertension, which is controlled with ramipril. He also has a family history of heart disease as his brother had a heart attack at 52 years of age. He is a current smoker of 15 cigarettes a day and drinks moderately.

Today, I have explained that, after cardiovascular screening, he is at moderate risk of developing CVD and as a result has been prescribed a statin. I have counselled him on statin use and have provided him with an information leaflet to take away with him. He is keen to consider lifestyle changes and we have discussed these at length.

QUESTIONS AND ANSWERS FOR CANDIDATE

Give three examples of physical signs that suggest hypercholesterolaemia.
- Tendon xanthomata
- Xanthelasma
- Corneal arcus

Give an example of another medication used to lower cholesterol.
- Ezetimibe prevents small-intestine absorption of cholesterol; it can be used with statins

What inherited condition can give patients very high cholesterol levels?
- Familial hypercholesterolaemia
- This is an inherited condition where patients have very high cholesterol levels, putting them at an increased risk of developing heart disease

A Case to Learn From

After presenting to hospital with an NSTEMI and undergoing angioplasty, a patient was started on a high-dose statin as part of secondary prevention protocol. However, he was very concerned about using statins as he had read a lot of negative press online about them. He refused to take statins despite counselling. It is important to remember that ultimately it is the patient's choice what medications they take, but our job to counsel them correctly.

Top Tip

When explaining the estimated risk of developing heart disease in the future, pictograms can help to illustrate and emphasise the percentage risk a person has. It is better than just quoting statistics as often they are easier for patients to understand.

STATION 4.4: EXPLAINING INHALER TECHNIQUE

SCENARIO

You are a junior doctor working in a primary care practice and have been asked to see Rosie Johnson, a 24-year-old woman, who has come in for an asthma review. Rosie has recently been diagnosed with asthma and has been prescribed a salbutamol inhaler to manage her symptoms. Please review her symptom control and explain the correct way of using an inhaler, both with a spacer and without.

CORE CONCEPT

- Patient understanding of the indications for their medications promotes good adherence and therefore better disease control
- Poor inhaler technique is common, leading to reduced drug delivery
- Technique should be checked before altering medication dosage
- If an inhaler or spacer is provided, use it to demonstrate the steps

Common Concerns

What about the side effects of steroids?	• The pump delivers the medication directly to the lungs where it is needed, and minimises delivery elsewhere, so any side effects are minimal. Also these steroids are very different from the type of steroids patients may have heard of that body builders use (catabolic steroids) and are far safer • The most common side effects are hoarseness of voice and fungal mouth infections
Do I need to carry one everywhere I go?	• The patient should always carry an inhaler, especially when exercising. Provide the patient with more than one if needed
My inhaler does not seem to have worked?	• Steroid inhalers, which act to prevent flare-ups, don't have an immediate effect when the asthma gets worse. The blue inhaler is a reliever so should work quickly. If not, the patient should come into hospital

GATHERING INFORMATION AND COMMUNICATIONS

This case has two parts:
1. Briefly reviewing how well controlled the patient's asthma is
2. Explaining correct inhaler and spacer techniques

REVIEWING SYMPTOM CONTROL

Ask the patient questions to establish if her symptoms have improved since starting the inhaler, specifically:
- Presence of wheeze
- Chest tightness
- Shortness of breath, especially if it limits her daily activities
- Effect on day-to-day life
- Frequency of inhaler usage
- Any new symptoms: Be aware of the side effects

EXPLAINING CORRECT INHALER AND SPACER TECHNIQUE

- Explain to the patient the importance of good inhaler technique and how it affects the efficacy of the medication
- Ask the patient first to show you how they use their inhaler
- Then explain in a step-by-step manner, demonstrating each step as you go
- Remember to keep the language very simple and easy to follow
- Inhaler technique:
  1. Check the expiration date.
  2. Ensure that the inhaler has been well shaken.
  3. Remove the inhaler cap.
  4. Sit up straight and lift the chin to open the airway.
  5. Breathe out completely.
  6. Place the inhaler between the teeth and form a good seal around it with the lips.
  7. Press the top of the inhaler whilst taking a slow deep breath in at the same time.
  8. Once the lungs are full, take the inhaler out of the mouth and hold the breath for around 10 s or as long as able to do so.
  9. Remove the inhaler and breathe normally again.

10. If repeat puffs are required, shake the inhaler well before using it again.
11. Once finished, replace the cap.
- Inhaler and spacer technique:
  1. Remove the inhaler cap and insert the inhaler into the end of the spacer.
  2. Breathe out completely and sit with an upright back.
  3. Put the spacer mouthpiece in between your lips and form a good seal.
  4. Press the top of the inhaler to release one puff of medicine into the spacer.
  5. Breathe in slowly through the spacer.
  6. Remove the spacer and hold your breath for around 10 s, or as long as able to do so.
  7. If repeat puffs are required, remove the inhaler from the spacer and shake it again before use.

DIFFERENT TYPES OF INHALER DEVICES IN ASTHMA

There are two main types of inhaler devices used in asthma:
1. Metered-dose inhaler (MDI)
2. Dry-powder inhalers

MDIs require good coordination to press the canister and inhale at the same time. Dry-powder inhalers only need to be inhaled to take in the medication. Table 4.4 outlines the differences between the two.

There are also combination inhalers which contain a long-acting bronchodilator and steroids; for example, budesonide/formeterol combination inhalers are also known as Symbicort.

TYPES OF SPACERS

All children should be using spacers. Like inhalers, spacers come in a variety of different types which fit on to different inhalers and are for different ages:
- Older children/adults: MDI with spacer
- 2–10 years old: MDI with spacer
- Under 2 years old: MDI with spacer and mask
  - Babyhaler: Spacer with mask; does not have to be upright; listen for five clicks
  - Volumatic: For greater than 2-year-old children (Fig. 4.1)
  - Aerochamber: Different-sized masks for infants, children and adults (Fig. 4.2)

Table **4.4** Drugs used in asthma inhalers and their differences

TYPE OF INHALER	EXAMPLE	INDICATION	TIME OF ONSET
Short-acting bronchodilators: Relievers	• Salbutamol • Terbutaline	• Use when symptoms occur	• Immediate effect
Steroid inhalers: Preventers	• Beclometasone • Fluticasone • Budesonide	• Use daily to prevent symptoms	• Not effective immediately
Long-acting bronchodilators	• Salmeterol • Formeterol	• Use in conjunction with steroid inhalers, to prevent symptoms	• Work for up to 12 h after the dose has been taken

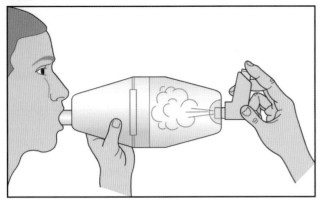

Fig. 4.1 Volumetric spacer.

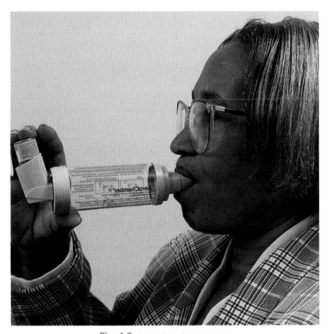

Fig. 4.2 Aerochamber spacer.

WASHING A SPACER

- Wash once a week in warm soapy water
- Leave to drip dry
- Do not put in dishwasher or wipe dry

Rare Side Effects of Inhaled Steroids

- Adrenal suppression: Non-specific symptoms like anorexia, abdominal pain, weight loss, headache, nausea and vomiting
- Skin: Easy bruising and thinning of skin
- Weakened immunity: Instruct the patient that they should inform their doctor if they feel unwell
- Development: In comparison with non-asthmatic children, children with asthma may have a later onset of puberty and growth retardation

PERSONALISED ASTHMA ACTION PLANS

All patients should have a personalised asthma action plan which they can follow at home (Fig. 4.3). These contain a lot of information which include a patient's daily inhalers, what they can do if their asthma is worsening and instructions on what to do in an emergency. The action plan is a core part of managing a patient's asthma and can be reviewed from time to time if a patient's control is deteriorating.

Present Your Findings

Miss Johnson is a 24-year-old woman who has recently been diagnosed with asthma. She has been prescribed a reliever inhaler but has found that her symptoms of shortness of breath and wheeze have persisted. Rosie has been struggling with how to use her inhaler and therefore, I explained and demonstrated the correct technique of using her inhaler.

As she is complaining of persisting wheeze and shortness of breath and has been using her inhaler more than three times a week, I have reminded her to follow her personalised asthma action plan. She will be reviewed again in 1 month to see if her asthma control has improved.

QUESTIONS AND ANSWERS FOR CANDIDATE

A hoarse voice, sore throat and fungal infection are the most common side effects from steroid inhalers. How can these be prevented?
- By using a spacer
- Rinsing out the mouth with water after inhaler use

Name three symptoms of an asthma attack.
- Severe breathlessness
- Inability to complete sentences in one breath
- Increasing wheeze
- Chest tightness
- Chest pain
- Dizziness

If a patient was having an asthma attack, what would you advise?
- Try to remain calm and sit up
- Take one puff of the reliever (blue) inhaler every 30–60 s up to a maximum of 10 puffs
- Call for help and call 999 if they feel worse at any point whilst using the inhaler or the attack is not relieved by 10 puffs

A Case to Learn From

A patient had very poorly controlled asthma, requiring an escalation of treatment. The team were very concerned about her increasing requirements and polypharmacy. Her technique was checked and found to be incorrect. Her symptoms vastly improved following a correct technique and her medication requirements reduced. Always check inhaler technique!

Every day asthma care:

My asthma is being managed well:

- With this daily routine I should expect/aim to have no symptoms

- If I have not had any symptoms or needed my reliever inhaler for at least 12 weeks, I canask my GP or asthma nurse to review my medicines in case they can reduce the dose.

- My personal best peak flow is:

My daily asthma routine:

My preventer inhaler (insert name/color):

....

I need to take my preventer inhaler every day even when I feel well.

I take .... puff(s) in the morning

and .... puff(s) at night.

My reliever inhaler (insert name/colour):

....

I take my reliever inhaler only if I need to

I take .... puff(s) of my reliever inhaler if any of these things happen:

- I'm wheezing • My chest feels tight
- I'm finding it hard to breathe • I'm coughing

Other medicines and devices (e.g spacer, peak flow meter) I use for my asthma every day:

 When A feel worse:

My asthma is getting worse if I'm experiencing any of these:

- My symptoms are coming back (wheeze, tightness in my chest, feeling breathless, cough).

- I am waking up at night.

- My symptoms are interfering with my usual day-to-day activities (eg at work, exercising).

- I am using my reliever inhaler three times a week or more.

- My peak flow drops to below: ....

⚠️ **URGENT! If you need your reliever inhaler more than every four hours, you need to take emergency action now. see section 3.**

What I can do to get on top of my asthma now:

If I haven't been using my preventer inhaler, I'll start using it regularly again or if have been using it:

- Increase my preventer inhaler dose to................ puffs................times a day until my symptoms have gone and my peak flow is back to my personal best

- Take my reliever inhaler as needed (up to .... puffs every four hours).

- Carry my reliever inhaler with me when I'm out.

⚠️ **URGENT! See a doctor or nurse within 24 hours if you get worse at any time or you haven't improved after seven days.**

Other advice from my GP about what to do if my asthma is worse (eg MART or rescue steroid tablets):

3 In an asthma attack:

I'm having an asthma attack if i'm experiencin any of these:

- My reliever inhaler is not helping or I need it more than every four hours.

- I find it difficult to walk or talk.

- I find it difficult to breathe.

- I'm wheezing a lot, or I have a very tight chest, or I'm coughing a lot.

- My peak flow is below: ....

What to do in an asthma attack

1. Sit up straight - try to keep calm.
2. Take one puff of your reliever inhaler (usually blue) every 30-60 seconds up to 10 puffs.
3. If you feel worse at any point OR you don't feel better after 10 puffs **call 999 for an ambulance.**
4. If the ambulance has not arrived after 10 minutes and your symptoms are not improving, repeat step 2.
5. If your symptoms are no better after repeating step 2, and the ambulance has still not arrived, **contact 999 again immediately.**

Important: this asthma attack advice not apply to you if you use a MART inhaler.

After an asthma attack

- If you dealt with your asthma attack at home, see your GP today.

- If you were treated in hospital, see your GP within 48 hours of being discharged.

- Finish any medicines they prescribe you, even if you start to feel better.

- If you don't improve after treatment, see your GP urgently.

What to do in an asthma attack if I'm on MART:

Fig. 4.3 An example of an asthma action plan.

 Top Tip

With children, suggest interesting ways to ensure the child uses their inhaler every day; for example, a star chart.

STATION 4.5: SMOKING CESSATION COUNSELLING

SCENARIO

You are a junior doctor working in a primary care practice and your next patient is Jennifer Roland, a 30-year-old woman, who wants help with quitting smoking. Please take a brief smoking history and counsel her regarding smoking cessation.

CORE CONCEPT

- Smoking can increase the risk of patients developing many life-threatening diseases. It also has an impact on other people exposed to smoking and has implications on children's health
- To help with smoking cessation, patients can use NRT or other medications
- Whilst quitting, patients can attend a local smoking cessation clinic, which will provide them with either one-to-one or group sessions to support their efforts
- When it comes to counselling patients to stop smoking, it is important to be non-judgemental and empathetic
- Patients may find it difficult to admit that they have failed to quit in the past and will need reassurance that this is common. Those who are successful in quitting smoking usually have had multiple attempts

Common Concerns

What about e-cigarettes?	• E-cigarettes can be helpful in those wanting to quit smoking, as they also contain nicotine but not tobacco, and are becoming increasingly common. They are much safer compared to cigarettes, but the full risks are unknown as they are new to the market. The risks will only be known later
Will using NRT be enough to stop smoking?	• Though NRT has been found to be very effective in helping people to stop smoking, it is not always enough on its own. For the best chances, NRT should be combined with willpower and attending a smoking cessation clinic
Will I get withdrawal symptoms from stopping so abruptly?	• Some people will experience withdrawal symptoms; for example, sweating, nausea and a sore throat. These tend to peak in the first few days but will settle over the next 2–4 weeks. NRT can help to reduce the effect of these symptoms

GATHERING INFORMATION AND COMMUNICATIONS

This case has two parts:
1. Taking a brief smoking history
2. Counselling the patient about smoking cessation

SMOKING HISTORY

• Age when started smoking
• Number of cigarettes smoked per day
• Who is around when smoking
Establish the patient's motivations to stop smoking:
• Any previous attempts and what actions were taken
• Reason for quitting now

SMOKING CESSATION ADVICE

First, explain to the patient the risks associated with smoking, both to their personal health and that of others.
• Smoking is associated with a number of serious illnesses that can reduce a person's life expectancy. These include:
  • Cancers, with the most well-known examples being lung and throat cancer

• Coronary heart disease, which puts patients at risk of heart attack, stroke, aneurysm and heart failure
• Chronic obstructive pulmonary disease (COPD)
Smoking also poses a threat to those who do not smoke themselves but are exposed to cigarette smoke by others. This is known as passive smoking and exposure to cigarettes can be particularly harmful to:
• Children: Can increase the risk of asthma, chest infections and, sudden infant death syndrome (SIDS)
• Pregnant women: Smoking during pregnancy can increase the risks of miscarriage, premature delivery, low birth weight and stillbirth. Those who smoke more than 10 cigarettes per day are considered high-risk and need to have consultant-led antenatal care
Then address smoking cessation and why it can be difficult to quit:
• The reduction in nicotine when stopping smoking can lead to withdrawal symptoms for some people, including:
  • Cravings to smoke
  • Anxiety
  • Irritability
  • Headache and dizziness
• It can be difficult to stop smoking as nicotine, one of the chemicals in cigarettes, is addictive
• Withdrawal symptoms tend to reach a peak after a day of stopping smoking. They gradually ease over 2–4 weeks
• Most people who have successfully stopped smoking have had multiple attempts
Try focusing on the ways smoking cessation may become easier:
• Get support! There is lots available, for example:
  • Inform family and friends of the plan to quit so that they can help with avoiding smoking
  • Sign up to a local smoking cessation clinic, which provides one-to-one and group support
  • Call the national smoke-free helpline where there are trained advisors to consult
  • Explore the free support available through apps, email or text message programmes
Following this, you can mention NRT as an adjunct to willpower:
• Most people use NRT to help them quit smoking, and this is recommended
• This is a way of getting nicotine into the body without smoking, helping to stop smoking by reducing the withdrawal symptoms

- NRT comes in lots of forms, including patches, gum, inhalers and sprays. There are higher doses aimed at those who smoke more than 18–20 cigarettes per day
- To have the best chances of quitting, use nicotine replacement for at least 2–3 months, gradually reducing the amount and how often it is used towards the end
- NRT should not be combined with other medications that are used to help with stopping smoking; for example, varenicline and bupropion

PRESCRIBED DRUGS FOR SMOKING CESSATION

 Drugs used in smoking cessation

Varenicline	- Prescription only - Partial nicotine agonist - Relieves withdrawal symptoms, as well as reduces cravings to smoke - Usually started 1 week before the stop date and taken for 12 weeks
Bupropion	- Prescription only - Antidepressant, but can be used for smoking cessation - Relieves withdrawal symptoms - Usually started 1–2 weeks before the stop date and taken for 7 weeks

 Present Your Findings

Miss Roland is a 30-year-old current smoker who smokes 10 cigarettes a day and has been doing so since she was 17, giving her a 6.5-pack year history. She had tried to quit smoking last year and would like to try again this year, as she is hoping to get pregnant.

Today I counselled her on the benefits of smoking cessation and have recommended that she use NRT whilst trying to quit. I have also referred her to the smoking cessation clinic, which she will attend next week.

❓ QUESTIONS AND ANSWERS FOR CANDIDATE

How do you calculate pack years?
- Number of years smoked multiplied by the average number of packs smoked per day
- 20 cigarettes are equivalent to one pack

Name five red-flag symptoms in a smoker that may suggest a lung malignancy.
- Haemoptysis
- Persistent cough
- Loss of appetite
- Unexplained weight loss
- Recurrent chest infections

Give three examples of cancers that smoking can predispose a patient to.
- Lung
- Bladder
- Stomach
- Oesophageal

 A Case to Learn From

A 58-year-old ex-smoker who presented with a long-standing cough, shortness of breath and wheezing on exertion was diagnosed with chronic obstructive pulmonary disease (COPD). Initially he did not believe the diagnosis because he had stopped smoking years ago, so he thought that he was no longer at risk. It is important to remember that the effects of smoking may not be seen until many years later, even if the patient has already stopped.

 Top Tip

Use motivational interviewing to get the patient to identify their reasons for giving up and identify the strengths they have to help ensure that they do. Remind them that it takes at least three goes for most people. Therefore, they should not feel disheartened if their first try is not successful.

STATION 4.6: CONSENT FOR ASCITIC DRAIN

SCENARIO

You are a junior doctor working on the medical admission unit and have been asked to see Perry Bard, a 59-year-old man, who has presented with increasing abdominal swelling and shortness of breath over the last 3 months. He is known to have liver cirrhosis. On examination of the abdomen, there is shifting dullness. Please take a brief history and gain Mr Bard's consent for an ascitic drain.

CORE CONCEPT

When asking for consent make sure to cover:
- What the procedure will entail
- Indications and benefits of the procedure
- Potential risks
- Assess the patient's capacity to make the decision

Common Concerns

Will it hurt?	• The procedure is carried out under local anaesthetic, therefore the patient may experience a small sharp scratch when the local anaesthetic is injected, but afterwards should not feel pain • After the procedure, the patient may be given simple painkillers; for example, paracetamoll
Once it's drained, will it come back?	• The build-up of fluid can be prevented through the use of diuretics and restricting salt intake. However, in time the fluid can build up again if the underlying condition progresses
What are the alternatives to having it drained?	If patients do not want to have their ascites drained, there are other options: • Continue to monitor and only drain if symptomatic • Manage with salt restriction and diuretics • Radiological procedures such as a transjugular intrahepatic portosystemic shunt (TIPS)

GATHERING INFORMATION AND COMMUNICATIONS

This case has two parts:
1. Taking a brief history
2. Gaining consent for an ascitic drain

HISTORY

In a patient presenting with new ascites, ask about:
• Onset and duration: Speed of onset and length of time the abdominal swelling has been present
• Associated abdominal pain: The presence of pain with tense ascites can be a sign of spontaneous bacterial peritonitis
• Peripheral oedema: Heart failure is an important cause of both peripheral oedema and ascites
• Shortness of breath: Tense ascites can splint the diaphragm, leading to respiratory symptoms

Before the procedure, also ask the patient about potential contraindications:
• Known coagulopathies or usage of anticoagulants
• Possibility of pregnancy in women
• Skin infection over the intended puncture site

CONSENT FOR AN ASCITIC DRAIN

It may help to establish the patient's current knowledge about ascitic drains and whether they have had one inserted before.

WHAT IS AN ASCITIC DRAIN?

• Placement of a small tube into the abdominal wall which will drain the fluid that has built up

What Will The Procedure Involve?
1. The patient will be asked to lie flat during the procedure.
2. The skin will first be cleaned and then numbed with a local anaesthetic.
3. A small needle will then be passed through the abdominal wall to create a hole, through which a tube is inserted. An ultrasound may be used at the same time to guide the needle.
4. The tube inserted will drain the fluid in the abdomen and will be attached to a collection bag.
5. The tube will be stitched or taped in place.
6. It may take several hours or more for all the fluid to be drained.

BENEFITS OF AN ASCITIC DRAIN
• Reduces the risk of peritonitis
• Symptomatic relief
• Diagnostic, to find out what has caused the swelling

RISKS
It is important to explain that an ascitic drain is a commonly performed procedure; however there are some risks associated with it. These include:
• Failure to insert the drain
• Damage to surrounding structures during drain insertion, including bowel perforation
• Bleeding
• Drain leakage
• Infection
• Need for repeat procedure

RISK FACTORS FOR THE DEVELOPMENT OF ASCITES
• Liver cirrhosis:
  • Alcohol consumption
  • Autoimmune diseases
  • Hepatitis exposure
• Malignancy:
  • History of smoking
  • Known malignancy
  • Exposure to asbestos

- Previous medical history:
  - Known heart failure
  - Pancreatitis

ASCITIC FLUID ANALYSIS

Once a sample of ascitic fluid has been collected, it should be sent for:

- Microbiology: Microscopy, culture and sensitivity (MCS)
- Haematology: Automated white cell count (WCC)
- Biochemistry: Albumin, protein, lactate dehydrogenase, glucose
- Cytology: Presence of malignant cells

 Present Your Findings

Mr Bard is a 59-year-old man with known liver cirrhosis who has presented today with worsening ascites.

I have explained the benefits and risks of having an ascitic drain inserted for symptomatic relief. He is happy to go ahead with the procedure and I have documented his verbal consent.

 QUESTIONS AND ANSWERS FOR CANDIDATE

Name three common causes of abdominal swelling.

- Fat
- Flatus
- Faeces
- Fetus
- Fluid

Which diuretics are first line in the management of ascites?

- Aldosterone receptor antagonists; for example, spironolactone

What is a TIPS?

- A TIPS is placed between the hepatic and portal veins to reduce portal hypertension and is most commonly used in refractory ascites

 A Case to Learn From

A patient was admitted under the gynaecology team with new abdominal bloating and difficulty passing stools. She was being investigated for a possible ovarian malignancy. On admission, her previously unreported alcohol abuse was elicited. On further investigation, it was ascertained that she had liver disease and subsequent ascites. Always take a thorough history.

 Top Tip

It is important to know whether your patient has transudate or exudative ascites, as this may change their management.

STATION 4.7: CONSENT FOR HERNIA REPAIR

SCENARIO

You are a junior doctor working on the surgical ward and have been asked to see Benjamin Penneck, a 62-year-old man, who has recently been diagnosed with an inguinal hernia. Please take a brief, relevant history and explain to him the available management options as well as the risks and benefits of surgical repair of the hernia.

CORE CONCEPT

- The only definitive management of a hernia is repair via surgery, which can be done either laparoscopically or by open surgery. The operation may involve the insertion of a prosthetic mesh to strengthen the abdominal wall, preventing recurrence. If done electively, the operation will be carried out as a day-case procedure
- The procedure can be performed under general, regional or local anaesthetic. The decision of which anaesthetic to use is made by the surgeon and the anaesthetist
- It is important to explain the benefits and risks of the operation to the patient, as whilst hernia repair is a common and relatively safe procedure, risks include: Infection, bleeding and hernia recurrence

 Common Concerns

Will my hernia come back?	• The risk of recurrence of a hernia is about 5% in 5 years, regardless of technique
What if I do not want an operation?	• The decision to operate is largely based on symptoms • Hernias that do not cause any symptoms can be safely monitored under follow-up, without significant risk of complications such as incarceration, strangulation and bowel obstruction • Once a hernia starts to cause discomfort, the risk of developing these complications increases and the risks of surgery are easier to justify
How long will I be in hospital?	• Most patients are able to go home either on the day of, or the day after, the operation

GATHERING INFORMATION AND COMMUNICATIONS

This case has three parts:
1. Taking a brief history specific to the hernia
2. Explaining the management options for an inguinal hernia
3. Counselling the patient on the risks and benefits of surgical repair of the hernia

HISTORY

Ask the following questions in a patient presenting with a suspected hernia:
- Onset and duration of the lump: Some hernias may spontaneously occur after heavy lifting or may have an insidious onset. Ascertain how long the lump has been present
- Associated ache or pain: Whilst a 'dragging' sensation is common with a hernia, pain may be associated with strangulation
- Size of the hernia and any changes: The sizes of hernias may be positional; many increase when standing and decrease when lying down
- Whether the hernia is reducible: If it is irreducible, strangulation is more likely to occur

MANAGEMENT OF A HERNIA

WHAT IS A HERNIA?

- A hernia can be thought of as a hole or a weak spot in the wall of the abdomen, where internal organs, for example, the intestine or the gut, partly come out through the hole and appear under the skin, causing a lump (Table 4.5)
- Hernias can potentially cause problems; for example, pain. The gut that is protruding can become kinked, compressed or blocked and, if the blood supply is also kinked or compressed, the gut may suffer and, rarely, may even burst

SURGICAL MANAGEMENT

- Surgery to prevent the complications of hernias from occurring

- It can be done as an open procedure with a cut in the groin or laparoscopically with keyhole. This depends on patient and hospital factors

Laparoscopic Repair

- Using a keyhole technique, a camera and some surgical instruments are inserted through several small cuts in the abdomen. Any tissues sticking out through the hernia are pulled back in through the hernia 'hole' and this hole in the wall of the abdomen can be repaired. A patch is then put over the original site of the hernia, to help reduce the chances of this happening again
- For a keyhole repair, a general anaesthetic is required
- In about 2% of cases, the procedure has to be converted to open surgery

Open Surgery

- A 10-cm cut is made in the groin, just above the swelling. The protruding gut is pushed back in, the hole is stitched over and a patch is placed over the site of the hole
- Open repair is commonly done under general anaesthetic, but can be done with regional anaesthetic

RISKS

- Hernia repairs are generally regarded as a safe procedure that is very commonly done in hospital

Short-Term Risks

- Infection: The mesh is a foreign body and if it gets infected, it may need to be removed and replaced
- Bleeding: Due to damage to blood vessels or gut
- Difficulty passing urine (postoperative urinary obstruction): May require a tube in the bladder to help drain urine
- Patches of numbness in the skin: Usually resolve
- Testicular pain (ischaemic orchitis): Usually resolves

Long-Term Risks

- May develop chronic pain (abdominal or scrotal): Due to nerve damage

Table 4.5	Information on different types of hernia
HERNIA TYPE	**COMMON DEMOGRAPHIC**
Inguinal hernia	• More common in males • Indirect – infants • Direct – elderly
Femoral hernia	• More common in females • More likely to strangulate
Umbilical hernia	• Obese, middle-aged patients
Incisional hernia	• Elderly patients with previous operations, usually within a year of operation
Spigelian hernia	• Hernia through the spigelian fascia • Rare • Often interparietal and at high risk of strangulation

- Recurrence of hernia: About 5% in 5 years, regardless of technique

RECOVERY

- The majority of patients are able to go home either the day of, or the day after, surgery
- As it is normal to experience discomfort around the incision sites for a few days after the operation, patients are therefore discharged home with pain relief
- Constipation may occur over the first few days after the operation; this can be prevented by drinking plenty of fluids and eating high-fibre foods
- The patient may be able to return to work after 1–2 weeks, but should avoid heavy lifting and strenuous activities for 4–6 weeks
- Patients should seek further help if any of the following occur:
  - *Abdominal* swelling and persistent pain
  - *Bleeding* around the incision sites
  - *Coughing* and shortness of breath
  - *Difficulty* passing urine
  - *Erythema* (redness) around the incision site

The above signs and symptoms can be remembered using the acronym mnemonic ABCDE.

OTHER GENERAL ADVICE REGARDING HERNIAS

Treat risk factors! Look for and treat causes of raised intra-abdominal pressure, such as:
- Obesity
- Ascites
- Constipation
- Chronic coughing from COPD

These won't help the hernia but may prevent it from getting any larger or prevent any more hernias developing.

 Present Your Findings

Mr Penneck is a 62-year-old man who has presented with a groin lump that appeared after he was helping his son move furniture 1 month ago. The lump is painless and can be reduced manually.

The groin lump was diagnosed as an inguinal hernia and the option of surgery was discussed with him. I have explained the risks and benefits of having surgery to repair the hernia and Mr Penneck is happy to consent to a laparoscopic repair.

❓ QUESTIONS AND ANSWERS FOR CANDIDATE

Anatomically, what is the difference between a direct and an indirect inguinal hernia?
- Indirect inguinal hernias usually occur due to the failure of the inguinal canal to close properly. Therefore, these pass through the internal ring,

lateral to the inferior epigastric artery and along the inguinal canal and come out at the external ring
- Direct inguinal hernias usually occur due to a weakness in the posterior wall of the inguinal canal. Therefore, these protrude through the posterior wall of the canal

Excluding an inguinal hernia, give three differential diagnoses for a lump presenting in the groin of a male patient.
- Femoral hernia
- Hydrocele
- Varicocele
- Abscess

What is a strangulated hernia?
- Strangulated means that blood vessels supplying the hernia contents become occluded at the neck, leading to ischaemia

 A Case to Learn From

When working in general medicine, an elderly woman with dementia was admitted from her care home with what appeared to be abdominal pain and increased agitation. Her primary care doctor was concerned about bowel obstruction. Only after thorough examination, including examining the hernial orifices, was a femoral hernia diagnosed. Always examine the hernial orifices when a patient presents with abdominal pain!

Top Tip

Infection and numbness are much less common after a laparoscopic repair.

 Top Tip

Bowel obstruction is not a risk, except with a transabdominal laparoscopic preperitoneal (TAPP) repair. Laparoscopic repairs which are total extraperitoneal (TEP) do not carry a risk of adhesion formation because the peritoneum is never entered.

STATION 4.8: DEALING WITH AN AGITATED PATIENT

SCENARIO

You are a junior doctor working in colorectal clinic and have been asked to see Bill Gates, a 65-year-old man. He is very angry because he was supposed to receive a computed tomography (CT) scan for bowel investigations over a month ago and hasn't heard anything about it. Please explore the concerns Mr Gates has.

CORE CONCEPT

- You should place your own safety first. Give clear boundaries to the patient if they are being inappropriately aggressive or rude. Do not approach the patient if it is unsafe to do so
- During the consultation, it is important to remain calm and allow the patient to vent their anger, if necessary, without interruption
- Validate their feelings and, together with the patient, come up with a shared plan regarding how to address any problems that have arisen
- An apology is very important. To reinforce this, it can be done at the beginning, middle and end of the consultation. It is not necessarily an admission of guilt or an invitation for a complaint. It merely acknowledges what has happened and the patient's justifiable anxiety

Common Concerns

If you were in my position, would you make a complaint?	• It is entirely up to the patient as to whether they would like to put in a formal complaint. In this situation, you should give them the details of the Patient Advice and Liaison Service (PALS) so that they can make a complaint if they would like to
I need to speak to a senior member of staff immediately.	• This may or may not be possible. However, if there is a manager or senior member of staff available then it may be useful to ask them to speak to the patient
Will you report what has occurred?	• All patient safety incidents, including any 'near misses', should be reported to enable investigation and work to be done to prevent future incidents. Local guidelines or processes will vary

GATHERING INFORMATION AND COMMUNICATIONS

This case has one part:
1. Exploring the patient's emotions

EXPLORING THE PATIENT'S EMOTIONS

- Ask open questions to establish why the patient is angry
- Do not assume that the patient is angry for the reasons you might be in his circumstance. Allow them to explain their specific concerns and address these individually and immediately. For example:

- Mr Gates may be well informed about his investigations. Talking about the disease is not as relevant as focusing the discussion on practically arranging to get the scan done
- Mr Gates may be desperate to have the CT scan because he understands nothing about the disease and associates the scan with finding out more information. In this case, counselling the patient about not just the CT scan, but also his disease, may help relieve anger
- Mr Gates may have worsening symptoms; for example, with worsening appetite, weight loss and tiredness. Anger may stem from feeling that his disease is getting worse, yet appearing to be ignored by the system. Identifying and managing his symptoms, talking about the disease and arranging the scan all need emphasis here
- Make sure you acknowledge and understand the patient's concerns. It may be helpful to summarise and repeat these concerns to the patient
- Allow the patient to talk and do not interrupt
- Active listening techniques, for example, maintaining eye contact, nodding and small verbal comments, may be useful, depending on the patient
- It is important to remain empathetic throughout the discussion. This builds rapport and may diffuse the situation
- Apologise to the patient and explain the steps that you will take to rectify the situation
- If the patient wishes to make a formal complaint, provide them with the details of the local PALS:
  - The patient is within their rights to complain and this should normally be done within 12 months
  - The chief executive of the hospital will reply as soon as reasonably possible
  - It can be done through several channels, including the local complaints manager and the primary care trust complaints manager (many hospitals will have a PALS and patients can be referred to this)
  - They may also complain directly to a professional body, such as the General Medical Council
  - Help on practically filing a complaint can be obtained from organisations; for example, the Citizens Advice Bureau

THINGS TO AVOID

Avoid:
- Focusing the consultation around attributing blame
- Being defensive
- Criticising the patient for his approach to the situation
- Interrupting or patronising the patient

- Giving no information. Even if you are not an expert, you may still be able to say something useful to the patient such as how you could get in contact with someone who can help

 Present Your Findings

Mr Gates is a 65-year-old man who has been waiting for a staging CT for his bowel cancer. He states that he has not yet received an appointment, which is making him anxious about his future treatment, especially as he has been having worsening symptoms.

To address his symptoms, I have increased his analgesia and given him an antiemetic. Furthermore, I have apologised for the delay and have arranged to call him in the next week to confirm the date for the scan.

QUESTIONS AND ANSWERS FOR CANDIDATE

Name three red-flag symptoms of colorectal cancer.
- Rectal bleeding
- Weight loss
- Change in bowel habit

Patients who are suspected of having cancer should be seen within what timeframe?
- 2 weeks

Name the two main staging systems used in colorectal cancer.
- Dukes' staging classification
- Tumour, node, metastasis (TNM) system

 A Case to Learn From

A patient was prescribed and given an antibiotic they were already known to be allergic to. After ensuring the patient was well and stopping the antibiotic, I immediately informed the charge nurse and the consultant what had happened. I apologised to the patient and their family, who were angry. I clearly documented what had happened, including the discussions, and filled in a critical incident form. When an error occurs, identify it, address it and try to suggest measures to prevent it happening again.

Top Tip

Always acknowledge the reasons why the patient is frustrated. This validates what they are going through, reassures them that you are listening and goes a long way towards building rapport.

STATION 4.9: BLOOD TRANSFUSION

SCENARIO

You are a junior doctor on the phone to a ward nurse who has called you urgently about a patient, Janet Blatt, who started a blood transfusion 2 h ago. The patient's temperature is now 37.7°C, blood pressure is 99/60 mmHg and the patient is anxious. Explore this further on the phone and identify what you would like the nurse to do and what you are going to do to further manage this patient.

CORE CONCEPT

A 'situation, background, assessment, recommendation (SBAR)' format is generally used for communication from nursing staff to medical staff:
- *Situation*: A brief summary of the problem, including the patient's details, locations and the concern
- *Background*: Relevant details about the patient's previous medical or surgical history and reason for admission
- *Assessment*: A summary of what you think has happened, as well as details of any pertinent investigation results and changes in observations
- *Recommendation*: What should happen next; for example, is a senior review required or is advice enough?

Do not hesitate to contact your senior colleagues if you require any assistance, advice or an independent review. Again, you can use the SBAR format when asking for advice.

In a patient who has deteriorated whilst having a blood transfusion, you will be concerned about:
- ABO incompatibility: Potentially catastrophic and occurs in the first few minutes
- Non-haemolytic transfusion reaction: Less dramatic but may occur at any time
- Transfusion-related acute lung injury (TRALI): More likely with fresh frozen plasma (FFP)
- Volume overload: Can be due to a rapid infusion of a large volume of blood
- Anaphylaxis: Allergic reaction to the blood products

If the patient is periarrest and is no longer able to maintain her airway, the nurse should call the on-call crash team whilst you are on your way.

Common Concerns

Have I been given the wrong blood?	• Although this is a possibility, there are very stringent policies and checking procedures in place to reduce this risk
Why can some of the risks happen if I am just receiving some blood?	• Everyone's blood is made up of a unique combination of blood cells with specific proteins on their surfaces. In the context of blood transfusion, the blood that you are receiving can be considered as a foreign body, as the donor blood's is not an exact match of the recipient's, so the body may begin to respond to it differently to how we'd expect
I am a regular blood donor; how will a blood transfusion affect me?	• Currently, if you have had a blood transfusion then you will no longer be able to donate blood. This is to reduce the risk of variant Creutzfeldt–Jakob disease (vCJD) being passed on by donors

GATHERING INFORMATION AND COMMUNICATIONS

This case has one part:
1. Managing post-blood transfusion complications

MANAGING POST-BLOOD TRANSFUSION COMPLICATIONS

Clarify any clinical concerns:
• Reason for transfusion
• What product was being transfused
• Presence of any symptoms
  Clarify any change in the observations, especially at:
• The start of the transfusion
• Any of the checkpoints (15, 30 and 60 min) in routine monitoring of the transfusion

This will help you establish the time course of events and point you in the direction of a diagnosis. For example, patient 1, being transfused after an acute intra-abdominal blood loss, awaiting theatre, may have deteriorated due to further bleeding, whereas this is less likely in patient 2, who is being transfused for long-standing anaemia secondary to chronic kidney disease.

Clarify any management already implemented by nursing staff:
• Stopping the transfusion
• Give intravenous (IV) fluids (if prescribed)

• The transfusion may need to be stopped, but this depends on the clinical scenario; for example, the presence of haemodynamic instability in an acute bleed

Assume now that the patient is having a non-haemolytic febrile transfusion reaction.

Whilst making your way to review the patient, you should ask the nursing staff to:
• Stop the transfusion and put up IV fluids through a clean giving set
• Give oxygen if saturations are below 94%
• Check the blood pack and patient details
• Administer paracetamol orally (if already written on the drug chart)
• Take bloods (if trained) for: Full blood count (FBC), urea and electrolytes (U&Es), group and save (to cross-match again) and a coagulation screen
• Phone the blood bank to inform them of the reaction and send the sample back to the blood bank
• Consider inserting a urethral catheter to monitor urine output

Then let the nursing staff know you are on your way to review the patient. This will depend on other clinical emergencies, but this patient must be reviewed as a clinical priority. Encourage nursing staff to contact you again if there are any further questions or concerns whilst you are making your way to review the patient.

PRESCRIBING BLOOD PRODUCTS

• Blood must be prescribed on the relevant chart. Hospitals will generally have a pathway document for blood transfusions
• Each unit must be prescribed separately

BLOOD PRODUCT ADMINISTRATION

• Two members of the medical or nursing team must check:
  • The patient's details
  • The blood pack
  • The patient's wristband
• Ensure that there is IV access and a clean giving set is used
• Each unit of red cells can be administered over 1–4 h. A faster rate may be required in emergencies

MONITORING DURING TRANSFUSION

• Baseline observations (heart rate, blood pressure, respiratory rate and temperature) are repeated again at 15, 30 and 60 min after the transfusion is started

SAFETY-NET ADVICE

Ask nurses to call the doctor if they observe:
• Changes from baseline observations
• Urticarial rash
• Features of anaphylaxis

MANAGEMENT OF COMMON COMPLICATIONS OF BLOOD TRANSFUSION

❗ Management of common complications of blood transfusion

DIAGNOSIS	PRESENTATION	ACTION	INVESTIGATIONS	MANAGEMENT
• Acute haemolytic reaction: ABO incompatibility	• Rapid spike in temperature to > 40°C (at the start of transfusion) • Hypotensive and tachycardic • Unwell, agitated, flushed • Pain (abdomen, chest and/or cannula site) • Bleeding from the cannula site	• Resuscitate the patient using an ABC approach • Stop the transfusion • Check that the correct blood was given by looking at the patient identification number and documentation • Inform the haematologist and blood bank • Send the blood transfusion bag back to the laboratory • May require senior help or intensive therapy/treatment unit (ITU) intervention	• Routine observations • Bloods: FBCs, U&Es, coagulation screen, group and save • Catheterise to monitor urine output • Dipstick the urine for blood	• Give saline through a new giving set
• Anaphylaxis	• Bronchospasm • Cyanosis • Tachycardic and hypotensive • Swelling • Rash	• Resuscitate the patient using an ABC approach • Stop the transfusion • Check that the correct blood was given by looking at the patient identification number and documentation • Inform the haematologist and blood bank • Send blood transfusion bag back to the laboratory • May require senior help or ITU intervention	• Bloods: FBC, U&Es, coagulation screen, group and save	• Adrenaline 0.5 mg 1:1000 intramuscular (IM) • Nebulisers if wheezy • Fast IV fluids to treat anaphylactic shock
• Non-haemolytic febrile transfusion reaction	• Slow-rising temperature approximately 60 min after transfusion commenced	• Resuscitate the patient using an ABC approach • Stop the transfusion • Check that the correct blood was given by looking at the patient identification number and documentation • Inform the haematologist and blood bank • Send blood transfusion bag back to the laboratory • May require senior input	• Monitor haemodynamic stability of patient • Bloods: FBCs, U&Es, coagulation screen, group and save	• Paracetamol 1 g • IV fluids through a new giving set
• Fluid overload	• Shortness of breath • Hypoxia • Tachycardia • Raised jugular venous pressure (JVP) • Bi-basal inspiratory crepitations	• Slow or stop the transfusion	• Monitor haemodynamic stability of patient • Bloods: FBCs, U&Es • ECG • Arterial blood gas (ABG) • Chest X-ray (CXR)	• Give oxygen, aiming for a saturation >94% • Diuretic therapy
• Urticarial reaction	• Urticarial rash on skin	• Resuscitate the patient using an ABC approach • Stop the transfusion • Check that the correct blood was given by looking at the patient identification number and documentation • Inform the haematologist and blood bank • Send blood transfusion bag back to the laboratory • Flush cannula with saline • Monitor urticarial progression	• Group and save	• Chlorphenamine 10 mg slow IV or IM

Present Your Findings

Mrs Blatt is a 60-year-old woman who was receiving 2 units of red blood cells for chronic anaemia. Her temperature increased to 37.7°C, her blood pressure dropped to 99/60 mmHg and the nurse reported that she began to feel anxious. I believe that she has had a non-haemolytic febrile transfusion reaction and have therefore asked the nurses to stop the transfusion and give her IV fluids through a new giving set whilst I make my way to the patient.

QUESTIONS AND ANSWERS FOR CANDIDATE

If a patient requiring a blood transfusion is at risk of volume overload, what can be done to reduce this risk?
- Furosemide can be given during the blood transfusion to reduce the risk of fluid overload

In pre-transfusion compatibility testing, what is the difference between a group and save and a group and cross-match?
- Group and save: The patient's blood is processed to identify the ABO and Rhesus D grouping and an antibody screen is carried out. The serum will also be kept in the blood bank for 48 h in case a further cross-match is needed
- Group and cross-match: The patient's serum is screened and tested directly for compatibility with available units in the blood bank. These cross-matched units of blood will be retained for 48 h

Which blood group is also known as the universal donor?
- O-negative blood is used in emergencies when the blood group of the patient is unknown
- This is because group O blood contains no antigens and therefore will not cause an ABO incompatibility reaction (Table 4.6)

A Case to Learn From

When on call, I was asked to review three different patients at the same time, who all sounded urgent: Chest pain, a temperature spike of 38.8°C and a patient who was tachycardic. Getting a good SBAR handover from the nurses not only allowed me to prioritise better who to see first, but also saved time when I reviewed the patient.

Top Tip

If you get the chance, try to go to the blood transfusion unit and observe from start to finish how a blood transfusion is conducted. I did so in my final year and the nursing staff were extremely helpful! They talked me through all the checks and showed me all the specific blood transfusion charts that they use on the unit, which could come up in an exam and were helpful for when I had to fill them in as a junior doctor.

STATION 4.10: COMMENCING WARFARIN THERAPY

SCENARIO

You are a junior doctor working in a cardiology clinic and have been asked to see Peter Jacobs, a 70-year-old man who was recently diagnosed with atrial fibrillation. He has been sent to your clinic, with a view to potentially starting warfarin therapy. Please counsel him about warfarin therapy and its implications.

CORE CONCEPT

Warfarin is a widely prescribed anticoagulant used in:
- Therapeutic management of venous thromboembolism (VTE): Including deep-vein thrombosis (DVT), pulmonary embolism (PE) and arterial thrombosis
- Prophylaxis: Secondary prevention of venous thrombosis, prevention of cardioembolic complications (indication in atrial fibrillation, mechanical or prosthetic heart valves)

Warfarin comes in a tablet which is usually taken every day. The dose of warfarin a patient takes can vary from day to day and is dictated by the international normalised ratio (INR), a blood test which tells you the 'thinness' of the patient's blood. A patient's target INR range will also vary depending on the reason they are on warfarin.

To help keep track of a patient's warfarin dose, patients will be given a 'yellow anticoagulant' record, which will contain:
- Indication for warfarin
- Target INR

 Table 4.6   Compatible recipient and donor blood groups

	BLOOD DONOR			
RECIPIENT	O	A	B	AB
O	☺	✖	✖	✖
A	☺	☺	✖	✖
B	☺	✖	☺	✖
AB	☺	☺	☺	☺

- Most recent INR values
- Most recent warfarin doses

Warfarin increases the risk of bleeding and patients are therefore advised to watch out for signs of bleeding, including haematuria, haematemesis, easy bruising and prolonged nose bleeds.

When counselling patients about medications, make sure to cover the following points:
- Indication for prescribing this drug
- What the drug is and how it works
- How often to take the medication and the dosage
- Side effects and contraindications
- What to do if side effects occur or a dose is missed

Common Concerns

Why would my dose of warfarin change?	• Each patient requires a different dose and the response to warfarin therefore needs to be monitored. It is guided by the INR, which is a blood test that measures the 'thinness' of the blood • The patient's target INR also depends on the indication of the warfarin and therefore may be different to other patients
How often do I need a blood test?	• The INR should be checked at least every 4 weeks, but it may need to be checked more frequently if it goes out of the range that is required to prevent clots
Are there known interactions with certain foods?	• Certain foods and natural health products or herbal remedies can affect warfarin levels. Some increase warfarin levels, for example, gingko biloba, whilst others reduce the warfarin effect, for example, ginseng • Vitamin K reduces the effect of warfarin. Foods rich in vitamin K, such as broccoli, Brussels sprouts and green leafy vegetables such as spinach, coriander and cabbage, can be taken in the usual amounts in a normal diet

GATHERING INFORMATION AND COMMUNICATIONS

This case has two parts:
1. Taking a brief and relevant history
2. Counsel the patient about warfarin

HISTORY

In the brief history, you should aim to find out why the patient has been commenced on warfarin:
- Any previous history of VTE
- Risk of developing clots
- Mechanical prosthetic valve

Before commencing patients on warfarin, you should rule out any potential contraindications to warfarin treatment. This includes:
- Full drug history: As warfarin is known to interact with many medications. Note that this also includes herbal medicines and supplements. Certain drugs will also increase bleeding risk with warfarin; for example, antiplatelet agents such as aspirin and clopidogrel. However, they do not necessarily affect the INR. Both the oral contraceptive pill and hormone replacement therapy should be stopped in patients with venous thromboembolic events
- Possible concurrent pregnancy: As warfarin can affect fetal development
- Presence of bleeding disorders: For example, haemophilia
- Previous history of bleeds: For example, upper gastrointestinal bleeds

COUNSELLING ON WARFARIN USE

WHY?

Explain why the patient is being asked to take warfarin:
- Diagnosis of atrial fibrillation, which is a condition that can increase the risk of blood clots forming in vessels supplying the heart and brain
- Taking warfarin will reduce this risk

WHAT?

Explain what warfarin is:
- A medication that thins the blood, reducing the risk of blood clots forming

WHEN?

Explain when the drug should be taken:
- Approximately the same time every day. It is advised to take it at 6 p.m. as this will allow the doctor to contact the patient if the dose needs reducing due to a high INR reading
- Warfarin tablets come in different strength and colour tablets: 1 mg (brown), 3 mg (blue) and 5 mg (pink). A supply of all of these is given to the patient to allow for dose adjustment

ANTICOAGULATION BOOK

Patients on warfarin are often given a 'yellow anticoagulation' book, which is a written record of their INR values and warfarin doses.

SAFETY-NET ADVICE

How this medication will impact the patient's life:

- Alcohol may increase the effects of warfarin, so patients should be counselled adequately about keeping their alcohol intake at a safe and stable level
- Patients should also be told to refrain from activities such as contact sports, due to an increased bleeding risk
- Warfarin can interact with many medications so check this before taking any other tablets
  Also remind the patient to watch out for:
- Bleeding or severe bruising
- Prolonged nose bleeds
- Coughing up or vomiting blood
- Passing foul-smelling black tar-like bowel motions
- Passing blood in the urine

MISSED DOSES

If a dose is missed:
- Take the missed dose as soon as possible and call the primary care doctor for advice. Do not double up the dose the next day if one dose is missed

TARGET INR

The INR is derived from the prothrombin time (PT), which is prolonged when there is a reduction in the activated forms of vitamin K-dependent coagulation factors. The INR is used only for patients on warfarin. The longer the PT, the longer the time for clot formation and therefore, the 'thinner' the blood is. So, the higher the PT, the higher the INR and the thinner the blood.

The target INR is dependent on the reason for being on warfarin in the first place (Table 4.7).

LENGTH OF WARFARIN THERAPY

The length of time the patient must take warfarin, like target INR, is also dependent on the indication (Table 4.8).

Present Your Findings

Mr Jacobs is a 70-year-old man who was recently diagnosed with atrial fibrillation, which was incidentally found by his primary care doctor. He has had no previous strokes or heart attacks. He is taking ramipril and simvastatin and has no known allergies. Today I counselled Mr Jacobs on starting warfarin and have given him a 'yellow anticoagulation' book. He will be seen in the warfarin clinic next week, where we will monitor his INR.

QUESTIONS AND ANSWERS FOR CANDIDATE

What is the mechanism of action of warfarin?
- It inhibits the conversion of vitamin K from its inactive to its active form, therefore reducing the activity of vitamin K-dependent coagulation factors

Which coagulation factors are dependent on vitamin K?
- Factor II
- Factor VII
- Factor IX
- Factor X

Give three examples of direct oral anticoagulants (DOACs).
- Dabigatran
- Edoxaban
- Apixaban
- Rivaroxaban

A Case to Learn From

A man was admitted into the medical assessment unit with a COPD exacerbation and had brought in his medications in a pill box. However, the patient mentioned in passing that he was also on warfarin. But as his warfarin was not included in the pill box, it was nearly missed out when it came to prescribing his regular medications. It is important to verify a full drug history and not make assumptions; for example, that all drugs will be in the pill box.

Table 4.8   Duration of treatment with warfarin

INDICATION	DURATION OF REGIMEN
VTE	• Calf DVT: 6 weeks • Provoked venous thromboembolism and low risk of recurrence: 3 months • Unprovoked venous thromboembolism: 6 months • Recurrent DVT or PE: Long-term
Atrial fibrillation	• Usually long-term • If cardioversion is indicated, maintain target INR at least 3 weeks before cardioversion
Mechanical prosthetic valves	• Long-term

Table 4.7   Examples of target INRs

Normal range	0.8–1.2
Atrial fibrillation	2–3
PE and DVT	2–3
Aortic mechanical valve	2–3
Mitral mechanical valve	2.5–3.5

Top Tip

Even if a patient states that they know the dose of warfarin they are taking, double check with their 'anticoagulation book' before prescribing because warfarin doses can change regularly based on the INR.

STATION 4.11: SICKLE CELL DISEASE DIAGNOSIS

SCENARIO

You are a junior doctor working in primary care and have been asked to see Mrs Carr, mother of Jacob Carr. Jacob is a 7-week-old newborn baby who was diagnosed with sickle cell anaemia following routine screening. His mother is keen to know more about the diagnosis. Please explain the diagnosis and answer any questions the parent may have.

CORE CONCEPT

- Sickle cell anaemia is an inherited disorder which alters the shape of the red blood cells. This predisposes the 'sickle' cells to blocking blood vessels, resulting in symptoms of pain as well as other problems that can affect most of the body
- Repeated blockages can also result in long-term complications
- In many countries, it is diagnosed at birth following the results of a heel prick test taken in the first week after birth
- Strategies can be put in place to reduce exacerbations, but patients need to be aware of how to manage pain and possible infections, as for most individuals, it will be a chronic, lifelong condition

Common Concerns

What are the chances that our future children will also have sickle cell anaemia?	• As two copies of the faulty gene are required to develop sickle cell anaemia, each child has a 25% chance of inheriting the condition (Fig. 4.4)
Is sickle cell disease life threatening?	• It is a serious condition which requires awareness of complications and early treatment to prevent life-threatening problems; for example, infection, acute chest syndrome and sudden severe anaemia. Although the disease is very variable, most patients are able to lead relatively normal lives most of the time
If I have sickle cell trait, how will it affect my health?	• Those who are only carriers of the sickle cell trait will not develop sickle cell disease

GATHERING INFORMATION AND COMMUNICATIONS

This case has two parts:
1. Taking a brief and relevant history
2. Counselling the patient about sickle cell disease

HISTORY

In most cases, those affected by sickle cell disease will be identified via newborn screening. Therefore before counselling the family, it may help to ask the following:
- Family history of sickle cell disease
- Any sickle cell disease testing during the pregnancy
- Current knowledge about sickle cell disease

When explaining a condition, it may be helpful to make sure that you have included everything by covering:
- What the condition is
- The potential short- and long-term complications
- The cause
- Available treatment

COUNSELLING ON SICKLE CELL DISEASE

WHAT?

Explain what sickle cell disease is:
- Sickle cell anaemia is a condition in which red blood cells become 'sickle'-shaped
- Normal red blood cells are shaped like doughnuts and are very flexible
- 'Sickle' shaped red blood cells are more likely to get stuck and block blood vessels, leading to pain, stroke and acute chest syndromes, amongst other complications
- Sickle cells are also more easily damaged than normal red blood cells and, therefore, do not last as long
- This results in anaemia as the body is unable to keep up with the demand of producing new red blood cells

AETIOLOGY

Explain the cause of sickle cell disease:
- Autosomal-recessive inheritance genetic condition. The child has inherited two copies of a faulty gene, one from each parent (Fig. 4.4)
- The affected gene produces an abnormal form of haemoglobin
- Haemoglobin is a protein found in red blood cells which carries oxygen around the body. The abnormal form of haemoglobin changes the shape of the red blood cell, turning it into the characteristic 'sickle' shape

COMPLICATIONS

Explain the potential complications of sickle cell disease:
- When sickle cells block a blood vessel, oxygen cannot reach the tissue

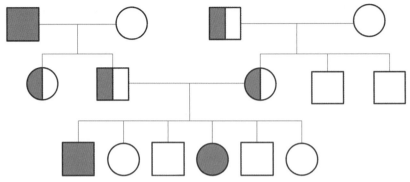

Fig. 4.4 Pattern of inheritance for sickle cell disease.

- The lack of oxygen causes a sharp sudden pain. These are called 'sickle cell crises'. Common sites include: Leg, back, abdomen, fingers (dactylitis). Crises can be triggered by:
  - *Cold*
  - *High* altitude
  - *Infection*
  - *Lack* of oxygen
  - *Dehydration*

  The above triggers can be remembered using the acronym CHILD.

  Between episodes of sickle cell crises, patients are usually symptom-free.
- Blockages can also cause organ damage:
  - Lung: Acute chest syndrome
  - Brain: Stroke
  - Kidney: Chronic kidney disease
  - Eye: Retinopathy
  - Spleen: Increased risk of infection, severe anaemia
- Sickle cell disease can also contribute to severe anaemia. Whilst those with sickle cell disease will normally have slightly low levels of red blood cells in their blood (anaemia), this can drop further and they may require a blood transfusion

MANAGEMENT

- Preventing crises:
  - Avoid known triggers of sickling (CHILD: See above acronym)
  - Emphasise the need for all childhood immunisations to be completed, including hepatitis B, meningitis and the annual flu vaccine
  - Give prophylactic antibiotics once the child is 3 months old
  - Hydroxyurea can reduce the occurrence of crises
  - Stem cell and gene therapy are emerging treatment options
- Treatment:
  - Painkillers
  - Antibiotics
  - Oxygen
  - Rehydration
- Blood transfusions are also used in the management of acute chest syndrome and severe anaemia

> **Q Present Your Findings**
>
> Jacob is a 7-week-old baby who has been diagnosed with sickle cell disease following the results of the heel prick test and of prophylactic antibiotics.
>
> I explained that it is a genetic condition affecting the red blood cells which can result in painful episodes and long-term complications. I have emphasised the need to complete all the childhood vaccinations. He will be followed up by a haematologist in a couple of weeks.

ANAEMIA IN SICKLE CELL DISEASE

Two processes that can lead to severe anaemia are:
- Splenic sequestration: Sickle cells are trapped in the spleen, causing it to enlarge and leaving fewer red blood cells circulating in the blood
- Aplastic crisis secondary to parvovirus infection: Parvovirus infection can cause the bone marrow to stop producing red blood cells

In these cases, patients require blood transfusions.

ACUTE CHEST SYNDROME

This is a severe complication that occurs when blood vessels in the lungs become blocked by sickling or in association with a chest infection. It typically occurs following a sickle cell crisis.

Symptoms include:
- Chest pain
- Fever
- Hypoxia
- Shortness of breath

Management includes:
- Pain relief
- Antibiotics
- Incentive spirometry
- Blood transfusion and exchange transfusion
- Fluids

❓ QUESTIONS AND ANSWERS FOR CANDIDATE

What is the difference between sickle cell disease and sickle cell trait?
- Sickle cell trait occurs in those who only inherit one copy of the gene. Most individuals with sickle cell trait are completely asymptomatic and do not

develop any of the complications associated with sickle cell disease.

Which antibiotic do patients with sickle cell anaemia take every day?
- Penicillin
- Erythromycin if they are penicillin-allergic

Name two examples of complications associated with repeated blood transfusions.
- Iron overload
- Alloimmunisation

 A Case to Learn From

A pregnant patient who was out of area presented to the acute assessment unit in the maternity hospital and did not have her notes with her. She presented with shortness of breath and some presyncope. A brief history was taken and she was sent to have a chest X-ray to rule out any obvious lung pathology. It wasn't until she returned from radiology that she disclosed she had sickle cell disease. This changed her management as it became important to check she wasn't anaemic. It is vital to ensure a full history is taken from patients, especially if you do not have access to their notes. In times of distress, patients may easily forget to disclose important clinical information without direct questioning.

 Top Tip

When explaining the chances of having a child with sickle cell disease to a couple who both have sickle cell trait, it really helps to draw a genetic diagram. This helps them to understand that the chances of inheritance are 25% and that this chance remains the same with each pregnancy.

STATION 4.12: CONSENT FOR HIV TESTING

SCENARIO

You are a junior doctor working in primary care and have been asked to see Anna Fredrick, a 19-year-old woman, who has attended asking for a human immunodeficiency virus (HIV) test. Please establish the level at which she is at risk of HIV and counsel her on HIV testing.

CORE CONCEPT

- HIV is a retrovirus which affects CD4 T cells and if left untreated can lead to acquired immunodeficiency syndrome (AIDS)
- HIV can be transmitted through:
  - Sexual intercourse: Vaginal, anal and oral
  - Infected blood
  - Needle sharing or accidental needlestick injuries
  - Mother to child (vertical) transmission

- Patients must be consented before a HIV test is carried out, though written consent is not required
- By knowing if they are HIV-positive, patients can:
  - Access treatment before the onset of symptoms, therefore prolonging their life
  - Take precautions to prevent further spread

 Common Concerns

If the test is positive, do I have to tell other people?	• It is recommended that you tell your current partner and any partners you've had since being infected, so that they too can be tested and begin treatment if necessary • There are certain circumstances in which you might be prosecuted for HIV transmission • Sexual health clinics have health advisors who can help you with this
If I test positive, does that mean I also have AIDS?	• AIDS and HIV are not the same thing • AIDS is an umbrella term covering a range of infections and illnesses that can develop from a weakened immune system as a result of HIV infection • Those who are HIV-positive may not develop AIDS • Often, it takes many years for the affected white cells to reach low enough levels that the immune system is affected, causing AIDS
I've heard that you can take emergency treatment for HIV; can I have some?	• Postexposure prophylaxis (PEP) can prevent HIV infection after a person has come into contact with it • For it to be effective, it must be started within 72 h of coming into contact with the virus and it is usually started if there is a very high risk of infection • Depending on the clinical situation, it may not be appropriate to start PEP

GATHERING INFORMATION AND COMMUNICATIONS

This case has two parts:
1. Taking a brief and relevant history to establish the patient's risk
2. Counselling the patient on HIV testing

HISTORY

Assess the risk of the patient by asking about the following risk factors:

- Sexual history:
  - Orientation: Must establish for males whether any same-sex relationships have occurred
  - Type of sex: Must establish if penetrative intercourse, with or without condoms, has occurred since the last HIV test
  - Sexual partner(s): Number of partners and, of those, the number known to be HIV-positive or at high risk
  - Condom usage: Never, not always or always
  - Other sexual activity: Recent sexual contact with sex workers
  - Sex abroad in high-risk countries: Country of origin, gender of partner, type of sex, barrier contraception
  - Sexual assault: In the past or recent
  - Diagnosis: Of other sexually transmitted infections
- Invasive procedures in non-sterile environments: For example, piercings or tattoos
- Blood transfusions: Overseas (and particularly from 1975 to 1985 in the UK)
- IV drug abuse: Where the patient would perform this, with whom and whether injecting equipment is shared
- Health problems: Opportunistic infections, immunocompromised states

  Also establish the patient's reasons for requesting a HIV test.

COUNSELLING ON HIV TESTING

WHAT?

Establish what the patient currently knows about HIV:
- What HIV is and briefly go through the lifecycle (Fig. 4.5)
- There is an increased risk of infection when white cell counts drop to a very low level
- Although incurable, HIV is treatable with antiretroviral drugs, which allow people to lead a near-normal life

HOW?

Explain the process of HIV testing:
- A blood test that detects specific antibodies against HIV

  Discuss the implications of a positive test result, which may include:
- A repeat blood test to confirm the diagnosis
- Informing other partners, contact tracing
- Preventing further spread
- Undergoing treatment

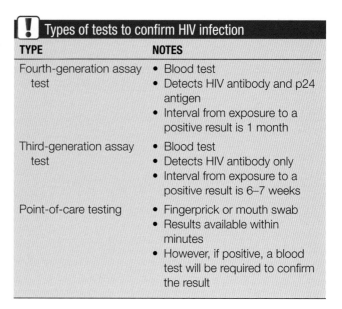

! Types of tests to confirm HIV infection

TYPE	NOTES
Fourth-generation assay test	• Blood test • Detects HIV antibody and p24 antigen • Interval from exposure to a positive result is 1 month
Third-generation assay test	• Blood test • Detects HIV antibody only • Interval from exposure to a positive result is 6–7 weeks
Point-of-care testing	• Fingerprick or mouth swab • Results available within minutes • However, if positive, a blood test will be required to confirm the result

Q Present Your Findings

Miss Fredrick is a 19-year-old student who wants to have a HIV test after having unprotected sex whilst on holiday in Spain last month. She does not know if her partner, who was also from the UK, was HIV-positive. She has no other risk factors. I have explained the HIV test and she is happy to undergo testing.

? QUESTIONS AND ANSWERS FOR CANDIDATE

What lifestyle advice can you give patients about preventing HIV transmission?
- Use condoms during sexual intercourse, as they are the most effective form of protection against HIV
- Do not share needles, syringes or other injecting equipment

Name two malignancies closely associated with HIV.
- Cervical cancer
- Kaposi sarcoma

Give three examples of opportunistic infections that are associated with HIV.
- *Pneumocystis jirovecii* pneumonia
- Tuberculosis
- Cytomegalovirus
- Cryptococcal meningitis
- Toxoplasmosis
- Histoplasmosis

 A Case to Learn From

A patient requested a HIV test 2 weeks after he had had unprotected sex abroad with a prostitute. His test result was negative, but he was advised that he might need repeat testing in a few weeks' time as, at only 2 weeks after the possible exposure, he was still in the window period. The window period refers to the time when a patient may still be infected with HIV despite testing negative.

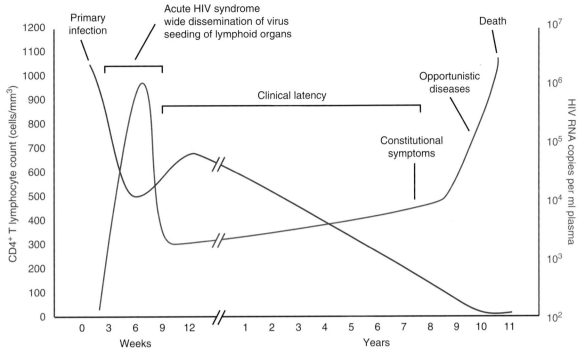

Fig. 4.5 Proposed timeline for HIV pathology.

 Top Tip

If you know that the patient is HIV-positive and you are likely to come into contact with any bodily fluids, make sure to cover yourself with enough personal protective equipment. For example, double glove when taking bloods or wear visors or goggles in theatre if you anticipate that blood may splatter.

STATION 4.13: POSTMORTEM DISCUSSION

SCENARIO

You are a junior doctor speaking to Laura Parker, daughter of one of your patients, Irene Parker. Mrs Parker died last week and the cause of death was pneumonia. A number of abnormal lesions were noted on a previous CT scan, which are not thought to be related to the cause of death but are of unknown origin. The family and medical team are interested to explore this further and your consultant has asked you to get authorisation for a hospital autopsy.

CORE CONCEPT

- Postmortems are carried out for two reasons: At the request of either the coroner or a hospital doctor to establish the cause of death
- If requested by the hospital doctor, consent needs to be obtained. If the patient has not expressed any views on having an autopsy, consent can be obtained from someone close to the patient
- Consent can be limited to only examining one area of the body

- Local rules for seeking authorisation for a postmortem may vary depending on the hospital. Most hospitals will require a death certificate to have been issued and others have policies regarding authorisation to be obtained by medical staff of at least a certain grade
- A witness will be required for the discussion. That person must be able to sign the authorisation form. This need not be a doctor and is often a nurse who may have known the family

Common Concerns

Can we still have an open casket?	• An open casket will still be possible if that is what the family or deceased patient would have wanted
Who can give consent to a hospital postmortem?	• The patient can either consent or refuse before death • They can also appoint a representative to do this on their behalf • If none of the above are present, consent can be given by someone close to the patient. This is someone who is in a qualifying relationship. Examples of qualifying relationships, in order are: Spouse or partner Parent or child Brother or sister Grandparent
Can I object to my relative's body being examined in a coroner's postmortem?	• If the coroner decides that a postmortem is required to identify the cause of death, consent is not required from the patient's family

GATHERING INFORMATION AND COMMUNICATIONS

This case has one part:
1. Gaining consent for a hospital autopsy

GAINING CONSENT FOR A HOSPITAL AUTOPSY

BACKGROUND INFORMATION

- Attempt to find out if the deceased patient had ever expressed any views on having an autopsy
- Try to ascertain what the relative understands by an autopsy; they may have many preconceived ideas

THE AUTOPSY

- Explain why you are seeking authorisation to perform an autopsy and what questions you are seeking to answer
- The examination may reveal information that helps the relatives to understand the circumstances around the death
- Roughly half of autopsies performed produce findings that are not suspected before the person died

RESPECTING THE DECEASED

- The examination will be carried out in a manner that is respectful to the deceased and the family's wishes
- Organs will not be retained without specific permission, but in some regions of the UK, small thumbnail-sized pieces of tissue will routinely be retained for microscopic examination
- Explain that the autopsy examinations can be limited to one area of the body or even to one organ, but that this will prevent any comment being made on any other disease processes elsewhere

RESPECTING PATIENT OR FAMILY WISHES

- Explain that this is not something that has to be agreed to and that permission can be refused. Be supportive of such a decision
- Explain that the family can withdraw authorisation at any time up until the examination has started
- The only caveat to these wishes is that a coroner can mandate a postmortem. In these cases, communication with the family about this and the reasons why is vital

AFTER MEETING WITH THE FAMILY

- Having established that the family are happy to give authorisation, complete the form by recording their wishes regarding the autopsy, particularly with respect to any limitations being placed on the examination, to tissue retention and eventual disposal
- The form must be signed and witnessed as required
- A copy of the form should be given to the relatives, along with any information booklets if they so wish
- The case notes, authorisation form and any required pathology request form should be passed to the mortuary without delay

POSTMORTEM SCANNING

Whilst postmortems usually involve the body being opened up and examined, there are some cases in which this is not carried out and, instead, the body is examined via CT or magnetic resonance imaging (MRI). This may be due to consent to a less invasive examination. However, this type of postmortem is still quite uncommon.

🔍 Present Your Findings

Mrs Parker died last week from pneumonia, but her last CT scan showed lesions in her lungs which were of unknown origin. I discussed the prospect of a hospital postmortem with her daughter and explained what happens at an autopsy.

I have reassured her that her mother's body will be treated with respect at all times and, depending on her wishes, only the lungs can be examined if this is what the family wishes. She is currently undecided what her mother would want so wants more time to decide and to discuss with her family. I have arranged to speak with her again later today.

❓ QUESTIONS AND ANSWERS FOR CANDIDATE

Give three examples of situations in which a death would need to be referred to the coroner.
- The cause of death is unknown
- Death was unnatural or suspicious
- Death occurred as the result of an accident
- Deaths during or shortly after detention in police or prison custody
- Deaths where the doctor did not see the patient either after death or within 14 days before death
- Death due to an industrial disease
- Suicides
- Deaths occurring during an operation or due to an anaesthetic

Give three examples of signs that you would be looking for whilst confirming death.
- No palpable pulses felt after 1 min of checking
- No breath or heart sounds on auscultation after 5 min of checking
- Both eyes fixed and dilated

Who can issue a death certificate?
- Ideally, a doctor who was involved in the patient's care during the last illness and who has seen the deceased within 14 days of death or after death can issue a death certificate

A Case to Learn From

As a student, I encountered a case in which a patient died whilst he was in prison. As a result, his case was referred to the coroner. When I asked the doctors about who could give consent to the postmortem, I was told that cases which required a postmortem under the coroner's instructions did not need consent. This is important to know so it can be explained to relatives.

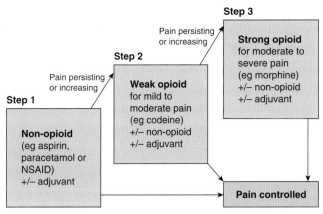

Fig. 4.6 WHO analgesic ladder.

 Top Tip

In complex cases, seek advice from a senior colleague or pathologist regarding what may be involved in answering specific questions; for example, there is no point in obtaining authorisation for a limited examination which excludes the head when the patient may have died of a neurological condition.

 Top Tip

Find out if the family want answers to specific questions. There may have been other health issues not directly relevant to the final illness which they would like clarified; for example, that a previously diagnosed and treated malignancy has not returned.

STATION 4.14: OPIATE COUNSELLING

SCENARIO

You are asked to see Alan Smith, a 62-year-old man, who is suffering from severe pain. He has a diagnosis of inoperable pancreatic cancer. You have found it difficult to control his pain and now feel that his analgesia should be increased. Please counsel him on the risks and benefits of morphine therapy and discuss other adjuncts to improve his symptoms.

CORE CONCEPT

- According to the World Health Organization (WHO) pain ladder, if a patient's pain is not controlled through non-opioids or weak opioids, a stronger opioid, such as morphine, may need to be used (Fig. 4.6)
- Patients may have concerns about using morphine, mainly due to fears of being addicted and suffering from side effects

When counselling patients about medication, make sure to cover the following points:

- Indication for prescribing this drug
- What the drug is and how it works
- How often to take the medications and the dosage
- Side effects and contraindications
- What to do if side effects occur or if a dose is missed

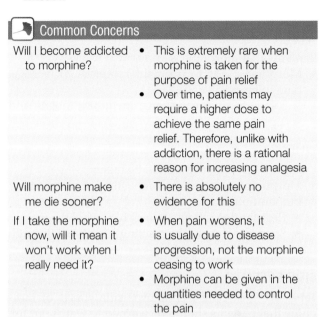

GATHERING INFORMATION AND COMMUNICATIONS

This case has two parts:
1. Taking a brief pain history
2. Counselling the patient about morphine

PAIN HISTORY

Enquire about:
- Pain:
  - *Site*
  - *Onset*
  - *Character* of pain
  - *Radiation*
  - *Associated* symptoms
  - *Timing* and duration
  - *Exacerbating* and relieving factors
  - *Severity*

The above can be remembered using the mnemonic SOCRATES.
- Previous analgesia used and the efficacy
- Any known drug allergies

It is also important to establish what worries the patient may have about starting morphine. Addressing these, even if they are not rooted in fact, increases the likelihood of patient compliance.

COUNSELLING ON MORPHINE USE

WHY?

Explain why the patient is recommended to take morphine:
- The reason for starting morphine; for example, symptomatic relief

WHAT?

Explain what morphine is and how it works:
- Morphine binds to μ opioid receptors to increase pain tolerance
- It comes in different forms, including tablets and syrups

WHEN?

Explain when the drug should be taken:
- Morphine can come in long-acting or short-acting preparations:
  - Regular doses (long-acting) to control the pain
  - Sporadic doses (short-acting) for breakthrough pain

SIDE EFFECTS

Table 4.9 lists some well-known side effects of morphine that patients should be warned to watch out for.

ALTERNATIVES

Discuss any adjuncts to improve the patient's symptoms:

- Adjuvant drugs are other medications which are beneficial in controlling certain types of pain, but are not primarily used in pain relief. Examples are listed in Table 4.10
- In this scenario, as Mr Smith has described symptoms of neuropathic pain, counselling him on the use of amitriptyline to manage his pain relief may be appropriate
- It is important to emphasise that the indication for this drug is to treat his pain and it does not imply that he has another condition

⚠ Examples of opiate drugs and their indication(s)

OPIATE	INDICATION
Morphine sulphate tablets (MST Continus)	Usually first-line for regular analgesia
Morphine sulphate solution (Oramorph)	Usually first-line for breakthrough analgesia
Buprenorphine and fentanyl	Available as patches in the management of severe chronic pain
Diamorphine	IM injection used in labour Anticipatory prescribing
Pethidine	IM injection used in labour

Table 4.9   Potential side effects of opioids

SIDE EFFECTS	INFORMATION
Constipation	• Virtually inevitable; use prophylactic laxatives, for example, senna, which is a stimulant laxative, or lactulose, which is a softener laxative
Nausea	• Fairly common in opiate-naïve patients; sometimes clears after 1 week but may recur after a dose increase • Cover with an antiemetic; for example, metoclopramide
Drowsiness	• Normally an acute problem, clearing within 1 week • If the patient is significantly drowsy, it may be a sign of opiate toxicity. In this case alternative opioids, for example, oxycodone should be considered
Myoclonus	• Seen especially in renal impairment • Consider reducing the dose or changing to another opioid • Consider administering midazolam, especially in the terminal phase
Hallucinations	• Can occur, especially if the dose is too high; therefore the dose can be reduced • Individuals may have vivid dreams, which is not always a problem

Table 4.10   Examples of adjuvant drugs and their uses

DRUG	INDICATION
Low-dose antidepressants For example, amitriptyline	Neuropathic pain
Anticonvulsants For example, carbamazepine and gabapentin	Neuropathic pain
Radiotherapy and chemotherapy	Bone pain
Bisphosphonates	Bone pain from metastatic disease

MORPHINE WITHDRAWAL

If patients who have been taking opiates for a long time suddenly stop, they may suffer from withdrawal symptoms. These include:
- Anxiety
- Agitation
- Sweating
- Nausea and vomiting
- Diarrhoea

OTHER ANALGESIC APPROACHES

- Discuss referral to an appropriative palliative care team (community or hospital) for further management as these teams may be able to offer more specialist support service
- Offer emotional and spiritual support through, for example, the chaplaincy or counselling services
- Relaxation techniques and creative therapies; for example, sensory monitoring and mindful-based therapy, may provide coping strategies that patients can use to augment their analgesia
- Acupuncture and aromatherapy
- Transcutaneous electrical nerve stimulation (TENS)

Present Your Findings

Mr Smith is a 62-year-old man who has been diagnosed with inoperable pancreatic cancer. His current pain regimen of codeine and paracetamol is ineffective, as he still has constant abdominal pain as well as intermittent episodes of shooting pain in his back.

As a result, I have discussed the benefits and risks of commencing morphine to manage his pain and have also suggested amitriptyline as an adjuvant for the neuropathic pain.

❓ QUESTIONS AND ANSWERS FOR CANDIDATE

Give three examples of signs or symptoms found in opiate overdose:
- Symptoms:
  - Confusion or drowsiness
  - Nausea and vomiting
  - Constipation
- Signs:
  - Pinpoint pupils
  - Respiratory depression

What is the name of the drug that is used to counteract an opioid overdose?
- Naloxone

If a patient is prescribed a total of 60 mg over 24 hours, what dose should their pro re nata (PRN) morphine be?
- 10 mg, as the PRN dose is usually equivalent to 1/6th of total 24-h dose

 A Case to Learn From

On the general surgical ward round, we reviewed a patient who had undergone a laparoscopic appendicectomy the previous day. She was complaining of severe pain and had difficulties mobilising and taking deep breaths as a result of the pain. When we checked the drug chart, we saw that she had not requested any of the Oramorph that she was prescribed for her breakthrough pain. The consultant explained the purpose of this and reminded her to ask for it if she was in pain. Later in the afternoon, her pain was well controlled and she was able to go home. Always ensure patients are aware to ask for as-required medication.

 Top Tip

When assessing a patient with chronic pain, do not forget to ask about the effect the pain may have on their mood and daily activities. A patient may say the pain is low in severity but it has a significant impact on their lifestyle. This is important to acknowledge and address.

STATION 4.15: BREAKING BAD NEWS

SCENARIO

You are a junior doctor working on the respiratory ward and have been asked to see Mrs Gardner. You admitted her husband last week; he was suffering from a chest infection, on a long-term background of colorectal cancer. Despite antibiotic therapy, he is now rapidly deteriorating and your consultant anticipates that Mr Gardner has days, if not hours, to live. Please have a discussion with Mrs Gardner regarding Mr Gardner's deterioration.

CORE CONCEPT

Breaking bad news is a difficult skill to master, especially within a short OSCE scenario. However, there are many different ways to do it successfully. Ensure that you are clear about the patient's situation, who exactly you are talking to and what you are trying to communicate.

The SPIKES technique is an effective method to structure breaking bad news:
- *Setting*: Speak to the relative in a quiet, private and bleep-free environment
- *Perception*: Establish what the patient already knows about the situation
- *Invitation*: Introduce the purpose of the discussion.
- *Knowledge*: This is the information you are telling the relative
- *Empathy*: Respond to the relative's reaction with empathy

- *Strategy* and *summary*: Provide the relative with written information if appropriate and an opportunity to speak again

GATHERING INFORMATION AND COMMUNICATIONS

This case has two parts:
1. Gauging what the relative already knows
2. Explaining the patient's current situation and risk of deterioration

RELATIVE'S INFORMATION

- Establish what the relative knows so far and what her current expectations are
- This will help you assess the information you need to convey and the language that is most appropriate. It will also highlight any initial misconception
- Early in the consultation, identify the concerns of the relative. These may not necessarily be the concerns you would have in a similar situation. For example, in this case, hypothetically Mrs Gardner may feel very guilty because she believes she gave her husband the chest infection. Until this guilt is addressed, it may be more difficult for her to focus on other discussions

EXPLAINING THE SITUATION

Convey the important information in small chunks and check that the relative has understood. For example:
- Explain that Mr Gardner has developed a chest infection, from which he is dying, despite maximal treatment with antibiotics
- The team caring for him think he has days, if not hours, to live regardless of what treatment is given
- Emphasise that he will still be monitored closely, but that you believe the aim of all further management should be making sure that he is as comfortable as possible
- State that any further tests would not change his outlook but might cause him unnecessary distress and so you do not think doing any more tests is in his best interests
- State that he will be put in a room without other patients, so that he and the family can have some privacy
- Make sure you regularly check that the relative understands what you are saying and ask if she has any questions
- Warning shots are useful!
Showing empathy is probably the most important part of the consultation and involves specifically dealing with how the relative reacts:
- If a relative becomes upset or angry, recognising this can be useful
- It is acceptable to allow a period of silence and to offer to talk further when the relative has had time to

think about the issues in more detail. Offer tissues if appropriate
- If the relative falls silent, it is tempting to fill the space with more reassurance, but you should respect the silence for a while
Relatives may want to discuss:
- Issues involving the process of dying, pain and loss of independence
- Wider issues with regard to family and money
Acknowledging and allowing the relative to express such emotions is often beneficial

DNACPR FORM

Depending on the scenario, it may be appropriate to introduce the concept of a DNACPR form. When discussing DNACPR forms, it is important to remember:
- The medical team, acting in the best interests of the patient, will ultimately decide whether resuscitation will be attempted, although agreement should be sought
- All DNACPR decisions should be discussed with the patient if they have capacity, unless it is thought the discussion will cause physical or psychological harm
- Doctors should also discuss the decision to attempt CPR with those close to the patient

Common Concerns

Does 'Do not attempt cardiopulmonary resuscitation' (DNACPR) mean that all treatment will be stopped?	• The DNACPR only applies to whether cardiopulmonary resuscitation (CPR) will be attempted in an event of a cardiopulmonary arrest. It does not mean that all other treatments will be stopped
What if I want to be resuscitated?	• Ultimately, the decision to attempt CPR lies with the medical team who will be acting in your best interests and who believe that CPR will not work in the individual situation. If you disagree with the decision after discussing it with the medical team, they can provide you with a second opinion
How will everyone know what my wishes are?	• All hospitals will have their own paperwork regarding this. It is our duty, as your clinicians, to disseminate information regarding treatment escalation and DNACPR to all those looking after you

ANTICIPATORY MEDICATIONS

The anticipatory medications listed in Table 4.11 are used to control patients' symptoms and keep them comfortable when they are deteriorating and are at the end of life.

Table **4.11** Anticipatory drugs and their indications

MEDICATION	INDICATION
Midazolam	Agitation and restlessness
Haloperidol	Nausea and vomiting
Hyoscine butylbromide	Excess chest secretions
Diamorphine hydrochloride	Pain relief

Present Your Findings

Today I spoke with Mrs Gardner and explained that her husband has deteriorated over the last few days, despite being on antibiotics for a chest infection. Initially, she was concerned that she had given him the chest infection after she had had a cold last week. I reassured her that this is not the case and that she should not feel guilty. She is concerned that he is dying and wishes for him to be kept comfortable now. I have explained that he will be moved to a side room so that they can have some privacy, but that he will remain closely monitored.

QUESTIONS AND ANSWERS FOR CANDIDATE

How long is a DNACPR form valid?
- Unless specified that it is to be reviewed at a certain date, a DNACPR form will be indefinitely valid. However, the form should be reviewed if the patient's clinical condition changes, or if the patient moves to a different healthcare setting; for example, discharged from hospital back to the community

Who can sign a DNACPR form?
- Any doctor with a full licence to practise can sign the DNACPR form but before this is done, the decision should be discussed with the responsible senior clinician, who should also sign the DNACPR form

What is an advance decision to refuse treatment form?
- An advance decision to refuse treatment form is a legally binding document made by a patient whilst they have capacity. The document specifies which treatments a patient would like to refuse in certain circumstances, if they are no longer able to make or communicate the decisions themselves. Examples of treatments that can be included are: Ventilation, antibiotics and CPR

A Case to Learn From

An elderly patient who had multiple comorbidities was admitted to the ward with an exacerbation of heart failure. During her admission, a DNACPR form was discussed with her and her husband. Her husband became upset as he believed that having the DNACPR form in place meant that she would stop all her active treatment. The consultant took the time to explain clearly that this was not the case, as the form is only in relation to CPR, not other treatments. This conversation may need to be repeated with family members several times during an admission.

Top Tip

Try to offload your bleep to a colleague before breaking bad news. A bleep that keeps ringing can detract from the attention you need to give to the patient. If this isn't possible, warn the relatives before starting the discussion but assure them that you will give them your full attention unless there is an emergency.

STATION 4.16: ETHICS

SCENARIO

You are a junior doctor working in the emergency department and have been asked to assess Evelyn Beech, a 79-year-old woman who has presented with back pain. During your examination, you see that she has multiple bruises on her back. When questioned, she confides that sometimes her carer gets frustrated with her. Please discuss your options with the examiner and what you would do in this situation.

CORE CONCEPT

When it comes to medical ethics, there are four key pillars:
- Non-maleficence: 'First do no harm'
- Beneficence: In all cases, aim to do good
- Justice: Treat all patients fairly
- Autonomy: Respect a patient's right to make their own opinions and allow them to do so
  In addition, there are also the three Cs:
- Confidentiality
- Consent
- Capacity

When discussing ethical dilemmas, refer to these overarching principles and use them to explore the issues and come to a conclusion.

Common Concerns

Can you promise not to tell anyone?	• You should not promise that you will not break confidentiality • Patients should be warned that their confidentiality may be broken in certain circumstances

I'm not sure if what I have been through is abuse?	• The HARK framework was developed to identify those who are victims of abuse and consists of four questions:
	  • Humiliation: Does your partner make you feel bad about yourself?
	  • Afraid: Have you been afraid of your partner?
	  • Rape: Are you ever forced to do anything you are not comfortable with?
	  • Kick: Does your partner physically hurt or threaten to hurt you?

Who will you report the abuse to?	• In every workplace there will be a person designated for domestic abuse who is responsible for taking the case further • They will assess the risk that the patient is in and, depending on the amount of risk, will facilitate and provide support to the patient • This may require referrals to other organisations; for example, social services and the police, if necessary

GATHERING INFORMATION AND COMMUNICATIONS

This case has one part:
1. Considering the four key pillars of medical ethics related to abuse.

ETHICAL DILEMMA CONSIDERATIONS

In the exam, you may be gathering information from the patient or discussing what you wish to explore further with the examiner. When discussing or exploring possible abuse with a patient, use open questions to find out the following:
• Length and frequency of the abuse
• Type of abuse

• Severity of the abuse
• Effect on the patient
• Identify other people at potential risk

As the doctor, outline the different options and explore the pros and cons of each before coming to a conclusion:
• Do nothing: This option would allow the doctor to maintain the patient's confidentiality and also respect her autonomy. However, it goes against the principles of non-maleficence and beneficence as the patient may experience more abuse
• Report the carer against the patient's wishes: This option, done with the patient's best interests in mind, goes against her autonomy and breaks confidentiality. This may result in a loss of rapport and trust between the patient and the doctor, and may lead to a breakdown of the doctor–patient relationship
• Encourage the patient to allow the doctor to report the abuser and take steps to remove herself from the situation: If the patient has capacity and insists that she does not want to leave, the doctor should respect this decision. However, the patient should be warned that her confidentiality may be broken if the doctor believes that she is at risk of significant harm

BREAKING CONFIDENTIALITY

Confidential information can be disclosed in the following circumstances:
• With the patient's consent
• Justifiable in the public interest:
  • To prevent a risk to national security or public health
  • To protect others from death or other serious harm
  • To prevent serious crime
• Ordered under the court of law

Present Your Findings

Mrs Beech is a 79-year-old woman who reported that she has suffered physical abuse from her carer. She does not want the doctor to tell others as she is afraid that her abuse may worsen if her carer found out.

When assessed, she has capacity to make this decision. Therefore, in this situation, I would try to convince the patient to allow me to report the case but would respect her decision if she did not want to. However, I would also let her know that there are certain situations in which I would break her confidentiality. A key example would be if I assessed her as being at high risk of harm. I have also given her details of where to seek support if she needs it.

QUESTIONS AND ANSWERS FOR CANDIDATE

Give three examples of types of abuse.
* Physical
* Emotional
* Sexual
* Neglect

Give three examples of risk factors for elderly abuse.
* Social isolation
* Lack of capacity
* Dependence on others

What does the term safeguarding mean and who is responsible for safeguarding?
* The term safeguarding means to protect vulnerable adults and children from harm. Though there may be a named lead within an organisation, safeguarding is everyone's responsibility

 A Case to Learn From

A patient with paranoid schizophrenia developed gangrene and required a leg amputation but the patient refused. The case was taken to court where it was decided to respect the patient's decision, showing that even though a person has a mental illness, it does not mean that they lack capacity. Remember that capacity is time- and decision-specific and if the patient has capacity then their decision must be respected, despite how unwise you feel their choice is.

Top Tip

During our career we will come across many ethical dilemmas. You will not be expected to deal with them by yourself. It is important to discuss these cases with senior colleagues. Most hospitals will also have an ethics board that can be a useful resource.

Data Interpretation

Content Outline

Never before have so many investigations been available to clinicians to help diagnose, monitor and treat diseases. Challenges arise in knowing which test to order, how to interpret the results and how to explain any findings to patients. This chapter will give you a variety of scenarios to practise and develop this key skill of data interpretation.

Some relevant background knowledge of the test requested is required and will be provided in the stations of this chapter. The key to data interpretation stations in OSCEs is to be able to apply the scientific knowledge surrounding an investigation to the clinical scenario you are faced with.

A flexible generic framework can provide a useful structure to follow. Remember to spend time gauging the clinical setting, who your patient is and their ideas, concerns and expectations. Ensuring you have a thorough and succinct method for history taking will also help you to be able to sieve through the information provided more easily.

Study Action Plan

- Unlike history taking or examination, it is difficult as a medical student to practise data interpretation skills on patients
- Ensure that your scientific knowledge is up to date before you practise
- Develop your own framework to guide your data interpretation. It is worth shadowing some junior doctors to observe different frameworks in action. However, remember always to adapt to each patient
- On the wards, there are hundreds of opportunities each day to interpret data. In pairs, practise reviewing test results and presenting findings to each other. Then ask one of the doctors if you can present to them. It is useful to practise under pressure!

STATION 5.1: FULL BLOOD COUNT

SCENARIO

You are a junior doctor on a primary care placement and have been asked to see Mrs Brown, a normally active 75-year-old woman, who has presented with an 8-week history of increasing lethargy. She appears quite pale. You take some blood tests and the results are reported as below. Please review the blood tests, explain the findings to Mrs Brown and formulate an appropriate management plan.

Results

COMPONENTS	RESULTS	REFERENCE RANGES WITH UNITS
Haemoglobin (Hb)	88 ↓	Males: 130–180 g/L Females: 115–165 g/L
Haematocrit (Hct)	0.3 ↓	Males: 0.4–0.54 L/L Females: 0.37–0.47 L/L
Red cell count (RCC)	3 ↓	Males: 4.5–6.5 × 10^{12}/L Females: 3.8–5.8 × 10^{12}/L
Mean cell volume (MCV)	50 ↓	80–95 fL
Mean corpuscular haemoglobin (MCH)	24 ↓	27–34 pg/cell
Mean corpuscular haemoglobin concentration (MCHC)	275 ↓	300–350 g/L
White cell count (WCC)	4	3.6–11.0 × 10^9/L
Platelets (Plt)	200	140–400 × 10^9/L
Neutrophils	2	1.8–7.5 × 10^9/L
Lymphocytes	3	1.0–4.0 × 10^9/L
Eosinophils	0.3	0.1–0.4 × 10^9/L
Basophils	0.07	0.02–0.10 × 10^9/L
Monocytes	0.5	0.2–0.8 × 10^9/L

DATA INTERPRETATION

Anaemia is a lower than normal RCC or a low Hb. It can be classified according to red cell volume or Hb concentration (Tables 5.1 and 5.2).

IRON METABOLISM

- A typical Western diet provides around 15 mg of iron a day; however only 5–10% of this is absorbed
- Two types of iron are found in food: Haem and non-haem iron
- Haem iron is found in meat and fish and is readily absorbed, whereas non-haem iron is found in vegetables, cereals and pulses and is not as readily absorbed
- Absorption of iron takes place in the duodenum and proximal jejunum. When absorbed, the iron is transported into the blood stream, where it is carried by transferrin
- About 75% of absorbed iron contributes to the synthesis of Hb. Hb transports oxygen in red cells. Red cells are synthesised in the bone marrow of long bones

RED CELL INDICES

Information on different measures of red cells

	DESCRIPTION
Hb	Four polypeptide chains, each of which is attached to a haem group
Hct	Packed red cell volume, i.e. the percentage volume of red cells in blood
MCV	Average red cell volume
MCH	Average amount of Hb in a red cell
MCHC	Average concentration of Hb in a red cell, i.e. the amount of Hb in a given volume of red cells

WHITE CELLS (TABLE 5.3)

- White blood cells are synthesised in the bone marrow. T and B lymphocytes are synthesised in the lymph nodes and spleen

Table 5.1 Classification of anaemia based on red cell volume

CLASSIFICATION	RED CELL SIZE	MCV	CAUSES
Microcytic	Abnormally small	Low	• Iron deficiency • Thalassaemia • Anaemia of chronic disease
Normocytic	Normal	Normal	• Anaemia of chronic disease • Acute blood loss
Macrocytic	Abnormally large	High	• Vitamin B_{12} deficiency • Folate deficiency • Increased alcohol • Liver disease • Pregnancy • Myelodysplasia

Table 5.2 Classification of anaemia based on Hb concentration

CLASSIFICATION	HB CONCENTRATION	MCH AND MCHC	CAUSES
Hypochromic	Low	Low	• Iron deficiency • Thalassaemia • Vitamin B_6 deficiency • Parasitic infestations; for example, hookworm • Bleeding
Normochromic	Normal	Normal	• Anaemia of chronic disease • Haemolytic anaemia • Bleeding • Aplastic anaemia
Hyperchromic	High	High	• Vitamin B_{12} deficiency • Folic acid deficiency

- WCC can be raised in infection, inflammation and malignancy and secondary to steroid treatment
- WCC may be reduced in pancytopenia, malignancy, chemotherapy, viral infections, severe infection, autoimmune disease, human immunodeficiency virus (HIV)/acquired immunodeficiency disease syndrome (AIDS) and hyposplenism

THIS CASE

The patient is presenting with signs and symptoms of anaemia. The blood tests show microcytic, hypochromic anaemia, suggestive of iron deficiency. It is important to explain the diagnosis to the patient but to also determine the cause.

Causes of Iron Deficiency Anaemia (IDA)

REDUCED SUPPLY OF IRON	INCREASED DEMAND
<ul><li>Insufficient dietary iron</li><li>Malabsorption: For example, coeliac disease, gastrectomy, gastritis</li><li>Chronic blood loss<ul><li>Gastrointestinal (GI) losses; for example, peptic ulcer disease, colitis, malignancy or haemorrhoids</li><li>Gynaecological causes; for example, menorrhagia, malignancy or haematuria</li></ul></li></ul>	<ul><li>Prematurity</li><li>Pregnancy</li><li>Growth spurts</li></ul>

Table 5.3   Key blood cells

CELL	TYPE	FUNCTION	CAUSES OF HIGH LEVELS	CAUSES OF LOW LEVELS
Neutrophil	Granulocyte	• Respond to bacterial and fungal infection	• Bacterial infection • Acute inflammation • Medications; for example, prednisolone • Chronic myeloid leukaemia	• Aplastic anaemia • Lupus • Vitamin B_{12} deficiency • Medications; for example, valproate
Lymphocyte	Agranulocyte	• T and B cells contain MHC antigen receptors and are involved in specific immune response	• Viral infection • Lymphoma • Post-splenectomy • Acute lymphoblastic leukaemia • Chronic lymphoblastic leukaemia	• Common cold • Radiation • Severe stress • Rheumatoid arthritis • Malnutrition • Viral infections
Eosinophil	Granulocyte	• Involved in allergic response and parasitic infections	• Allergic rhinitis • Hodgkin's lymphoma • Acute myelogenous leukaemia	• Excess alcohol consumption • Cushing's disease
Basophil	Granulocyte	• Responsible for short-term inflammatory and allergic response	• Hypothyroidism • Myeloproliferative disorders • Autoimmune inflammation	• Hyperthyroidism • Infections • Anaphylaxis
Monocyte	Agranulocyte	• Involved in antigen presentation • Macrophages phagocytose foreign material • Dendritic cells are found in skin, lungs and the GI tract and are exposed to environmental pathogens	• Chronic infection • Sarcoidosis • Autoimmune disorders	• Chemotherapy • Any infection
Platelets	Derived from megakaryocytes which are produced in the bone marrow	• Clot formation	• Primary thrombocytosis • Secondary to anaemia, malignancy, infection or surgery	• Idiopathic thrombocytopenic purpura • Viral infections • Haematological malignancy • Drug-induced; for example, heparin

RELEVANT PATIENT INFORMATION

You suspect that this patient has IDA. Ask about known medical conditions, relevant treatments and any hospital admissions.

History Of Presenting Complaint
- Haematemesis
- Haemoptysis
- Melaena
- Fresh per rectum (PR) bleeding
- Haematuria
- Menorrhagia/postmenopausal bleeding
- Jaundice

Previous Medical/Surgical History
- Any chronic disease
- Previous abdominal operation, especially if it resulted in short-bowel syndrome

Drug History
- Non-steroidal anti-inflammatory drugs (NSAIDs)
- Steroids
- Antidepressants
- Direct oral anticoagulants (DOACs)
- Warfarin
- Antiplatelet medication

Social History
- Poor diet
- Alcohol or drug history
- Smoking
- Occupation

 Present Your Findings

We sent off a blood sample to investigate the cells in your blood. It shows that you are anaemic, which means that a substance called haemoglobin, which carries oxygen around your body, is low. Haemoglobin is found in red blood cells. Your red blood cells are smaller than they should be, which suggests that you do not have enough iron in your system. This could explain why you are tired and pale. I would like to organise more tests to find the cause of your anaemia. These will include more blood tests and a special camera test to look into your stomach and bowel. This will help us to treat you appropriately. Have you any questions?

❓ QUESTIONS AND ANSWERS FOR CANDIDATE

What are the clinical features of IDA?
- Pallor (e.g. seen in conjunctiva or palmar creases)
- Angular stomatitis
- Glossitis
- Dyspnoea
- Lethargy
- Chest pain
- Palpitations
- Orthostatic hypotension/syncope

Give three test you could do to investigate IDA.
- Blood film: To evaluate the cells in the blood, looking at quantity, shape, size and colour

- Iron studies: Serum iron, ferritin, transferrin, transferrin saturation to check for any deficiencies

What is the treatment for IDA?
- Treat the underlying cause
- Oral replacement; for example, ferrous fumarate
- Iron infusion
- Blood transfusion if unstable due to anaemia or if very severe and symptomatic

 A Case to Learn From

A 62-year-old woman on a surgical ward had a major postoperative GI haemorrhage of 2000 mL. However, at the time of bleeding, her Hb was 82 g/L, which was the same as her pre-operative Hb. During a major haemorrhage, the Hb may not have fallen as the blood has not had time to dilute. The urea, however, had risen (from blood being digested), indicating that her Hb would in fact be a lot lower, as clinically suspected.

💡 **Top Tip**

In actively bleeding patients, it is important to send an FBC, coagulation screen and cross-match as soon as possible. There may not be an immediate drop in Hb; however, even if normal, it is useful to know the baseline. A normal Hb in a patient with major bleeding should not preclude transfusion. Replace blood with blood. Repeat the FBC intermittently for monitoring.

STATION 5.2: UREA AND ELECTROLYTES (U&E)

SCENARIO

You are a junior doctor on a general medicine placement and have been asked to see Mrs Smith, a 70-year-old woman, who was admitted with gastroenteritis. The nursing staff are concerned that she has not passed urine in 12 h. She has a background of type 2 diabetes, hypertension and osteoarthritis in her spine. You take some blood tests and the results are reported as below. Please review the results, explain the findings to Mrs Smith and formulate an appropriate management plan.

🚶 **Results**

COMPONENTS	RESULTS	REFERENCE RANGES WITH UNITS
Sodium	136	135–145 mmol/L
Potassium	5.7 ↑	3.5–5.5 mmol/L
Chloride	100	95–110 mmol/L
Bicarbonate	25	22–29 mmol/L
Urea	10 ↑	2.5–6.5 mmol/L
Creatinine	130 ↑	60–120 µmol/L
Estimated glomerular filtration rate (eGFR)	45 ↓	>60 mL/min/1.73 m²

DATA INTERPRETATION

Physiology and causes for increased and decreased levels of each U&E component

	PHYSIOLOGY	INCREASED	DECREASED
Sodium	• Sodium is the main extracellular cation. It has functions in fluid balance, acid–base balance and the generation of an action potential • Primarily it is passively reabsorbed at the proximal convoluted tubule • A small amount is reabsorbed at the distal convoluted tubule and collecting duct	Hypervolaemic: • Usually iatrogenic; for example, hypertonic saline infusions Euvolaemic: • Diabetes insipidus • Drugs; for example, proton pump inhibitors, selective serotonin receptor inhibitors (SSRIs) Hypovolaemic: • Dermal losses; for example, burns • GI losses; for example, vomiting and diarrhoea • Renal losses; for example, AKI/ CKD, loop diuretics	Hypervolaemic: • Heart failure • Liver failure • Nephrotic syndrome Euvolaemic: • Syndrome of inappropriate antidiuretic hormone secretion • Addison's disease • Hypothyroidism Hypovolaemic: • GI losses; for example, vomiting and diarrhoea • Renal losses; for example, AKI/ CKD, loop diuretics
Potassium	• Potassium is the main intracellular cation. It has functions in maintenance of the membrane potential, acid–base balance and the generation of an action potential • It is actively reabsorbed in the proximal convoluted tubule and thick ascending limb of loop of Henle, and is secreted in the distal convoluted tubule	• AKI/CKD • Acidosis • Trauma Iatrogenic: • Potassium infusions, oral potassium-sparing diuretics; for example, spironolactone Artefact: • Haemolysis • Prolonged tourniquet time	• Vomiting • Diuretics • Diabetic ketoacidosis (DKA)
Chloride	• Chloride is the main anion in extracellular fluid. It is involved in fluid balance and acid–base balance	• Dehydration • Cushing's syndrome • CKD • Hyperventilation	• Vomiting • Loop diuretics • Congestive cardiac failure (CCF) • Addison's disease • COPD
Bicarbonate	• Bicarbonate is filtered freely at the glomerulus and reabsorption primarily occurs at the proximal convoluted tubule	• Cushing's syndrome • CKD • Hyperaldosteronism • COPD	• Diabetic ketoacidosis • Addison's disease • Lactic acidosis
Urea	• Urea is the primary breakdown product of protein catabolism, formed in the liver via the urea cycle. It is freely filtered at the glomerulus but not actively reabsorbed	Prerenal: • GI bleed • Protein catabolism (trauma, surgery, starvation) • Increased dietary protein • Reduced renal perfusion Renal: • Acute tubular necrosis • Glomerulonephritis • Hypertensive/diabetic nephropathy • Autoimmune disease Postrenal: • Obstruction	• Pregnancy • Malnutrition • Chronic hepatic disease

Physiology and causes for increased and decreased levels of each U&E component—cont'd

	PHYSIOLOGY	INCREASED	DECREASED
Creatinine	• Creatinine is a waste product of muscle breakdown	• Renal failure • Muscle breakdown • Increased muscle bulk • Increased dietary protein • Hypothyroidism • DKA • Drugs; for example, steroids	• Reduced muscle mass (including elderly, female sex) • Low-protein diet • Hyperthyroidism
eGFR	• The glomerular filtration rate can be estimated by measuring the renal clearance of a substance which is freely filtered at the glomerulus but is not reabsorbed, is not secreted by the nephron and not metabolised • In clinical practice, this is calculated using creatinine clearance		• AKI • CKD

Signs and symptoms, investigations required and management of abnormal sodium and potassium levels

	SYMPTOMS	INVESTIGATIONS	MANAGEMENT
Hyponatraemia	Early signs and symptoms: • Headache • Anorexia • Nausea and vomiting • Lethargy Advanced signs and symptoms: • Confusion • Agitation • Seizures • Focal neurological deficits • Cheyne–Stokes respiration • Coma	• Serum osmolality • Urine osmolality • Urinary sodium Consider: • Thyroid function tests (TFTs) for hypothyroidism • Short Synacthen test for Addison's disease • Brain natriuretic peptide (BNP) for heart failure • Liver function tests (LFTs) for liver failure	• Depends on serum osmolality, urine sodium, fluid status and presence/absence of symptoms Hypovolaemic: • Fluid replacement. The rate is dependent on the symptoms Euvolaemic: • If symptomatic, hypertonic saline and diuretics • If asymptomatic, fluid restriction • Fluid restriction Hypervolaemic: • Treat the underlying cause, and it usually includes fluid restriction
Hypernatraemia	Depending on cause: • Thirst • Polyuria • Polydipsia • Lethargy • Confusion • Oliguria • Dry mouth	• Send urgent repeat U&Es • Check blood glucose level • Request urine and serum osmolality if diabetes insipidus is suspected	• Depends on the underlying cause, which may require separate treatment • Correct dehydration • Correct hypovolaemia
Hypokalaemia	• Weakness • Constipation • Leg cramps • Breathing difficulties	• Send urgent repeat U&Es • Perform an urgent electrocardiogram (ECG) • Check magnesium level	• Depends on the underlying causes and severity • Stop any drugs that cause increased potassium loss; for example, diuretics and laxatives • Potassium replacement (oral or intravenous (IV)) • Consider magnesium replacement if required

Continued

	SYMPTOMS	INVESTIGATIONS	MANAGEMENT
	Signs and symptoms, investigations required and management of abnormal sodium and potassium levels—cont'd		
Hyperkalaemia	• Muscle weakness • Palpitations • Paraesthesia • Hypoxia	• Send urgent repeat U&Es • Obtain rapid reading on blood gas. This is less accurate than U&Es, but it should not delay treatment particularly if symptoms/ECG changes are present	• Stop all potassium infusions, oral replacements, potassium-sparing diuretics, NSAIDs and other drugs containing potassium; for example, laxatives • Treat severe hyperkalaemia urgently. Use your trust protocol and hyperkalaemia kit Treatment includes: • 10 mL 10% calcium gluconate IV over 2 min, to stabilise the cardiac membrane • 10 units Actrapid in 50 mL 50% dextrose IV over 5 min to drive the potassium intracellularly • 10 mg salbutamol nebulised to drive potassium intracellularly • Dialysis may be required if refractory • Monitor blood glucose and U&Es regularly posttreatment

THIS CASE

This patient has become hypovolaemic due to gastroenteritis and her kidneys are insufficiently perfused. As a result, she is oliguric and her U&Es show a raised creatinine and urea, and low eGFR, indicative of acute kidney injury (AKI). She is hyperkalaemic, which is likely secondary to the AKI.

AKI DEFINITION AND CAUSES

Causes of AKI

PRE-RENAL	RENAL	POSTRENAL
• Hypovolaemia: Bleeding, GI losses • Sepsis • Renovascular disease: Peripheral vascular disease • Oedematous states: CCF, liver failure	• Acute tubular necrosis: Secondary to prolonged prerenal cause, nephrotoxic drugs/contrast, ischaemia, rhabdomyolysis • Glomerulonephritis: Lupus, granulomatosis with polyangiitis • Interstitial nephritis: Drug reaction, autoimmune disorder	• Obstruction: Renal calculi, blood clot, hypertrophied prostate, tumour

• Oliguria (<0.5 mL/kg/h) for > 6 consecutive hours
or
• Rise in creatinine > 26 μmol/L in 48 h
or
• Rise in creatinine × 1.5 from baseline

RELEVANT PATIENT INFORMATION

You suspect that this patient has hypovolaemia. Ask about known medical conditions, relevant treatments and any hospital admissions.

HISTORY OF PRESENTING COMPLAINT

• Duration of nausea and vomiting
• Ability to tolerate oral fluids

PAST MEDICAL/SURGICAL HISTORY

• Pre-existing renal disease; for example, renal failure
• Hepatic disease which may predispose to hepatorenal syndrome; for example, liver cirrhosis
• Hypertension, with the complication of hypertensive nephropathy
• Diabetes, with the complication of diabetic nephropathy
• Atherosclerotic disease, therefore predisposing towards renal artery stenosis

MEDICATION HISTORY

Drugs which are nephrotoxic can be remembered through the mnemonic DAAMN:

- *Diuretics*, especially loop diuretics; for example, furosemide
- *Angiotensin*-converting enzyme inhibitors (ACEi) are in fact renoprotective in CKD. The reason they are harmful in patients with prerenal failure is their inhibition of compensatory rise in blood pressure, due to the activation of the renin–angiotensin–aldosterone system in hypotension, leading to ongoing hypotension and hypoperfusion. Always restart ACEi in CKD patients once acute illness has resolved. Alpha receptor blockers are a good alternative if ACEi cannot be tolerated
- *Aminoglycosides/aciclovir*
- *Metformin*
- *NSAIDS*; for example, ibuprofen

 Present Your Findings

One of the blood tests that we took was of your kidney function. It shows that your kidneys have become damaged due to dehydration, as you have lost a lot of fluid through vomiting and diarrhoea. This can usually be reversed by rehydration, so I would like to give you some fluids into the vein. I would encourage you to take sips of fluid as tolerated.

I would also like to insert a catheter into your bladder as this will tell us how much urine you are producing every hour, which helps to monitor how well your kidneys are working. Some of your medications, including those for your high blood pressure, diabetes and back pain, have been withheld as they may damage your kidneys further.

Lastly, I would like to carry out a tracing of your heart as one of the salts in your blood is slightly high and this can have an effect on your heart. Have you any questions?

❓ QUESTIONS AND ANSWERS FOR CANDIDATE

What is the maximum rate of routine potassium infusion peripherally?
- 10 mmol/h

What are the indications for renal dialysis?
These can be remembered through the mnemonic AEIOU:
- *Acidosis*: pH < 7.2, base excess < 10
- *Electrolyte* abnormalities: Persistent hyperkalaemia > 7 mmol/L
- *Intoxication*; for example, overdose of BLAST drugs:
  - *Barbituates*
  - *Lithium*
  - *Alcohol*
  - *Salicylates*
  - *Theophylline*
- *Overload*: Refractory pulmonary oedema
- *Uraemia*

Give some initial investigations that might be helpful in AKI.
- FBCs and C-reactive protein: Raised inflammatory markers may suggest sepsis as a cause
- Bone profile, U&Es, and magnesium: Deranged electrolytes on U&Es may be associated with deranged

bone profile and magnesium. It also shows albumin, which if low, may indicate nephrotic syndrome
- Lipid profile: If considering nephrotic syndrome
- Creatinine kinase (CK): Consider if there is a possibility of rhabdomyolysis
- Autoantibodies: Antineutrophil cytoplasmic antibodies (ANCA), antinuclear antibody (ANA), antiglomerular basement membrane, antistreptolysin O titer if considering a renal cause
- Venous blood gas: To exclude acidosis/alkalosis
- Urine dipstick: Infection/intrinsic renal disease
- Ultrasound scan (USS) kidneys and renal tracts

 A Case to Learn From

A 63-year-old man who was normally fit and well was admitted after feeling generally unwell for 3 months with flu-like symptoms, recurrent infections and night sweats. He was septic, hyponatraemic and had an AKI. The hyponatraemia and AKI were attributed to dehydration; however, autoantibodies were reported to be raised a few days later. This prompted a renal biopsy which confirmed the diagnosis of granulomatosis with polyangiitis with involvement of renal vasculature. Always consider a wide differential diagnosis.

💡 **Top Tip**

Ensure you do not take blood from the arm in which an infusion is going through, as this may give rise to abnormal results, as any fluid in the infusion can dilute the blood.

STATION 5.3: LIVER FUNCTION TESTS

SCENARIO

You are a junior doctor on a general surgery rotation and have been asked to see Mrs King, a 44-year-old woman, who was admitted with constant right upper quadrant pain, fever and vomiting. Over the past few months she has noticed colicky pain after eating fatty food. Her husband noticed that her skin and sclera now look quite yellow. You take some blood tests and the results are reported as below. Please review the results, explain the findings to Mrs King and formulate an appropriate management plan.

🏃 **Results**

COMPONENT	RESULTS	REFERENCE RANGES WITH UNITS
Total bilirubin	38 ↑	< 20 mg/dL
Alanine aminotransferase (ALT)	35	5–40 U/L
Aspartate aminotransferase (AST)	22	5–40 U/L
Gamma-glutamyl transferase (GGT)	270 ↑	<65 U/L
Alkaline phosphatase (ALP)	350 ↑	25–130 U/L
Albumin	42	35–50 g/dL

DATA INTERPRETATION (TABLE 5.4)

Function of the liver:
- Synthesis of clotting factors
- Synthesis on immunoglobulins
- Synthesis of proteins; for example, albumin
- Synthesis of iron and copper-binding proteins
- Formation of bile
- Drug metabolism
- Detoxification; for example, alcohol and ammonia
- Storage of glycogen, iron and fat-soluble vitamins

THIS CASE

This patient has had ongoing symptoms of biliary colic. Her symptoms have acutely worsened, including pyrexia, right upper quadrant pain and jaundice, demonstrating Charcot's triad, which is consistent with ascending cholangitis. Her LFTs show raised GGT and ALP, and her husband describes clinical jaundice. This suggests a stone has moved into the CBD, causing obstructive jaundice.

Causes of obstructive jaundice

HEPATIC	INTRAHEPATIC	EXTRAHEPATIC
• Obstruction of flow of conjugated bilirubin	• Primary biliary cirrhosis • Primary sclerosing cholangitis	In the lumen: • CBD stone • Mirrizi's syndrome • Clot In the wall of the biliary tree: • Cholangiocarcinoma • Biliary stricture Extrinsic: • Tumour in head of pancreas • Lymph node

RELEVANT PATIENT INFORMATION

You suspect this patient has choledocolithiasis and ascending cholangitis. Ask about known medical conditions, relevant treatment and any hospital admissions.

HISTORY OF PRESENTING COMPLAINT

- Temporal relationship of symptoms to consumption of fatty food
- Pale stools or dark urine
- Any recent rapid weight loss can trigger gallstone formation

PAST MEDICAL/SURGICAL HISTORY

- Ileal resection
- Diabetes
- Weight loss surgery

- Previous cholecystectomy (does not exclude recurrence of gallstone in CBD stump)
- History of inflammatory bowel disease

MEDICATION HISTORY

- Paracetamol
- Any new drugs: Many medicines affect LFTs
- Recent antibiotics

RISK FACTORS FOR GALLSTONES

These can be remembered as the five Fs:
- *Fat*
- *Female*
- *Forties* (age 40–49 years)
- *Fertile*
- *Family* history

Investigations to consider if LFTs are abnormal

BLOODS	OTHER
• Coagulation screen: To test synthetic function • Hepatitis screen • HIV test • Paracetamol level: To exclude overdose • Ferritin: High in haemochromatosis • α_1-antitrypsin: Positive in α_1-antitrypsin deficiency • Ceruloplasmin: Wilson's disease • Epstein–Barr virus (EBV) and cytomegalovirus (CMV) serology • Anti-mitochondrial antibodies: Positive in primary biliary cirrhosis • ANA, smooth-muscle antibody and ANCA: Primary sclerosing cholangitis, associated with inflammatory bowel disease • Anti-smooth muscle antibody (+ ANA): Autoimmune hepatitis	• USS abdomen: First-line radiological investigation for gallstones. Will also show liver texture and ascites and look at the patency of the portal vein • Computed tomography (CT) or magnetic resonance imaging (MRI): To exclude malignancy/abscess • Magnetic resonance cholangiopancreatography (MRCP): May be indicated following USS to detect stones in the CBD • Biopsy: For tissue diagnosis

OTHER CONSIDERATIONS IN LIVER FAILURE

- Hepatorenal syndrome: Cirrhosis, ascites and renal failure
- Bleeding: Reduced synthesis of clotting factors. Raised portal venous pressure secondary to cirrhosis may cause oesophageal varices, which may lead to massive haematemesis if they rupture

Table 5.4   Physiology and causes for abnormal levels and patterns of abnormality of each LFT component

	PHYSIOLOGY	ABNORMALITIES	PATTERN
Bilirubin	• Breakdown product of haem catabolism • Most circulating bilirubin is unconjugated and bound to albumin. This is insoluble in water • Bilirubin is conjugated to a soluble form in the hepatocytes, which is then secreted into the bile • It is raised in jaundice	Conjugated hyperbilirubinaemia: • Hepatocellular pathology: Hepatitis, neonatal jaundice, drugs • Defective biliary excretion from hepatocytes: Dubin–Johnson syndrome, Rotor syndrome • Intrahepatic or extrahepatic cholestasis Unconjugated hyperbilirubinaemia: • Overproduction: Haemolysis (haemolytic anaemia, haematoma, sickle cell crisis) • Defective bilirubin uptake: Right heart failure, drugs • Defective conjugation: Gilbert's syndrome	
ALT AST	• An enzyme found primarily in the cytoplasm of hepatocytes • Small amounts are present in the kidney, skeletal muscle and myocardium • Raised ALT is a measure of hepatocyte damage • An enzyme which is found in hepatocytes, primarily in the mitochondria • Also found in the myocardium, skeletal muscle, kidneys and brain. Therefore raised levels are seen in cardiac and hepatic pathology, as well as muscle injury • It is less specific to liver disease than ALT	Elevated levels of both ALT and AST suggest hepatocellular damage: • Hepatitis: Alcoholic, viral, autoimmune, non-alcoholic steatohepatitis • Many drugs; for example, statins, paracetamol, NSAIDS, antibiotics, illicit drugs • Genetic conditions: Haemochromatosis, Wilson's disease • Ischaemia	Comparing the degree of elevation of transaminases can aid diagnosis: • ALT rises faster than AST in acute liver pathology • ALT > AST in chronic liver disease, except when cirrhosis present • 2:1 rise in AST:ALT is consistent with alcoholic liver disease • ALT is often initially > 1000 in acute stone obstruction, then rapidly decreases
GGT ALP	• An enzyme found in hepatocytes and biliary system epithelium • Elevated levels suggest biliary tract obstruction rather than hepatocellular damage • An enzyme which is found in hepatic canaliculi • It is more widespread than the liver enzymes above, and can be found in bones, the GI tract, kidneys and placenta	Elevated levels of both GGT and ALP suggest cholestasis. Intrahepatic: • Primary biliary cirrhosis • Primary sclerosing cholangitis • Congestive hepatopathy (secondary to heart failure. May also have moderate rise in transaminases) Extrahepatic: • Common bile duct (CBD) stone • Tumour in the biliary tree/head of pancreas • Biliary stricture	• GGT can be raised in any liver pathology • GGT may be raised with even small quantities of alcohol. It is raised in alcoholism • Raised ALP with normal GGT suggests bone disease; for example, osteomalacia, Paget's disease, malignancy • ALP is usually normal in acute stone obstruction of the CBD • ALP may be raised in the third trimester of pregnancy
Albumin	• Albumin is the primary protein found in plasma; it is synthesised in the liver and is therefore a good indicator of liver function • It binds to many drugs, hormones and ions • It is a major contributor to colloid osmotic pressure in vasculature • It may be normal in acute liver failure	High: • Dehydration Low: • Malnutrition • Nephrotic syndrome • Liver failure • Inflammation	N/A

- Hypoglycaemia: Reduced glycogen storage capacity
- Hepatic encephalopathy: A spectrum of neuropsychiatric disorders caused by accumulation of nitrogenous waste
- Wernicke–Korsakoff syndrome: Wernicke's encephalopathy caused by thiamine deficiency in chronic alcohol dependence may progress to the irreversible Korsakoff's psychosis
- Spontaneous bacterial peritonitis: Infection of ascitic fluid

Present Your Findings

We sent off a blood sample to investigate the condition of your liver. It shows that there is a blockage in the tube connecting your liver to your bowel, probably due to a gallstone. This means that a substance called bile, which aids digestion, cannot move from the gallbladder into the bowel. This is why your skin looks quite yellow and you have been feeling unwell. It is likely that the blockage has caused infection, which is why you have a temperature.

I would like to order a scan to confirm the presence of a gallstone in this tube and another to see if there are gallstones in the gallbladder.

I will initially treat you with fluids into the vein, antisickness medication, pain relief and antibiotics; however you may need a procedure to release the stone from the tube. This is called endoscopic retrograde cholangiopancreatography. Do you have any questions?

❓ QUESTIONS AND ANSWERS FOR CANDIDATE

What are the features of gallstones on USS?
- Acoustic shadow
- Thickened gallbladder wall caused by inflammation
- Duct dilatation if the stone is in the CBD

Name five clinical manifestations of chronic liver disease.
- Jaundice
- Spider naevi
- Gynaecomastia
- Ascites
- Caput medusa
- Liver flap (asterixis)
- Dupuytren's contracture
- Leukonychia
- Finger clubbing
- Palmar erythema
- Body hair loss
- Hepatomegaly: Hepatitis, fatty liver disease
- Splenomegaly

What is the management of cholecystitis?
Conservative:
- Antibiotics
- IV fluids if vomiting
- Analgesia
- Antiemetic

Interventional radiology:
- Percutaneous cholecystostomy: If empyema or mucocele suspected, or if the patient is unstable with biliary sepsis

Surgical:
- Laparoscopic or open cholecystectomy: Often carried out after the acute phase has settled, within 6 weeks of presentation

A Case to Learn From

An elderly patient presented with LFTs suggestive of obstruction, presumed to be secondary to a CBD stone. Of note, her Hb was also low. No stone was detected on MRCP. She became haemodynamically unstable and required a transfusion. On further imaging it became clear that she had bled into her gallbladder and the previously noted obstruction had been due to a clot in the CBD. This highlights the importance of considering wider differential diagnoses.

Top Tip

Always measure amylase in patients presenting with right upper quadrant pain, as pancreatitis is both an important cause of upper abdominal pain and a complication of gallstones.

STATION 5.4: COAGULATION SCREEN

SCENARIO

You are a junior doctor in the emergency department (ED) and have been asked to see Mr Barr, a 73-year-old man, with a background of atrial fibrillation (for which he is on warfarin) and ischaemic heart disease. He was commenced on antibiotics for a urinary tract infection 3 days ago. He has presented with lethargy, dizziness and haematemesis. You did some blood tests, the results of which are now back. Please review the blood tests, explain the findings to Mr Barr and formulate an appropriate management plan.

🏃 Results

COMPONENT	RESULTS	REFERENCE RANGE
Prothrombin time (PT)	22 ↑	11–13 s
Activated partial thromboplastin time (APTT)	40 ↑	23–32 s
Fibrinogen	4	1.5–4.0 g/L
International normalised ratio (INR)	8.0 ↑	2.0–3.0

DATA INTERPRETATION (TABLE 5.5)

The blood sample is collected in a bottle containing an anticoagulant, such as citrate, to prevent clotting, thus enabling different components of the coagulation pathway to be investigated in the laboratory. Calcium is added in the lab to reverse the anticoagulant.

HAEMOSTASIS

Vessel Wall

Upon injury, endothelial cells release several mediators to initiate haemostasis, including adenosine diphosphate (ADP), tissue factor and endothelins.

Platelet Plug

Various molecules trigger platelet activation and aggregation upon vessel wall injury, including exposed collagen in the vascular wall, ADP, thrombin and thromboxane A_2. Glycoproteins found on the surface of the platelets enable them to adhere to the damaged endothelium and each other.

Activation of platelets leads to an increase in size and change in shape and they become irregular with surface projections. Exocytosis of granules containing mediators – for example, ADP, thromboxane A_2 and serotonin – occurs, recruiting and activating more platelets by positive feedback. This leads to formation of a platelet plug.

COAGULATION CASCADE

Extrinsic Pathway

Activation of factor VII by tissue factor, which is found in the exposed subendothelial tissue, triggers the coagulation cascade.

Intrinsic Pathway

Exposure to collagen in damaged epithelium activates factor XII, which leads to sequential activation of factors XI, IX and VIII.

COMMON PATHWAY

The two pathways merge at the activation of factor X by activated factors VII and VIII to prothrombinase

Table 5.5   Physiology and causes of abnormal levels of each component

	PHYSIOLOGY	CAUSES OF ABNORMAL LEVELS
PT	• PT measures the extrinsic pathway of the coagulation cascade • In the laboratory, a reagent known as thromboplastin (phospholipid and tissue factor) is added to the blood and this binds to factor VII. This complex then triggers the coagulation cascade • The time taken for the time to clot is measured, giving the PT	Elevated levels Iatrogenic: • Early warfarin therapy Coagulation factor deficiency: • Congenital factor VII deficiency • Vitamin K deficiency Other: • Early sepsis • Liver disease
APTT	• APTT measures the intrinsic pathway of the coagulation cascade • In the laboratory, an APTT reagent containing phospholipid (without tissue factor, hence the term 'partial thromboplastin time') and an activator of the intrinsic pathway are added to the blood to activate the intrinsic pathway • The time taken for the blood to clot gives the APTT	Elevated levels Iatrogenic: • Massive transfusion • Unfractionated heparin treatment Coagulation factor deficiency: • Haemophilia A and B (factor VIII and IX deficiency respectively) • Factor XI and XII deficiency Other: • Disseminated intravascular coagulation (DIC) • Liver disease • Antiphospholipid syndrome
Both PT and APTT	As above	Iatrogenic: • Warfarin therapy (PT more affected) • Dabigatran therapy (coagulation screen does not correlate well with levels of other DOACs) Coagulation factor deficiency: • Vitamin K deficiency Other: • DIC
Fibrinogen	• Fibrinogen is also known as factor I • It is a protein synthesised in the liver; it is converted to fibrin by thrombin in the coagulation cascade	Elevated levels: • It may be high in an acute infection or inflammation Low levels: • It may be low in liver failure and DIC

(factor Xa). Factors Xa and Va (found on the surface of activated platelets) convert prothrombin to thrombin, which in turn will activate fibrinogen to fibrin.

Thrombin also activates parts of the intrinsic pathway to amplify the process.

Fibrin fibrils form a mesh and stabilise the platelet plug, forming a thrombus.

THIS CASE

This patient has presented with an acute upper GI bleed and a coagulation screen confirmed raised PT and APTT. It is important to resuscitate the patient, determine the cause of the bleed and inform the patient of the diagnosis and management plan.

CAUSES OF INCREASED ACTION OF WARFARIN

This can be remembered through the mnemonic O DEVICES:
- *Omeprazole*
- *Disulfiram*
- *Erythromycin*
- *Valproate*
- *Isoniazid*
- *Ciprofloxacin* and *cimetidine*
- *Ethanol* (acutely)
- *Sulphonamides*

RELEVANT PATIENT INFORMATION

You suspect this patient has an acute upper GI bleed. Ask about known medical conditions, relevant treatment and any hospital admissions.

PAST MEDICAL/SURGICAL HISTORY
- Congenital clotting factor deficiency; for example, haemophilia A or B
- Acquired deficiency of clotting factors; for example, liver failure and acquired haemophilia
- Autoimmune disease; for example, antiphospholipid syndrome

HAEMOPHILIA

Haemophilia A is an X-linked recessive condition, resulting from congenital deficiency of factor VIII, with a prevalence of 1:5000 males.

Haemophilia B is an X-linked recessive condition, resulting from congenital deficiency of factor IX, with a prevalence of 1:35,000 males.

Haemophilia may result in spontaneous bleeds, bleeding on minor trauma or prolonged bleeding in situations where some bleeding is anticipated; for example, surgery. These may be life-threatening depending on the severity of the disease, which is determined by the level of the affected clotting factor in the blood. Haemarthrosis and soft-tissue bleeds are common features.

DISSEMINATED INTRAVASCULAR COAGULATION

DIC is a condition resulting from either acute or chronic systemic processes which promote abnormal and excessive activation of the coagulation system and platelets, leading to occlusion of microvasculature by fibrin thrombi. This consumes platelets and clotting factors, thereby leading to a pro-haemorrhagic state.

ANTIPHOSPHOLIPID SYNDROME

Antiphospholipid syndrome is a prothrombotic auto-immune disorder associated with raised antiphospholipid antibodies, and adverse pregnancy outcomes for both mother and fetus in pregnant women.

MEDICATION HISTORY
- Anticoagulants; for example, warfarin, DOACs and heparin
- Antiplatelets
- Steroids
- SSRIs
- NSAIDs

Present Your Findings

We sent off a blood test to determine how long your blood takes to clot, which can help point towards why you have bled. It shows that your blood is taking longer to clot than it should. This is likely to be due to an interaction between the antibiotics you have been taking and your warfarin, which increased the activity of warfarin. This is why you have vomited blood.

I will initially treat you with fluid into the vein; however you may also need a blood transfusion. Your warfarin will be stopped for the time being and you will be treated with a vitamin K infusion to reverse the warfarin and another medication containing substances to help your blood clot. We will likely have to do a camera test to look into your stomach to see if we can stop any ongoing bleeding. Do you have any questions?

QUESTIONS AND ANSWERS FOR CANDIDATE

What are the indications for a coagulation screen?
- Suspicion of bleeding disorder
- Active bleeding
- Paracetamol overdose
- To assess synthetic function in liver disease
- Monitoring for DIC during blood transfusion
- Before surgery

What are the onsets of action of oral and IV vitamin K?
- Oral: 24 h
- IV: 2 h

Why is it preferable to reverse anticoagulation with a prothrombin complex concentrate (PCC) rather than fresh frozen plasma (FFP) in an emergency?

- Reversal using PCC is associated with faster reduction in INR, reduction in adverse effects such as volume overload and reduced requirement for red cell transfusion than FFP

A Case to Learn From

A patient on the GI ward had a variceal bleed. He was initially transfused with O-negative packed red cells and the massive haemorrhage protocol was activated. At baseline, his coagulation screen was slightly deranged; however, during the haemorrhage, his PT and APTT became more prolonged and he was given FFP as part of the protocol. It is important to remember that a patient with significant blood loss may need platelet transfusion, FFP and cryoprecipitate in addition to packed red cells.

Top Tip

Some trusts now have point-of-care testing for clotting screening. This is usually in major theatres where the incidence of emergency massive haemorrhage is higher. Rapidly available results allow for swift management of bleeding.

STATION 5.5: THYROID FUNCTION TESTS

SCENARIO

You are a junior doctor on a primary care placement and have been asked to see Mx Freesia, a 46-year-old non-binary person who has presented feeling tired all the time with a history of unintentional weight gain. They saw your colleague last week who took some bloods and the results are now back. They are known to have hypertension. Please review the blood tests, explain the findings to Mx Freesia and formulate an appropriate management plan.

Results

COMPONENT	RESULTS	REFERENCE RANGES WITH UNITS
Thyroid-stimulating hormone (TSH)	14 ↑	0.5–5.7 mU/L
Free thyroxine (T4)	28 ↓	70–140 mmol/L

DATA INTERPRETATION

In the UK, initial TFTs often only include TSH and T_4. The levels of these hormones can help diagnose thyroid disorders (Table 5.6).

Table 5.6   Signs and symptoms, investigations required and management of hypo-and hyperthyroidism

	SIGNS AND SYMPTOMS	INVESTIGATIONS	MANAGEMENT
Hypothyroidism	• Weight gain • Reduced appetite • Constipation • Dry skin • Cold intolerance • Loss of outer third of the eyebrows • Thin hair • Bradycardia • Hypertension • Hypercholesterolaemia • Heavy menstrual bleeding • Subfertility • Reduced libido • Lethargy • Muscle aches • Memory impairment • Depression • Delayed relaxation of reflexes	• Antithyroid peroxidase antibody (TPO) • Antithyroglobulin antibody • Imaging if indicated	• Levothyroxine
Hyperthyroidism	• Weight loss • Diarrhoea • Increased appetite • Heat intolerance • Sweating • Palpitations: Tachycardia, atrial fibrillation • Fatigue/hyperactivity • Mood swings/irritability • Thyroid eye disease (Grave's disease): Proptosis, lid lag • Goitre/thyroid nodule • Fine tremor • Oligomenorrhoea/ amenorrhoea	• TSH receptor antibody • TPO • Antithyroglobulin antibody • Ultrasound • Fine-needle aspiration of any nodules • Isotope scan	• Antithyroid drugs: For example, carbimazole or propylthiouracil • Beta-blockers: For symptomatic relief • Radioactive iodine: Contraindicated in pregnancy/ breastfeeding. • Thyroidectomy

Physiology and causes of increased and decreased levels of each component

	PHYSIOLOGY	INCREASED	DECREASED
TSH	• Thyrotrophin-releasing hormone from the hypothalamus stimulates the secretion of TSH from the pituitary gland. TSH acts on receptors in the thyroid gland to release T4 and Triiodothyronine (T3) from the follicular cells • These hormones act via nuclear receptors and have many roles, including in neurodevelopment and metabolism	• Hypothyroidism • Subclinical hypothyroidism • TSH-secreting tumour	• Hyperthyroidism • Hypothalamic or pituitary disorder • Subclinical hyperthyroidism
T_4	• T_4 is released alongside T_3 from the thyroid gland • T_4 is released in higher quantities and is converted into the more active hormone, T_3, once it reaches its target organ	• Hyperthyroidism • TSH-secreting tumour	• Hypothyroidism

THIS CASE

The patient is presenting with signs and symptoms of hypothyroidism. The blood tests have confirmed this, with a raised TSH level and low T_4 level. It is important to explain the diagnosis to the patient but also to determine the cause.

COMMON CAUSES OF HYPOTHYROIDISM

- Autoimmune hypothyroidism: The most common cause in the developed world includes:
  - Atrophic thyroiditis
  - Hashimoto's thyroiditis
  - Postpartum thyroiditis
- Medications: For example, amiodarone or lithium
- Pituitary disorders
- Radioactive iodine therapy
- Congenital hypothyroidism
- Head and neck radiation therapy

RELEVANT PATIENT INFORMATION

You suspect this patient has hypothyroidism. Ask about known medical conditions, relevant treatments and any hospital admissions.

MEDICATION HISTORY

- Amiodarone
- Lithium
- Interferon

FAMILY HISTORY

- Hypo- or hyperthyroidism
- Diabetes
- Hypertension

Present Your Findings

One of the blood tests we took was of your thyroid function. The thyroid is a gland in your neck that performs many functions. The tests show that your thyroid may be underactive, so not working well enough. This is called hypothyroidism. This would explain your symptoms of tiredness and weight gain. What I would like to do now would be to start you on a thyroid hormone tablet which is taken in the morning and is a lifelong treatment.

Also, I will take a further blood test to check for thyroid antibodies. This will help us to determine why your thyroid gland is not working as well as expected. It is important that you get your thyroid levels checked every year. Have you any questions?

QUESTIONS AND ANSWERS FOR CANDIDATE

What are the causes of thyrotoxicosis?
- Graves' disease
- Toxic adenoma
- Toxic multinodular goitre
- Carcinoma
- Thyroiditis
- Medications: For example, amiodarone and lithium

What are the pregnancy-related changes in the thyroid?
- There are many hormonal changes in pregnancy, including:
  - Increased thyroid-binding globulin: Due to this, there is an increase in T_3 and T_4 levels
  - Reduced TSH levels in the first trimester: Due to this, women with known hypothyroidism require an increase in their thyroxine dose, initially around 25–50 mcg
- Any woman with known thyroid disease should be referred to specialist obstetricians in their pregnancy

- Women with known thyroid disease require regular thyroid function assessment during pregnancy to ensure that they are euthyroid
- Postnatal thyroid function checks are also important

Why might a patient have low/normal T₄ and slightly raised TSH?

- Subclinical hypothyroidism: TFTs should be repeated in 3–6 months. If TSH is consistently above 10 mU/L, treatment with levothyroxine should be considered.
- After surgery or radioactive iodine treatment: Deemed to be 'compensatory'
- Non-compliance with treatment: A patient who does not adhere well to treatment may start taking their T₄ shortly before having their TFTs monitored. This may be enough to normalise T₄ but not to suppress TSH

 A Case to Learn From

A postpartum woman presented to her GP when her periods did not recommence. She was also fatigued and having trouble losing weight. Blood tests showed low T₄ and TSH. Through further history taking it transpired that she had suffered a significant postpartum haemorrhage after delivery of her baby. Further bloods showed low prolactin, and the woman was referred to endocrinology for further investigations for suspected Sheehan's syndrome. It is important to be mindful of problems upstream of the thyroid gland as causes of abnormal results.

DATA INTERPRETATION

 Top Tip

It is important to perform TFTs in any patient with unexplained tachycardia, new-onset atrial fibrillation, or as a part of the confusion screen.

STATION 5.6: BONE PROFILE

SCENARIO

You are a junior doctor on a primary care placement and have been asked to see Mrs Stone, a 68-year-old woman, who has presented with fatigue, constipation and dyspepsia. She saw your colleague last week who took some bloods and the results are now back. Please review the blood tests, explain the findings to Mrs Stone and formulate an appropriate management plan.

Results

COMPONENT	RESULTS	REFERENCE RANGES WITH UNITS
Adjusted calcium	2.95	2.2–2.6 mmol/L
ALP	130	35–120 u/L
Phosphate	0.6	0.8–1.4 mmol/L
Albumin	40	35–50

Physiology of and causes of increased and decreased level of each component of a bone profile

	PHYSIOLOGY	INCREASED LEVELS	DECREASED LEVELS
Calcium	Calcium: • 99% of the calcium in the body is found in bones. In the circulation, 50% of calcium is bound to proteins, for example, albumin, 10% complexed with anions and 40% is in the ionised form. The latter is the most physiologically important form • Calcium is important for nerve conduction, muscle contraction, blood clotting and cell signalling Adjusted calcium: • Since 50% of circulating calcium is bound to protein, changes in protein levels can result in falsely high or low calcium levels. A formula is applied to the measurements to correct for this	Excessive parathyroid hormone (PTH) secretion: • Primary hyperparathyroidism • Tertiary hyperparathyroidism • Ectopic PTH secretion Malignancy: • Myeloma • Lymphoma • Bony metastases • Multiple endocrine neoplasia 2 and 3 Excess vitamin D: • Excess intake • Granulomatous disease; for example, tuberculosis (TB), sarcoidosis Excess calcium intake: • Milk-alkali syndrome Drugs: • Thiazide diuretics • Vitamin A toxicity • Lithium Endocrine disease: • Thyrotoxicosis • Addison's disease • Acromegaly Other: • Familial hypocalciuric hypercalcaemia • Paget's disease with fracture or bed rest • Immobility • Prolonged tourniquet time	High phosphate: • Phosphate supplements • Tumour lysis syndrome • Chronic renal disease Hypoparathyroidism: • Post-thyroidectomy/parathyroidectomy • Congenital deficiency; for example, Di George's syndrome • Severe hypomagnesaemia • Idiopathic hypoparathyroidism Vitamin D deficiency: • Osteomalacia/rickets • Vitamin D resistance Drugs: • Calcitonin • Bisphosphonates Other: • Acute pancreatitis • Hypoalbuminaemia • Malabsorption • Massive transfusion • Hyperventilation can cause transient hypocalcaemia

Continued

Physiology of and causes of increased and decreased level of each component of a bone profile—cont'd			
	PHYSIOLOGY	**INCREASED LEVELS**	**DECREASED LEVELS**
Phosphate	• 85% of the phosphate in the body is found in bones. The remainder is primarily intracellular. • It is an important component of adenosine triphosphate (ATP), deoxyribonucleic acid (DNA) and cell membranes	Reduced excretion: • Severe renal impairment. Furthermore, phosphate is not efficiently removed at dialysis, therefore phosphate-binding therapy is often required • Hypoparathyroidism Extracellular shift: • Rhabdomyolysis • Tumour lysis syndrome • Diabetes (deficiency of insulin) Pseudohyperphosphataemia: • Haemolysed sample Increased reabsorption: • Vitamin D therapy • Acromegaly • Bisphosphonates	Reduced oral intake: • Poor diet Reduced absorption: • Vitamin D deficiency • Malabsorption Intracellular shift: • Refeeding syndrome • Insulin (including DKA treatment) • Respiratory alkalosis Increased urinary excretion: • Hyperparathyroidism • Renal tubular defects • Fanconi syndrome

THIS CASE

The patient is presenting with signs and symptoms of hypercalcaemia. The blood tests have confirmed this. It is important to explain the diagnosis to the patient, but also determine to the cause.

RELEVANT PATIENT INFORMATION

You suspect that this patient has hypercalcaemia. Ask about known medical conditions, relevant treatments and any hospital admissions.

MEDICATION HISTORY

• Vitamin D therapy
• Calcium therapy
• Thiazide diuretics
• Vitamin A therapy
• Prolonged lithium therapy

FAMILY HISTORY

• Parathyroid adenoma/hyperplasia/carcinoma
• Familial hypocalciuric hypercalcaemia
• Endocrine disease: Addison's disease, hyperthyroidism, acromegaly

Signs and symptoms, investigations required and management of abnormal calcium and phosphate levels			
	SIGNS AND SYMPTOMS	**INVESTIGATIONS**	**MANAGEMENT**
Hypercalcaemia	Bones: • Arthritis • Osteomalacia/rickets • Osteoporosis • Osteitis fibrosa cystica Stones: • Renal calculi • Nephrogenic diabetes insipidus • Uraemia Gastrointestinal symptoms: • Constipation • Anorexia • Nausea and vomiting • Peptic ulcer disease • Dyspepsia • Pancreatitis Neurological/Psychiatric • Lethargy • Confusion • Personality change • Coma Other: • Hypercalcaemia can also shorten QT interval, prolong PR and broaden QRS on the ECG, leading to arrhythmias and cardiac arrest	• ECG/telemetry • PTH • FBC • LFTs, specifically ALP • U&Es • Vitamins D and A • TFTs • Short Synacthen test • Insulin-like growth factor-1 and oral glucose tolerance test (acromegaly) • Imaging; for example, CT chest, abdomen and pelvis to detect and stage malignancy	• The mainstay of treatment is hydration with IV fluids, which reduce calcium concentration via dilution. Furthermore, increasing the intravascular volume increases renal clearance of calcium • Bisphosphonates should be considered in accordance with trust protocol to aid reduction in calcium, by inhibiting osteoclast activity • Furosemide may be used to inhibit tubular reabsorption of calcium

⚠ Signs and symptoms, investigations required and management of abnormal calcium and phosphate levels—cont'd

	SIGNS AND SYMPTOMS	INVESTIGATIONS	MANAGEMENT
Hypocalcaemia	• Paraesthesia (particularly perioral and digits) • Muscle spasms (Trousseau's sign is carpopedal spasm) • Confusion • Increased smooth muscle tone (laryngospasm, cramps) • Heart failure • Prolonged QT on ECG • Tetany • Seizures	• May need uncuffed sample (no tourniquet) to prove true hypocalcaemia • Magnesium • Vitamin D • U&Es (CKD) • PTH (hypoparathyroidism) • Amylase (pancreatitis) • CK (rhabdomyolysis) • ECG (prolonged QT)	• Oral or IV (calcium gluconate) replacement • Correct magnesium • Vitamin D replacement
Hyperphosphataemia	• Often asymptomatic • Bone pain • Itch • Deposition of calcium phosphate in tissues; for example, blood vessels (causing hypertension), joints (causing joint pain) and skin • Symptoms of associated hypocalcaemia	• U&Es (CKD) • Magnesium • PTH (hypoparathyroidism) • Vitamin D • Imaging if malignancy suspected	• Correct calcium if low (hypoparathyroidism) • Restrict dietary phosphate (CKD) • Phosphate binders (CKD)
Hypophosphataemia	• Usually asymptomatic • Poor appetite • Bone pain, osteopenia • Muscle weakness • Confusion • Coma • Death	• U&Es (renal tubular disease may cause electrolyte abnormalities) • LFTs (high ALP if phosphate chronically low) • Vitamin D • PTH • Arterial blood gas (ABG) (may show respiratory alkalosis; for example, caused by salicylate poisoning) • Plasma protein electrophoresis • X-rays of areas of deformity (rickets) • 24-h urine collection. (Refeeding syndrome, respiratory alkalosis and reduced GI absorption) • Dual-energy X-ray absorptiometry scan • Genetic tests; for example, for Fanconi syndrome	• Oral/IV phosphate replacement • May need calcium/vitamin D replacement • Treatment of the underlying cause

PARATHYROID HORMONE

- PTH, also known as parathormone, is secreted from chief cells in the parathyroid glands in response to falling calcium levels
- It raises calcium level and reduces phosphate level by:
  - Increasing osteoclastic resorption of bone
  - Increasing synthesis of 1,25-cholecalciferol (calcitriol), which leads to increased intestinal absorption of calcium
  - Increasing renal tubular reabsorption of calcium
  - Increasing excretion of phosphate by reducing tubular reabsorption

 Present Your Findings

One of the blood tests that we took measured some of the minerals in your blood. It showed that your calcium is high. While calcium is important for healthy bones and for nerves and muscles to work, if there is too much in your blood, it can be harmful.

You have four tiny glands in your neck called parathyroid glands, which produce a hormone which raises calcium levels in the blood. If this hormone is overproduced, it can raise calcium levels above normal. I would like to take another blood test to see if too much of this hormone is being made. If it is, we will scan your neck to look at your parathyroid glands. If there is an abnormality it is likely you will need an operation on your neck to remove at least one parathyroid gland. Have you any questions?

❓ QUESTIONS AND ANSWERS FOR CANDIDATE

What is the role of PTH in calcium and phosphate regulation?

- PTH, also known as parathyroid hormone, is secreted from chief cells in the parathyroid glands in response to falling calcium levels

What are the complications of parathyroid surgery?

- Hypocalcaemia: Following parathyroidectomy, there is often a relative hypoparathyroidism leading to increased deposition of calcium in bone, increased renal excretion of calcium (provided the patient is not in end-stage renal failure) and reduced intestinal absorption of calcium
- Recurrent laryngeal nerve damage: May present with hoarseness postoperatively. If damaged bilaterally, airway obstruction requiring intubation may result
- Haematoma in pretracheal space: Can cause airway compromise and requires urgent evacuation. Suture cutters should be kept by the bedside

postoperatively to be used in the event of life-threatening airway compromise

What are the causes of hyperparathyroidism?

- Primary hyperparathyroidism:
  - Parathyroid adenoma
  - Parathyroid carcinoma
- Secondary hyperparathyroidism:
  - Secondary hyperparathyroidism is hypersecretion of PTH in response to chronic hypocalcaemia; for example, due to renal failure, liver disease, malabsorption
  - It is associated with normal serum calcium
- Tertiary hyperparathyroidism:
  - Tertiary hyperparathyroidism is hyperplasia of the parathyroid and autonomous PTH secretion due to long-standing secondary hyperparathyroidism

 A Case to Learn From

A patient on a surgical ward had a parathyroidectomy for a parathyroid adenoma and later that night reported perioral and digital paraesthesia. Examination was unremarkable and she was Chvostek's- and Trousseau's-negative. A repeat bone profile showed hypocalcaemia.

I encouraged her to drink a glass of milk whilst awaiting the result. Trust protocol was followed with regard to replacing calcium; in this case oral replacement was sufficient. It is important to measure calcium regularly post-parathyroidectomy/thyroidectomy and notify your seniors of any abnormalities.

Top Tip

Electrolyte abnormalities often coexist, so if one is identified then others should be checked. Check magnesium in hypocalcaemic patients. Low magnesium will need to be replaced, otherwise calcium will be difficult to normalise.

STATION 5.7: ARTERIAL BLOOD GAS

SCENARIO

You are a junior doctor in the ED and have been asked to see Mrs Freesia, a 72-year-old woman who presented with shortness of breath and swollen legs. On examination, you note that she is tachypnoeic, has a raised jugular venous pressure and fine bi-basal crepitations on chest auscultation. She had a myocardial infarction (MI) 5 years ago.

You have obtained an ABG. Please review the result, explain the findings to Mrs Freesia and formulate an appropriate management plan.

🏃 Results

COMPONENT	RESULTS	REFERENCE RANGES WITH UNITS
pH	7.36	7.35–7.45
Arterial oxygen partial pressure (PaO_2)	8.0 ↓	10–14 kPa
Arterial carbon dioxide partial pressure ($PaCO_2$)	4.7	4.6–6.0 kPa
Oxygen saturation (SaO_2)	88% ↓	> 94%
Bicarbonate (HCO_3^-)	25	24–28 mmol/L
Base excess (BE)	1.0 ↑	–2.0 ± 2.0

DATA INTERPRETATION

METHOD FOR INTERPRETING ABG RESULTS

Assess oxygenation and ventilation (Table 5.7).

The PaO_2 gives an indication of oxygen uptake. When assessing the PaO_2 it is vitally important to consider the PaO_2 at the same time.

Assess the pH:
- Low (<7.35) indicates acidosis
- High (> 7.45) indicates alkalosis
- Tight control of pH is achieved by excretion of acid and buffering by bases; for example, bicarbonate
Is the pH explained by the CO_2 (Table 5.8)?
- CO_2 is an acidic gas. This means that:
  - High levels of CO_2 will cause the blood pH to be acidotic
  - Low levels of CO_2 will cause the blood pH to be alkalotic
- For example, if the pH indicated acidosis and the CO_2 levels were high, this would imply that the

Table 5.7 Differentiating between type 1 and type 2 respiratory failure

RESPIRATORY FAILURE	CAUSE	PaO_2	$PaCO_2$
Type 1	Failure to oxygenate	< 8 kPa	Normal/low
Type 2	Failure to ventilate	< 8 kPa	> 6 kPa

Table 5.8 ABG interpretation based on pH and $PaCO_2$

pH	CO_2	DIAGNOSIS
↓	↑	Respiratory acidosis
↑	↓	Respiratory alkalosis

Table 5.9 ABG interpretation based on pH and HCO_3^-

pH	HCO_3^-	DIAGNOSIS
↓	↓	Metabolic acidosis
↑	↑	Metabolic alkalosis

acidosis was due to the excess CO_2 and therefore, the cause of the acidosis was respiratory
- If the pH indicated acidosis and the CO_2 levels were low, this would imply that the cause of the acidosis was not respiratory and therefore, further questions would need to be asked (see below)

If the pH is not explained by the $PaCO_2$, is it explained by the HCO_3^- (Table 5.9)?
- HCO_3^- is alkaline and acts as a buffer. This means that:
  - Low levels of HCO_3^- in the blood indicate acidosis as it is 'consumed' in the setting of metabolic acidosis
  - High levels of HCO_3^- in the blood will cause the blood pH to be alkalotic
- For example, if the pH indicated acidosis and the HCO_3^- levels were low, this would imply that the acidosis was explained by the HCO_3^- and therefore the cause of the acidosis was metabolic

To help you determine the cause of a patient's metabolic acidosis, the anion gap can be calculated.

$$\text{Anion gap} = (Na^+ + K^+) - (Cl^- + HCO_3^-)$$
$$\text{Normal range}: 6 - 16\ mmol/L$$

Normal range: 6 - 16 mmol/L.

THIS CASE

This patient is presenting with signs and symptoms of pulmonary oedema. The ABG supports this as the patient is hypoxic. It is important to carry out prompt initial management and explain the diagnosis to the patient but also to determine the cause (Table 5.10).

CAUSES OF PULMONARY OEDEMA

CARDIOGENIC

CCF due to:
- Acute coronary syndrome
- Valvular heart disease: Severe aortic stenosis, acute aortic or mitral regurgitation
- Acute arrhythmia
- Hypertensive crisis
- Cardiomyopathy
- Cardiac tamponade

Table 5.10 Physiological changes and causes of the different types of ABG abnormalities

TYPE OF ABNORMALITY	pH	PaCO$_2$	HCO$_3^-$	COMPENSATION	CAUSES
Respiratory acidosis	↓	↑	↔	Increased HCO$_3^-$	• Hypoventilation • Lung pathology • Asthma (life-threatening exacerbation) • COPD • Pneumonia • Pulmonary oedema • Pulmonary embolism (PE) • Obesity • Myasthenia gravis • Guillain–Barré syndrome • Chest well defects • Medications; for example, opioids and sedatives
Respiratory alkalosis	↑	↓	↔	Decreased HCO$_3^-$	• Hyperventilation • Stroke • Intracranial bleed • Meningitis
Metabolic acidosis	↓	↔	↓	Decreased CO$_2$	Causes of a high anion gap: • DKA • Lactic acidosis • Uraemia • Aspirin overdoseCauses of a normal anion gap: • Diarrhoea • Addison's disease • Renal tubular acidosis • Pancreatic fistulaCauses of a low anion gap: • Hypoalbuminaemia • Multiple myeloma
Metabolic alkalosis	↑	↔	↑	Increased CO$_2$	• Vomiting • Burns • Diarrhoea • Hypokalaemia • Conn's syndrome

NON-CARDIOGENIC

- Renal failure
- Liver failure
- PE
- Acute respiratory distress syndrome
- Iatrogenic fluid overload
- Sepsis
- Pneumonia
- High altitude
- Trauma
- Drugs; for example, opioids

RELEVANT PATIENT INFORMATION

You suspect that this patient has pulmonary oedema. Ask about known medical conditions, relevant treatments and any hospital admissions.

DRUG HISTORY

- Opioids
- Chemotherapy
- Diuretics

FAMILY HISTORY

- Ischaemic heart disease
- Cardiomyopathy
- Venous thromboembolism
- Renal failure
- Liver failure

COMPENSATION

When there has been deviation from the normal blood pH, the body activates pathways to try to compensate for the deviation and attempts to bring the pH back within normal range.

- The lungs compensate for a metabolic disturbance by altering the levels of carbon dioxide. This is generally rapid and can occur within minutes
- The kidneys compensate for a respiratory disturbance by controlling the levels of bicarbonate ions. This is generally slower and takes from a few days to a week to occur

A patient can be uncompensated. This usually implies an acute event; the body has not had time to adapt to the change in pH.

A patient can be partially compensated. This implies that the pH is out of the normal range and the body is making an attempt to compensate for the disturbance. For example, there may be a respiratory acidosis (raised carbon dioxide), and a small metabolic alkalosis (raised bicarbonate) to compensate. However, the compensation is only partial and the patient remains acidotic.

A patient can be fully compensated. This implies the pH is within normal range but other values are still abnormal in order to correct the underlying disturbance. This implies a chronic process.

It is important to remember that, in general, overcompensation does not happen. The body brings the pH back within normal range.

It is also possible to have a mixture of causes for acid–base imbalances; for example, acidosis could be caused by both exacerbation of COPD as well as lactic acidosis secondary to sepsis.

ASSESSING OTHER ANALYTES

An arterial sample can provide a rapid indication of important analytes; for example, haemoglobin and potassium. This can assist in diagnosis and guide early intervention. These can also be obtained from a venous blood gas.

 Present Your Findings

One of the blood tests that we took was to look at levels of oxygen and carbon dioxide in your blood. The tests show that the levels of oxygen in your blood are not as high as they should be, and the swelling of your legs and crackles in your chest suggest this could be because you have fluid in your lungs.

What I would like to do now is to send off more blood tests, get a chest X-ray and a tracing of your heart. If your shortness of breath and low oxygen levels are due to fluid in your lungs, you will be treated with medications that make you get rid of fluid by passing more urine, and we will continue to give you oxygen. We will also arrange a scan of your heart to check if this might be what is causing a fluid build up

QUESTIONS AND ANSWERS FOR CANDIDATE

Why is Allen's test performed before an ABG?

- To test the patency of the radial and ulnar arteries to ensure circulation to the hand will not be compromised when performing an ABG

What can you do to preserve an ABG sample if it cannot be analysed straight away?

- The sample can be stored on ice, allowing it to be analysed within 2 h

What is meant by the hypoxic drive?

- Central chemoreceptors in the medulla detect changes in CO_2 levels in the blood. Detection of high levels of CO_2 triggers an increase in depth and rate of respiration, and vice versa
- Patients retaining CO_2, for example, those with COPD, have chronically raised CO_2, causing the central chemoreceptors to become desensitised
- In this case ventilation is driven by hypoxia, which is detected by peripheral chemoreceptors in the aortic arch and carotid bodies
- Applying a high fraction of inspired oxygen (FiO_2) to these patients may cause them to lose the hypoxic drive and therefore may lead to respiratory arrest

 A Case to Learn From

A patient with known type 2 respiratory failure had a drop in his oxygen saturation in blood plasma (SpO_2) to 80% after dialysis. He was not symptomatic of this. An ABG showed he had an SaO_2 of 95%. It transpired that he was hypotensive after having fluid removed on dialysis and was peripherally vasoconstricted secondary to this, therefore giving a falsely low oxygen saturation reading. ABGs give a more accurate measure of oxygenation than pulse oximetry.

 Top Tip

It is important to record what supplementary oxygen the patient was on when the ABG was taken to enable accurate interpretation.

STATION 5.8: ELECTROCARDIOGRAM

SCENARIO

You are a junior doctor on an emergency medicine placement and have been asked to see Mr Fredrickson, a 65-year-old man who has presented with central crushing chest pain and diaphoresis. He has type 2 diabetes and his mother had stents inserted due to 'heart trouble'. Glyceryl trinitrate spray has not helped the patient. An ECG performed by the ambulance crew, which arrived with Mr Freesia, showed ST depression in leads V2–V6. They performed a second ECG en route to the hospital, which is shown in Fig. 5.1. Please review the ECG, explain the findings to Mr Freesia and formulate an appropriate management plan.

RESULTS

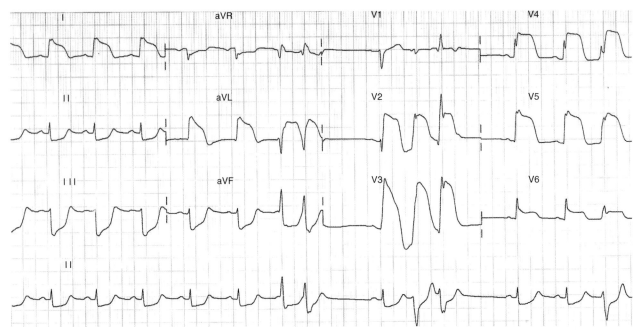

Fig. 5.1 Second ECG for Mr Fredrickson.

DATA INTERPRETATION

INTERPRETING AN ECG (TABLE 5.11)

You should consider the following when interpreting an ECG. It is also a useful checklist for you to ensure that you have not missed anything when presenting an ECG:

- Patient details: Name, date of birth
- Time and date of ECG
- Calibration
- Paper speed
- Heart rate
- Heart rhythm
- Cardiac axis
- Wave morphology
- Segments and intervals
- The context of the ECG: Clinical information; for example, the patient's haemodynamic stability, current signs and symptoms, electrolyte abnormalities, etc.

It is useful to compare with an old ECG as this enables you to identify new changes which may need further investigation or treatment.

WAVEFORMS

P Wave

- Represents atrial depolarisation
- Best seen in leads II and V1
- Normally less than three small squares (120 ms)

PR Interval

- Measured from the beginning of the P wave to the beginning of the QRS complex
- It represents the time taken for transmission of the impulse from the atria to the ventricles
- Normal is 3–5 small squares (120–200 ms):
  - Short PR interval: Sinus tachycardia, Wolff–Parkinson–White syndrome
  - Prolonged PR: Heart block, hyperkalaemia

⎍ Table 5.11 Information on the ECG paper	
TIME IS MEASURED HORIZONTALLY	**VOLTAGE IS MEASURED VERTICALLY**
One small square represents: • 1 mm on the paper • 0.04 s • 40 ms	Two large squares represent: • 10 mm • 1 mV
One large square represents: • 5 mm on the paper • 0.2 s • 200 ms	To check that the ECG is calibrated: • Look at the left-hand side of the paper for a rectangular trace, which should be 10 mm tall
Five large squares is equivalent to 1 s	

QRS Complex

- QRS represents the spread of depolarisation through the ventricles
- Normally < 3 small squares (120 ms)
- Q wave:
  - First negative deflection before the R wave; may or may not be visible
  - Caused by depolarisation of the septum with the current travelling away from the electrode
- R wave:
  - First positive deflection of the QRS
  - Increases in height from V1 to V5
- S wave:
  - Negative deflection following the R wave

T Wave

- Represents ventricular repolarisation
- Usually same polarity as QRS
- Always inverted in aVR and often inverted in III and V1

HEART RATE

If Regular Rhythm

- Count the number of large squares between one R–R complex (ventricular rate)
- Divide this number into 300
- For example, if there were four large squares between two consecutive R waves, 300/4 = 75, therefore the heart rate is 75 bpm

If Irregular Rhythm

- Count the number of R waves in 30 large squares (6 s) and multiply by 10
- For example, if there were 22 R–R intervals on the 10-s rhythm strip, the heart rate is 22 × 6 = 132 bpm

A heart rate >100 bpm is tachycardia and a heart rate <60 bpm is bradycardia.

INTERPRETATION OF THE RHYTHM

Irregular or regular?

- A regular rhythm will have constant R–R intervals, whereas an irregular rhythm will not
- If an irregular rhythm follows a predictable pattern it is regularly irregular. If not, it is irregularly irregular. If unclear, mark the R waves on a separate piece of paper and move the paper along to see if it matches

Does the impulse originate in the atria or the ventricles?

- QRS duration <120 ms (narrow-complex):
  - Focus of arrhythmia is supraventricular as a narrow QRS implies efficient conduction along the atrioventricular (AV) node, bundle of His and ventricles
- QRS >120 ms (broad complex):
  - Focus of arrhythmia comes from within the ventricles
  - Exception: Bundle branch block (BBB) or an aberrant pathway, which results in inefficient ventricular depolarisation and thus a broad QRS

RHYTHM

Sinus Rhythm (Fig. 5.2)

- Regular atrial tachycardia (QRS <120 ms) (Table 5.12)
- Irregular atrial tachycardia (QRS <120 ms) (Table 5.13)
- Ventricular tachycardia (VT) and ventricular fibrillation (VF) (QRS >120 ms) (Table 5.14)
- Bradycardia (Table 5.15)

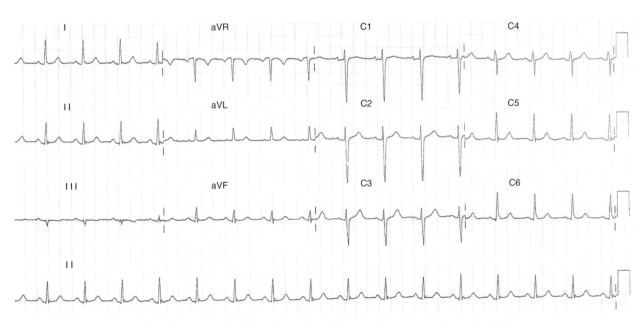

Fig. 5.2 Sinus rhythm. Regularly regular with normal P waves preceding each QRS.

Table 5.12   Causes and ECG patterns of regular atrial tachycardia

RHYTHM NAME	CAUSES	RHYTHM	P WAVES	QRS	ADDITIONAL INFORMATION
Sinus tachycardia	• Fever • Sepsis/shock • Exercise • Pain	Regular	Normal	Narrow	
Atrial flutter (Fig. 5.3)	• Hypertension • Ischaemia • Cardiomyopathy • Valve dysfunction	Regular. Although it can be irregular if there is variable AV node block.	None. The baseline appears 'saw toothed' due to the presence of flutter waves	Narrow	Flutter waves: • Rate typically around 300 bpm with 2:1 AV block (due to physiological response of AV node) • This would give a ventricular rate of 150 bpm • Rate may be normal or bradycardic, especially if already on rate control treatment

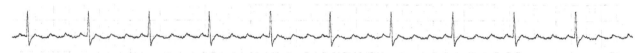

Fig. 5.3 Atrial flutter. 4:1 ratio of flutter waves to ventricular beats.

Table 5.13   Causes and ECG patterns of irregular atrial tachycardia

RHYTHM	CAUSES	RHYTHM	P WAVES	QRS	ADDITIONAL INFORMATION
Sinus arrhythmia	• Often unknown	• Regularly irregular	• Normal P waves preceding each QRS	• < 120 ms	• Constant PR interval
Sinus rhythm with ectopic beats	• Alcohol • Caffeine • Recreational drugs	• Regular background rhythm • Occasional beats appear before the next normal beat is expected	• Abnormal P wave followed by QRS indicates an atrial ectopic beat. • Absent P wave and isolated QRS indicates a ventricular ectopic beat	• < 120 ms (except ventricular ectopics)	• Atrial ectopics: If P wave is concealed by preceding T wave, it can give a peaked appearance • Ventricular ectopics: Usually followed by a compensatory 'pause' as the ventricle is refractory until the next sinus impulse
Atrial fibrillation (Fig. 5.4)	• Hypertension • Coronary artery disease • MI • Congenital cardiac defects • Hyperthyroidism • Valve dysfunction	• Irregularly irregular	• No P waves	• < 120 ms	• Heart rate may be normal, rapid or bradycardic, especially if already on rate control treatment

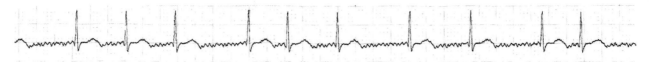

Fig. 5.4 Atrial fibrillation. Irregularly irregular with no visible P waves.

| | Table 5.14 | Causes and ECG patterns of VT and ventricular VF |

RHYTHM NAME	CAUSES	RHYTHM	P WAVES	QRS	ADDITIONAL INFORMATION
VT (Fig. 5.5)	• Cardiomyopathy • Ischaemic heart disease • Cardiac failure • Periarrest	• Regular	• May be present, but no relationship with QRS	• Broad	Can be: • Monomorphic (all abnormal complexes look the same) • Polymorphic; for example, torsades de pointes
VF (Fig. 5.6)	• Often unknown • Associated with known cardiac disease	• Irregular	• No P waves	• Broad, no organised complexes	• The heart is no longer beating effectively. This rhythm is not compatible with life

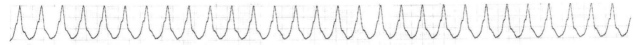

Fig. 5.5 Ventricular tachycardia. Regular wide-complex tachycardia.

Fig. 5.6 Fine ventricular fibrillation. Irregularly wide-complex tachycardia. There will be no pulse/cardiac output!

| | Table 5.15 | Causes and ECG patterns of various types of bradycardia |

RHYTHM	CAUSES	P WAVES PRESENT?	EVERY P WAVE FOLLOWED BY QRS?	PR INTERVAL	QRS
Sinus bradycardia	• Myocarditis • Hypothyroidism • Extreme fitness • MI • Medications	• Yes	• Yes	• Normal	• Normal
First-degree heart block (Fig. 5.7)	• AV nodal disease • Myocarditis • Acute MI • Electrolyte imbalances	• Yes	• Yes	• Prolongation of the PR interval	• Normal
Second-degree heart block: Mobitz type I, also known as Wenckebach	• Congenital heart block • MI • Coronary artery disease • Hypokalaemia	• Yes	• No	• Progressive lengthening of the PR interval until a beat is dropped from a non-conducted P wave	• Typically narrow
Second-degree heart block: Mobitz type II	• Congenital heart block • MI • Coronary artery disease • Hypokalaemia	• Yes	• No	• Constant PR interval, but occasionally the P wave is not conducted (not followed by QRS)	• May be broad
Third-degree heart block (Fig. 5.8)	• Congenital heart block • MI • Coronary artery disease • Hypokalaemia • Medications	• Yes (unless in atrial fibrillation)	• No	• No relation between P and R wave	• May be broad

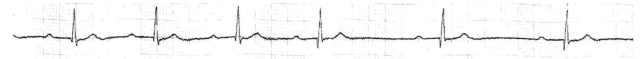

Fig. 5.7 First-degree heart block. Prolonged PR interval, but no dropped beats.

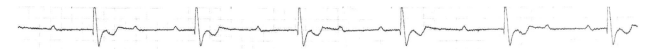

Fig. 5.8 Third-degree heart block. No relationship between atrial (P-wave) and ventricular (QRS-complex) activity.

Table 5.16   Classification of axis deviation

LEFT-AXIS DEVIATION	NORMAL RANGE	RIGHT-AXIS DEVIATION
• < –30° • Lead I positive • Lead II negative Causes: • Conduction defect • Left ventricular hypertrophy	• –30° to +90° • Lead I positive • Lead II positive	• > +90° • Lead I negative • Lead II positive Causes: • Right ventricular hypertrophy

CARDIAC AXIS (TABLE 5.16)

- Cardiac axis is the overall direction of spread of depolarisation
- It is measured from a reference point, 0°, which is at the same position as lead I
  An axis above this line is denoted by a negative number of degrees and if below, by a positive number of degrees.
- A crude way to determine the axis is by looking at leads I–II. A lead is positive if there is a greater positive deflection in the QRS than negative deflection, i.e. the R wave is taller than the S wave. A negative lead has a greater negative deflection
- Leads I and II should be positive
- In right-axis deviation, the direction of spread of depolarisation is shifted slightly to the right, producing a negative deflection in lead I, while lead II remains positive
- In left-axis deviation, the spread of depolarisation shifts above lead I (visualise this area of the axis corresponding to the left ventricular wall), whereas lead II is mainly negative

WAVEFORM MORPHOLOGY

P WAVE

P-wave morphology and causes

MORPHOLOGY	CAUSE
No P wave or fibrillatory waves	Atrial fibrillation
No P waves and 'saw tooth' pattern	Atrial flutter
Flattened P waves	May be a sign of hyperkalaemia
Broad or bifid P wave	P mitrale, reflecting an enlarged left atrium
Tall P wave > two small squares	P pulmonale, reflecting an enlarged right atrium

QRS COMPLEX

- Pathological Q waves: Suggest an old ST elevation MI (STEMI). These are either more than one small square wide or have a voltage (height) > 25% of that of the R wave. In an evolving MI, they may develop on serial ECGs and suggest a completed infarct
- A broad QRS complex: May be due to BBB or VT

BUNDLE BRANCH BLOCK (TABLE 5.17)

- In the conduction system, the bundle of His divides into the right and left bundle branches
- BBB is most easily recognised on leads V1 and V6

T WAVE

- Ischaemic T-wave changes: Inverted, flattened, bi-phasic, peaked
- Hyperkalaemia: Tall, tented T waves
- T-wave inversion occurs across several leads: In the same myocardial territory – myocardial ischaemia becomes more likely

ST SEGMENTS

- This represents the time between the end of ventricular depolarisation and the beginning of repolarisation. It is sensitive to ischaemia
- Important changes to identify include ST elevation or depression
- Perform serial ECGs on patients with chest pain to observe for an evolving MI
- In the presence of LBBB, the ST segments cannot be accurately interpreted
  Causes of ST elevation include:
- STEMI: Represents a transmural (full-thickness) infarct (Table 5.18)

Table 5.17   Comparison of left and right BBBs

LEFT BUNDLE BRANCH BLOCK (LBBB)	RIGHT BUNDLE BRANCH BLOCK (RBBB)
Left ventricle depolarises after the right ventricle	Right ventricle depolarised after the left ventricle
Causes broad QRS with a 'W' morphology in V1 and an 'M' morphology in V6	Causes broad QRS with an 'M' morphology in V1 and a 'W' morphology in V6
WiLLiaM	**MoRRoW**
Causes:	Causes:
• MI	• Normal variant
• Hypertension	• MI
• Conduction system fibrosis	• PE
• Cardiomyopathy	• Cor pulmonale
	• Congenital heart disease
	• Cardiomyopathy

Table 5.18   STEMI anatomical relations

LOCATION OF INFARCTION	ST ELEVATION IN LEADS	AFFECTED ARTERY (S)
Anteroseptal MI	V1–V4	Left anterior descending artery
Extensive anterior STEMI	V1–V6, I, AVL	Left main stem
Anterolateral STEMI	I, AVL, V5, V6	Left coronary artery, circumflex
Inferior STEMI	II, III, AVF	Right coronary artery or left circumflex
Posterior MI	Tall R wave V1–3, with ST depression	Left circumflex or right coronary artery

- The ST elevation is localised to the ischaemic territory; there may be reciprocal ST depression
- The PR interval is normal
- Pericarditis: Widespread 'saddle'-shaped ST elevation with no reciprocal ST depression and with PR depression

Causes of ST depression include:
- Horizontal:
  - Myocardial ischaemia
  - Evolving MI
  - Non-ST elevation MI (NSTEMI)
- Downsloping:
  - Myocardial ischaemia
  - Digoxin 'reverse tick' appearance of ST segment
  - BBB
  - Hypokalaemia
- Upsloping: Usually physiological

U WAVES

- Defined as the wave following the T wave, but before the P wave
- Can be caused by: Hypokalaemia, hyperthyroidism, central nervous system disease

THIS CASE

This patient is presenting with signs and symptoms of a STEMI. The ECG has confirmed what is an anterior STEMI. This patient needs urgent management and cardiology referral.

RELEVANT PATIENT INFORMATION

You suspect this patient is having an MI. Ask about known medical conditions, relevant treatments and any hospital admissions.

ASSOCIATED SYMPTOMS

- Nausea
- Sweating
- Shortness of breath
- Presyncope

PAST MEDICAL HISTORY

- Angina
- Previous MI, including whether the patient had stents inserted before
- Diabetes
- Hypercholesterolaemia
- Hypertension
- Peripheral vascular disease or stroke

FAMILY HISTORY

- Cardiovascular disease

SOCIAL HISTORY

- Smoking
- Exercise
- Diet
- Level of function and usual exercise tolerance

Present Your Findings

Since you have developed chest pain, an ECG was performed. This is a test which shows the electrical impulses in your heart, which cause your heart to beat. Your ECG shows changes associated with a heart attack. This means an artery (blood vessel) in your heart is blocked, therefore blood with oxygen and nutrients cannot reach part of your heart muscle, causing damage. This is why you have had chest pain.

You will shortly be brought to the cardiology ward and we want to insert stents into the blocked artery in your heart, which will open the artery and allow blood to flow through it again.

In the meantime, we will take a sample of blood and give you painkillers, antisickness medication and tablets to prevent further excessive blood clotting. Do you have any questions?

❓ QUESTIONS AND ANSWERS FOR CANDIDATE

What ECG changes are associated with MI?
- ST segment elevation or depression
- T-wave changes: Inverted, peaked, flattened
- Poor R-wave progression (R waves usually get progressively taller from V1 to V6)
- Pathological Q waves
- New left BBB
- The ECG can be normal

What is the immediate treatment of acute coronary syndrome?
Reassure, provide high flow via non-rebreathe mask if $SpO_2 < 94\%$, prescribe morphine (IV 1–10 mg titrated to avoid respiratory depression and an antiemetic), aspirin (300 mg chewed), nitroglycerine and clopidogrel (300 mg or ticagrelor 180 mg).

What ECG are changes associated with hyperkalaemia?
- PR prolongation
- Flattened P waves
- Broad, bizarre QRS
- Tall, tented T waves (early sign)

A Case to Learn From

A 69-year-old woman on a medical ward reported heartburn and requested something to relieve her symptoms. She had a background of bronchiectasis, CCF and CKD and was admitted with an infective exacerbation of bronchiectasis. She had become slightly more breathless throughout the day. Since MI can present as heartburn, an ECG was performed and this

A Case to Learn From—cont'd

showed T-wave inversion in V1–V3, which had not been present on her previous ECG. This required further investigation and she was subsequently found to have had an NSTEMI. This illustrates the importance of considering alternative diagnoses and atypical presentations of common conditions.

💡 Top Tip

In an OSCE it is easy to focus on the first abnormality you see on an ECG. Develop your own system for interpreting ECGs and work through it each time you interpret one. You may wish to point out the most obvious abnormality, but then go on to interpret the rest of the ECG systematically. This tells the examiner that you can spot a striking abnormality, but also ensures that you do not miss anything.

STATION 5.9: CEREBROSPINAL FLUID (CSF)

SCENARIO

You are a junior doctor on an acute medicine placement and have been asked to see Mr Smith, a 19-year-old man who has presented with fever, headache, muscle aches, photophobia and general malaise. After a CT brain was carried out, you performed a lumbar puncture. On inspection, the CSF was clear. The results of the CSF are now back, as is the plasma glucose you sent. Please review them, explain the findings to Mr Smith and formulate an appropriate management plan.

🏃 Results

COMPONENTS	RESULTS	REFERENCE RANGES WITH UNITS
Predominant cell type	Lymphocytes	Lymphocytes
WCC	900 ↑	0–4/µL
Protein	0.8 ↑	0.2–0.4 g/L
Glucose	4	Half to two-thirds of plasma glucose

Plasma glucose: 6.0 mmol.

DATA INTERPRETATION

🏃 Likely diagnosis based on CSF results

DIAGNOSIS	APPEARANCE	PREDOMINANT WHITE CELL TYPE	WCC (/µL)	PROTEIN (G/L)	GLUCOSE
Normal	Clear	Lymphocytes	0–4	0.2–0.4	Half to two-thirds that of plasma glucose
Viral meningitis	Clear	Lymphocytes	50–1000	0.4–1.0	More than half of plasma glucose

Likely diagnosis based on CSF results—cont'd

DIAGNOSIS	APPEARANCE	PREDOMINANT WHITE CELL TYPE	WCC (/µL)	PROTEIN (G/L)	GLUCOSE
Bacterial meningitis	Turbid	Neutrophils	100–10,000	> 1.0	Less than half of plasma glucose
Tuberculous meningitis	Turbid If left to settle for hours, a fibrin web may develop	Lymphocytes	50–1000	1.0–5.0	Less than half of plasma glucose
Fungal meningitis (usually in immunosuppressed patients)	Clear/ turbid May develop fibrin web	Lymphocytes	50–500	0.1–0.5	Less than two-fifths of plasma glucose

MENINGITIS

This is an inflammatory process of the meninges and CSF.

Note: V that viral meningitis is the commonest type of aseptic meningitis. Aseptic meningitis may also be caused by TB, fungi, parasites, autoimmune disease or malignancy.

CEREBROSPINAL FLUID

CSF bathes the brain and spinal cord. It is produced by the choroid plexus in the lateral, third and fourth ventricles.
Its functions include:
- Buoyancy: Ensures that the brain floats in the cranial cavity, avoiding pressure damage to the inferior aspect of the brain
- Shock absorber
- Maintenance of physiological intracranial pressure
- Nourishment of the brain
- Electrolyte balance
- Removal of toxic metabolites

THIS CASE

This patient has presented with signs and symptoms of meningitis. Initial CSF results indicate viral meningitis, with lymphocytes being the predominant cell type, raised protein and elevated glucose levels. It is important to explain the diagnosis to the patient but also to determine the cause.

CAUSES OF VIRAL MENINGITIS

COMMONEST (85%)

- Enterovirus; for example, echovirus, coxsackie, poliovirus

OTHER

- Varicella zoster
- Herpes simplex virus
- EBV
- CMV
- HIV
- Mumps

RELEVANT PATIENT INFORMATION

Explore the patient's full medical history for evidence to support your differential diagnosis of meningitis (Table 5.19) and to help determine the causative organism.

VIRAL

- Enterovirus: Contacts with diarrhoea (faecal–oral transmission) or with infected person's eye/nose/mouth secretions
- Herpes simplex virus: Contact with infected bodily fluid; for example, kissing, using a glass or cutlery previously used by infected person

BACTERIAL

Causes of bacterial meningitis by age

Neonatal–3 months	• Group B streptococcus • *Escherichia coli* • *Listeria monocytogenes*
Young children	• *Neisseria meningitidis* • *Streptococcus pneumoniae* • *Haemophilus influenzae*
Teenagers–adults	• *Neisseria meningitidis* • *Streptococcus pneumoniae*
Elderly	• *Neisseria meningitidis* • *Streptococcus pneumoniae* • *Listeria monocytogenes*

- *Streptococcus pneumoniae*: Recent infections; for example, pneumonia, otitis media, sinusitis
- *Neisseria meningitidis*: Residence at boarding school/hostels, recent outbreaks
- *Listeria monocytogenes*: Ingestion of unpasteurised dairy foods or processed/cold cooked meats, particularly if pregnant, neonate or elderly
- *Staphylococcus aureus*: Skull fracture, recent neurosurgery

FUNGAL

- Patients taking immunosuppressants; for example, steroids, chemotherapy medications or patients who have a diagnosis of HIV

Table 5.19   Differential diagnosis

DIAGNOSIS	APPEARANCE	WCC	PROTEIN	GLUCOSE	OTHER
Subarachnoid haemorrhage (SAH)	Blood-stained, then xanthochromia (yellow) after 12 h	Raised	Raised	Normal	Raised red blood cell count
Multiple sclerosis	Clear	None or raised	Raised	Normal or mildly increased	
Guillain–Barré syndrome	Clear	None	Raised	Normal	Oligoclonal bands on electrophoresis

Present Your Findings

The sample of fluid we took from around your spinal cord confirms that you have meningitis, which is inflammation of the lining of the brain and spinal cord. In your case it is likely caused by a virus, which is usually a less severe condition than meningitis caused by bacteria.

The reason you were given antibiotics is because bacterial meningitis can worsen rapidly and waiting to find out if this was the cause before treating would be very dangerous.

We will keep you hydrated and comfortable by giving you fluids into the vein, pain relief and antisickness medication. We will continue the antibiotics until we get one more test back, which is where they look to see if there is any bacteria growing in the spinal fluid. Antiviral medications can be effective against certain types of viruses, so we will treat you with these until we know the particular virus causing your infection.

QUESTIONS AND ANSWERS FOR CANDIDATE

Why is CT brain often performed before lumbar puncture?
- This is to identify patients with an intracranial mass effect. Performing a lumbar puncture in these patients is contraindicated as it may cause tonsillar herniation (coning)

Which vaccine-preventable disease can potentially cause meningitis?
- Meningococcal disease

What are some contraindications to performing a lumbar puncture?
- Raised intracranial pressure
- Coagulopathy or low platelet count
- Cutaneous infection at lumbar puncture site

A Case to Learn From

A 55-year-old man presented to the ED with a thunderclap headache and CT brain showed no abnormality. Since 5% of SAH do not show on CT, he was admitted to the acute medical ward for observation and further investigations. As per guidelines, a lumbar puncture was carried out 12 h after the onset of symptoms. It showed xanthochromia, a yellow discoloration due to the presence of bilirubin from the breakdown of red cells in the CSF, confirming SAH. CT scans do not pick up all SAHs.

Top Tip

A lumbar puncture should ideally be performed before antibiotics are administered if meningitis is suspected. However, it should not delay antibiotic treatment. Proceed with antibiotics before lumbar puncture if delay is anticipated.

STATION 5.10: PLEURAL FLUID

SCENARIO

You are a junior doctor on the respiratory ward and have been asked to see Mr Green, a 76-year-old man who has a temperature, worsening dyspnoea and tachypnoea. On examination you note reduced left-sided expansion in addition to a stony dull percussion note and reduced breath sounds on the left side.

You have sent some blood tests and a sample of pleural fluid for analysis. Please review the results, explain the findings to Mr Brown and formulate an appropriate management plan.

Results

COMPONENT	RESULTS	REFERENCE RANGE WITH UNITS
Pleural fluid protein	35 ↑	10–20 g/L
Serum protein	60	60–80 g/L
Pleural fluid lactate dehydrogenase (LDH)	98 ↑	<50% of plasma LDH (u/L)
Serum LDH	150	100–250 u/L
Cell count and differential count	900/mm³	<1000 white cells/mm³
Gram stain	Nil	Nil
Cytology	Nil	
Glucose	2.2 ↓	4–6 mmol/L
pH	7.2 ↓	7.60–7.66

DATA INTERPRETATION (TABLE 5.20)

1. Determine whether it is a transudate or exudate:

	Table 5.20	Likely diagnosis based on investigation results for pleural fluids

INVESTIGATION	POTENTIAL DIAGNOSIS
Cell count and differential cell count (the percentage of each type of white cell)	Infection and malignancy
Gram stain and culture	Infection
Cytology	High: Malignancy (only detects 60% of malignant effusions)
Glucose	Low: Infection, malignancy
pH	Low: Infection, malignancy

Two methods can be used to differentiate between transudates and exudates:
- Protein content of pleural fluid
  - > 30 g/L protein= exudate
  - < 30 g/L protein= transudate
  - This method is not completely accurate but may be used as a guide
- Light's criteria:
  - The effusion is an exudate if:

Pleural fluid to serum protein ratio > 0.5, i.e. pleural fluid protein more than double serum protein

or

Pleural fluid LDH to serum LDH ratio > 0.6

or

Pleural fluid LDH greater than two-thirds of the upper limit of normal serum LDH
  - Elevated protein and LDH = exudate
  - This method is more accurate
2. Initial pleural fluid laboratory investigations (Table 5.21)
3. Gross examination of pleural fluid (Table 5.22)

THIS CASE

This patient is presenting with signs and symptoms of a complex parapneumonic effusion. The pleural fluid analysis supports this diagnosis. It is important to carry out prompt management and explain the diagnosis to the patient.

	Table 5.21	Other laboratory investigations to consider

INVESTIGATION	POTENTIAL DIAGNOSIS
Amylase	High: Pancreatitis
Hct	> 1%: Pneumonia, trauma, cancer, PE ≥ 50% of the blood Hct: Haemothorax
Triglycerides	> 110 mg/dL: Chylothorax
Ziehl–Neelsen stain	TB
N-terminal-prohormone BNP	> 1500 pg/mL: Congestive heart failure

Causes of Effusion

	TRANSUDATE	EXUDATE
Commonest causes	Think 'failure': • Heart: CCF • Liver: Cirrhosis, ascites • Renal: Nephrotic syndrome	Think MIP: • *Malignancy*: Lung, breast • *Infarction*: PE • *Pneumonia*
Other causes	Think HUMP: • *Hypothyroidism* • *Urinothorax* • *Meig's* syndrome (seen in ovarian cancer) • *Peritoneal* dialysis	Think CHAPP: • *Chylothorax* • *Haemothorax* • *Autoimmune*: Systemic lupus erythematosus (SLE), rheumatoid arthritis • *Post-MI* (Dressler's syndrome) • *Post* coronary artery bypass graft

	Table 5.22	Gross examination of pleural fluid

GROSS EXAMINATION	POTENTIAL CAUSE
Bloody	• Trauma • Pneumonia • Cancer • PE • Haemothorax
Cloudy	• Pneumonia • Chylothorax • Pseudochylothorax
Foul odour	• Anaerobic infection

RELEVANT PATIENT INFORMATION

You suspect this patient has a pleural effusion. Ask about known medical conditions, relevant treatments and any hospital admissions.

DRUG HISTORY

Drugs That May Cause Effusions
- Hydralazine
- Nitrofurantoin
- Methotrexate
- Ovarian stimulation therapy
- Methysergide
- Beta-blockers
- Amiodarone
- Phenytoin

FAMILY HISTORY

- Heart failure
- Kidney failure
- Liver failure
- Venous thromboembolism (VTE)

- Hypothyroidism
- Ovarian cancer

ADDITIONAL INFORMATION

OTHER INVESTIGATIONS TO CONSIDER

- Interferon, adenosine deaminase and *Mycobacterium tuberculosis* polymerase chain reaction can be used to investigate for TB
- Tumour markers may be requested if malignancy is suspected
- Contrast-enhanced CT scans can aid diagnosis of empyema, lung abscess and malignancy
- If malignancy is suspected and other investigations are inconclusive, percutaneous pleural biopsy of pleural nodules should be performed
- Thoracoscopy should be performed for direct visualisation of pleura if the pleural aspirate was non-diagnostic and malignancy is suspected

 Present Your Findings

We carried out a variety of tests on the sample of fluid that was taken from your chest. The tests suggest that the fluid in your chest is due to an infection.

We will treat you with antibiotics into your vein; however antibiotics alone will not get rid of the fluid and so we need to insert a tube into your chest to drain it. We will also continue to treat you with nebulisers, oxygen and chest physiotherapy.

❓ QUESTIONS AND ANSWERS FOR CANDIDATE

By what mechanisms can pleural fluid accumulate?
Transudates:
- Increased pulmonary hydrostatic pressure, associated with CCF
- Decreased colloid osmotic pressure, associated with hypoalbuminaemia, liver cirrhosis
- In these cases, there is no abnormality of the pleural membrane or capillary wall permeability
Exudates:
- Inflammation causes disruption of the pleural membrane and increased capillary wall permeability, allowing protein to leak out into the pleural space

What is the difference between a simple parapneumonic effusion and an empyema?
Simple parapneumonic effusion:
- Inflammation causes increased capillary permeability, allowing leakage of fluid into the pleural space. The fluid in the effusion is not itself infected
- Features of the fluid include:

- Grossly clear
- No organisms
- Low WCC
- Normal pH, LDH and glucose
- May be treated with antibiotics
Empyema:
- Further formation of fibrin and infection of the fluid in the effusion
- Features include:
  - Pus in the pleural space
  - Raised LDH
  - Low glucose
  - Low pH
  - May have positive Gram stain and culture
- Cannot be treated with antibiotics alone; it also requires drainage, and may require surgery

What are the features of an effusion on chest X-ray?
- Blunting of the costophrenic angles
- Homogeneous opacification and fluid level, manifesting as a meniscus
- Bilateral effusions are more likely to be transudates. Unilateral effusions are more likely to be exudates

 A Case to Learn From

A patient on a gynaecology ward with recurrence of an ovarian malignancy developed shortness of breath, tachypnoea and reduced oxygen saturations. CXR revealed a right-sided pleural effusion. A pleural tap was carried out to determine the aetiology of the effusion, as she had risk factors for many potential causes, including: Meig's syndrome, hospital-acquired pneumonia, effusion secondary to lung metastases and PE. The cause was infective and rapid access to initial results aided prompt appropriate management.

 Top Tip

If permitted, a blood gas machine can potentially be used to analyse a pleural fluid sample, as it gives rapid results of many analytes; for example, pH, glucose, haematocrit and lactate.

STATION 5.11: ASCITIC FLUID

SCENARIO

You are a junior doctor on a hepatology placement and have been asked to see Mr Can, a 65-year-old man who has presented with abdominal swelling. One of your colleagues performed an ascitic tap and sent the fluid for analysis. The results are now back. He is known to have alcoholic liver disease. Please review the results, explain the findings to Mr Can and formulate an appropriate management plan.

Results

	RESULTS	REFERENCE RANGES WITH UNITS
Ascitic fluid albumin	3 g/dL	<4 g/dL
Serum albumin	5 g/dL	3.5–5.5 g/dL
Total protein	3.5 g/dL	<4 g/dL
Glucose	7 g/L	7–10 g/L
Amylase	150 u/L	140–400 u/L
Bilirubin	0.7 mg/dL	0.7–0.8 mg/dL
Triglycerides	10 mL/dL	<110 mL/dL
Differential WCC	150 cells/mm³	<300 cells/mm³

DATA INTERPRETATION (TABLE 5.23)

1. Calculate the serum ascites albumin gradient (SAAG) (Table 5.24)
   - This is the preferred method used to characterise ascites, rather than traditional classification of transudate or exudate based on protein and LDH.
   - The SAAG = (serum albumin) – (albumin level of ascitic fluid)
   - It is used to determine if ascites is secondary to portal hypertension
   - It is based on the balance between hydrostatic and colloid osmotic pressures
2. Initial laboratory investigations (Table 5.25)
3. Gross examination of ascitic fluid (Table 5.26)

THIS CASE

This patient is presenting with signs and symptoms of ascites. Due to his background of alcoholic liver disease, cirrhosis is a likely cause. This is supported by a SAAG > 1.1 mg/dL, and the absence of other abnormal biochemical markers. It is important to explain the diagnosis to the patient and to formulate a management plan.

Table 5.23   Differential WCC and potential causes

PREDOMINANT WHITE CELL	POTENTIAL CAUSE
Neutrophils	• Pneumonia • Empyema • PE • Pancreatitis
Lymphocytes	• Malignancy • TB • Post-coronary artery bypass graft • Chylothorax
Eosinophils	• Pneumothorax • Haemothorax

Table 5.24   SAAG values and relationship with portal hypertension

SAAG	GRADIENT	SECONDARY TO PORTAL HYPERTENSION?
>1.1 mg/dL	High	Yes
<1.1 mg/dL	Low	No

Table 5.25   Other laboratory investigations to consider

COMPONENTS	POSSIBLE DIAGNOSIS
Glucose	Low: • Spontaneous bacterial peritonitis • TB • Malignancy
Amylase	High: • Ascites secondary to pancreatitis/ pancreatic trauma
Bilirubin	High: • Biliary leak
Triglycerides	High: • Malignancy • TB • Parasitic infection
Differential WCC	Neutrophilia (>250 cells/mm³): • Spontaneous bacterial peritonitis Lymphocytosis: • TB
Culture/Gram stain	• Microorganisms
Cytology	• Malignant cells

Table 5.26   Gross examination of ascitic fluid

COLOUR	POSSIBLE DIAGNOSIS
Straw	• Cirrhosis
Milky (chylous)	• TB • Parasitic infection • Malignancy • Cirrhosis • Lymphatic obstruction
Blood-stained	• Malignancy • TB • Trauma • Perforated ulcer • Haemorrhagic pancreatitis
Turbid	• Bacterial infection • Pancreatitis • Bowel perforation

Causes of Ascites

HIGH SAAG	LOW SAAG
• Cirrhosis • CCF • Nephrotic syndrome • Hepatic metastases • Chronic hepatitis • Budd–Chiari syndrome • Portal vein thrombosis	• TB • Pancreatitis • Intra-abdominal/pelvic malignancy • Biliary ascites • Myxoedema

RELEVANT PATIENT INFORMATION

PAST MEDICAL HISTORY

- Alcohol excess
- Malignancy

- Cardiac: CCF, MI, cardiomyopathy, valvular disease
- Hepatitis
- Renal disease
- Autoimmune disease; for example, systemic lupus erythematosus
- Venous thromboembolism
- Hypothyroidism
- TB

FAMILY HISTORY

- Cardiac disease; for example, MI, cardiomyopathy, CCF
- Intra-abdominal or pelvic malignancy
- TB

 Investigations to consider to confirm the cause

INVESTIGATION	INTERPRETATION
Urine dipstick	Proteinuria may suggest nephrotic syndrome
Urinary albumin to creatine ratio	Quantifies proteinuria
ECG	To look at the activity of the heart: • Ischaemic changes • Axis deviation • Ventricular strain, which may indicate heart failure
Echocardiogram	Heart failure
Liver screen (hepatitis screen, EBV, CMV, autoantibodies)	Hepatic pathology
Abdominal ultrasound	Confirms ascites It may show: • Fatty liver • Cirrhosis • Evidence of malignancy
Portal vein Doppler	Portal vein thrombosis

Present Your Findings

The results of the tests we carried out on the fluid from your tummy are back and show that the most likely explanation for the fluid gathering in your tummy is alcohol-related liver damage. We will scan your tummy to confirm this.

We will treat you with medication to help you get rid of fluid by passing more urine, and we have to restrict your salt intake. This should offload the fluid in your tummy; however if this is not sufficient, then we may consider putting a drain into your tummy. It is also important for you to think seriously about stopping drinking alcohol and I would like to have a chat with you about this when you feel a bit better.

❓ QUESTIONS AND ANSWERS FOR CANDIDATE

What is spontaneous bacterial peritonitis?

- Infection of peritoneal fluid with no evidence of an intra-abdominal or surgically treatable cause

What are the causes of generalised abdominal swelling?

- The five Fs:
  - Fat
  - Fluid
  - Flatus
  - Faeces
  - Fetus

What is refractory ascites?

- Ascites that fails to respond to salt restriction and maximum/maximum tolerated diuretic therapy

🐘 A Case to Learn From

A 49-year-old man with no significant past medical history presented with fever, abdominal pain and vomiting, initially thought to be gastroenteritis. However, abdominal distension and shifting dullness were evident on examination and ultrasound confirmed ascites. A diagnostic tap was performed and he was treated empirically for spontaneous bacterial peritonitis. The history was revisited and the patient then admitted to drinking a bottle of wine at least 5 nights a week for the past 3 years. Sometimes when you have a diagnosis, revisiting the history can lead to new information that previously was not disclosed.

💡 Top Tip

Paracentesis can cause hypotension and hypoalbuminaemia due to the loss of protein-rich fluid. Therefore, it is important to follow trust protocol regarding the rate at which to drain and albumin supplementation.

STATION 5.12: SYNOVIAL FLUID

SCENARIO

You are a junior doctor in the ED and have been asked to see Mr Brady, a 65-year-old man who has presented with a red, hot and swollen knee. One of your colleagues obtained a synovial fluid aspirate from the knee and sent it for analysis. The results are now back. He is overweight and takes medication for hypertension. Please review the results, explain the findings to Mr Brady and formulate an appropriate management plan.

 Results

COMPONENTS	RESULTS	REFERENCE RANGE WITH UNITS
Crystals	Monosodium urate ↑	Nil
WCC	2000/mm³ ↑	<200/mm³
% Polymorphonuclear neutrophils (PMN)	56% ↑	<25%
Colour	Yellow ↑	Colourless
Clarity	Cloudy ↑	Clear
Viscosity	Low ↓	High
Gram stain	Negative	Negative

Examples of synovial fluid results for different aetiologies

	NON-INFLAMMATORY	INFLAMMATORY	SEPTIC	HAEMORRHAGIC
Colour	Yellow	Yellow	Purulent	Bloody
Clarity	Clear	Clear-cloudy	Turbid	Bloody
Viscosity	High	Low	Low	Variable
Cell count	<2000/mm³	2000–75,000/mm³	>60,000/mm³	Raised red cells
% PMN	<25%	>50%	>75%	Variable
Crystals	Nil	Gout: Monosodium urate Pseudogout: Calcium pyrophosphate dihydrate	Nil	Nil
Culture/Gram stain	Nil	Nil	Organisms on Gram stain, positive culture	Nil

THIS CASE

This patient is presenting with signs and symptoms of gout. This has been confirmed by the presence of monosodium urate crystals in the synovial fluid.

Causes of Joint Effusion

	NON-INFLAMMATORY	INFLAMMATORY	SEPTIC	HAEMORRHAGIC
Causes	• Osteoarthritis • Trauma • Chronic gout • Chronic pseudogout • SLE	• Rheumatoid arthritis • Psoriatic arthritis • Reiter's syndrome • Acute gout • Acute pseudogout • SLE • Viral arthritis	• Septic arthritis	• Trauma • Fracture • Haemophilia • Malignancy

RELEVANT PATIENT INFORMATION

DRUG HISTORY

- Thiazide diuretics
- Aspirin
- Ciclosporin and chemotherapy drugs

PAST MEDICAL HISTORY

Indicating Hyperuricaemia

- End-stage renal disease
- Alcoholism
- Haematological malignancy
- Obesity
- Psoriasis
- Diet: High intake of purines; for example, asparagus, liver, kidney, anchovies and mussels

Indicating Acute Flare of Gout

- Trauma: May be minor; for example, knock to the joint
- Surgery
- Recent illness
- Stress

Phases of Gout

- Asymptomatic hyperuricaemia
- Acute gout
- Intercritical gout
- Chronic tophaceous gout

Present Your Findings

The results of the tests on the fluid from your knee are back and show that you have gout. This means that there are crystals and inflammation in your knee joint. We will treat you with anti-inflammatory medication in the first instance. Some people cannot tolerate these, and if that is the case for you, we can try a medication called colchicine or alternatively steroids.

You can also help yourself by resting your knee and avoiding any trauma to it; for example, knocking it. You may find that ice packs also ease the pain. You may need long-term treatment to prevent further attacks and we can have a chat about other factors that may contribute to gout; for example, your diet, medications and alcohol intake.

Differential Diagnosis

CAUSE	PRESENTATION	INVESTIGATION	MANAGEMENT
Infected joint	• Fever • Painful, red, hot, swollen joint • Stiffness	• Aspiration • FBCs and CRP • Blood cultures • X-ray	• Dependent on the cause, but commonly flucloxacillin as *Staphylococcus* is a common causative pathogen
Crystal arthropathy; for example, gout, pseudogout	• Painful, red, swollen joint	• Aspiration and synovial fluid microscopy	• Dependent on the type of crystal arthropathy
Haemarthrosis	• Painful, red, hot swollen joint • Stiffness • Excessive bruising near the affected joint	• Aspiration • X-ray	• Dependent on the cause, usually conservative • Patients with a bleeding disorder may require clotting factor replacement
Osteoarthritis	• More common in women • Pain on movement • Worse at the end of the day • Pain at rest • Stiffness • May be associated with bony swelling	• X-ray	• Analgesia; for example, paracetamol, NSAIDs • Weight loss • Consider surgery
Fracture	• Pain on weight bearing	• X-ray	• Dependent on the type of fracture
Reactive arthritis	• Swollen, painful stiff joints, commonly the hands and feet	• X-ray • FBC, CRP and ESR	• Regular exercise • Physiotherapy • Analgesia; for example, NSAIDs • Medical therapy; for example, steroids • Consider surgery

? QUESTIONS AND ANSWERS FOR CANDIDATE

Describe the crystals found in gout and pseudogout.
- Gout: Monosodium urate crystals: These are needle-shaped and negatively birefringent under polarised light microscopy
- Pseudogout: Calcium pyrophosphate dehydrate: These are small, rhomboid-shaped crystals that are positively birefringent

What are the risk factors for septic arthritis?
- Joint prosthesis
- IV drug abuse
- Pre-existing joint pathology
- Joint surgery
- Joint injections
- Diabetes
- Immunodeficiency

What are the X-ray features of gout?
- Punched-out erosions
- Tophaceous deposits
- Intraosseous lesions
- Sclerotic, overhanging edges
- Preservation of joint space
- Absence of osteopenia
- Periarticular soft-tissue swelling

 A Case to Learn From

An elderly man on the ward was recovering from severe sepsis and two upper GI bleeds. He was beginning to recover renal function after being dialysis-dependent during the acute phase of his illness. He developed a red, hot, swollen knee and was unable to weight bear. Due to his history of gout, this was a likely differential. However, there was concern regarding haematogenous spread of infection and, to exclude septic arthritis, a sample of fluid was aspirated. This confirmed gout. Even when gout is likely, have a low threshold for considering sepsis in a swollen joint.

 Top Tip

Carry out an USS of the joint before aspiration to exclude bursitis.

STATION 5.13: PEAK FLOW AND SPIROMETRY

SCENARIO

You are a junior doctor on a respiratory placement and have been asked to see Mrs Smith, a 60-year-old woman who has presented with shortness of breath, chronic cough and reduced exercise tolerance. She has smoked 30 cigarettes a day for 45 years. She saw your colleague last week who ordered some investigations and the results are now back. Please review the results, explain the findings to Mrs Smith and formulate an appropriate management plan.

Results

	RESULTS (% PREDICTED)	REFERENCE RANGE (% PREDICTED)
Forced expiratory volume in 1 s (FEV$_1$)	60% ↓	>80%
Forced vital capacity (FVC)	90%	>80%
FEV$_1$/FVC	0.67 ↓	>0.7
Peak expiratory flow rate (PEFR)	85%	>80%

DATA INTERPRETATION (TABLE 5.27)

Spirometry is a method of assessing lung function by measuring the volume of air that can be expelled on forced expiration after maximal inspiration (Fig. 5.9). It contributes to the diagnosis of respiratory disorders.

PEFR is the maximal flow rate of air during forced expiration after maximal inspiration. It is used to diagnose and monitor asthma.

Lung volumes and PEFRs are compared against predicted values for someone of that patient's age, sex and height and are expressed as 'percentage of predicted' values (Fig. 5.9). PEFRs can also be expressed as a percentage of that patient's own best reading.

OBSTRUCTIVE DISORDERS (TABLE 5.28)

- Obstructive airways diseases are characterised by increased resistance to expiratory air flow due to narrowed airways
- This leads to relatively prolonged expiration and therefore reduced FEV$_1$. FVC is normal or minimally reduced. This gives a decreased FEV$_1$/FVC
- Examples include: COPD (an umbrella term encompassing chronic bronchitis and emphysema) and asthma

RESTRICTIVE DISORDERS

- Restrictive airway diseases are characterised by reduced compliance or inadequate expansion of the

Table 5.27 Spirometry measurements and definitions

SPIROMETRY MEASUREMENTS	DEFINITION
FEV$_1$	The volume of air expelled in the first second of forced expiration
FVC	The maximum volume of air that can be exhaled after maximal inspiration
FEV$_1$/FVC	The ratio of FEV$_1$ to FVC expressed as a decimal

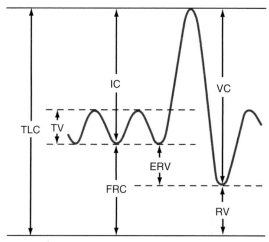

Fig. 5.9 Different measurements of lung volumes. TLC= total lung capacity, TV = tidal volume, FRC = functional residual capacity, IC= inspiratory capacity, ERV = expiratory residual volume, RV = residual volume, VC = vital capacity

Table 5.28 Obstructive versus restrictive disorders

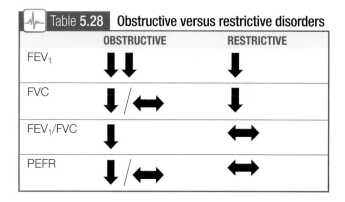

	OBSTRUCTIVE	RESTRICTIVE
FEV$_1$	⬇⬇	⬇
FVC	⬇ / ⬌	⬇
FEV$_1$/FVC	⬇	⬌
PEFR	⬇ / ⬌	⬌

lungs. This leads to a proportionate reduction in both FEV$_1$ and FVC, and therefore a normal/raised FEV$_1$/FVC
- Examples include: Pulmonary fibrosis, asbestosis and neuromuscular defects affecting the chest wall

THIS CASE

The patient is presenting with symptoms suggestive of COPD. Spirometry has shown an obstructive pattern, with a decreased FEV$_1$, normal FVC, reduced FEV$_1$/FVC and reduced PEFR, therefore supporting this diagnosis.

Table 5.29   MRC dyspnoea scale

GRADE	DEGREE OF BREATHLESSNESS ACCORDING TO LEVEL OF ACTIVITY
1	Not troubled by breathlessness except on strenuous exercise
2	Short of breath when hurrying or walking up a slight hill
3	Walks slower than contemporaries on level ground because of breathlessness or has to stop for breath when walking at own pace
4	Stops for breath after walking about 100 m or after a few minutes on level ground
5	Too breathless to leave the house or breathlessness when dressing or undressing

CAUSES OF COPD

- Tobacco smoking
- Alpha-1 antitrypsin deficiency
- Occupational exposure to irritants, such as dust, flour, coal, etc.
- Air pollution

RELEVANT PATIENT INFORMATION

You suspect this patient has COPD. Ask about known medical conditions, relevant treatments and any hospital admissions.

FAMILY HISTORY

- COPD
- Alpha-1 antitrypsin deficiency
- Asthma

SOCIAL HISTORY

- Tobacco smoking
- Exposure to second-hand smoke
- Occupational exposure to dust, fumes or chemicals

The diagnosis of COPD is made based on clinical signs and symptoms and supported by an obstructive pattern on spirometry. The Medical Research Council (MRC) dyspnoea scale is a useful tool to assess severity of dyspnoea, which is one of the most important features of COPD (Table 5.29).

Present Your Findings

The tests of your breathing that we carried out show that you are not able to blow air out of your lungs as quickly as we would expect. This is likely to be due to a chest condition called chronic obstructive pulmonary disease, or COPD, which means that the tubes that carry air from your mouth and nose to your lungs become narrowed and the pockets of air trapped in your lungs become bigger. These changes are what have been causing you to feel breathless.

This is related to smoking, so the most important thing you can do to help yourself is to stop smoking. We can chat more about this and come up with a plan to help you with that. We can also relieve your symptoms with inhalers and it is important that you get some vaccinations to help protect you from chest infections.

QUESTIONS AND ANSWERS FOR CANDIDATE

Why might you obtain inconsistent spirometry readings?
- Inadequate or incomplete inhalation
- Inadequate seal formed by lips around the mouthpiece
- Incomplete exhalation
- Coughing
- Poor understanding or communication of instructions

How can PEFR measurement help determine severity of asthma?
See Table 5.30.

Describe the choices of inhaled therapy for patients with stable COPD.
- Short-acting beta agonists as required for symptomatic relief
- If the patient is still breathless or suffering frequent exacerbations despite short-acting beta agonists as required, consider maintenance therapy (e.g. Long-acting beta-2 agonist, inhaled corticosteroid or long-acting muscarinic agonist)

A Case to Learn From

An elderly woman who had a 50-pack year history of smoking developed severe hospital-acquired pneumonia after abdominal surgery. Serial ABGs were performed over a period of days and showed raised CO_2, which did not reduce significantly despite clinical improvement, and low bicarbonate. It was suspected that she had undiagnosed COPD and after her acute illness was resolved, she was referred for spirometry. In patients with a chest infection, always consider an underlying respiratory condition.

Top Tip

To obtain reliable, consistent readings, explain the instructions for performing spirometry and peak flow clearly, allow patients to demonstrate their technique and repeatedly encourage them to exhale fully whilst they are performing the manoeuvre.

 Table 5.30   PEFR measurements paired with respective level of severity

% OF BEST/PREDICTED	SEVERITY
>75%	Mild
50–75%	Moderate
33–50%	Acute severe
<33%	Life-threatening

STATION 5.14: CHEST X-RAY

SCENARIO

You are a junior doctor on a medical placement and have been asked to see Mrs Black, a 63-year-old woman, with a history of COPD. She has had a sudden onset of increased shortness of breath and right-sided pleuritic chest pain. A CXR was carried out and the results have returned (Fig 5.11). Please review the film, explain the findings to Mrs Black and formulate an appropriate management plan.

DATA INTERPRETATION

To interpret CXRs, you should develop a system. Table 5.31 gives a suggested system; however you may tweak it to suit yourself, as long as you ensure you cover all areas.

THIS CASE

The patient is presenting with signs and symptoms of a pneumothorax. The CXR has confirmed this). It is important to explain the diagnosis to the patient.

Causes of pneumothorax

CAUSES OF PNEUMOTHORAX	EXAMPLES
Spontaneous	• Primary • Secondary
Iatrogenic/trauma	• Pleural tap • Transbronchial biopsy • Central venous line insertion • Mechanical ventilation • Pacemaker insertion
Obstructive lung disease	• Asthma • COPD
Infection	• Pneumonia • TB • Cystic fibrosis
Connective tissue disease	• Marfan syndrome • Ehlers–Danlos syndrome

RELEVANT PATIENT INFORMATION

You suspect this patient has a pneumothorax. Ask about known medical conditions, relevant treatments and any hospital admissions.

Table 5.31 Method used to interpret a CXR

	AREA	DETAILS
1	Projection	• Somewhere on the film you should see something that indicates whether it is anteroposterior (AP) or posteroanterior (PA). If not, assume it is PA and say so • AP films are more difficult to interpret and are usually only performed on haemodynamically compromised patients. If you cannot remember which one is standard view, remember AP is in 'crAP', so PA is standard • If you are asked to justify why a film is PA, remember that the arms are raised up during PA films, so the scapulae are pulled almost fully out of the lung fields. In AP films, the patient is unwell so you can see a humerus down either side of the film and scapulae in the lung fields
2	Patient details	• These will be on the film (unless anonymised for the exam) • Say the name, age/date of birth and when the film was taken
3	Technical quality	• Check that you can see both lung apices, both lateral sides of the ribcage and both costophrenic angles on the film • It is unlikely that in the exam they will give you a film that does not show the entire lungs, but some parts are occasionally missed in practice

4	Rotation, inspiration, penetration (RIP)	• Rotation:
		  • Heads of the clavicles (medial ends) should be equidistant from the spinous processes of the vertebral bodies
		• Inspiration:
		  • PA films are taken in held deep inspiration
		  • Count the ribs to assess inspiratory effort. The last rib to count is the one going through the diaphragm
		  • Six anterior ribs or 10 posterior ribs indicate adequate inspiratory effort
		  • More ribs, particularly with flattened diaphragms, indicate airway obstruction; for example, COPD. Fewer ribs indicate poor inspiration
		• Penetration:
		  • Assume adequate penetration when you can just see the vertebral bodies behind the heart
		  • Underpenetrated means you cannot see behind the heart and overpenetrated means you will be able to see the vertebral bodies overly clearly
		• Rotated, underinspired or under/overpenetrated films hinder accurate assessment

Continued

Table 5.31 Method used to interpret a CXR—cont'd

	AREA	DETAILS

5	Obvious abnormalities	• If you can see obvious abnormalities, say so and describe them:
		  • Which lung?
		  • Which zone (upper, middle or lower)? If possible, suggest which lobe it is likely to be. Remember that this is not always obvious without a CT
		  • Size
		  • Shape: Well or poorly demarcated
		  • Density/texture: Uniform, patchy, dense, cotton wool-like
		  • If there is anything else in the abnormality; for example, air bronchograms or fluid levels, then mention these too

6	Systematic review of the film	• Initially assess from about 120 cm away to see difference in lung shadowing/obvious masses, then reassess close up • It doesn't matter what system you have as long as you stick to one and don't miss any areas. A useful system is ABCDD (airway, breathing, circulation, diaphragm, delicates) Airway: • Whether the trachea is central Breathing: • Start in the apices and work down to the costophrenic angles, comparing both lungs to look for differences. Ensure that you inspect the apices, hila, mediastinum and costophrenic angles • The left hilum should never be lower than the right (except in dextrocardia) and they should both be the same density • Look around the edge of the lung fields, assessing for pneumothoraces Cardiac: • Cardiomegaly: Defined as the heart shadow being more than half the width of the chest cavity on a PA film • Heart borders: If the left and right heart borders are not clearly visible, consolidation or collapse should be considered • Cardiophrenic angles: Should be clear. Masses or pericardial cysts can obliterate this space • Behind the heart: Look for any abnormalities; for example, lung masses Diaphragm: • Hemidiaphragms: Both should be visible and not flattened. The right hemidiaphragm is normally slightly higher than the left due to the position of the liver • Costophrenic angles: Should be clearly demarcated and check if they contain any fluid • Look for air under the diaphragm. A gastric air bubble on the left is normal Delicates: • Bones: Look for fractures and any rib space narrowing, suggesting collapse • Look for gas in the soft tissues (black areas) as a surgical emphysema Review areas: Double check the following areas at the end, since they are easy to miss on initial viewing: • Apices • Hila • Behind the heart • Costophrenic angles • Around the pleura/edge of the lung fields, assessing for pneumothoraces and pleural thickening • Under the diaphragm • Also comment on man-made abnormalities; for example, lines, pacemakers or nasogastric tubes
7	Summary	• Summarise your findings and give a differential list. Think about the history as well as the findings when making your differentials

FAMILY HISTORY

• Asthma
• COPD
• Connective tissue disorders
• Cystic fibrosis

XR DIAGNOSIS	XR DETAILS
Pneumonia (Fig. 5.10)	• Dense or patchy consolidation, usually one-sided • May contain air bronchograms • In the lower zones it may be difficult to distinguish from effusions, so both should be on your differential list • It is important to know which lobes touch the heart and diaphragmatic borders since loss of clarity of the borders indicates the affected lobe: • Diaphragms: Left and right lower lobes • Right heart border: Right middle lobe • Left heart border: Lingual • If in doubt about the lobe, describe it as upper/middle/lower zone
Pleural effusions (Figs 5.11 and 5.12)	• Look for loss of the costophrenic angles, a homogeneous opacification and fluid level which manifests as a meniscus • Bilateral effusions are more likely to be exudates • Pleural aspiration helps identify the cause of the effusion • To assess if heart failure is the cause, remember ABCDEF • A: *Alveolar* (interstitial) shadowing • B: Kerley *B* lines (little white horizontal dashes, usually in the lateral lower edges) • C: *Cardiomegaly* (cardiothoracic ratio of greater than 50% on a PA film) • D: Upper-lobe *diversion* (prominent upper-lobe vasculature) • E: *Effusions* • F: *Fluid* in the horizontal fissure
Pneumothorax (Fig 5.13)	• Loss of lung markings in the peripheral lung fields • You may also identify a discrete lung edge • If under tension, there may be tracheal/mediastinal deviation away from the pneumothorax and flattening of the ipsilateral dome of the diaphragm. A tension pneumothorax should never be diagnosed on CXR! It is a medical emergency, is diagnosed clinically and treated immediately with needle thoracocentesis
Lobar collapse (Figs 5.14 and 5.15)	• Look for loss of volume • Narrowing of the space between the ribs compared to the opposite side • A raised hemidiaphragm ipsilaterally • There may be tracheal and mediastinal shift towards the collapsed side • Left upper lobe: Veil sign. The whole lung field looks like it is covered by a veil • Left lower lobe: Sail sign. Sharp line like the edge of a sail at the same angle as the left heart border • Right upper lobe: Hazy right upper lobe, with raised horizontal fissure and the abnormality well demarcated by the fissure • Right middle lobe: Loss of the right heart border, but can be difficult to differentiate from consolidation • Right lower lobe: Hard to differentiate from effusion. Normally there is complete loss of diaphragmatic border due to haziness while the right heart border is normally clear

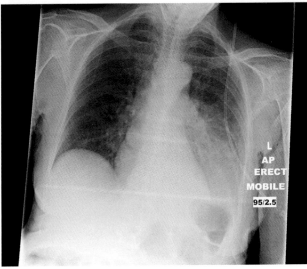

Fig. 5.10 Left lower-lobe consolidation. Note the left hemidiaphragm is obscured but the left heart border is well defined. Therefore, the consolidation must be in the lower lobe.

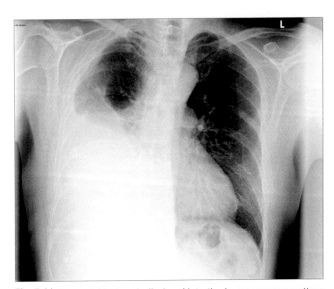

Fig. 5.11 Large right pleural effusion. Note the homogeneous pattern of the opacity obscuring the right hemidiaphragm and heart border, and the crisp upper border of the effusion. An effusion of this size will be approximately 3–4 L in volume.

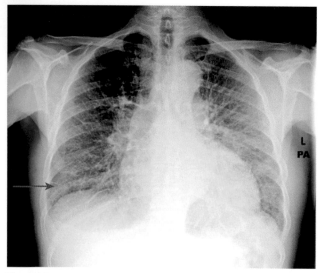

Fig. 5.12 Heart failure. Note the cardiomegaly, upper-lobe venous diversion and Kerley B lines (arrowed).

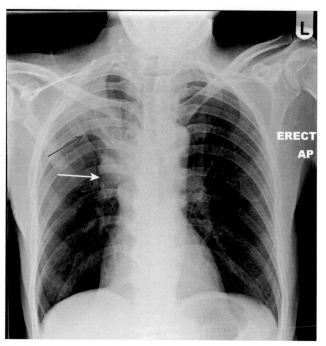

Fig. 5.14 Right upper-lobe collapse (pink arrow) with a right hilar mass (white arrow).

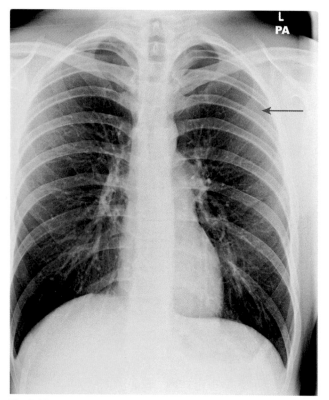

Fig. 5.13 Subtle left apical pneumothorax. This pneumothorax is not easy to see at first glance but note the visible lung margin in the left apex (arrowed) and the loss of lung markers beyond this.

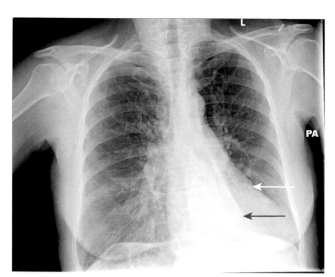

Fig. 5.15 Left lower-lobe collapse with evidence of the sail sign (pink arrow). Left heart border shown (white arrow).

CAUSES OF IMPORTANT FINDINGS ON CXR

! Important XR findings and common causes

XR FINDINGS	CAUSE	

Demarcated lesions (single or multiple) (Figs 5.16–5.18)	Causes of a single coin lesion:
	• Malignant tumour
	  • Bronchial
	  • Single pulmonary metastasis
	• Infection
	  • Pneumonia
	  • Abscess
	  • TB
	  • Hydatid cyst
	• Benign tumour
	  • Hamartoma
	  • Schwannoma
	  • Infarction
	  • Rheumatoid nodule
		Causes of cavitating lung lesions:
		• Abscess
		  • *Staphylococcus* or *Klebsiella*
		• Neoplasm
		  • Usually squamous cell
		• Cavitation
		  • Around a pneumonia
		  • TB
		• Infarction
		  • Rheumatoid nodules (rare)

Numerous calcified nodules	• Infection: TB, histoplasmosis, chickenpox • Inhalation: Silicosis • Chronic renal failure • Lymphoma: Following radiotherapy • Chronic pulmonary venous hypertension	
Bilateral hilar enlargement	• Sarcoid, berylliosis • Tumours: lymphoma, bronchial carcinoma, metastases • Infection: TB, recurrent chest infections, AIDS	
Hilar lymphadenopathy (Fig. 5.19)	• Neoplastic: Spread from bronchial carcinoma, lymphoma • Infective: TB • Sarcoidosis (rarely unilateral)	

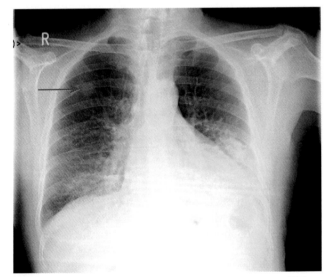

Fig. 5.16 There is loss of the hemidiaphragm and a heterogeneous opacification in the left lower zone, signifying left lower-lobe consolidation. Also note the single coin lesion in the right upper zone (arrowed).

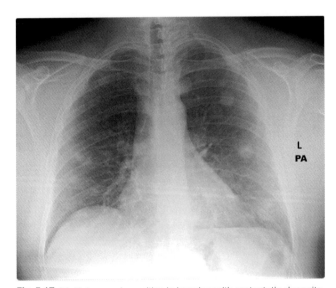

Fig. 5.17 Multiple round opacities in keeping with metastatic deposits.

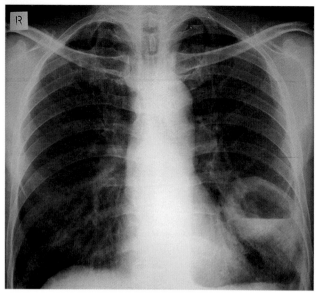

Fig. 5.18 Circular lucent area in left lower zone with surrounding 'wall' and air–fluid level. Common causes are infection (abscess or pneumonia) and neoplasia.

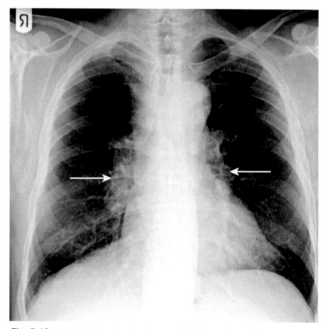

Fig. 5.19 Bilateral hilar lymphadenopathy in keeping with sarcoidosis.

Present Your Findings

People with COPD often have enlarged air sacs in their lungs called bullae, and sometimes these can burst, causing an air leak from your lung into your chest. This air leak means that your lung cannot expand properly. The X-ray we took of your chest shows that this has happened to you, which is why you suddenly became very short of breath.

We will continue to treat you with oxygen and will also have to put a tube into your chest through your ribs to drain this air away, which will help your breathing. Have you any questions?

QUESTIONS AND ANSWERS FOR CANDIDATE

What are the causes of a single coin lesion?
- Malignant tumour: Bronchial, single pulmonary metastasis
- Infection: Pneumonia, abscess, TB, hydatid cyst
- Benign tumour: Hamartoma, schwannoma
- Infarction
- Rheumatoid nodule

What are the causes of cavitating lung lesions?
- Abscess (*Staphylococcus* or *Klebsiella*)
- Neoplasm (usually squamous cell)
- Cavitation around a pneumonia/TB
- Infarct
- Rheumatoid nodule (rare cause)

What are the causes of bronchiectasis?
- Structural: Kartagener's syndrome, obstruction (carcinoma, foreign body)
- Infection: Childhood pertussis/measles, TB, pneumonia
- Immune: Hypogammaglobulinaemia, allergic pulmonary aspergillosis
- Metabolic: Cystic fibrosis
- Idiopathic: Secondary to stasis

A Case to Learn From

It is important to get a CXR after procedures involving the thorax/neck, such as central venous catheterisation, pacemaker insertion and removal of chest drain, to exclude pneumothorax. An elderly woman had a permanent pacemaker inserted but she did not have a routine CXR after her procedure. Later that night she desaturated and became tachypnoeic. Her CXR showed a large pneumothorax requiring a chest drain. This could have been identified and treated earlier.

Top Tip

Inverting the image (if viewing on a digital viewer) can make pneumothoraces more obvious.

STATION 5.15: ABDOMINAL X-RAY

SCENARIO

You are a junior doctor on a surgical placement and have been asked to see Mr Adams, a 65-year-old man, who has presented with abdominal pain and distension, vomiting and no bowel movements for 3 days. He has a history of an appendicectomy at 22 years old. An Abdominal X-ray (AXR) was carried out and the results are back (Fig 5.24). Please review the film, explain the findings to Mr Adams and formulate an appropriate management plan.

DATA INTERPRETATION

To interpret AXRs, you should develop a system. Table 5.32 gives a suggested system; however you may tweak it to suit yourself, as long as you ensure you cover all areas.

Table 5.32   Method used to interpret an AXR

	AREA	DETAILS
1	Projection	• The standard AXR is taken AP in the supine position, so assume this is the case unless told otherwise
2	Patient details	• These will be listed on the film (unless anonymised for the exam) • Say the name, age/date of birth and when the film was taken
3	Technical adequacy	• Make sure the entire abdomen is present on the film • Ideally, the region from the diaphragm down to past the pubis should be visible
4	Obvious abnormalities	• Abnormalities are not always obvious on initial viewing but if, for example, there is a dilated loop of large bowel measuring 12 cm in diameter, comment on this before conducting your systematic review

5	Systematic review of the film	• Assess the bowel. When looking at the bowel it is important to identify:
		   • Large or small bowel
		   • Size of bowel
		   • Cause of abnormalities
		   • Extraluminal and intraluminal content (note that air is black, faeces is mottled grey)
		 • Liver, spleen and gallbladder
		 • Abdominal aorta
		 • Kidney stones
		 • Bones
		 • Foreign bodies: Mention clips from previous surgery and any indwelling lines

6	Summary	• Summarise your findings and give a differential list. Think about the history as well as the findings when making your differentials

THIS CASE

The patient is presenting with signs and symptoms of bowel obstruction. The AXR has confirmed small bowel obstruction (Fig 5.20) It is important to explain the diagnosis to the patient but also to determine the cause.

CAUSES OF BOWEL OBSTRUCTION (TABLE 5.33)

The mnemonic HAT can be useful:
• Hernia
• Adhesions
• Tumour

RELEVANT PATIENT INFORMATION

You suspect this patient has bowel obstruction. Ask about known medical conditions, relevant treatments and any hospital admissions.

PAST MEDICAL/SURGICAL HISTORY

• Hernia
• Inflammatory bowel disease
• Previous abdominal or pelvic surgery
• Malignancy

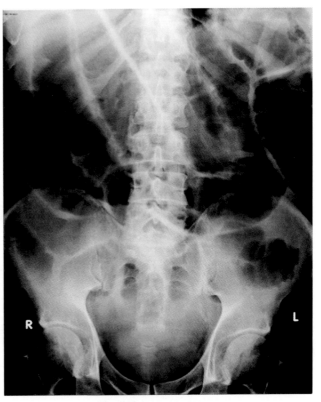

Fig. 5.20 Mr Adam's X-ray.

Table 5.33 | **Differentiating between small-bowel and large-bowel obstruction**

SMALL-BOWEL OBSTRUCTION (FIG. 5.21)	LARGE-BOWEL OBSTRUCTION (FIG. 5.22)
• The cause is most likely either adhesion or a hernia • Evidence of previous surgery, such as surgical clips, may suggest adhesion • Looking at the inguinal hernial orifices is essential for identifying inguinal hernias	• The level of the obstruction is normally clear • Malignancy commonly causes large-bowel obstruction. This requires further imaging for identification • The other cause not to be missed on the AXR is a caecal or sigmoid volvulus. These usually twist inwards, so they appear like balloons in the midline of the film • If the small bowel is also enlarged, then the ileocaecal valve is incompetent. In the short term, this is a good thing, since it reduces the risk of perforation of the large bowel

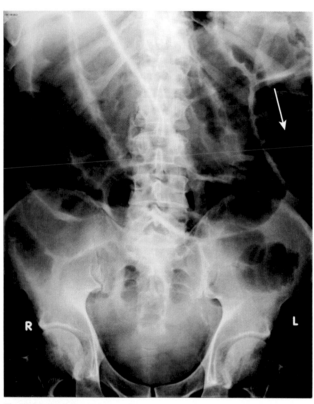

Fig. 5.21 Mr Adam's X-ray. Small-bowel obstruction. Note the central position of the distended bowel loops and the valvulae conniventes (arrowed).

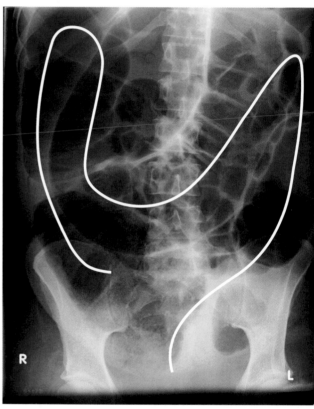

Fig. 5.22 Large-bowel obstruction with associated small-bowel dilatation.

⚠	**Important features of an AXR not to miss**	
ASPECT OF AXR	**XR DETAILS**	
Large bowel	• The large bowel is usually the easiest to identify as it classically runs around the outside of the abdomen, so start by looking for the large bowel • Apart from its position, the large bowel can also be identified by haustra, which are horizontal lines that only partially cross the width of the large bowel • The large bowel should be no wider than 5 cm, except the caecum, which can be up to 8 cm • Identify the rectum; it usually contains air • Follow this around to the left edge to the sigmoid colon and up the descending colon to the splenic flexure • Follow the transverse colon. Often, this hangs down through the middle of the film before rising again to the hepatic flexure • Follow the ascending caecum from the hepatic flexure down to the caecum • If you follow the entire large bowel around, then identifying the small bowel is easy as it is the remaining part of the intestine	

! Important features of an AXR not to miss—cont'd

ASPECT OF AXR	XR DETAILS
Small bowel	• The small bowel normally lies more centrally and should be no more than 3 cm in diameter. The small bowel can also be identified by the valvulae conniventes, which are lines that traverse the full width of the small bowel • Remember that in a 'normal' AXR the large and small bowel can often be difficult to see clearly. Instead a 'non-specific bowel gas pattern' is usually seen. The small and large bowel become much easier to recognise when there is bowel dilatation from mechanical obstruction or an ileus
Extraluminal gas (pneumoperitoneum) (Fig. 5.23)	• The best evidence of perforation is free air under the diaphragm. Note that a gastric air bubble under the left diaphragm is normal. Always ask for an erect CXR to assess for this • On the AXR, air under the diaphragm may be visible so comment on this if you see it • Rigler's sign is where you can clearly see both sides of the bowel wall. Normally only the inner wall of the bowel is visible. This is due to the contrast of the inner wall against air present inside the bowel. Therefore, when air is also outside the bowel, you can see the outside of the bowel wall as well • 'Football sign' is a round area of air, usually towards the top of the film, mainly found in neonates • Always look for perforation, even without evidence of bowel obstruction. Perforation can occur in gallstone disease, inflammatory conditions such as Crohn's disease, appendicitis or trauma
Oedema of the bowel wall (Fig. 5.24)	• Thumbprinting is thickening of the bowel wall caused by oedema. It is so named because it looks like someone has punched their thumb into it in several places. This gives a wavy pattern and occurs in inflammatory bowel disease and ischaemic colitis • If you see a massively enlarged colon, always question if this is inflammatory bowel disease-related (particularly ulcerative colitis) toxic megacolon
Liver, spleen and gallbladder	• Look at the size of the liver and spleen • Look for gallstones within the gallbladder • Remember that the majority of gallstones are radiolucent and will not be seen on X-ray
Kidneys	• Look for calcification along the renal tract. With practice the kidneys can be visualised on most AXRs (T12–L2) • Stones classically obstruct the renal pelvis, pelvoureteric junction and vesicoureteric junction • There may be stones within the bladder itself • Beware of phleboliths (calcified pelvic vessels), which are common. If you do not look at their position carefully, you may mistake them for renal or bladder stones
Bones	• Look for pelvic and hip fractures • Look at the spine. Often, osteoporotic fractures can be seen, as well as scoliosis and metastatic deposits
Abdominal aorta. (Fig. 5.25)	• Always look for the aorta and iliac vessels. • Often the aorta is calcified, so the two edges can be seen and measured. An aorta < 3 cm is normal, but if it is > 3 cm, then this suggests an aneurysm and requires further investigation and possible surgery • If you are suspecting dissection, look closely at the psoas muscle shadows that are normally present on AXR films • If they are absent, this suggests blood in the intraperitoneal cavity

🔍 Present Your Findings

Due to the symptoms you have described, we suspected that you might have a bowel obstruction, which means that there is a blockage in your bowel. The X-ray we took confirmed a blockage in your small bowel. We will need to do some blood tests and a chest X-ray and may need further scans to find the cause of the blockage.

For now, we will treat you with pain relief and antisickness medication and we will have to keep you nil by mouth, which means you will not be able to eat or drink, so we will give you fluids into a vein. We will also have to put a fine tube through your nose into your tummy to drain the contents of your stomach, as they cannot move through your system due to the blockage and the tube will stop you from vomiting. Hopefully you will get better on this treatment, but there is a possibility that you might need an operation, so I will ask a surgeon to come and see you. Have you any questions?

❓ QUESTIONS AND ANSWERS FOR CANDIDATE

What features on AXR is indicative of a sigmoid volvulus?
• The 'coffee bean sign'
• Convergence of the lower margins of the distended loops in the left iliac fossa
• A dilated loop of bowel extending from the left iliac fossa to the left flank overlying the descending colon

In patients with ulcerative colitis, which potentially life-threatening complication is usually assessed with serial abdominal X-rays?
• Toxic megacolon

How much radiation does an AXR use compared to a CXR?
• An AX-ray uses 30–50 times more radiation than a CXR

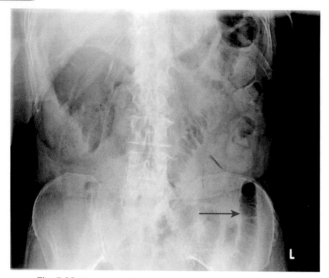

Fig. 5.23 Pneumoperitoneum demonstrating Rigler's sign.

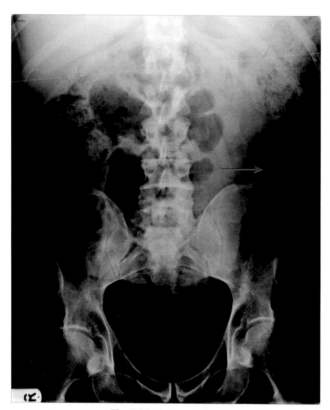

Fig. 5.24 Thumbprinting.

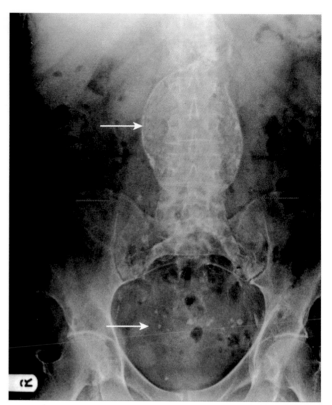

Fig. 5.25 Non-specific bowel gas pattern. Large calcified abdominal aorta (white). Psoas shadows are visible (pink). Incidental phleboliths (grey).

Top Tip

If bowel perforation is suspected, an AXR and an erect CXR should be carried out in the first instance. The patient should be positioned as upright as tolerated for around 15 min before the erect CXR to allow detection of pneumoperitoneum.

STATION 5.16: ORTHOPAEDIC X-RAY

SCENARIO

You are a junior doctor on an emergency placement and have been asked to see Mrs Cotton, an 84-year-old woman, who has presented with left-hip pain, shortening and internal rotation following a fall in her garden. She has a history of polymyalgia rheumatica. A hip X-ray was carried out and the results are back (Fig 5.26). Please review the film, explain the findings to Mrs Cotton and formulate an appropriate management plan.

DATA INTERPRETATION

To interpret orthopaedic X-rays, you should develop a system. Table 5.34 gives a suggested system; however you may tweak it to suit yourself, as long as you ensure you cover all areas.

There are specific extra bits to look at in each joint (see individual joints) (Figs. 5.27–5.37):

A Case to Learn From

A 52-year-old woman presented with severe left iliac fossa pain, nausea and diarrhoea. An erect CXR and AXR were carried out; however findings were non-specific. A CT scan with IV contrast was requested and this showed thickening of the sigmoid colon, likely due to sigmoid colitis. It is important to remember that where ischaemic bowel is suspected, an AXR and erect CXR should be carried out to investigate for signs of ischaemia; for example, pneumatosis intestinalis, bowel obstruction, mucosal thickening and perforation. However, CT is more sensitive than AXR at detecting pneumatosis intestinalis and is often required.

Data Interpretation CHAPTER 5

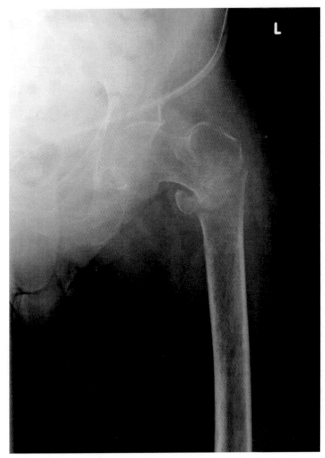

Fig. 5.26 Mrs Cotton's hip X-ray.

	Table 5.34	**Method used to interpret an orthopaedic XR**
	AREA	**DETAILS**
1	Projection	• At least two views: 'One view is one too few' • Normally, AP and lateral views • For some sites, such as the scaphoid, where fractures are difficult to detect, it is routine procedure to obtain more than two views • For some patients in whom the clinical suspicion is high, but it is not evident on the usual two views, additional views may be requested; for example, internal rotation views of the hip • If the shaft of a long bone is fractured, it is imperative to X-ray the joint above and below because of the potential for fracture or dislocation at these sites
2	Patient details	• Name, date of birth/age, when the film was taken (unless anonymised for the exam)
3	Technical adequacy	• The film needs to show all the joints in question from at least two different angles • It needs to be exposed correctly so that the bone and soft tissues can be seen and differentiated

4	Systematic review of the film	• Review the bone for fractures, subluxations and dislocations:
		  • If no fractures are obvious, look around the edges of all the bones for fractures
		  • New fractures appear as black lines through the cortex and may have callus around the bone
		  • If a fracture results in bone fragments that overlap, the result is an area of increased X-ray absorption and thus a whiter area on the X-ray

🏃 Features to note when interpreting cervical spine films

ADEQUACY	NORMAL ANATOMY			COMMENTS
	LATERAL VIEW	AP VIEW	PEG VIEW	
At least three views: • Lateral: Which must show all seven cervical vertebrae and the top of the first thoracic vertebra • AP • Open-mouth AP/peg view: To view C1 and C2	Vertebral alignment (arcuate lines-should be smooth and unbroken): • Anterior spinal line: Goes along the anterior margins of the vertebral bodies • Posterior spina line: Goes along the posterior margins of the vertebral bodies • Spinolaminar line: Joins the bases of the spinous processes Vertebral bodies: • From the third cervical vertebra downwards, the vertebral bodies should have a regular rectangular shape • There should be no wedging, i.e. the height of the anterior and posterior aspects of the vertebral bodies should be equal • The intervertebral discs should be the same size Prevertebral soft tissues: • The distance between the anterior spinal line and the edge of the prevertebral soft tissues should be < 7 cm between C1 and C4 and < 22 cm between C5 and C7 • An increase in these distances suggests the presence of a haematoma and thus an important injury	Alignment: • The spinous processes should follow a straight line. The alignment may look abnormal with asymmetric bifid spinous processes Spacing: • The spinous processes should be roughly equidistant. The intervertebral disc spaces should be a uniform height	Alignment: • The lateral masses of C1 and C2 should line up Spacing: • The peg should be equidistant from the lateral masses of C2	Fractures: • Look for deformity in the lines of the vertebrae on both AP and lateral views. Any sign that a vertebra has 'stepped out' could be a fracture and requires further imaging • Roughly 10% of patients with a cervical spine fracture have a second non-contiguous vertebral column fracture

aThese curves should be smooth and unbroken.

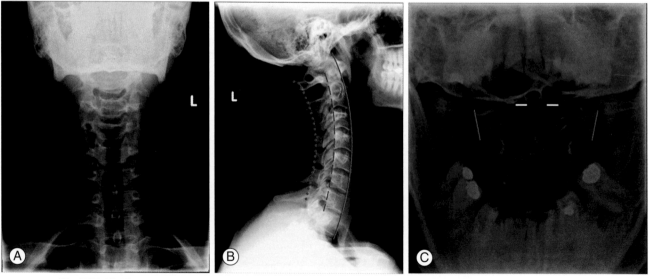

Fig. 5.27 (A) AP cervical spine radiograph (normal), (B) Lateral cervical spine radiograph showing anterior spinal (solid line), posterior spinal (dashed line), spinolaminar (dotted line) lines and (C) Peg view radiograph showing the odontoid peg equidistant from the lateral masses of C1 (white lines) and normal alignment of C1/2 (pink lines).

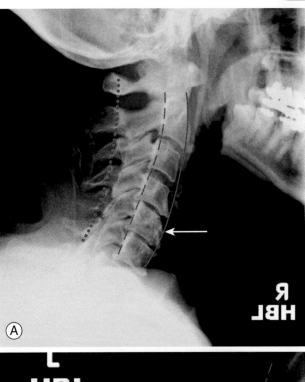

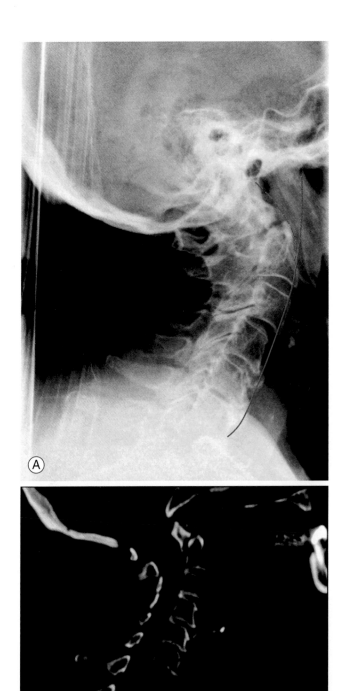

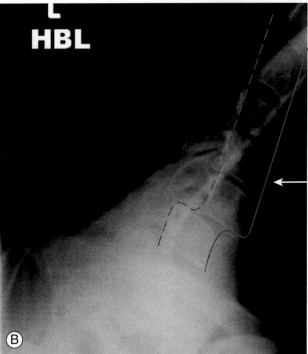

Fig. 5.28 (A) Lateral radiograph showing disruption to the arcuate lines (solid and dotted line) due to a fracture through the odontoid peg. Degenerative changes of the lower cervical spine. Note that this lateral view is inadequate as the C7/T1 junction cannot be visualised. The patient proceeded to CT and (B) Sagittal view radiograph showing the fracture through the odontoid peg. The odontoid peg is displaced posteriorly relative to the body of C2.

Fig. 5.29 (A) Only C1–C6 can be seen on this lateral view. There is a possible fracture through C5 vertebral body (arrowed). and (B) Swimmer's view shows C7 and T1 junction. The C5 fracture can be clearly seen (arrowed) but disruption of the arcuate lines is now also evident due to anterior subluxation of C6 on C7.

Features to note when interpreting thoracic and lumbar spine films

COLUMNS OF THE SPINE	NORMAL ANATOMY		COMMENTS
	LATERAL VIEW	AP VIEW	
The three columns of the spine should be assessed: Anterior: • Anterior longitudinal ligament and the anterior two-thirds of the vertebral body and the anterior part of the annulus fibrosus Middle: • Posterior third of the vertebral body, the posterior part of the annulus fibrosus and the posterior longitudinal ligament Posterior: • Posterior ligaments and bone arch Instability is present if two of the three columns are disrupted (breaks, steps or kinks)	Alignment: • Smooth, unbroken contour to the lumbar spine • No breaks, steps or kinks in any of the three columns Vertebral bodies: • Anterior and posterior margins should be equal in height • Posterior margin is normally slightly concave	Alignment: • The spinous processes should follow a straight line Pedicle: • The pedicles from L1 to L5 become slightly wider apart	Fractures: • Look at the height of the vertebral bodies, comparing each side and comparing above and below, as crush/osteoporotic wedge fractures are common • Most fractures will be evident on the lateral film Stability: • If a fracture is present, comment on whether the abnormality is stable or unstable (by assessing the columns of the spine as above) Spacing: • Joint space narrowing is common in the spine and may cause nerve root compression Others: • Kyphosis, which is anterior convexity, i.e. outward curvature of the spine. Normally there is a thoracic and sacral kyphosis • Lordosis, which is anterior concavity, i.e. inward curvature of the spine. Normally there is a cervical and lumbar lordosis • Scoliosis, which is side-to-side curvature of the spine • Osteoporosis, which is also common in the spine

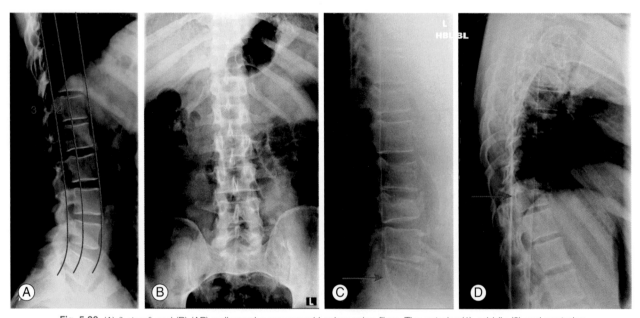

Fig. 5.30 (A) (Lateral) and (B) (AP) radiographs are normal lumbar spine films. The anterior (1), middle (2) and posterior (3) columns are shown on the lateral film, (C) Radiograph shows multiple compression fractures (T12, L2 and L3). To identify which vertebrae are involved, count up from the L5 vertebra (arrowed pink) and (D) This radiograph shows a vertebral compression fracture at T11 with anterior wedging (arrowed pink). There is also evidence of subluxation of T10 on T11 of approximately 25%.

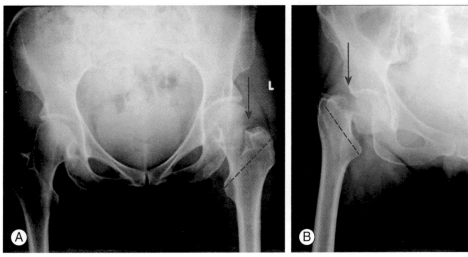

Fig. 5.31 Intracapsular neck of femur fractures (the dotted line signifies the boundary between intra- and extracapsular fractures). (A) Minimally displaced fracture, which can be fixed with cannulated screws; (B) the more commonly encountered displaced fracture, which needs hemiarthroplasty fixation.

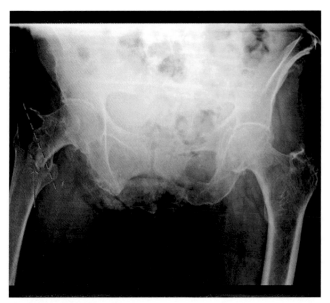

Fig. 5.32 Extracapsular neck of femur fractures (the dotted line signifies the boundary between intra- and extracapsular fractures).

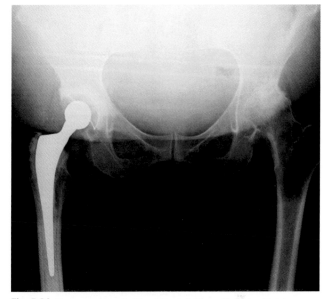

Fig. 5.34 Severe osteoarthritis of the left hip, with loss of joint space, subchondral sclerosis, cysts and osteophytes. There is also a right total hip replacement.

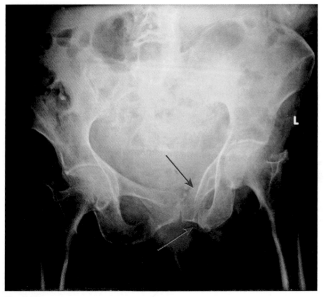

Fig. 5.33 Superior and inferior left-sided pubic rami fractures (pink arrows).

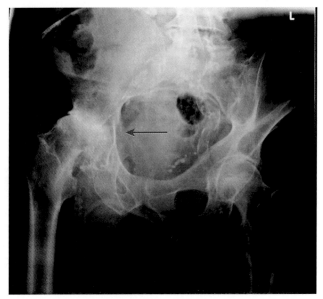

Fig. 5.35 Severe osteoarthritic change, this time affecting the right hip but in addition there is a right-sided acetabular fracture (arrowed).

HIP FILM

- Probably the most likely orthopaedic film you will be shown)
- Look for signs of a fracture (Table 5.35), or other possible pathology (Table 5.36)

KNEE RADIOGRAPH

Fractures

- Most are easily seen
- A fat–fluid level, detectable on a horizontal-beam lateral X-ray, signifies a lipohaemarthrosis and may be the only sign of an intra-articular fracture
- The majority of tibial plateau affects the lateral plateau. Look for an area of depression/increased density

Soft-Tissue Injuries

- Injury to ligaments or menisci usually causes no abnormality on X-ray
- Effusions can be seen as a soft-tissue density deep to the quadriceps tendon

Osteoarthritis

- Joint space narrowing
- Osteophyte formation
- Subchondral sclerosis
- Bony cyst formation

⌁ Table 5.35   Interpreting neck of femur fractures

NECK OF FEMUR FRACTURES

- Most neck of femur fractures are displaced and easy to detect
- Characterise the site of the fracture as this affects management and prognosis
1. Draw a line between the greater and lesser trochanters
2. A fracture proximal to this line is intracapsular
3. A fracture distal to this line is extracapsular (roughly speaking)

INTRACAPSULAR (FIG. 5.31)	EXTRACAPSULAR (FIG. 5.32)
• Subcapsular or transcervical • There is risk of disruption to the blood supply to the head of the femur • This fracture type usually requires some form of arthroplasty (total or hemiarthroplasty, depending on premorbid mobility), unless there is minimal displacement, in which case cannulated screws can be considered	• Intertrochanteric or subtrochanteric • No risk of avascular necrosis • These fractures are typically treated with internal fixation (a dynamic hip screw for intertrochanteric and gamma nail for subtrochanteric)

⌁ Table 5.36   Features to look closely at/for when you cannot identify a fracture

FEATURES	DETAILS
Disruption to the cortex.	Look for a step, buckle or gap.
Interrupted trabecular pattern.	Trabecular pattern refers to the arrangement of the trabecular of bone in relation to marrow spaces.
A transverse region of sclerosis.	Caused by impacted fracture.
Shenton's line.	Normally a smooth curve drawn along the inferior edge of the superior pubic rami and the medial side of the femur and femoral neck. If Shenton's line shows a sudden sharp angle, the fracture is nearby.
Changes on the lateral view.	These are more easily missed than on the AP view.
Acetabular and pubic rami fractures.	These can present with similar symptoms to neck of femur fractures. If the pelvis is broken in one place, it must actually be broken in another place as well (same as polo mints!).
Other.	Look for any signs of osteoarthritis (reduced joint space, subchondral sclerosis, subchondral cysts, osteophytes) and observe the pelvis and vertebrae for fractures and osteoporosis.

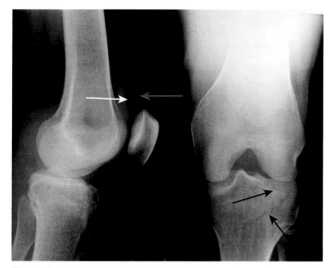

Fig. 5.36 (A) The lateral horizontal-beam X-ray demonstrates a fat–fluid level, with blood showing as the denser fluid (white arrow) and fat adjacent to this (pink arrow). (B) The AP X-ray demonstrates a fracture of the proximal tibia with intra-articular involvement (black arrows).

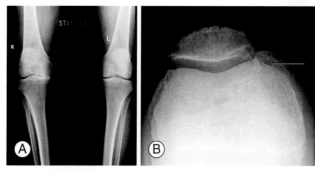

Fig. 5.37 These X-rays show osteoarthritis of the right knee. The AP (left) shows loss of joint space and subchondral sclerosis. The skyline patellar view (above) shows degenerative change with a marginal osteophyte formation (arrowed) on the femoral surface of the patella and distal femur. The joint space is reasonably preserved.

THIS CASE

This patient is presenting with signs and symptoms of a right fractured neck of femur. This is confirmed by her X-ray, which shows a displaced intracapsular neck of femur fracture.

RELEVANT PATIENT INFORMATION

You suspect this patient has a neck of femur fracture. Ask about known medical conditions, relevant treatments and any hospital admissions.

MEDICATION HISTORY

- Steroids
- Depot progestogen contraception
- Thyroid replacement
- Gonadotrophin-releasing hormone agonists
- Aromatase inhibitors, used as breast cancer treatment
- Androgen deprivation therapy, used as prostate cancer treatment
- Proton pump inhibitors
- Antiepileptics
- Diuretics
- Calcium/vitamin D and bisphosphonates may indicate a previous diagnosis of osteoporosis

PAST MEDICAL/SURGICAL HISTORY

- Osteoporosis

- Inflammatory conditions which may require exogenous steroid therapy; for example, inflammatory bowel disease, asthma, polymyalgia rheumatica, systemic lupus erythematosus
- Malignancy, pathological fracture
- Falls
- Previous fractures

FEATURES USED TO DESCRIBE FRACTURES (TABLE 5.37)

Being able to provide an accurate description of a fracture is vital for conveying the correct information to other members of the team.

SUBLUXATION VERSUS DISLOCATION

The difference between these two terms may not appear obvious in the first instance:
- Subluxation: When the normal anatomy of the joint is disrupted but some contact remains between the articular surfaces of the joint (Fig. 5.36)
- Dislocation: Complete disruption of the joint with no contact between the joint surfaces (Fig. 5.39)

Present Your Findings

Since your hip has been painful and resting in an unusual position since your fall, we suspected that you had broken your hip. The X-ray we took confirmed this.

Due to the type of fracture you have, you will need an operation to fix it. It is likely that a nail will be used to repair the fracture. In the meantime, we will give you pain relief and keep your leg and hip immobilised. After the operation you will need to have some rehabilitation, including a period of physiotherapy to get you back on your feet. Have you any questions?

Table 5.37 Summary of the terminology used to describe fractures

FEATURE	DETAILS	
Bone	Which bone is involved?	
Site	Which part of the bone is fractured? • Proximal third • Middle third • Distal third • Intra-articular	
Fracture pattern	Simple	Skin is intact (or open: Skin is not intact)
	Comminuted	More than two fragments of bone
	Impacted	When bone fragments are driven into each other
Type	Transverse	Perpendicular to the long axis of the bone
	Oblique	Angled less than 90° to the long axis of the bone
	Spiral	Curving around the bone
	Greenstick	Occurs in children, is a break in one cortex with the other cortex remaining intact, often associated with angulation
Displacement	• Relationship of the distal fragment to the proximal fragment • Non-displaced or anterior, posterior, medial, lateral displacement • It is essential to use both films to assess this	
Angulation	The movement of the distal fragment relative to the proximal bone in degrees	
Rotation	• Measured along the longitudinal axis of the bone • Generally detected on clinical examination but may be diagnosed on X-rays • Requires knowledge of the normal anatomical alignment • Either internal or external rotation • Important to assess all long-bone fractures for rotation	
Shortening	Compare to other side	
Joint space	May be smaller than it should be; asymmetrical or foreign bodies may be present	
Joint cartilage	Look for outline symmetry and any fractures on the surface of the bones	
Bone lucency	• If most of the bone is radiolucent (dark), this suggests osteoporosis • Radiolucency just around the joint suggests an inflammatory/infected joint • Radiopaque (bright) areas are rare (Paget's, osteoporosis, sclerotic bone metastases)	

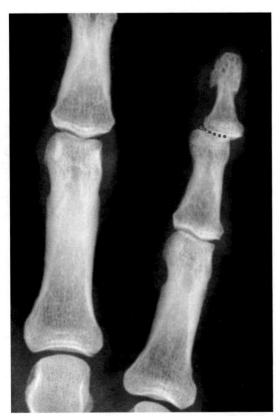

Fig. 5.38 Ulnar subluxation of the distal phalynx of the fifth digit. The dotted pink line highlights the contact that remained between the articular surfaces.

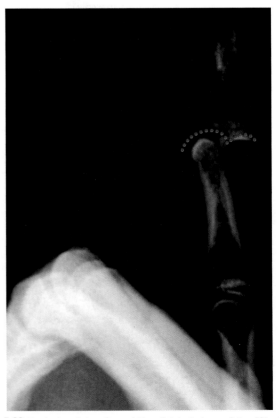

Fig. 5.39 Posterior dislocation of the distal phalynx of the fifth digit. The dotted lines highlight the two articular surfaces, which are not in contact.

❓ QUESTIONS AND ANSWERS FOR CANDIDATE

Where is the typical location for pain following a scaphoid fracture?

- The anatomical snuffbox, formed by the boundaries of extensor pollicis longus, extensor policis brevis and abductor pollicis longus

What must you remember to do if a single cervical spine fracture is identified?

- Look for a second vertebral fracture. Around 10% of patients with a cervical spine fracture have a second non-contiguous vertebral fracture
- Always review cervical spine X-rays with a senior doctor, as they can be difficult to interpret

What is a Lisfranc injury?

- It is a complex injury where there is disruption of the Lisfranc ligament which attaches from the second metatarsal base to the medial cuneiform. X-ray shows disruption of the normal alignment between the first and second metatarsals and the intermediate cuneiforms respectively

 A Case to Learn From

An elderly man fell on the ward and had tenderness of his left hip but no shortening or rotation. His hip X-ray showed no fracture. The next day he was unable to weight bear and his pain was persisting, so a CT was requested as it was the weekend at a small district general hospital, and an MRI was not feasible. This showed a left non-displaced extracapsular fracture. X-ray will often show a fracture; however normal X-ray does not exclude pathology. If there are persistent or worsening symptoms an MRI should be obtained, and if not possible within 24 h then at least a CT should be obtained.

 Top Tip

Avoid using eponymous names, such as Colles' fracture, unless you are certain, as these names are for very specific fractures and are often misused.

STATION 5.17: CT HEAD

SCENARIO

You are a junior doctor on an emergency medicine placement and have been asked to see Mr May, an 84-year-old man, who has presented with a headache of sudden onset, left-sided hemiparesis and left-sided brisk reflexes. A CT head has been performed (Fig. 5.40). Please review the scan, explain the findings to Mr May and formulate an appropriate management plan.

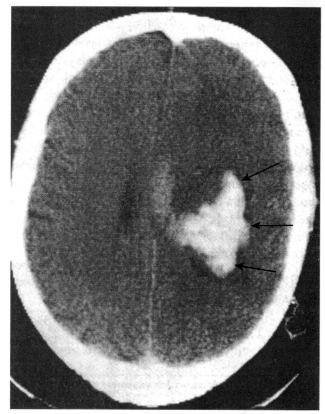

Fig. 5.40 Mr May's CT scan.

DATA INTERPRETATION

THE CT IMAGE

- The standard CT image is the axial (transverse) image
- The patient is supine and images are viewed as though looking from the patient's feet toward their head
- Therefore the left side of the image corresponds to the right side of the body

WINDOWING

- The attenuation of a tissue on CT (the shade of grey it appears) is similar to the density of that tissue and is represented by the Hounsfield unit (HU)
- There are several different automatic windowing presets – for example, lung, abdomen/soft tissue, bone and brain – which are optimised to identify abnormalities in the respective organs/tissues (Table 5.38)

CONTRAST

- Establish whether contrast was used and if so, the mode of delivery (IV, oral, rectal or a combination)
- The use of iodinated contrast material further enhances the contrast differences between structures and tissues, which aids image interpretation

Table 5.38   Information on windowing presets

TISSUE DENSITY	X-RAY ABSORPTION BY TISSUE	HOUNSFIELD INDEX	SHADE OF GREY ON SCAN
Low	Low: X-rays pass through tissue	Low	Dark (air is black)
High	High: X-rays absorbed by tissue	High	Light (cortical bone is white)

- Consider any potential risk of contrast nephropathy and interactions with medications – for example, metformin – when requesting a contrast-enhanced CT
- Consider the patient's allergies when requesting a contrast-enhanced CT. Those with other allergies/atopy and cardiac disease are most at risk and may require premedication with antihistamines or steroids

REVIEW AREAS

The mnemonic 'Blood Can Be Very Bad' is a useful tool to ensure you review the important areas (Table 5.39).

HAEMORRHAGE (TABLE 5.40)

- Acute haemorrhage is high-attenuation (i.e. bright)
- As blood ages, it becomes less dense and its attenuation drops; for example, a chronic subdural haemorrhage will have a similar density/attenuation as the CSF
- Haemorrhage can be intra-axial (i.e. within the brain parenchyma), extra-axial (i.e. within the space between the brain and the skull) or both
- Intra-axial haemorrhage may be the result of several different disease processes; for example, a haemorrhagic stroke, a bleed into an underlying lesion; for example, a tumour or vascular malformation, trauma or venous sinus thrombosis. Further imaging, for example, CT angiogram or venogram or MRI, may often be required to clarify its aetiology
- Extra-axial haemorrhage includes subarachnoid, subdural and extra/epidural haemorrhages (Figs 5.41–5.44)
- The role of CT in acute stroke is to identify a haemorrhage or an alternative cause for the clinical findings; for example, a space-occupying lesion. It is less useful for diagnosing an acute ischaemic stroke as the CT findings of an ischaemic stroke are usually only visible at least 6 h after the stroke started. An ischaemic stroke is usually diagnosed on clinical grounds once CT has deemed a haemorrhagic stroke or alternative causes are less likely

Table 5.39   Important areas to review on a CT scan

AREA	DETAILS
Blood	Look for evidence of: • Intra-axial haemorrhage • Subarachnoid haemorrhage • Subdural haemorrhage • Intraventricular haemorrhage
Cisterns	These are collections of CSF and must be reviewed for BAE: • *Blood* • *Asymmetry* • *Effacement* There are four cisterns to be checked: • Circummesencephalic • Sylvian • Quadrigeminal • Suprasellar
Brain	Look for: • Sulcal effacement (loss of normal sulcal-gyral pattern, which is a sign of raised intracranial pressure) • Inconsistencies of grey–white-matter differentiation • Structural shifts/herniation • Hypodense (air, oedema)/hyperdense (blood) areas
Ventricles	Check the lateral, third and fourth ventricles for: • Asymmetry • Effacement • Haemorrhage • Dilatation (hydrocephalus)
Bone	Look for fractures, which are best seen on 'bone' window

CT HEAD (TABLE 5.41)

- One of the most commonly requested CT scans
- They are very quick to perform but sensitive to patient movement. The patient must be able to lie still
- Common indications include:
  - Acute stroke: To identify haemorrhagic stroke or other pathology; for example, a space-occupying lesion
  - Trauma: To identify intracranial haemorrhage (extradural, subdural, subarachnoid and parenchymal) and fractures
  - Abnormal neurological signs/symptoms: To identify space-occupying lesions; for example, metastases, primary tumours, abscesses
- Most CT head scans are performed without IV contrast. The use of IV contrast is usually decided by the radiologist. There are three types (phases) of contrast-enhanced CT head scans, depending on the delay between administering the IV contrast and acquiring the CT scan (Table 5.42)

TYPE OF HAEMORRHAGE	SITE OF BLEEDING	CLINICAL PRESENTATION	CAUSES	CT FEATURES
Intra-axial (Fig. 5.41)	Within the brain parenchyma	• Headache • Loss of consciousness • Features of space-occupying lesion; for example, seizures/ vomiting/focal neurological deficit	• Haemorrhagic stroke • Bleed into underlying lesion; for example, tumour, trauma.	• High attenuation in the brain parenchyma
Acute subarachnoid (Fig. 5.42)	Between pia mater and arachnoid mater	• Sudden onset • Severe headache • Seizures • Focal neurology • Vomiting • Neck stiffness (meningism)	• Ruptured aneurysm (90%) • Trauma • Vascular malformation • Extension of intraparenchymal haemorrhage • Idiopathic	• High attenuation in the subarachnoid space (CSF spaces and cisterns around the circle of Willis/brainstem, Sylvian fissure, cortical sulci and ventricles) • Resultant hydrocephalus • CT angiogram will often demonstrate an aneurysm
Acute subdural (Fig. 5.43)	Between arachnoid mater and dura mater	• Gradual onset • Headache • Confusion • Seizures • Focal neurology	• Traumatic rupture of bridging veins • Commonest in neonates, infants and elderly	• High-attenuation crescent-shaped collection over brain surface (usually cerebral hemispheres) • Resultant mass effect (midline shift, effacement of adjacent ventricle/ CSF space, herniation)
Acute extradural (Fig. 5.44)	Between dura mater and skull	• Headache • Focal neurology • Loss of consciousness • Initial lucent period is typical	• Traumatic arterial bleeding (most commonly the middle meningeal artery in the temporal region)	• High-attenuation biconvex collection (egg-shaped) overlying the brain • Frequently associated with skull fractures • Resultant mass effect

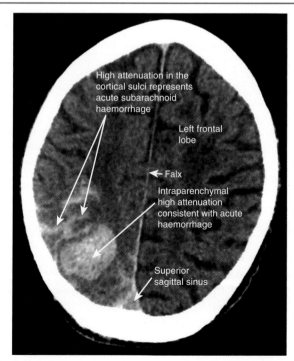

Fig. 5.41 Axial slice from a non-contrast CT head demonstrating an intraparenchymal acute haematoma (with some acute blood within the adjacent subarachnoid space). The cause of the haemorrhage is unclear on this image. It may be due to an underlying tumour or vascular malformation. However, these can only be identified on imaging once the haematoma has resolved (usually a delayed MRI scan (wait at least 6 weeks) is required).

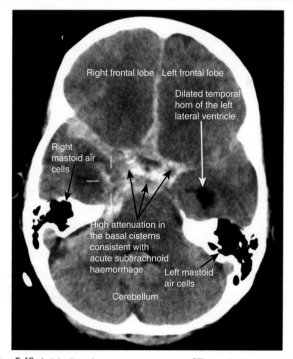

Fig. 5.42 Axial slice from a non-contrast CT head demonstrating high attenuation in the basal cisterns and surrounding CSF spaces, consistent with an acute subarachnoid haemorrhage. The dilated temporal horn of the left lateral ventricles is just visible, in keeping with hydrocephalus.

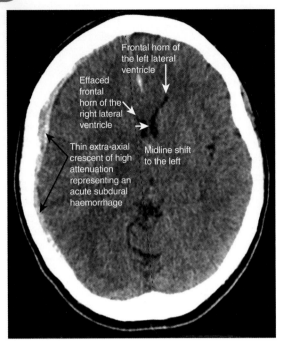

Fig. 5.43 Axial slice from a non-contrast CT head demonstrating a thin crescent-shaped collection overlying the right cerebral hemisphere, consistent with an acute subdural haemorrhage. Despite its relatively small size, there is evidence of mass effect, with a shift of the midline to the opposite side.

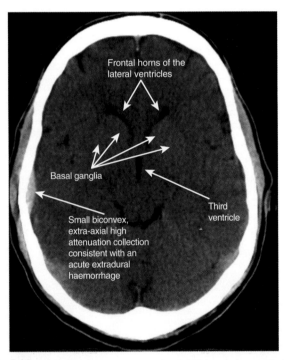

Fig. 5.44 Axial slice from a non-contrast CT head demonstrating a small biconvex high-attenuation collection overlying the right temporal lobe, in keeping with an acute extradural haemorrhage.

THIS CASE

This patient is presenting with signs and symptoms of an intracerebral haemorrhage and a CT brain confirmed an intraparenchymal haemorrhage.

RELEVANT PATIENT INFORMATION

PAST MEDICAL/SURGICAL HISTORY

- Previous stroke
- Recent bleeds, including: Haemoptysis, haematemesis, haematuria, PR bleed, epistaxis
- Cardiovascular disease
- Malignancy
- Trauma
- Known disorders of coagulation
- Alcohol excess

MEDICATION HISTORY

- Anticoagulants: Most recent INR if on warfarin, and when the last dose was taken
- Antiplatelets: For example, aspirin and clopidogrel
- Metformin: Be aware of the risk of lactic acidosis with contrast
- Diuretics, ACEi, NSAIDS: Increase risk of contrast nephropathy
- Illicit drugs: For example, amphetamines

Present Your Findings

Since you developed weakness and a headache today, we carried out a scan of your head to find the cause. Unfortunately, it has shown that you have had a stroke caused by a bleed on your brain.

The first thing we need to do is reverse your warfarin to help stop any bleeding and prevent further bleeding. We will give you some medication to reduce your blood pressure slowly. I will also contact my colleagues in neurosurgery, who specialise in the brain and nerves, as their ward is the best place for your care going forward. They may also discuss the possibility of an operation on your head to remove any clots or repair bleeding vessels, but not everyone needs this. After this initial treatment we can have a chat about ongoing care, which will involve some physiotherapy and occupational therapy. Have you any questions?

❓ QUESTIONS AND ANSWERS FOR CANDIDATE

What are the criteria for immediate request for CT head following a head injury in adults?

- Glasgow Coma Scale (GCS) < 13 on initial assessment in the ED

Table **5.41** Details on important abnormalities seen on CT head scans

CT HEAD FINDINGS	DESCRIPTION	CAUSE	OTHER CT DETAILS

Space-occupying lesions. (Fig. 5.45)	• Masses can arise within the brain parenchyma (Fig. 5.45) or the surrounding space between the brain and the skull	• The most common parenchymal masses are metastases. Primary tumours which commonly metastasise to the brain include:
		  • Lung cancer
		  • Breast cancer
		  • Genitourinary tract tumours
		  • Melanoma
		• There are a variety of primary brain tumours which are much less common than metastases.
			• There is often associated oedema (low-attenuation) in the white matter surrounding brain tumours, which can lead to mass effect
			• Contrast-enhanced CT and MRI are often helpful for further assessment

Mass effect (Fig. 5.45)	• Displacement of the soft tissue of the brain secondary to an increase in intracranial pressure due to an intracranial pathological process; for example, space-occupying lesions or haemorrhage	• Mass effect can result from:
		  • Space-occupying lesions (Fig. 5.45)
		  • Areas of haemorrhage
		  • Localised oedema or generalised cerebral oedema, which can occur after prolonged hypoxia
			• There may be effacement of the normal CSF spaces; for example, the ventricles or sulci, midline shift to the opposite side (Fig. 5.43) and herniation; for example, cerebellar tonsillar herniation

Hydrocephalus	• Hydrocephalus is dilatation of the ventricular system • It can be obstructive or communicating	• Obstructive hydrocephalus is caused by a blockage to the flow of CSF between the ventricles. This is usually a mass but can occur with SAH and meningitis. There will only be dilatation of the ventricles upstream of the blockage • Communicating hydrocephalus is the result of a problem with reabsorption of CSF by the arachnoid granulations, usually caused by a SAH or meningitis. There is dilatation of the entire ventricular system	• Dilatation of the temporal horn of the lateral ventricle is usually the earliest sign of hydrocephalus (Fig. 5.44)
Loss of normal grey–white-matter differentiation (Fig. 5.46)	• The myelinated sheaths of normal white matter make it less attenuating than grey matter (cortex), and it therefore is darker in appearance. The boundary between normal grey and white matter should be visible on CT • If there is oedema affecting the grey and white matter, this normal boundary becomes obscured (Fig. 5.46). This is known as loss of grey–white-matter differentiation	• It can occur as an early sign of an ischaemic stroke	

PHASE	TIMING OF CT	INDICATION
Arterial-phase scan (angiogram) (Fig. 5.47)	• CT acquired when the majority of the IV contrast is within the arterial system	• Usually performed to look for an aneurysm in cases of SAH
Venous-phase scan (venogram) (Fig. 5.48)	• CT acquired when the majority of the IV contrast is within the venous system	• Usually performed to look for thrombosis of the venous sinuses, which can cause haemorrhage in unusual areas and headaches
Delayed phase (Fig. 5.49)	• CT acquired 5–10 min after the IV contrast is administered. By this time, the contrast is 'within' the brain parenchyma	• Used to identify abnormal areas of enhancement; for example, primary and secondary tumours and abscesses

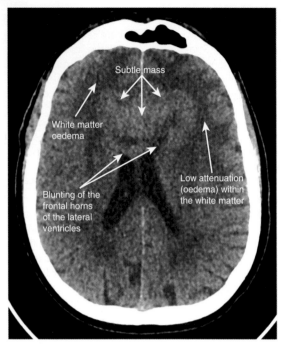

Fig. 5.45 Axial slice of a non-contrast CT head, which shows a subtle mass in both frontal lobes. There is surrounding white-matter oedema and blunting of the anterior horns of the lateral ventricles due to mass effect.

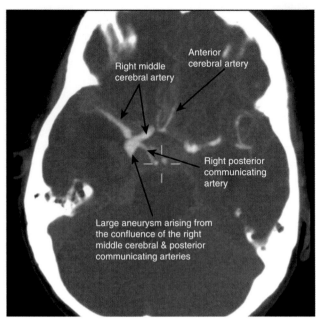

Fig. 5.47 Axial slice from a CT angiogram performed in the same patient with the acute subarachnoid haemorrhage shown in Fig. 5.53. It shows a large aneurysm arising from the right side of the circle of Willis.

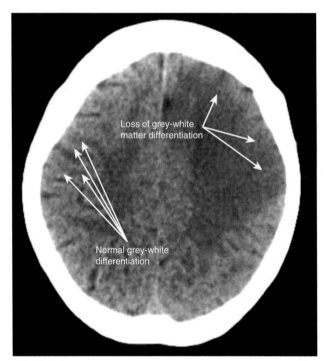

Fig. 5.46 Axial non-contrast CT head image. This shows a subtle abnormality of an acute ischaemic stroke. The difference between the grey matter of the cortex (higher attenuation = lighter) and the white matter (lower attenuation = darker) is visible in the right cerebral hemisphere. This is not the case in the anterior and midportion of the left hemisphere. Such a finding represents loss of the grey–white-matter differentiation and is caused by grey- and white-matter oedema. The commonest cause of this is an acute ischaemic infarct.

- GCS < 15 at 2 h after the injury on assessment in the ED
- Suspected open or depressed skull fracture
- Any sign of basal skull fracture (haemotympanum, 'panda' eyes, CSF leakage from the ear or nose, Battle's sign)
- Posttraumatic seizure
- Focal neurological deficit
- More than one episode of vomiting
- Amnesia for events more than 30 min before impact

Explain contrast nephropathy.

- Use of IV contrast poses the risk of acute tubular necrosis, leading to contrast nephropathy The risk is higher in patients with acute or chronic renal failure, diabetes and myeloma. Prehydration with IV fluids can reduce the risk; check your trust protocol. There is usually a cut-off renal function below which CT scanning is a relative contraindication. For patients below this cut-off, the options are:
  - Postponing the scan
  - Non-contrast CT
  - Alternative imaging; for example, MRI/USS
  - If the clinical benefit of making a diagnosis based on the contrast-enhanced CT outweighs the risk, it may be appropriate to proceed with the scan and manage any resulting renal impairment

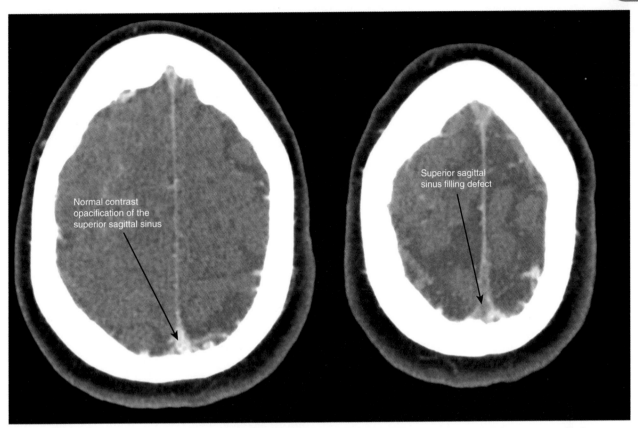

Fig. 5.48 Axial slices from a CT venogram showing abnormal areas in the superior sagittal sinus which are not opacified by contrast (filling defects), in keeping with dural venous sinus thrombosis.

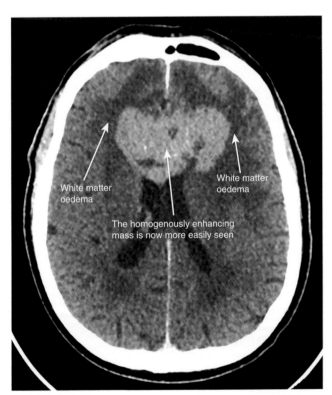

Fig. 5.49 Axial slice of a delayed-phase contrast-enhanced CT. The extent of the tumour is much more easily assessed on the contrast-enhanced scan, and any other tumour deposits will also be more easily seen.

Describe three contraindications or relative contraindications to CT scanning.

- Significant allergy to iodinated contrast
- Caution in unstable patients: This was previously an absolute contraindication, but there has been a move towards early scanning and accurate diagnosis. The patient should be resuscitated as much as possible without delaying the scan and will require a surgical/medical anaesthetic escort
- Relative contraindication include: Young people, pregnant women, those who have had multiple CTs

A Case to Learn From

An elderly man with a history of thrombocytopenia sustained a head injury by falling out of bed. He had a GCS of 13 from a baseline of 14–15. Although this did not meet conventional criteria for a scan, a CT brain was carried out, and a bleed was found. Guidelines ought to be adapted to the clinical picture, and patients with a low platelet count are at higher risk of bleeding.

Top Tip

Due to the high dose of radiation used in a CT scan, it is important to consider an alternative form of imaging which does not use ionising radiation in patients who are young, pregnant or undergoing multiple CTs.

6 Practical Skills

Content Outline

Practical skills can be nerve-wracking to perform in an exam setting. They not only require technical skill, but also demand good communication skills. Every practical skill comes with its own set of challenges. Practice makes perfect. We hope this chapter gives you an overview of some key skills along with the framework for passing your exams.

Many universities and hospitals have dedicated clinical skills-training sessions in clinical skills rooms. Make use of these to practise with the models that you will see in your exams. The key aspects of any practical skill are maintaining infection control, patient dignity and communication.

Keep in mind that everyone makes mistakes, particularly with skills you may not have had the opportunity to practise as much. If you make a mistake in the OSCE, deal with it in the same manner you would in clinical practice – identify the problem, explain it to the patient and address it appropriately.

Protocols for certain procedures will vary with local and national guidelines. Follow those that are applicable within your university or NHS trust.

Study Action Plan

- Shadow junior doctors and nursing staff. Ask if you can watch them perform practical skills. Your hospital is also likely to have a 'skills lab' with mannequins and equipment that you can use to practise
- Discuss any practical skill observed with the practitioner performing them. Nurses are often more than happy to teach you skills such as catheterisation and phlebotomy
- Sharing hints and tips from colleagues is also useful. Make the time to do this as you will each pick up different skills from observing different clinicians

STATION 6.1: INTERMEDIATE LIFE SUPPORT

SCENARIO

You are the junior doctor working in the emergency department (ED). You have been asked to follow up on Mr Bencini, a 33-year-old man, who was admitted following a motor vehicle accident. You notice that the patient has suddenly become unresponsive and the senior emergency nurse asks you to help resuscitate him. Please carry out intermediate life support (ILS) and follow any instructions given by your examiners throughout this station.

GENERAL ADVICE

- Always call the in-hospital cardiopulmonary resuscitation (CPR) team for assistance; this will lead to a better outome
- Ideally the patient should be lying on a flat hard surface as this increases the efficiency of the CPR
- An internationally used pneumonic to keep in mind when initiating ILS is the *DRS ABCD* (danger, response, shout, airway, breathing, circulation, defibrillation) approach

EQUIPMENT CHECKLIST

- Gloves
- Suction apparatus
- Watch or clock
- Crash trolley, including drugs and defibrillator
- Defibrillator pads or electrocardiogram (ECG) electrodes
- Oxygen supply and bag valve mask

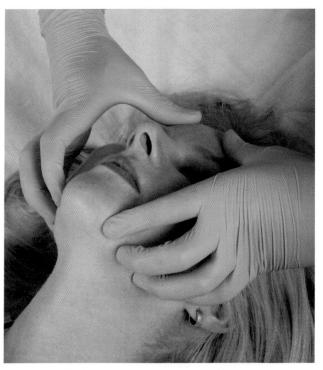

Fig. 6.1 The 'head tilt, chin lift' manoeuvre.

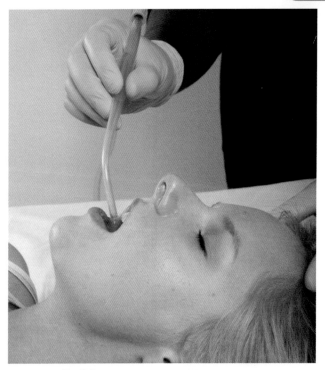

Fig. 6.2 Suction may help to clear the airway.

BASIC LIFE SUPPORT

- *Danger*: Your own safety is vital. Look out for hazards that might put you at risk
- *Response*: Shake the dummy lightly and shout, 'Hello, can you hear me?', whilst applying a painful stimulus
- *Shout*: Shout for help in the event of an unresponsive patient
- *Airway*:
  1. Look for signs of airway obstruction and remove any visible foreign bodies.
  2. If there is no concern about spinal injury, perform a 'head tilt, chin lift' manoeuvre (Fig. 6.1).
  3. Use suction apparatus or reposition the patient on to their side if you are concerned about foreign bodies in the airway (Fig. 6.2).
- *Breathing* and *circulation*:
  1. Simultaneously:
     Look for chest movement for 10 s.
     Listen for breath sounds for 10 s.
     Feel the carotid pulse for 10 s.
  2. In clinical practice if in doubt, call the crash team and start CPR.
  3. Start chest compressions (Fig. 6.3):
     Position: Directly over the bottom half of the sternum
     Rate: 100–120/min
     Depth: One-third of the depth of the chest. In most adults this equates to 5–6 cm
  4. After 30 chest compressions, give two breaths using a bag valve mask device connected to high-flow oxygen (Fig. 6.4).

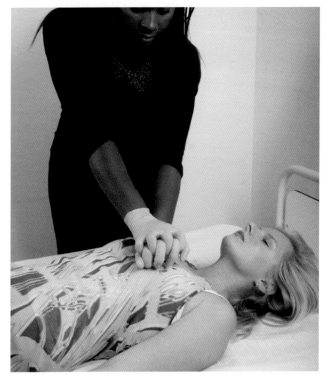

Fig. 6.3 Use both hands to perform chest compressions on an adult.

  5. Make sure you maintain a patent airway, otherwise the bag valve ventilation will not work. The use of airway adjuncts may be required; for example, a nasopharyngeal airway.
  6. Continue compressions and breaths at a rate of 30:2 respectively.
- *Defibrillation* (Fig. 6.5):

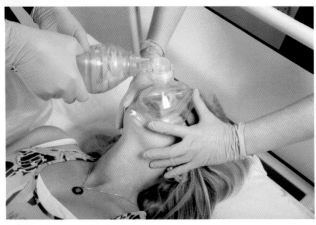

Fig. 6.4 If possible, use two people to operate a bag valve mask.

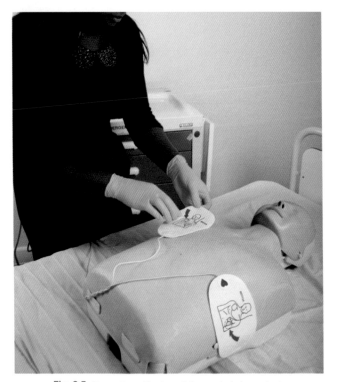

Fig. 6.5 Correct positioning of the pads is important.

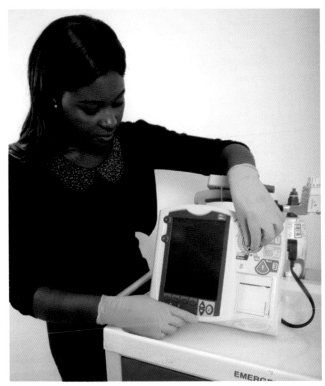

Fig. 6.6 Familiarise yourself with the defibrillator used at your trust.

7. The principal purpose of the rhythm check is to determine whether it is shockable or non-shockable.

SHOCKABLE RHYTHMS

- Pulseless ventricular tachycardia (pVT): Regular, broad-complex tachycardia (Fig. 6.7)
- Ventricular fibrillation (VF): Irregular with varying amplitude and frequency (Fig. 6.8)

MANAGEMENT OF SHOCKABLE RHYTHMS

1. State clearly: 'This is VF/pVT; this is a shockable rhythm'. Note to check for a pulse in the case of ventricular tachycardia.
2. Immediately instruct your colleague to resume chest compressions.
3. Turn the defibrillator to 150–200 J biphasic (150–360 J for subsequent shocks).
4. Press the charge button and state you are doing so: 'Charging.'
5. Instruct all members of the resuscitation team to 'stand clear' except for the individual performing chest compressions.
6. Remove any oxygen masks and/or equipment.
7. Once charging is complete, instruct your colleague who is performing chest compressions also 'stand clear.'
8. Press the shock button, stating 'shocking' just before you do so.
9. Immediately resume chest compressions and ventilation at a ratio of 30:2 for 2 min without pausing to reassess the rhythm or to look for signs of life.

1. Ensure that your colleagues continue with effective CPR, rotating at least every 2 min.
2. Turn on the defibrillator and apply the self-adhesive pads.
3. One pad is placed below the right clavicle and the second is placed in the V6 position in the left midaxillary line.
4. Ensure that CPR is continued whilst the pads are placed.
5. Once the pads are connected, charge the defibrillator, asking all (except the person performing CPR) to stand clear. Ensure that any oxygen supply is moved away.
6. Once charged, ask your team member to stop CPR so that you can assess the rhythm on the defibrillator display (Fig. 6.6).

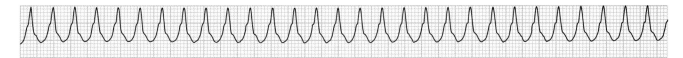

Fig. 6.7 Pulseless VT rhythm strip.

10. After a further 2 min, cease chest compressions and perform a second rhythm check.
11. Repeat steps 1–8 if the patient is still in a shockable rhythm.

COMMON DRUGS GIVEN DURING SHOCKABLE CARDIAC ARREST

After the third shock, administer:
- Adrenaline 1 mg intravenously (IV) or interosseously (IO)
- Amiodarone 300 mg IV/IO

After subsequent alternate shocks (every 3–5 min), administer:
- Adrenaline 1 mg IV/IO
- Amioderone 150 mg IV/IO should be given after the 5th shock

NON-SHOCKABLE RHYTHMS

- Pulseless electrical activity (PEA): Organised electrical activity but no pulse
- Asystole: No electrical activity

MANAGEMENT OF NON-SHOCKABLE RHYTHMS

1. State clearly: 'This is PEA/asystole; this is a non-shockable rhythm'.
2. Immediately instruct your colleague to resume chest compressions.
3. Administer 1 mg adrenaline IV/IO as soon as possible.
4. Continue CPR at a ratio of 30:2.
5. Pause compressions to perform a rhythm check after 2 min.
6. Repeat steps 1–5 if the patient is still in a non-shockable rhythm and no pulse is palpable.

COMMON DRUGS GIVEN DURING NON-SHOCKABLE CARDIAC ARREST

As soon as IV/IO access is obtained, administer:
- Adrenaline 1 mg IV/IO

After subsequent alternate CPR cycles (every 3–5 min), administer:
- Adrenaline 1 mg IV/IO

FINAL STEPS

- Postresuscitation care is initiated once the patient is out of a shockable rhythm, is displaying a rhythm consistent with organised electrical activity and has a pulse. This will involve high dependency unit (HDU)/intensive therapy unit (ITU) staff input

- The decision to stop CPR is discussed with the CPR team and is usually made by the most senior clinician present
- It is vital to document the CPR attempt and whether it was successful or not
- It is important to note the drugs given and how many cycles of CPR were given

REVERSIBLE CAUSES OF CARDIAC ARREST

🏃 Reversible causes of cardiac arrest	
CAUSE	**MANAGEMENT**
Hypoxia	The patient will be given 100% oxygen by bag and mask. Once an anaesthetist arrives, they can intubate the patient, securing the airway and ensuring optimal oxygenation
Hypovolaemia	Any fluid loss can be replaced IV. If the patient is septic and grossly vasodilated, vasopressors can also be used. Surgery will ultimately be required to control persistent haemorrhage
Hypothermia	Use a low-reading rectal thermometer to confirm the diagnosis. Ways to rewarm include using a blanket, Bair Hugger, giving warmed fluids IV, catheterising and filling the bladder with warmed fluids, peritoneal lavage and cardiopulmonary bypass
Hypo/hyperkalaemia (and other metabolic disturbances)	This should be found on venous gas. In the case of hyperkalaemia, calcium chloride should be administered IV in order to protect the myocardium
Toxins	Attempt to identify potential toxins. Check the patient's notes and ask staff. Treat accordingly; for example, naloxone for opiate toxicity
Thrombosis (coronary or pulmonary)	Follow local guidance for the management of acute coronary syndrome and massive pulmonary embolism
Tension pneumothorax	Insert a large-bore cannula into the second intercostal space, midclavicular line on the affected side and tape in place
Cardiac tamponade	Treat with pericardiocentesis

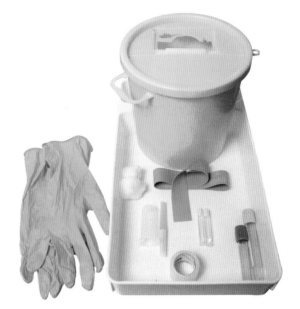

Fig. 6.8 VF rhythm strip.

QUESTIONS AND ANSWERS FOR CANDIDATE

When would you administer amiodarone during a resuscitation attempt?
- In the event of a shockable rhythm, after the third shock has been administered and after the fifth

How does the use of an advanced airway alter the ratio of compression:ventilation breaths?
- Compressions are performed continuously and are only interrupted for rhythm checks when an advanced airway has been sited
- Ventilation breaths are usually given at a rate of 10 breaths/min

How would you manage hypothermia?
It is important to warm the patient slowly. Some options are:
- Blankets
- Bair Hugger
- Giving warm fluids IV
- Catheterising and filling the bladder with warmed fluids
- Peritoneal lavage
- Cardiopulmonary bypass

A Case to Learn From

It is important to take into consideration how someone, medically trained or not, may feel if they observe a cardiac arrest with CPR. When I was a final-year medical student on a cardiology ward, there was a cardiac arrest during a ward round and everyone went to help. Unfortunately, the patient died. It was only afterwards when the nurse in charge asked me if I felt all right that it occurred to me that it can be an emotional and distressing experience. Don't be afraid to speak up to ask for help or counselling to deal with such incidents.

Top Tip

The rhythm may change between shockable and non-shockable throughout the resuscitation attempt. If this is the case, then remember to go to the beginning of the algorithm for whichever rhythm you are working on.

STATION 6.2: VENEPUNCTURE

SCENARIO

You are the junior doctor in primary care. Your next patient is Mr Fredrick, a 50-year-old man, who is having his renal function monitored after having recently started a diuretic medication. Please prepare your

Fig. 6.9 Tray of equipment required for venepuncture.

equipment and perform a venepuncture, explaining your steps to the examiner.

GENERAL ADVICE

- Check patient identification and gain valid consent
- Check whether the patient has any allergies
- Check whether the patient is needle-phobic
- Check whether the patient has lymphoedema, an atrioventricular (AV) fistula or has had a mastectomy

EQUIPMENT CHECKLIST

- Tray: Either single-use, disposable sterilised tray or a decontaminated plastic tray that is cleaned pre/post-procedure (Fig. 6.9)
- Single-use disposable apron
- Non-sterile gloves
- Disposable tourniquet
- Skin-cleansing solution (2% chlorhexidine gluconate (CHG) and 70% isopropyl alcohol (IPA) (for example, ChloraPrep))
- Venepuncture needle
- Vacutainer
- Blood bottles
- Cotton wool
- Tape
- Sharps bin: Should always be taken to the point of care

PERFORMING THE VENEPUNCTURE

PREPARATION

1. Wash hands.
2. Assemble equipment:

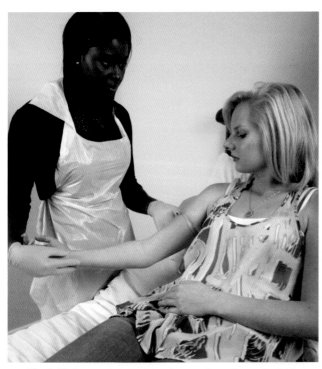

Fig. 6.10 Ensure the tourniquet is away from the sterile field.

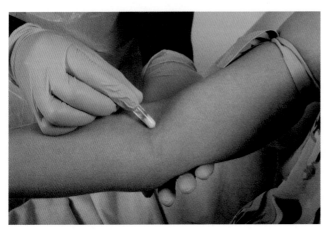

Fig. 6.11 Ensure the skin is cleaned properly.

- Attach the Vacutainer to the venepuncture needle
- Place the blood bottles in draw order
- Cut a piece of tape to size

DRAWING BLOOD

1. Clean hands, don non-sterile gloves and apply a single-use disposable apron.
2. Place the tourniquet 7–10 cm proximal to the proposed insertion point (Fig. 6.10).
3. Select a vein: It should feel 'bouncy'. If not, it is either inadequately filled or, if rigid, it may be thrombosed.
4. Loosen the tourniquet.
5. Clean the site: Clean for 30 s with ChloraPrep using an up-and-down, back-and-forth friction technique (Fig. 6.11). Allow to dry fully.
6. Retighten the tourniquet.

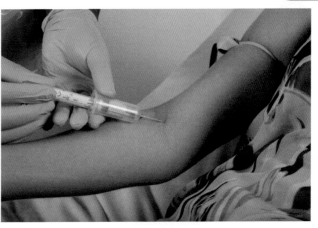

Fig. 6.12 Make sure you collect blood in the order of draw.

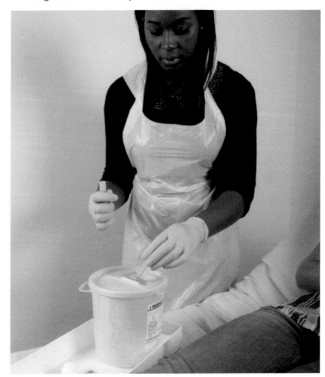

Fig. 6.13 Take the sharps bin to the bedside with you.

7. Puncture the vein using a non-touch technique (NTT), warning the patient of a 'sharp scratch'.
8. Draw blood (Fig. 6.12) and invert the bottles an appropriate number of times.
9. Remove the tourniquet.
10. Immediately dispose of any sharps (Fig. 6.13).
11. Apply pressure to the puncture site with cotton wool for 2 min or until the bleeding stops (Fig. 6.14).
12. Secure with tape.
13. Label the bottles at the bedside (Fig. 6.15).

FINAL STEPS

- Dispose of equipment and clean the tray
- Inform the patient to let a member of staff know if the site is painful, continues to bleed or if they have any other concerns
- Explain that the patient can remove the dressing after a couple of hours

- Remove your gloves and wash your hands
- Send the samples to the pathology lab

⚠ Blood bottles shown in draw order

TUBE COLOUR	DETAILS	WHAT IT CAN MEASURE	NUMBER OF TIMES TO INVERT
Blood cultures	Blue: Aerobic 5 mL Purple: Anaerobic 5 mL	• Blood culture • Sensitivity	3–4
Light blue	Sodium citrate: 2.7 mL	• International normalised ratio (INR) • Prothrombin time (PT) • Activated partial thromboplastin time (APTT)	3–4
Red	Plain: 10 mL	• Hepatitis status • Rubella serology • Virology • CA 125 • Coeliac screen	5–6
Gold	Serum-separating tube (SST): 5 mL	• Thyroid function tests (TFTs) • Liver function tests (LFTs) • Hormones • Lipids/cholesterol • Urea and electrolytes (U&Es) • Creatinine kinase (CK) • Digoxin, paracetamol and gentamicin levels • Amylase • Beta human chorionic gonadotrophin (β-hCG)	5–6
Green	Lithium heparin: 6 mL	• Amino acids • Parathyroid hormone (PTH) • Cortisol	8–10
Lavender	Ethylenediaminetetraacetic acid (EDTA): 3 mL	• Full blood count (FBCs) • Haemoglobin A_{1c} (HbA_{1c}) • Erythrocyte sedimentation rate (ESR)	8–10
Pink	EDTA: 6 mL	• Group and save • Cross-match • Blood group	8–10
Grey	Fluoride oxalate: 2 mL	• Glucose • Ethanol	8–10
Royal blue	EDTA: 5 mL	• Trace elements • Zinc • Copper • Selenium • Manganese • Lead	8–10

Note that colours may change between hospitals and trusts.

❓ QUESTIONS AND ANSWERS FOR CANDIDATE

What is the order of draw for taking FBCs, β-hCG and clotting?
1. Clotting
2. β-hCG
3. FBCs

Give three causes of hyperkalaemia.
- Drugs; for example, potassium-sparing diuretics, angiotensin-converting enzyme inhibitors (ACEi)
- Diabetic ketoacidosis
- Metabolic acidosis
- Renal insufficiency
- Burns

What is CK and when would you request it?
- CK is an enzyme that is important in tissues that consume adenosine triphosphate (ATP) rapidly
- It is used as a marker of damage of CK-rich tissue but is not specific to a tissue type. Therefore, it can be raised in rhabdomyolysis, acute kidney injury and myocardial infarction

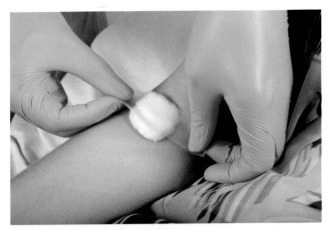

Fig. 6.14 Ask the patient to apply pressure, if they are able to.

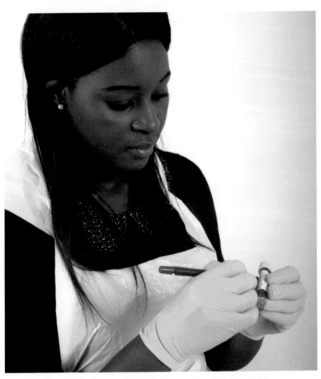

Fig. 6.15 Correctly label the bottles at the bedside.

 A Case to Learn From

During an on-call shift, a nurse had asked the on-call doctor to take some bloods from a patient. After he successfully got the bloods, he was bleeped to do something elsewhere on another ward. One hour later, he was bleeped by the nurse from before, saying that the same patient was now complaining of arm pain. When the doctor arrived, he realised that he had left the tourniquet on the patient's arm when he left the ward. Always dispose of your equipment properly and have a mental checklist before you leave the patient's bedside.

 Top Tip

It is often easier to approach a vein at the junction where two veins join, as it is more stable.

STATION 6.3: INTRAVENOUS CANNULATION AND SETTING UP A GIVING SET

SCENARIO

You are the junior doctor on call and the surgical ward has contacted you to see Mrs Jones, a 50-year-old woman, who was admitted with small-bowel obstruction. She is dehydrated and requires IV fluid; however, she does not have a cannula sited. Please prepare your equipment, site an IV cannula and start IV fluids, explaining your steps to the examiner

GENERAL ADVICE

- Ask the patient if they have an arm preference
- Consider if there are any predisposing medical or surgical conditions that would not allow use of a specific arm or blood vessel; for example, renal fistula, cellulitis or mastectomy
- Check for allergies, such as to CHG
- Position the patient comfortably and lay the patient down if they have suffered vasovagal episodes with needles in the past

EQUIPMENT CHECKLIST

EQUIPMENT FOR INTRAVENOUS CANNULATION

- Tray: Either single-use, disposable sterilised tray or a decontaminated plastic tray that is cleaned pre/post-procedure
- Sharps bin
- Two pairs of non-sterile gloves
- Single-use apron
- Skin-cleansing preparation
- 21G needle (though for drawing up medications, a blunt draw-up needle is preferred)
- 10-mL 0.9% saline ampoule for flush
- Sterile cap or bung for syringe
- Cannula
- Sterile adhesive dressing
- Cotton wool
- Disposable tourniquet
- Tape (if you fail to site the cannula you will need some tape and cotton wool to place over the puncture site)

ADDITIONAL EQUIPMENT FOR SETTING UP INTRAVENOUS FLUIDS

- IV fluid; for example, 1 L 0.9% saline
- Gravity administration set: Giving set
- Drip stand
- Non-sterile gloves

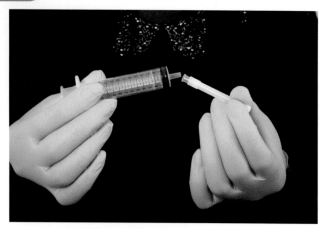

Fig. 6.16 Attaching the needle to the syringe.

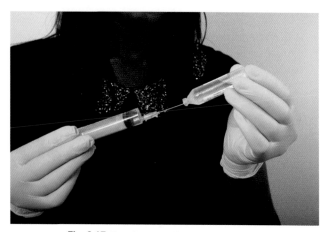

Fig. 6.17 Drawing up saline into the syringe.

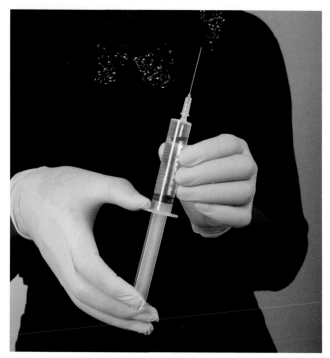

Fig. 6.18 Expelling air from the syringe.

PERFORMING INTRAVENOUS CANNULATION

PREPARING THE FLUSH

1. Clean your hands and put on non-sterile gloves.
2. Attach the 21G needle to the 10-mL syringe (Fig. 6.16).
3. Remove the top from the 0.9% saline and draw 10 mL up into your syringe (Fig. 6.17).
4. Expel any air from the syringe by tapping it and advancing the plunger (Fig. 6.18).
5. Discard the needle into the sharps bin and attach a sterile cap to the syringe.
6. Place the flush into the equipment tray alongside the other cannulation equipment.
7. Remove your gloves.

INSERTING THE CANNULA

1. Remove the cannula from its packaging and open the sterile dressing pack.
2. Position the patient's arm comfortably.
3. Place the tourniquet approximately 7–10 cm proximal to the site of insertion (Fig. 6.19).
4. Select a vein and then loosen the tourniquet.
5. Wash your hands and put on a new pair of non-sterile gloves and apron.
6. Clean the insertion site using skin-cleansing solution; clean for 30 s and allow to air dry (Fig. 6.20).

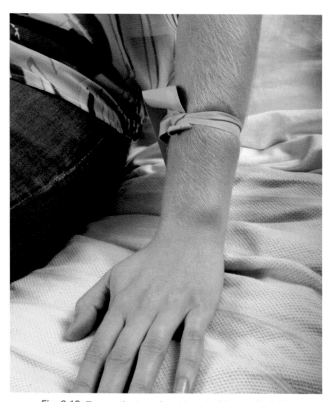

Fig. 6.19 Ensure the tourniquet is out of the sterile field.

7. Retighten the tourniquet.
8. Maintain traction on the vein that you have selected beneath the insertion site and insert the cannula at approximately 45° using an NTT (Fig. 6.21). Warn the patient of a 'sharp scratch'.
9. Advance the cannula until flashback is obtained (Fig. 6.22). Do not repalpate the aseptic area of the skin at any point during the procedure unless you are wearing sterile gloves.

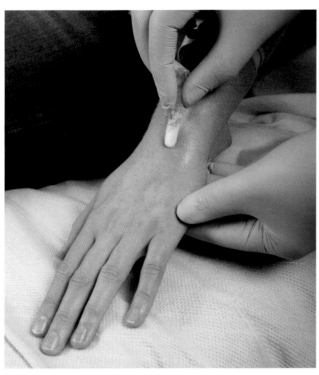

Fig. 6.20 Cleaning the cannula insertion site.

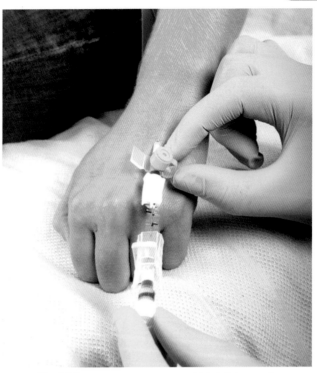

Fig. 6.22 Advance the cannula until it is fully inserted.

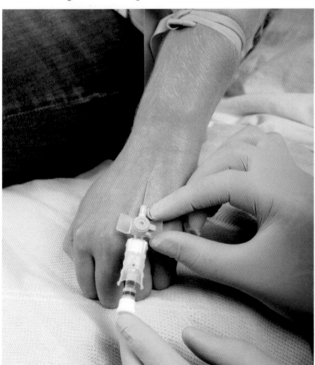

Fig. 6.21 Inserting the cannula using an NTT.

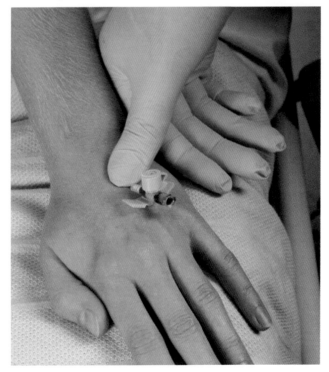

Fig. 6.23 Remove the needle and press firmly over the plastic cannula tubing to occlude it.

10. Once flashback is seen, advance the cannula slightly (1–2 mm). This ensures that the cannula tubing is within the vein before you advance it forward, over and off the needle.
11. Hold the needle still and advance the cannula over it, all the way into the vein. No part of the cannula tubing must be seen at the point of entry.
12. Release the tourniquet.

13. Occlude the vein and cannula with firm pressure whilst removing the needle (Fig. 6.23).
14. Dispose of the needle straight into the sharps bin.
15. Depending on trust policy, attach a cap, bung or IV extension set (which requires separate preparation) on to the end of the cannula (Fig. 6.24).
16. Wipe away any blood that may have leaked around the cannula with cotton wool.

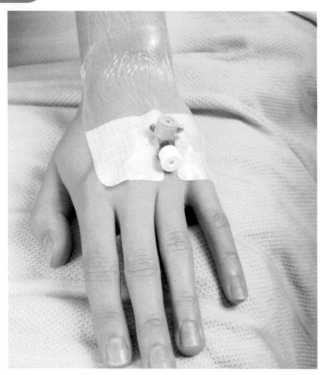

Fig. 6.24 Secure the cannula in place.

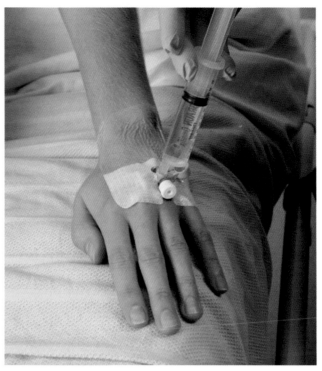

Fig. 6.25 Always flush the cannula after insertion.

17. Apply sterile adhesive dressing.
18. Write the date and time on the cannula dressing label.

FLUSHING THE CANNULA

1. Flip open the coloured cap of the cannula (however, if an IV extension set is applied, you would flush the cannula through this and not the coloured cap).
2. Remove the sterile cap from the saline flush syringe and attach the flush to the cannula.
3. Slowly flush the cannula with 5–10 mL saline, checking that the fluid does not leak into the surrounding tissues, causing swelling (Fig. 6.25).
4. Explain to the patient that they might feel coldness running up their arm as you are flushing the cannula.
5. Remove the syringe and replace the coloured cap.
6. Dispose of the syringe into the sharps bin.

SETTING UP A GIVING SET

1. Wash your hands.
2. Clean the tray according to local policy.
3. Clean your hands again.
4. Put on a pair of non-sterile gloves.
5. Check the fluid with the examiner:
   - Type and volume of fluid on the bag match the prescription
   - Any additives required
   - Expiry date
   - Check the bag integrity and that it has not leaked

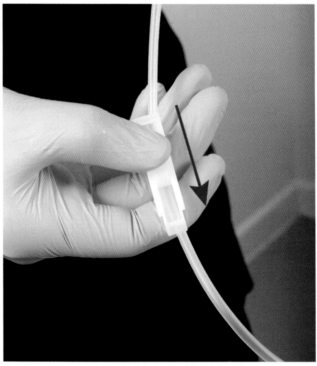

Fig. 6.26 Always turn the control wheel to the off position before starting.

6. Remove the bag of fluid from the outer packaging and hang it on to the drip stand.
7. Remove the giving set from the outer packaging and roll the flow control wheel down to the off position. The off position is where the tube is clamped, ensuring that the fluid does not run through the line, onto the floor (Fig. 6.26).

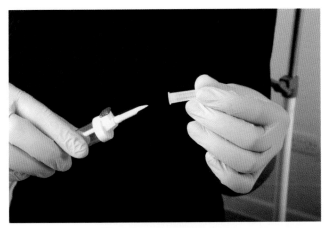

Fig. 6.27 Expose the trocar.

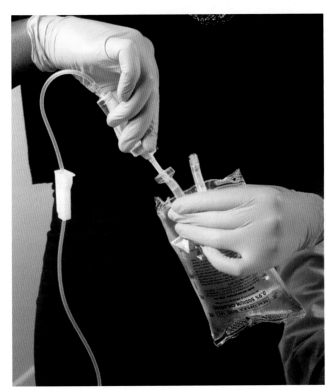

Fig. 6.28 Push and twist to insert the trocar.

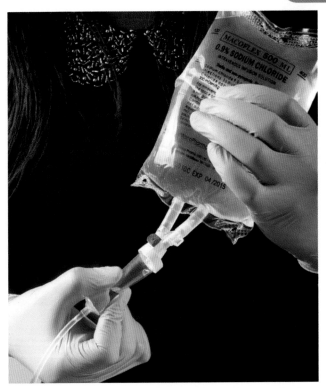

Fig. 6.29 Prepare the chamber of the giving set by squeezing it.

FINAL STEPS

- Decontaminate the tray as per local policy
- Remove your gloves and wash your hands
- Complete a cannula insertion record and place it in the notes
- Explain to the patient that if they have any pain or redness at or around the cannula site, or if they have any other concerns, they should speak to a member of staff

TYPES OF CANNULA

Information on different-coloured cannulas and their respective sizes and indication(s)

CANNULA COLOUR	CANNULA GAUGE	INDICATION FOR USE
Brown/orange	14	• Rapid infusion • Emergency
Grey	16	• Rapid infusion • Obstetrics
White/green	18	• Blood transfusion • Fluid infusion • Certain medications; for example, amiodarone
Pink	20	• Scheduled blood transfusion • Fluids • Bolus medications
Blue	22	• Fluids • Bolus medications
Yellow	24	• Paediatrics

8. Remove the cap from the fluid bag by twisting it and then remove the protective cover from the trocar of the giving set (Fig. 6.27). The trocar is a sharp hollow cylinder that pierces the fluid bag to provide a connection between the fluid and the giving set.
9. Insert the trocar into the bag of fluid by pushing hard and twisting (Fig. 6.28). This is easiest done by holding the fluid bag upside down.
10. Turn the fluid bag the correct way round and squeeze the chamber at the top of the giving set until it is half full of fluid (Fig. 6.29).
11. Slowly open the flow control wheel of the giving set so that the fluid flows continually and slowly down the line to the end.
12. Reset the flow control wheel to the closed position.
13. Hang the fluid bag back on to the drip stand. You are now ready to connect it to a cannula.

QUESTIONS AND ANSWERS FOR CANDIDATE

Name three complications of performing peripheral IV cannulation.
- Infection
- Bruising
- Thrombosis
- Pain
- Swelling of the surrounding tissues

In an emergency scenario, how could you maximise the rate at which you administer IV fluid?
- Insert the largest cannula size possible
- Increase the drip stand height
- Squeeze the fluid bag or apply a pressurised cuff
- Insert a second cannula

Name three signs that would suggest that a patient's cannula is not working correctly.
- Pain
- Swelling of surrounding tissue
- Erythema
- Flow of fluid slower than expected
- Inability to flush the cannula

 A Case to Learn From

During an intrapartum emergency, a patient had a cannula placed in both antecubital fossae. The next day she was still requiring IV medication but was a lot better. She was struggling to breastfeed her daughter as the cannulas were affecting her holding and positioning the baby. Following discussion, she agreed to having both cannulas removed and a new one placed in the back of her hand so she could feed her baby more comfortably. Always consider the comfort of the patient, as well as the clinical picture.

 Top Tip

Take more than one cannula with you to the bedside. Be prepared in case you miss!

STATION 6.4: ARTERIAL BLOOD GAS

SCENARIO

You are the junior doctor on call and the respiratory ward has contacted you to see Mr Frederick, a 60-year-old patient, who was admitted with an infective exacerbation of chronic obstructive pulmonary disease (COPD). He is unwell with a high temperature and respiratory rate. His oxygen saturations have fallen. You are asked to do an arterial blood gas (ABG), for which he has given you verbal consent. Please prepare your equipment and complete this procedure, explaining your steps to the examiner.

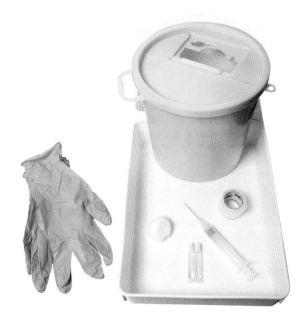

Fig. 6.30 Equipment checklist for performing an ABG.

GENERAL ADVICE

- Check whether your patient is on any anticoagulant medications, as this can increase the risk of bleeding and bruising
- Ideally, the patient would be breathing room air for a minimum of 20 min before taking the sample. If this is not possible, then we should know what oxygen supplementation (and by extension, the fraction of inspired oxygen (FiO_2)) the patient is receiving, as this needs to be taken into account when interpreting the results

EQUIPMENT CHECKLIST (FIG. 6.30)

- Tray: Either single-use, disposable sterilised tray or a decontaminated plastic tray that is cleaned pre/post-procedure
- Sharps bin
- Non-sterile gloves
- Single-use apron
- Skin-cleansing preparation
- ABG set
- Cotton wool
- Tape

PERFORMING A RADIAL ARTERIAL BLOOD GAS PUNCTURE

PALPATING THE RADIAL ARTERY

1. Ensure that the patient is comfortable with their forearm lying on a flat surface.
2. If necessary, hyperextend the wrist over a folded towel. Palpate the radial artery with your index and

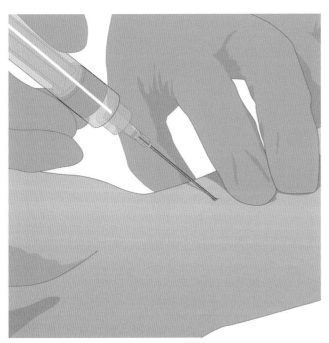

Fig. 6.31 Method A: The ABG needle is inserted distal to the index finger.

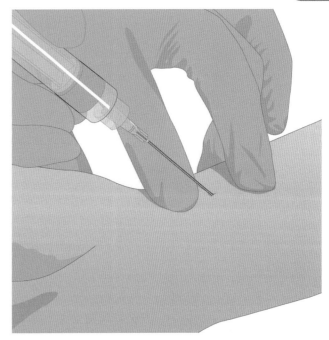

Fig. 6.32 Method B: The ABG needle is inserted between the palpating fingers.

middle fingers to determine a good position for the puncture.

SKIN PREPARATION

1. Wash your hands and put on non-sterile gloves and apron.
2. Clean the puncture site according to local trust policy, usually for 30 s, and allow it to dry.

SAMPLE COLLECTION

Method A

1. Place your index and middle fingers proximally to the puncture site by 1–2 cm.
2. Hold the needle and syringe like a pencil, bevel up.
3. Insert the needle at 45° just distal to your index finger (Fig. 6.31).

or:

Method B

1. Separate your index and middle fingers by 2–4 cm over the intended puncture site.
2. Hold the needle and syringe like a pencil, bevel up.
3. Insert the needle at 45° between your index and middle fingers (Fig. 6.32).

Then:

1. Advance the needle into the radial artery.
2. Obtain the sample, usually 3 mL.
3. Withdraw the needle.
4. Apply pressure to the puncture site using cotton wool and secure it with tape.
5. Direct pressure should be applied until the bleeding has stopped.
6. Dispose of the needle into the sharps bin.

7. Gently mix the sample by inverting the syringe up and down.

FINAL STEPS

- Inform the patient to let a member of staff know if the site is painful, continues to bleed or if they have any other concerns
- Explain that they can remove the dressing after a couple of hours
- Take the blood sample to the nearest blood gas analyser
- Once analysed, dispose of the syringe into a sharps bin
- Remove your gloves and wash your hands
- Document the procedure and findings in the patient's notes

ALLEN'S TEST

- Allen's test should be performed before taking a radial arterial blood sample
- The test checks the patency of the radial and ulnar arteries, ensuring that the circulation to the hand will not be compromised when the procedure is performed

MODIFIED ALLEN'S TEST

1. Ask the patient to open and close their hand to form a fist for 30 s.
2. Whilst the hand is elevated, occlude both the radial and ulnar arteries (Fig. 6.33).
3. With the hand still elevated, ask the patient to open the hand, which should be pale.

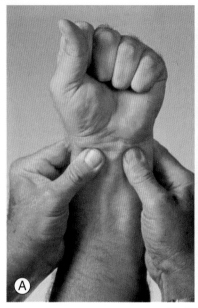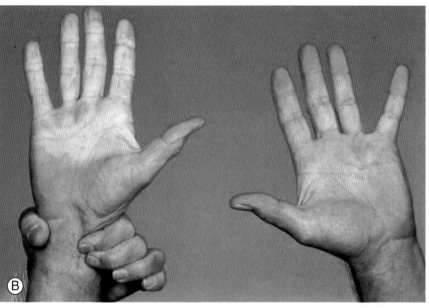

Fig. 6.33 The doctor is occluding both the radial and ulnar arteries.

4. Release the pressure from the ulnar artery and observe any colour changes.
   - A normal negative result: Hand colour returns to normal within 5–10 s, suggesting good ulnar blood supply to the hand. The radial arterial blood sampling can therefore be safely performed
   - An abnormal positive result: Hand colour does not return within 5–10 s, suggesting poor ulnar artery supply. The radial arterial blood sampling cannot be safely performed on this arm

❓ QUESTIONS AND ANSWERS FOR CANDIDATE

Name three complications of performing an arterial puncture.
- Infection
- Bleeding
- Bruising
- Thrombosis
- Pain
- Pseudoaneurysm formation

Which other arteries can commonly be used to take an arterial blood sample?
- The femoral and brachial arteries

What if the sample cannot be analysed straight away?
- The sample must be stored on ice and analysed within 2 h of obtaining the sample

 A Case to Learn From

When performing an ABG, the syringe stopped filling. I realised that I had gone through the artery so when I pulled the needle back it was fine and the syringe continued to fill. Don't give up!

💡 Top Tip

In patients with 'difficult to palpate' arteries, try marking on the skin with a pen the location of the artery prior to cleaning. This may help you locate the puncture site once you have prepared the skin.

STATION 6.5: MALE URETHRAL CATHETERISATION

SCENARIO

You are the junior doctor on-call and the surgical ward has contacted you to see Mr Miller, a 70-year-old man, who was admitted with abdominal pain and an inability to pass urine. Following an examination, you diagnose acute urinary retention. He has given you verbal consent for catheterisation. Please prepare your equipment and complete this procedure, explaining your steps to the examiner.

GENERAL ADVICE

- Always confirm consent verbally before starting
- Always use a chaperone
- Having an assistant makes the procedure easier to perform
- Lay the patient flat on a bed and ask him to expose himself from the belly button to the knees, covering the genital area with a blanket
- Ensure that you use the correct catheter

EQUIPMENT CHECKLIST (FIG. 6.34)

- Procedure trolley
- Sharps bin

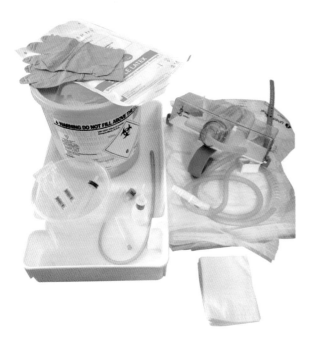

Fig. 6.34 Equipment checklist for catheterisation.

- Disposable bag for rubbish
- Catheterisation pack: Disposable dish, plastic pots, swabs and a sterile drape
- Sterile water or 0.9% saline sachets: According to trust policy
- Two pairs of sterile gloves
- Local anaesthetic (LA) gel or lubricant: According to trust policy
- 21G needle
- 10-mL syringe
- Sterile water syringe: Often predrawn up in a catheter pack
- Large incontinence pad
- Single-use disposable apron
- Male catheter
- Catheter bag: Urometer or leg bag, depending on which is appropriate for the patient
- Sterile universal container

PERFORMING MALE URETHRAL CATHETERISATION

PREPARE THE PROCEDURE TROLLEY

1. Wash hands.
2. Clean trolley according to trust policy.
3. Place the sharps bin on the bottom of your trolley.
4. Open the disposable rubbish bag and attach it to the side of your trolley.
5. Using an NTT, open the catheterisation pack on to the centre of the trolley.
6. Then open the packaging and drop LA gel, gloves and catheter into the aseptic field.
7. Do the same with the sterile water if predrawn up. If not preprepared, draw up the sterile water using a 21G needle and a 10-mL syringe, with the help of your assistant. After use, place the needle into the sharps bin.

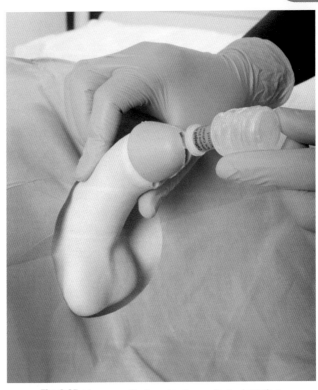

Fig. 6.35 Use anaesthetic gel before catheter insertion.

PREPARE THE PATIENT

1. Take your trolley to the bedside.
2. Ensure that the patient is correctly positioned and keep him covered until just before the procedure.
3. Put an incontinence pad under the patient.
4. Wash your hands and put on a single-use apron and a pair of sterile gloves.
5. Ask your assistant to remove the blanket.
6. Place a sterile drape with a central hole over the penis, leaving the penis exposed.

ASEPSIS AND ANAESTHESIA

1. Ask your assistant to empty the sterile water sachets into a plastic pot on your trolley.
2. Soak the swabs in water.
3. Hold the penis with your non-dominant hand and retract the prepuce/foreskin. This hand is contaminated and should now not touch the aseptic trolley.
4. With your dominant hand, clean the penis in circles, beginning at the urethra and moving progressively outwards. Repeat this at least three times.
5. Dispose of the swabs in the disposable rubbish bag.
6. With your non-dominant hand, apply some upwards traction to the penis and with your dominant hand insert the tip of the LA gel syringe into the urethral meatus (Fig. 6.35).
7. Administer the entire syringe, allowing some to coat the glans.
8. Leave the LA gel for 5 min to take effect.
9. Remove your gloves, wash your hands and put on a second pair of sterile gloves.

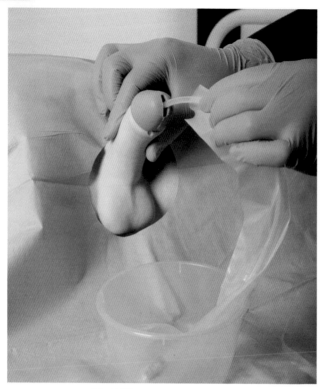

Fig. 6.36 Inserting the catheter.

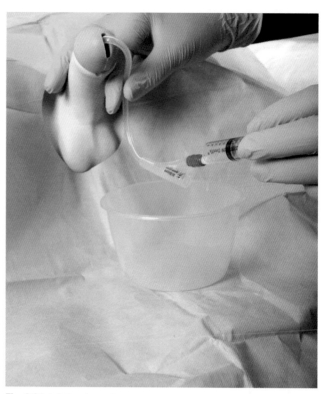

Fig. 6.37 Inflating the catheter balloon using sterile water into the side port.

◇ Table **6.1**	**Information on catheters**	
	MALE	**FEMALE**
Size	Generally 14 Charrière (Ch)	Generally 12 Ch
Length	Standard is approximately 40 cm	Standard is approximately 25 cm
Material	• Silicone or hydrogel: Lasts up to 3 months • Coated latex: Lasts up to 4 weeks	

INSERTING THE CATHETER (FIG. 6.36 AND TABLE 6.1)

1. Place a disposable dish between the patient's legs so that once the catheter is inserted, urine does not spill on to the bed.
2. Hold the base of the penis with your non-dominant hand and apply gentle upward traction.
3. Hold the catheter between the thumb and forefinger of your dominant hand.
4. Gently insert the catheter into the urethral meatus using an NNT, touching only the packaging. This is done by inserting directly from the sterilised packaging.
5. Advance the catheter using steady and gentle pressure until urine is seen. A catheter should never be forced.
6. Once urine is seen draining, advance the catheter by a further 2–3 cm.
7. If no urine is seen draining, advance the catheter the full length of the tube.

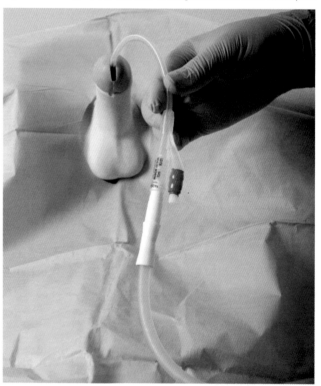

Fig. 6.38 Attaching the catheter to the drainage bag.

8. Attach the sterile water syringe to the balloon port of the catheter and insert 10 mL slowly. Stop if there is pain or high resistance (Fig. 6.37).
9. Attach the catheter to the catheter bag by removing the cap from the catheter bag tubing and plugging the plastic end into the end of the catheter (Fig. 6.38).
10. Replace the prepuce.

11. If there is a leg bag, attach it to the patient. If there are larger collection bags, then attach them to the patient's bed.
12. Clean the patient, remove the incontinence pad and ensure dignity by replacing the blanket.
13. Dispose of waste.
14. Clean the trolley according to trust policy.
15. Remove your gloves and wash your hands.

FINAL STEPS

- Tell the patient to report any pain or concerns to the nursing staff
- Document the procedure in the patient's notes
- Ensure a member of nursing staff knows the patient now has a urinary catheter

DOCUMENTING THE PROCEDURE
Document under the following headings:
- Consent
- Name of chaperone
- Date and time of insertion
- Reason for insertion
- Size, length and material of catheter
- Ease with which catheter passed
- Colour of urine drained
- Volume of sterile water inserted into the balloon
- Residual volume of urine: Volume 5–10 min after insertion
- Complications
- Details of follow-up and/or removal

QUESTIONS AND ANSWERS FOR CANDIDATE

What is the role of a three-way catheter?
- To provide continuous irrigation as well as drainage

When would a three-way catheter be used?
- Following bladder or upper urinary tract surgery
- Initial management of haematuria with large clots

Name three potential risks of male urethral catheterisation.
- Infection
- Bladder spasm
- Trauma
- Paraphimosis
- Inability to place a catheter

 A Case to Learn From

An inpatient with known dementia became very agitated overnight. Due to his dementia, he was not able to communicate the problem. Thorough care plans by the nursing staff showed that he had not had his bladder drained during the day and subsequent examination and bladder scan demonstrated urinary retention. He settled soon after urethral catheterisation. Remember to always consider urinary output and fluid balance when reviewing agitated patients.

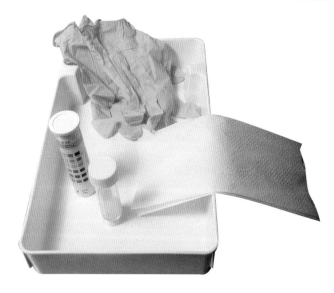
Fig. 6.39 Equipment checklist to perform urinalysis.

Top Tip

If you are unsure how many millilitres to use to inflate the balloon, then have a look on the catheter pack as there will always be specific instructions.

STATION 6.6: URINALYSIS

SCENARIO

You are the junior doctor in primary care. Your next patient is Mrs Manpreet, a 35-year-old woman, who presents with abdominal pain and vomiting. She has been going to the toilet more often than normal and is concerned that her urine is foul smelling. She has brought a urine sample with her. Please prepare your equipment, perform a urine dipstick and then discuss the results with her.

GENERAL ADVICE

- Where possible, it is important to obtain a fresh urine sample for analysis
- Ensure that when you interpret the urinalysis findings, you take into consideration the patient's history, signs and symptoms
- If you are going to throw away the urine sample after urinalysis, ensure this is into a sluice, and not a domestic sink

EQUIPMENT CHECKLIST (FIG. 6.39)

- Tray: Either single-use, disposable sterilised tray or a decontaminated plastic tray that is cleaned pre/post-procedure
- Non-sterile gloves
- Urine reagent strips
- Clinical waste bin
- Patient sample in a sterile urine pot

| Table 6.2 | How to interpret the appearance and smell of a urine sample |

APPEARANCE	INFERENCE
Red	• Haematuria • Food; for example, beetroot • Medications; for example, rifampicin
Cloudy	• Infection
Faeculent	• Colovesical fistula • Contaminated sample
SMELL	**INFERENCE**
Foul	• Infection
Sweet	• Diabetic ketoacidosis
Faeculent	• Colovesical fistula • Contaminated sample

PERFORMING URINALYSIS

OBTAINING A MIDSTREAM URINE SAMPLE (IF NOT PROVIDED)

1. Give the patient a sterile urine pot.
2. Ask them to collect a sample of midstream urine as described here.
3. Ask them to clean their external genitalia with water and tissue.
4. Ask the patient to pass a small amount of urine into the toilet.
5. Then, without stopping the flow of urine, ask them to catch a sample into the sterile pot.
6. They should immediately place the cap on to the sterile pot to reduce the chance of contamination.
7. Advise the patient that they can continue emptying their bladder into the toilet.

PERFORMING A URINE DIPSTICK

1. Wash your hands.
2. Put on non-sterile gloves.
3. Inspect the urine sample (Table 6.2).
4. Remove the cap of the sterile pot and note any odour.
5. Check the expiry date of the dipstick container and remove one dipstick.
6. Place the urine dipstick into the urine sample for 2–3 s, ensuring that all the reagents on the dipstick are immersed in urine (Fig. 6.40).
7. Remove the dipstick.
8. Place the dipstick horizontally on to a flat surface to ensure the chemicals do not mix (Fig. 6.41).
9. Leave the dipstick for the specified amount of time (found on the dipstick container).
10. Look at each reagent patch on the dipstick in turn. With each reagent, look at the corresponding colour on the dipstick container. There will be a colour code on the container so that you can interpret the results (Fig. 6.42).
11. Identify if the finding is normal or abnormal for each reagent patch.

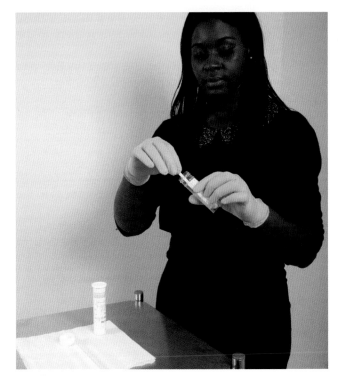

Fig. 6.40 Immersing the urine dipstick into the urine sample.

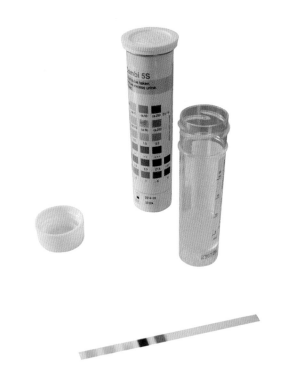

Fig. 6.41 Placing the urine dipstick on to a flat surface.

FINAL STEPS

• If the sample needs to be sent to the laboratory, label the pot and accompanying form with the patient and clinical details
• Remove your gloves and wash your hands
• Document the findings in the patient's notes

INTERPRETATION OF URINALYSIS

🏃 How to interpret each reagent patch of a dipstick

POSITIVE FINDING	INFERENCE
Blood	• Haematuria • Haemoglobinuria • Menstrual blood
Ketones	• Diabetic ketoacidosis • Starvation • Dehydration
Nitrites	• Suggests bacterial infection
Leukocytes	• Suggests inflammation and possible bacterial infection
Protein	• Renovascular, glomerular or tubointerstitial renal disease • Pre-eclampsia • Nephrotic syndrome • Benign, due to exercise or postural
Glucose	• Diabetes • Pregnancy • Medications, such as steroids
Specific gravity	High: • Dehydration • Heart failure • Liver failure • Syndrome of inappropriate antidiuretic hormone Low: • Diabetes insipidus • Increased fluid intake
pH	Alkaline: • Urinary tract infection (UTI) with urea-splitting organisms (*Proteus*) Acidic: • Urinary stones composed of uric acid and cysteine

❓ QUESTIONS AND ANSWERS FOR CANDIDATE

What methods are available for collecting urine samples in a baby?
• Clean catch urine: Waiting for urination with a sterile pot after the nappy has been removed and the surrounding area has been cleaned
• Suprapubic aspiration under ultrasound guidance
• Catheter sample

What are urinary Bence Jones proteins?
• Immunoglobulin light chains found in the urine, suggestive of multiple myeloma

What urine test needs to be requested for a pregnant woman who has a positive urine dip for protein only?
• Urinary protein-to-creatinine ratio. This helps diagnose pre-eclampsia

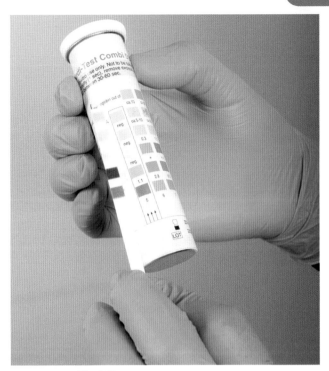

Fig. 6.42 Interpreting the urine dipstick.

📖 A Case to Learn From

A urine pregnancy test must be performed in all fertile women presenting with abdominal pain, even if the patient says she is not sexually active. A patient was listed for an emergency laparoscopy for abdominal pain under the general surgeons. It wasn't until a pregnancy test was performed on the ward that she was found to be pregnant and subsequently an ectopic pregnancy was diagnosed. She still had a laparoscopy performed but it was carried out by the gynaecologists, who removed her ectopic pregnancy and her fallopian tube.

💡 Top Tip

Don't throw away a urine sample after the dipstick is done. Wait until a decision is made as to whether it needs to be sent for further tests, especially in children where dipsticks can be more misleading.

STATION 6.7: INSTRUMENTS

SCENARIO

There are a number of instruments in front of you. Please take one, tell me its name and what you know about it.

GENERAL ADVICE

• If you are given a choice, start with the instrument you are most familiar with. This will help you to

gain confidence and momentum before you approach more difficult items
- Take the item and hold it in your hands
- Try and keep good eye contact with the examiner when discussing the instruments
- Try and keep to a structure. The following framework can be applied to almost any instrument:

1. Name and type of instrument
2. Indications for use
3. Example of clinical situation where you have seen it used
4. Complications with using the instrument
5. Contraindications to instrument use

COMMON INSTRUMENTS

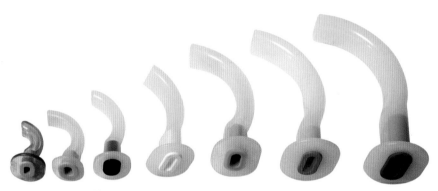

Fig. 6.43 Ensure you are familiar with all airway adjuncts.

Detail on oropharyngeal airway (FIG. 6.43)

Name	• Oropharyngeal airway, otherwise known as a Guedel airway, is an example of a non-definitive airway adjunct
Indication	• This device helps to maintain a patent airway in an unconscious patient to facilitate ventilation
Example of clinical situation instrument is used in	• I have seen it used in the ED and in the anaesthetic department. The correct size is chosen by measuring the distance from the incisors to the angle of the mandible. It is then held with two forefingers and a thumb at the thick plastic attached to the oval disc. During insertion, the Guedel airway is held in a position where the spout points towards the operator and the bend in the device is away from the operator. The device is rotated 180° as it descends past the hard palate. The approach reduces the risk of pushing the tongue backwards
Complications	• Trauma to the oropharynx • Upper-airway obstruction • Stimulation of the gag reflex resulting in vomiting
Contraindications	• Active airway reflexes • Active bleeding

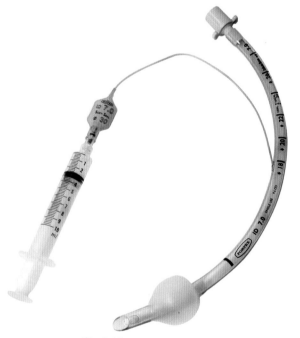

Fig. 6.44 Endotracheal tube.

Detail on endotracheal tube (FIG. 6.44)

Name	• Endotracheal tube. This is a cuffed endotracheal tube and is an example of a definitive airway
Indication	• This device is used in anaesthetics and in intensive care patients during intubation and ventilation of unconscious patients
Example of clinical situation instrument is used in	• I have seen it used during elective operating lists. It is inserted into the trachea under direct vision with the use of a laryngoscope to identify the glottis. After insertion the balloon cuff is inflated using air and a syringe to keep the tube in place and to prevent aspiration of gastric contents into the respiratory tract
Complications	• Tube misplacement • Trauma to teeth, gums or lips • Pulmonary aspiration of gastric contents • Oesophageal or tracheal perforation • Subglottic stenosis • Vocal cord paralysis
Contraindications	• Cervical spine injury: Immobilisation makes intubation difficult

Nasogastric tube (FIG. 6.45)

Name	• Nasogastric tube, of which there are fine- and wide-bore
Indication	• Fine-bore tubes are typically used for enteral feeding. Wide-bore tubes are typically used to provide gastric decompression in patients with bowel obstruction or following upper gastrointestinal surgery
Example of clinical situation instrument is used in	• I have seen a fine-bore feeding tube used on the stroke ward in patients with an unsafe swallow. The distance required to insert the tube is sized by measuring the distance of the tube from the nostril to the xiphisternum, passing via the tragus of the ear. The leading 10 cm is lubricated and advanced along the base of the nasal cavity in an upright patient. The patient is asked to sip water using a straw when the tube reaches the posterior pharynx. Drinking helps the introduction of the tube into the oesophagus. The tube is inserted the sized distance and then a little more to ensure correct positioning. Position is confirmed by testing some aspirate with pH paper and taking a chest X-ray
Complications	• Damage to the nasal turbinates • Malposition
Contraindications	• Base-of-skull fracture • Severe mid-face trauma • Recent nasal surgery • Oesophageal varices • Oesophageal obstruction • Coagulation abnormalities

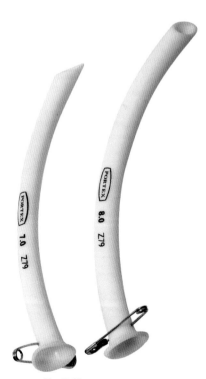

Fig. 6.45 Nasogastric tube.

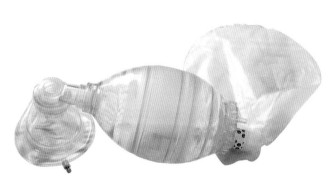

Fig. 6.46 Bag valve mask.

Bag valve mask (FIG. 6.46)

Name	• Bag valve mask
Indication	• This is used to provide positive-pressure ventilation. It is used to oxygenate and ventilate patients who are not breathing or breathing inadequately
Example of clinical situation instrument is used in	• I have seen it used in the ED during the acute care of a patient before a definitive airway was implemented. The bag valve mask can be connected to oxygen but also works independently and is self-filling. The mask is triangular and its tip should be placed just over the bridge of the patient's nose. The larger portion of the mask should be placed between the lower lips and the chin to provide a good seal. Although one person can operate the device, it is better with two: One person holding the mask in place and the other squeezing the bag to provide ventilation
Complications	• Aspiration • Hypoventilation • Hyperventilation
Contraindications	• Complete upper-airway obstruction • Facial fractures

Otoscope (FIG. 6.47)

Name	• Otoscope, of which there are four types: Direct, indirect, pneumatic and operating
Indication	• It is used by health professionals to examine the external auditory canal and tympanic membrane for ear pathology
Example of clinical situation instrument is used in	• I have seen the direct otoscope used in the ED on a patient with a suspected ear perforation. It is typically held in the same hand as the side of the face that the ear is on, i.e. if examining the left ear, then hold it with the left hand. It is held in the same way as a pen, with the fingers placed on its neck next to the eyepiece and the speculum facing away from the operator. After activating the light source and inspecting the external auditory canal and surrounding areas, the pinna is manually retracted superiorly and posteriorly with the other hand. The otoscope is gently introduced into the ear canal
Complications	• Trauma to ear canal
Contraindications	• None

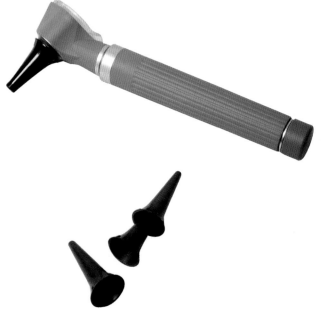

Fig. 6.47 Otoscope.

FINAL STEPS

• If you have some extra time you could discuss related instruments or ask the examiners if they have any other questions

Common Clinical Instruments

AIRWAYS	LINES	COLORECTAL
• Laryngeal mask airway • Tracheostomy • Nasopharyngeal airway	• Central venous line • Hickman line • Swan–Ganz catheter	• Rigid sigmoidoscope • Flexible sigmoidoscope • Proctoscope • Laparoscopic ports
ORTHOPAEDIC	**GYNAECOLOGY**	**OBSTETRICS**
• Dynamic hip screw • Joint prostheses • Intramedullary nail	• Cusco's speculum • Vaginal wall speculum • Pipelle tube	• Forceps • Ventouse • Rampley forceps

❓ QUESTIONS AND ANSWERS FOR CANDIDATE

In which direction should you pull the ear during an otoscopic examination in adults and why?
- The auricle of the ear should be pulled upwards and backwards in order to move the acoustic meatus in line with the auditory canal, aiding visualisation

Can you use oropharyngeal airways on children?
- Yes, and they can be inserted directly with inversion and/or with a tongue depressor

What device can be safely used to provide rescue breaths during CPR?
- Pocket face mask
- Bag valve mask

 A Case to Learn From

Never use a fine-bore nasogastric tube until the position has been confirmed. Even if you think the insertion is good, the tube can sometimes be coiled in the back of the mouth or in the chest!

 Top Tip

If you are struggling to insert a nasogastric tube, ask the patient to lean forwards slightly.

STATION 6.8: SUTURING

SCENARIO

You are a junior doctor in the ED. You have been asked to see Mr Harrison, a 27-year-old man, who has a small wound to his right forearm that requires suturing. Please prepare your equipment and complete this procedure, explaining your steps to the examiner.

GENERAL ADVICE

- Assess the wound to see if it requires referral to senior or specialist colleagues
- It may be useful to order an X-ray where retained or deep foreign bodies are suspected
- Assess the neurovascular supply to the region and involve senior staff if wounds involve tendons, nerves or large vessels
- A plastic surgery referral is essential for complex facial laceration, especially those involving the vermilion line (the border between the lips and skin)

EQUIPMENT CHECKLIST

WOUND-CLEANING EQUIPMENT

- Sterile gloves
- Single-use apron
- Sterile wound-dressing pack

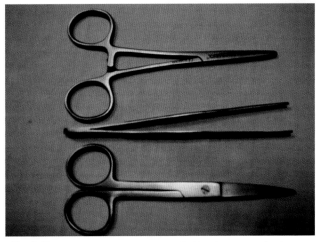

Fig. 6.48 From top to bottom: Needle holder, forceps and scissors.

- Iodine solution and/or sterile water
- Gauze

APPROPRIATE ANALGESIA – LOCAL ANAESTHETIC

- Tray: Single-use, disposable sterilised tray or a decontaminated plastic tray that is cleaned pre/post-procedure
- Sharps bin
- Lidocaine with 1/200,000 adrenaline (to minimise bleeding, but don't use adrenaline on extremities due to vasoconstrictive effect)
- 5 mL syringe
- 21G needle, to draw up LA
- 25G needle, to administer LA

SUTURING EQUIPMENT

- Sterile gloves
- Needle holder
- Toothed forceps
- Scissors
- Suture(s): For example, 4/0 synthetic, non-absorbable monofilament with a curved needle
- Sterile dressing

EXTRAS TO CONSIDER

- An assistant
- Tetanus injection

SUTURING

WOUND PREPARATION

1. Wash your hands and put on a single-use apron and a pair of sterile gloves
2. Remove large visible debris from the wound
3. Use sterile water to soak the gauze and clean the wound gently
4. Administer the LA (see below)
5. Further clean the wound with gauze soaked in iodine solution (this would sting a lot if done before LA administration)
6. Dry the wound with clean gauze

LOCAL ANAESTHETIC ADMINISTRATION

1. Check the LA dose and expiry date with a second person.
2. Draw up 5 mL LA using the 21G needle.
3. Detach the 21G needle without resheathing it and discard it into the sharps bin.
4. Attach the 25G needle and inject the LA into the skin and soft tissues around the wound in a circular fashion. Use the 'aspirate and infiltrate' technique to ensure that you are not inadvertently in a vessel.
5. LA can take 5–10 min to reach full effect; therefore, always test sensation with forceps before you start suturing.
6. Remove your first pair of sterile gloves.

SUTURING

1. Put on a pair of new sterile gloves.
2. Hold the needle holder in your dominant hand with your thumb and ring finger (Fig. 6.49).
3. Hold the toothed forceps in your non-dominant hand using a pen grip (Fig. 6.50).
4. Remove the needle and suturing from the packaging with the needle holder and reposition the needle using the forceps (Fig. 6.51).
5. Bring your thumb and ring finger together to lock the needle into the needle holder; several clicks should be heard.
6. The first suture should be in the centre of the wound.
7. With the forceps, gently manipulate the wound's edge.
8. Insert the needle perpendicular to the skin's surface approximately 5 mm from the wound edge (Fig. 6.52).
9. Advance the needle through the wound in a circular arc, aiming to exit in the middle of the wound (Fig. 6.53).
10. Grasp the needle with the forceps, taking care not to blunt the tip of the needle.
11. Release the needle from the needle holder.
12. Withdraw the needle with the forceps and regrip in the correct position with the needle holder.
13. Pull the suture through, leaving about 4 cm of suture length.

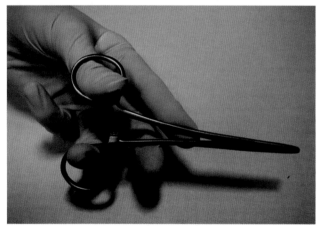

Fig. 6.49 Holding the needle holder.

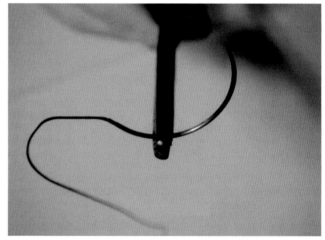

Fig. 6.51 Holding the needle.

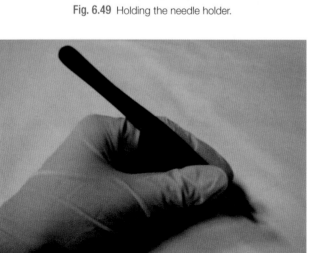

Fig. 6.50 Holding the forceps.

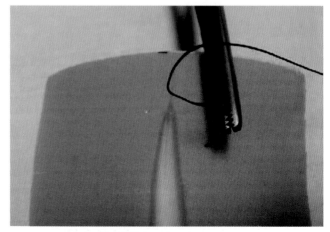

Fig. 6.52 Inserting the needle.

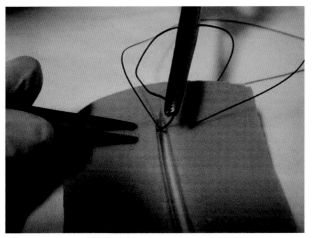

Fig. 6.53 Exiting the wound.

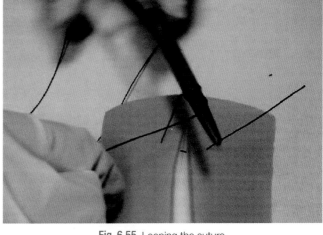

Fig. 6.55 Looping the suture.

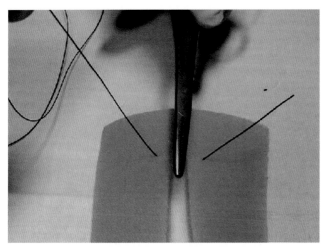

Fig. 6.54 The first 'V'.

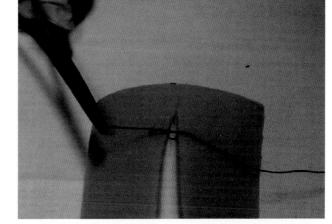

Fig. 6.56 The first knot.

14. Reinsert the needle from within the wound and aim to exit about 5 mm from the wound edge.
15. Once again, grasp the needle with the forceps, release from the needle holder and pull the suture material through.

TYING A SURGICAL KNOT

1. Place the needle holder (now not holding the needle) between the two ends of the suture thread that are forming a 'V' (Fig. 6.54).
2. Loop the thread attached to the needle around the needle holder three times in a clockwise fashion. Keep hold of this long end of the suture (Fig. 6.55).
3. Grasp the very tip of the short end of the suture with the needle holder. Pull the two ends of sutures in opposite directions at right angles to the wound, forming the first knot (Fig. 6.56).
4. Form a 'V' shape with the two ends of the suture and again, place the needle holder between the two ends (Fig. 6.57).
5. Loop the thread attached to the needle around the needle holder twice in an anticlockwise fashion.
6. Grasp the very tip of the short end of the suture material with the needle holder. Pull the two ends

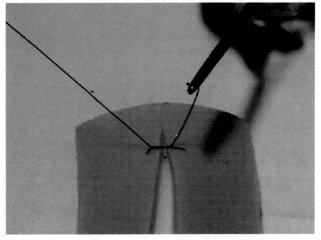

Fig. 6.57 The second 'V'.

of the sutures in opposite directions at right angles to the wound. This is the second knot (Fig. 6.58).
7. Follow steps 1–3 above to lay down the third knot.
8. Reposition your knots so that they are not lying over the wound (Fig. 6.59).
9. Cut the ends of the suture, leaving approximately 5 mm on each end (Fig. 6.60).

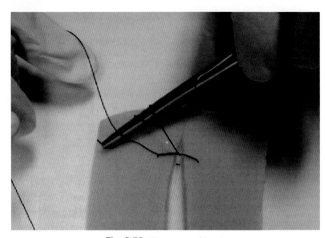

Fig. 6.58 The second knot.

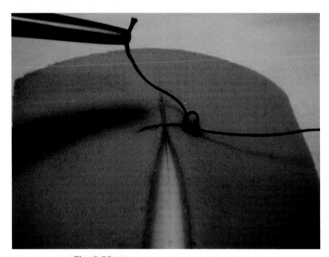

Fig. 6.59 Correct positioning of your knot.

10. Repeat the suturing and knot-tying steps until the whole wound is sutured. Sutures should be placed 5–10 mm apart from each other (Fig. 6.61).
11. Immediately dispose of the needle into the sharps bin when suturing is finished.

FINAL STEPS

- Apply a dressing over the wound, if required
- Administer a tetanus booster if the patient has not had one in the past 10 years or if the wound is contaminated
- Advise the patient to keep the wound dry whilst showering and washing
- Educate the patient on signs of wound infection:
  - Redness
  - Soreness
  - Discharge
  - Swelling
- Make sure that the patient is aware that the sutures are dissolvable or non-dissolvable. If they are non-dissolvable, make sure they understand how and when they should be removed
- Document the procedure under the following headings:
  - Consent and any chaperone present
  - Details of site of laceration and wound assessment
  - Any referrals made
  - Amount of LA used
  - Wound suturing performed on patient: Type of suture and number of sutures
  - Complications
  - Estimated blood loss
  - Any subsequent tests ordered
  - Details of follow-up and wound after care

❗ Details on the different types of sutures

ABSORBABLE	NON-ABSORBABLE	MONOFILAMENT	POLYFILAMENT
• They are naturally dissolved by the body and hence do not need to be removed • They are more likely to leave a pronounced scar when used on skin • They may be useful in children who are expected to be distressed during suture removal	• They are less tissue-reactive and therefore leave less scarring • They are typically used for skin suturing and are removed in a healthcare setting during a wound check	• They are recommended for skin closures • They have a decreased risk of infection compared to polyfilament	• They are made of many strands of thread twisted together • They are easier to tie than monofilament • The microspaces in between the threads allow for easier bacterial colonisation compared to monofilament

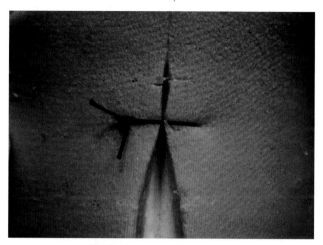

Fig. 6.60 An interrupted suture.

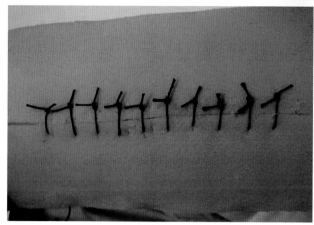

Fig. 6.61 A series of uninterrupted sutures closing the wound.

❓ QUESTIONS AND ANSWERS FOR CANDIDATE

Name two possible alternatives to suturing.
- Steri-Strips
- Staples
- Tissue adhesives (glue)

When are non-absorbable skin sutures removed?
- Sutures will normally be removed in 7–14 days, or 4–5 days if on the face
- Sutures can be removed by primary care doctors, practice nurses or district nurses. It does not have to be in a hospital

When is a mattress suture indicated?
- A mattress suture can be vertical or horizontal
- When the skin edges are difficult to evert. They provide good dermis-to-dermis contact and can be used in conjunction with simple interrupted sutures
- When a wound is not holding together; for example, if the wound edges are under tension

🔖 A Case to Learn From

It is important to understand which size of suture you require for different parts of the body. I was asked to suture a small cheek laceration and soon realised that 2/0 suture was far too big. I asked for senior advice and ended up using 6/0, a much smaller suture and needle!

💡 Top Tip

Each successive knot should be laid down in opposite directions as this pattern prevents the suture unravelling.

7 Obstetrics and Gynaecology

Content Outline

Obstetrics and gynaecology placements offer the student a fantastically broad range of subjects and skills. In many cases they are caring for not one but two patients: the mother and fetus. It is one of the few specialities which still involves a true mix of medicine and surgery.

It is also an excellent area in which to see multidisciplinary work, involving midwives, anaesthetists, specialist nurses, oncology teams and radiology staff. You will have the opportunity to improve communication skills, taking histories from women in clinics, wards and delivery suite. You should also use this time to improve your examination skills and should aim to end the rotation feeling confident in obstetric and gynaecological examination, as well as having the skill to put the woman at ease during such procedures.

Study Action Plan

- Get the most out of your time on the delivery suite. Introduce yourself to the midwife in charge on arrival and expect to put the hours in. If you work as part of the team you will gain more out of your time and hopefully get the privilege of delivering your first baby!
- Attend fetal medicine clinics and early pregnancy clinics. The staff there often have to break bad news to patients and you can learn how to do this in a sensitive manner
- Try to shadow the clerking doctor on gynaecology admissions and ask if you can take the histories and examine the patients with them
- Make sure you arrive early if you are due to be in theatre. Introduce yourself to the surgical team and ask if you can examine the patients. Many hospitals require patients to sign a separate consent form for this; ensure you know where these are kept. Theatre sessions are a good opportunity to test your anatomy knowledge, whether you are scrubbed at a major abdominal case or watching the screens during laparoscopy

STATION 7.1: HISTORY: HEADACHE IN PREGNANCY

SCENARIO

You are a junior doctor on the labour ward and have been asked to see Leanne Jones, a 36-year-old woman, who has presented with a headache. She is 36 weeks pregnant. Please take a history from Miss Jones, present your findings and formulate an appropriate management plan.

Cardinal Symptoms

Thunderclap onset

Focal neurological signs or symptoms

Changes with posture

Headache that wakes the patient up

Precipitated by exertion or Valsalva manoeuvre

Risk factors for cerebral venous sinus thrombosis

Jaw claudication or visual disturbance

Neck stiffness

Fever

New-onset headache in a patient with human immunodeficiency virus (HIV) or history of cancer

HISTORY OF PRESENTING COMPLAINT

- Site: Frontal, bilateral, unilateral
- Onset: Sudden or insidious
- Character: Throbbing, pulsating, pressure, unilateral or bilateral
- Radiation: Radiation to neck or jaw

- Associations: Jaw claudication, aura (reversible symptoms in alteration of speech, vision, power, sensation or balance)
- Timing: Any clear pattern seen, occurs at a specific time of day or week, relationship to work hours or stressors
- Exacerbating or relieving factors: Postural differences, avoiding light, exacerbation by exertion, helped or not by simple analgesia
- Severity: How bad the pain is on a scale of 1–10

ASSOCIATED SYMPTOMS

Other symptoms to enquire about include:
- Nausea: With or without vomiting
- Visual disturbance: Constant, on moving head or gaze, at certain times of the day
- Weakness or paraesthesia: Focal or generalised
- Neck stiffness: Localised or general
- Fever: Duration and grade
- Epigastric pain: Can be associated with pre-eclampsia

CURRENT OBSTETRIC HISTORY

- Scans to date: Dating scan, anomaly scan, placental site, any additional scans and why
- Complications: Admissions to hospital, previous bleeding
- Rhesus status: Should be taken at booking

PAST OBSTETRIC HISTORY

- Pregnancies to date: Year, livebirth, miscarriage, termination, mode of birth and birth weight
- Complications: Pre-eclampsia, haemorrhage, infections

PAST MEDICAL AND SURGICAL HISTORY

- General: Ask about known medical conditions, relevant treatments and any hospital admissions
- Headaches prior to this: Did the patient have migraines or headaches while taking oral contraceptives?
- Vaccination history: This is important as infections, for example, measles, may occur in the unvaccinated population
- Malignancy: Any headache in a patient with previous cancer is a red-flag symptom
- Infections: Any headache in a patient with human immunodeficiency virus (HIV) is a red-flag symptom

MEDICATION HISTORY

Enquire about prescribed and over-the-counter medications, including any recent changes. Allergies should also be included with the specific reaction noted. In this scenario be aware of:
- Medications that can cause headache: For example, nifedipine

- Analgesia use: For example, paracetamol, codeine
  It is also important to ask what analgesia the patient has used until presentation and the response.

SOCIAL HISTORY

Social history includes enquiring about occupation, residence, lifestyle (diet, exercise, smoking, alcohol, substance abuse) and recent travel. Additionally, in this scenario, consider:
- Smoking: A key reversible risk factor for pre-eclampsia
- Living arrangements: Use this as an opportunity to enquire about domestic violence and ensure there is no headache from a head injury

FAMILY HISTORY

Enquire about any significant family history, including:
- History of pre-eclampsia in first-degree relatives, as the risk is significantly increased

SYSTEMS REVIEW

On systems review, particularly pertinent questions to the above case may include questions regarding thrombosis, pre-eclampsia or infections. These include:
- Fever: Relating to infection
- Risk factors for venous thromboembolism (VTE): Swollen calves, shortness of breath, palpitations

Risk Factors for Pre-Eclampsia

- Nulliparity
- Extremes of reproductive age
- Previous pre-eclampsia
- First-degree relative with pre-eclampsia
- Pre-existing renal disease or hypertension
- Obesity
- Diabetes mellitus
- Multiparity with new partner

HEAD IMAGING IN PREGNANCY

- Fetal exposure to radiation from a head Computed tomography (CT) is < 0.005 mGy:
  - Background cumulative dose of radiation during pregnancy is 50 mGy
- Avoid iodine-based contrast if possible:
  - Gadolinium-based contrast is safe
  - Postnatal women can safely continue to breastfeed after the use of either contrast
- Try to avoid Magnetic resonance imaging (MRI) in the first trimester:
  - Risk of acoustic noise damage and hyperthermia
- Remember that the safety of the mother comes first at all times

Differential Diagnosis

CONDITION	CLINICAL PRESENTATION	INVESTIGATIONS	MANAGEMENT
Migraine	• Unilateral • Pulsating • Moderate to severe pain • May be accompanied by an aura • Disabling • Associated with: Nausea, vomiting, photophobia or sensitivity to sound	• Usually unnecessary, clinical diagnosis	• Analgesia
Tension headache	• Bilateral • Tightening • Mild to moderate pain • Not usually disabling • May have photophobia or sensitivity to sound • Pericranial tenderness	• Usually unnecessary, clinical diagnosis	• Analgesiaw
Medication overuse headache	• Constant • Dull • Present most days	• Accurate history taking • Rule out other causes	• Supportive withdrawal of analgesic drug, for at least 1 month • Warn patient that symptoms may rebound
Pre-eclampsia	At least two of: • Bilateral • Pulsating • Aggravated by physical activityIn addition: • Hypertension and proteinuria • The headache typically gets worse and better as pre-eclampsia does	• Full blood count (FBCs) • Urea and electrolytes (U&Es) • Clotting profile • Liver function tests (LFTs) • Uric acid • Cardiotocography (CTG) • Urine protein:creatinine ratio	• Analgesia • Treat hypertension • Consider magnesium sulphate infusion if at risk of seizures • Consider delivery
Cerebral venous thrombosis	• No specific features of headache • Papilloedema • Focal neurological deficits • Decreased Glasgow Coma Scale (GCS) • Seizures • Psychosis	• MRI with magnetic resonance venography (MRV)	• Low-molecular-weight heparin (LMWH) • Urgent referral to neurologists and neurosurgeons
Subarachnoid haemorrhage	• Thunderclap headache • Occipital in position • Vomiting • Seizures • Neck stiffness • Focal neurology	• CT scan • Lumbar puncture	• Urgent referral to neurosurgeons • May need clot evacuation

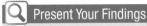

Present Your Findings

Miss Jones is a 36-year-old woman who presented with a headache at 36 weeks pregnant. The headache is bilateral and tightening in character. She has no focal neurological symptoms apart from this. She is generally fit and well and her pregnancy has been uncomplicated to date.

I feel the most likely diagnosis is a tension headache, with differentials being migraine and pre-eclampsia.

I would like to examine Miss Jones fully and perform a full set of observations, including blood pressure. I would like to take blood to check her FBCs, U&Es and LFTs and arrange a urine dip, looking for evidence of proteinuria.

❓ QUESTIONS AND ANSWERS FOR CANDIDATE

How common are headaches in pregnancy?
• Around a third of women will suffer from headaches in pregnancy

• Commonly headaches will be tension headaches or migraines

How common is pre-eclampsia?
• Between 2 and 3% of women develop pre-eclampsia
• If women have pre-existing hypertension, the number is nearer 15%

If you felt a head CT was necessary, how would you counsel the patient?
• Explain that the benefit is that we can give her more information about her headache to aid treatment if required
• Explain that the risk of radiation to the fetus is very small

A Case to Learn From

A woman on the postnatal ward developed a sudden-onset headache on day 1 following an emergency caesarean section. Initially she was thought to have a postdural puncture headache from her epidural but was still closely monitored given the broad range of differentials. She rapidly deteriorated and had a GCS of 8 an hour later. On CT, a massive subarachnoid haemorrhage was diagnosed. It is important to review patients with severe headache regularly, as the neurological picture can evolve quickly and patients can become unstable in a very short period of time.

 Top Tip

Always consider the patient as a whole and do not be guided by tests alone. If the woman has borderline blood pressure but very brisk reflexes, clonus and a mild headache, then she probably has pre-eclampsia. A full systematic examination is the only way not to miss clues.

STATION 7.2: HISTORY: REDUCED FETAL MOVEMENTS

SCENARIO

You are a junior doctor on the Obstetric Assessment Unit and have been asked to see Carol Grant, a 35-year-old woman, who has presented with reduced fetal movements. She is 34 weeks pregnant. Please take a history from Miss Grant, present your findings and formulate an appropriate management plan.

 Cardinal Symptoms

Absent movements
No response to usual triggers
Abdominal pain
Vaginal loss: Blood or amniotic fluid

HISTORY OF PRESENTING COMPLAINT

FETAL MOVEMENTS

- Normal pattern of movements: Frequency, strength
- Current movements: Frequency, strength
- Most recent movements: Date and time that movements were last felt
- Exacerbating or relieving factors: Lying down, cold drinks, sugary snacks

ASSOCIATED SYMPTOMS

Other symptoms to enquire about include:
- Concurrent illness: Viral, diarrhoea and vomiting, history of trauma
- Vaginal loss: Discharge, bleeding
- Pain: Abdominal pain, tightening sensation, pressure

CURRENT OBSTETRIC HISTORY

- Scans to date: Dating scan, anomaly scan, placental site, any additional scans and why
- Complications: Admissions to hospital, previous reduced movements
- Rhesus status: Should be taken at booking

PAST OBSTETRIC HISTORY

- Pregnancies to date: Year, livebirth, miscarriage, termination, mode of birth and birth weight
- Complications: Pre-eclampsia, haemorrhage, infections

PAST MEDICAL AND SURGICAL HISTORY

- General: Ask about known medical conditions, relevant treatments and any hospital admissions
- Abdominal surgery: Including caesarean sections and myomectomy
- Diabetes: A known risk factor for stillbirth
- Infections: Any immunosuppression can be a risk factor for stillbirth

MEDICATION HISTORY

Enquire about prescribed and over-the-counter medications, including any recent changes. Allergies should also be included with the specific reaction noted. In this scenario be aware of medications that:
- Increase bleeding risk: For example, aspirin or LMWH
- Alter blood sugar levels: Insulin

SOCIAL HISTORY

Social history includes enquiring about occupation, residence, lifestyle (diet, exercise, smoking, alcohol, substance abuse) and recent travel. Additionally in this scenario, consider:
- Smoking: A key reversible risk factor for pre-eclampsia and it increases the risk of stillbirth
- Drug use: Cocaine
- Living arrangements: Use this as an opportunity to enquire about domestic violence and ensure there is no abdominal injury

FAMILY HISTORY

Enquire about any significant family history, including:
- History of pre-eclampsia in first-degree relatives, as the risk is significantly increased

SYSTEMS REVIEW

On systems review, particularly pertinent questions to the above case may include questions regarding maternal physical well-being, that could affect fetal movements. These include:

- Fever: Relating to infection
- Dehydration: Secondary to viral illness or complications of other conditions; for example, diabetic keto-acidosis (DKA)
- Itching: Obstetric cholestasis, a liver disorder in pregnancy that is a risk factor for stillbirth

Risk Factors for Stillbirth

MATERNAL	FETAL	PLACENTAL
Age <20 or >40 years	Intrauterine growth restriction	Abruption
Obesity	Congenital anomalies	Cord prolapse
Social deprivation	Intrapartum causes	Cord entanglement
Smoking	Postmaturity	
Drug use	Fetal haemolytic disease	
Black and Asian ethnicity	Chromosomal abnormalities	
Pre-eclampsia	Infection	
Diabetes mellitus	Multiple pregnancies	
Obstetric cholestasis		
Systemic lupus erythematosus		
Thrombophilia		
Hypoperfusion; for example, sepsis		

INVESTIGATIONS IN STILLBIRTH

! Maternal investigations in stillbirth

Infection	• Temperature • Vaginal swab for group B streptococcus (GBS) • Bloods for toxoplasmosis, parvovirus, cytomegalovirus, rubella, *Listeria* and CRP
Fetomaternal haemorrhage	• Kleihauer
Pre-eclampsia	• Blood pressure • Urine dip • FBCs • Renal function • LFTs
Diabetes	• HbA1c • Blood glucose
Obstetric cholestasis	• Bile acids
Thrombophilia	• Anticardiolipin antibodies • Lupus anticoagulant • Antinuclear antibodies
Thyrotoxicosis	• Thyroid function tests (TFTs)

Fetal investigations in stillbirth

Postmortem	• Needs written consent
If postmortem declined	• Skin biopsy for karyotyping • Can consider X-rays or MRI if relevant

Placental investigations in stillbirth

Infection	Swabs from the surface
Karyotyping	Sent as a resected piece
Pathology	Histological analysis

Differential Diagnosis

CONDITION	CLINICAL PRESENTATION	INVESTIGATIONS	MANAGEMENT
Stillbirth	• Absent fetal movements	• Listen to the fetal heart with Pinard or Doppler • If absent, confirm with ultrasound scan as soon as possible	• Condolences to the family • Discuss mode of birth and investigations
Single episode of reduced movements, now resolved	• A period of reduced movements, now normal	• CTG	• Arrange growth scan if the patient has not had one within 2 weeks • Advise patient to present if there are any further episodes
Maternal illness	• May have dehydration secondary to fever, intercurrent illness or complications of an ongoing condition; for example, diabetes	• CTG • Maternal observations • Consider bloods: FBCs, U&Es and C- reactive protein (CRP)	• Rehydrate the mother • Monitor the fetus

Present Your Findings

Miss Grant is a 35-year-old woman who is 34 weeks pregnant and has presented with reduced fetal movements for 6 h. This is her first pregnancy and the pregnancy has been uncomplicated until now with normal scans, screening tests and blood pressure. Her movements have been normal since coming to hospital and the CTG shows normal fetal heart activity. She is well in herself and has no underlying health problems.

As her movements are now normal, I am going to discharge her from hospital, but I have arranged for a growth scan and advised her to return to hospital if this occurs again.

❓ QUESTIONS AND ANSWERS FOR CANDIDATE

What would you do if a fetal heart could not be located when the patient arrived?

- Explain that you could not hear the heart beat, but that you were going to leave the patient to get an ultrasound scan
- This should be performed in a single room, by a doctor, midwife or sonographer who is competent to do so
- If there is no fetal heart activity, this should be explained to the patient clearly and a second practitioner should confirm the findings as soon as possible

Do movements reduce at term?

- No, baby's movements do not reduce at term.
- The nature of the movements may change, but not the frequency

Why should a growth scan be arranged for women if they have reduced fetal movements?

- Measuring the women's symphysis–fundal height (SFH) is not accurate enough to use as a measure of fetal well-being in women with reduced fetal movements

 A Case to Learn From

A woman presented to the Obstetric Assessment Unit with 24 h of reduced fetal movements. She had been reassured by hearing her baby's heart beat at home with a home Sonicaid, but a friend had told her to attend the hospital. On arrival, the CTG showed a fetal bradycardia, which did not recover. An emergency caesarean section was carried out and a baby girl was delivered in poor condition. When talking to patients, make sure you inform them that home Sonicaids can provide false reassurance and they should not be used.

 Top Tip

Reduced fetal movements is a common presentation that can have many causes. One of these is domestic violence, so make sure you screen for it with every woman you review.

STATION 7.3: HISTORY: ANXIOUS PREGNANT WOMAN

SCENARIO

You are a junior doctor in the antenatal clinic and your next patient is Georgina Gordon, a 32-year-old woman who has been referred with increasing anxiety. She is 30 weeks pregnant and this is her first pregnancy. Please take a history from Miss Gordon and formulate an appropriate management plan.

 Cardinal Symptoms

Obsessional ideas

Lack of engagement with services

Denial of pregnancy

Suicidal ideation

Thoughts of harming the baby

HISTORY OF PRESENTING COMPLAINT

- Anxiety trigger: Specific worry or general anxiety
- Duration: Days, weeks or months, constant or intermittent
- Triggers: Lack of sleep, hospital appointments, arguments with friends or family
- Alleviating factors: Talking therapies; for example, counselling or cognitive behavioural therapy (CBT), medication, exercise, alternative treatments; for example, reiki, acupuncture
- Severity: Self-harm, suicidal ideation

ASSOCIATED SYMPTOMS

Other symptoms to enquire about include:
- Physical features: Shortness of breath, sweatiness, palpitations and tremors

CURRENT OBSTETRIC HISTORY

- Scans to date: Dating scan, anomaly scan, placental site, any additional scans and why
- Complications: Admissions to hospital, previous bleeding
- Rhesus status: Should be taken at booking

PAST OBSTETRIC HISTORY

- Pregnancies to date: Year, livebirth, miscarriage, termination, mode of birth, birth weight
- Complications: Pre-eclampsia, haemorrhage, infections
- Mental health history in pregnancies and postnatally: 'Baby blues', postnatal depression, anxiety and psychosis

PAST MEDICAL AND SURGICAL HISTORY

- General: Ask about known medical conditions, relevant treatments and any hospital admissions
- Mental health
  - If the patient had been known to mental health services before at any stage of life
  - History of eating disorders
  - Previously diagnosed with any mental health conditions
  - Previous admissions as an inpatient, whether voluntarily or under the Mental Health Act

MEDICATION HISTORY

Enquire about prescribed and over-the-counter medications, including any recent changes. Allergies should also be included with the specific reaction noted.

In this scenario ask about:

- Medications tried in the past for mental health and their response
- Any previous use of electroconvulsive therapy (ECT) and its effect

SOCIAL HISTORY

Social history includes enquiring about occupation, residence, lifestyle (diet, exercise, smoking, alcohol, substance abuse) and recent travel. Additionally in this scenario, consider asking in detail about:

- Social support: Does she have a good social support network; for example, friends and family? Is there a history of domestic violence?
- Stressors: For example, housing situation, immigration status, language barriers and other additional stressors are associated with worse outcome for mothers and babies
- Occupation: Expectations of workplace, hours involved, shift work
- Substance use: Smoking, alcohol and drug use that may increase anxiety and paranoia; for example, cannabis

- Previous involvement with social services: As a child or an adult
- History of childhood abuse: If this has not been disclosed before, be aware that this may need to be reported if children remain at risk

FAMILY HISTORY

It is important to ask about family history when assessing mental health risk to pregnant women. In particular:

- Family members (first-degree) with postnatal depression or psychosis
- Family members (first-degree) with bipolar disorder

SYSTEMS REVIEW

Remember to ask about physical manifestations of anxiety:

- Neurological: Headaches, dizziness
- Cardiovascular: Palpitations, chest pain, syncope
- Respiratory: Shortness of breath
- Gastrointestinal: Bloating, constipation, diarrhoea, nausea

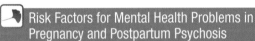

Risk Factors for Mental Health Problems in Pregnancy and Postpartum Psychosis

- First-degree relative with postpartum psychosis
- Bipolar disorder
- Schizophrenia
- New-onset psychological disturbance during pregnancy
- Single parent or poor couple relationship
- Low levels of social support
- Recent stressful life events
- Socioeconomic disadvantage
- Teenage pregnancy
- Early emotional or childhood abuse
- Unwanted pregnancy

Differential Diagnosis

DISEASE	CLINICAL PRESENTATION	INVESTIGATIONS	MANAGEMENT
Thyrotoxicosis	• Excess sweating • Heat intolerance • Weight loss • Palpitations • Diarrhoea	• TFTs	• Radioactive iodine • Beta-blockers
Anaemia	• Shortness of breath • Pallor • Dizziness	• FBCs	• Iron or blood transfusion • B_{12} injections if it is B_{12} deficiency anaemia
Cardiac arrhythmias	• Palpitations • Shortness of breath	• Electrocardiogram (ECG) • Electrolytes • TFTs	• Dependent on the type of cardiac arrhythmia
Drug withdrawal	Withdrawal symptoms: • Tremor • Agitation • Confusion	• Toxicology screen • ECG	• Dependent on the substance withdrawn from

Concerns With Mental Health In Pregnancy

From UK data:

- 23% of the women who died had a mental health-related cause
- One in seven maternal deaths were due to suicide
- Almost one-quarter were known to social services
- 17% were known to have a history of domestic abuse
- If the women who died had become ill at the time when the report was published, only 25% would have access to the highest standard of perinatal mental healthcare
- Unfortunately, 44% of women were found to have had care that, if improved, would have improved the outcome

 Present Your Findings

Miss Gordon is a 32-year-old woman who is currently 30 weeks pregnant in her first pregnancy. She has presented with new-onset symptoms of anxiety. Her main anxiety is around childbirth and what to expect. She has found herself losing sleep over this and her partner is also concerned. She has no previous mental health history of note and no significant family history. Her partner is very supportive, and she has family living nearby with whom she has felt able to share her concerns.

She has no red-flag symptoms at this time.

I have arranged for Miss Gordon to access CBT and discussed some pregnancy support groups. I will see her again in 2 weeks to see how she is managing but have given her and her partner telephone numbers to call if they think that she is deteriorating before that time.

? QUESTIONS AND ANSWERS FOR CANDIDATE

How should suicidal ideation be explored?

Some useful questions are:

- Have you ever felt so low/anxious/depressed/panicked that you have considered harming yourself or ending your own or your baby's life?
- If yes, do you have a plan for how you would do this?
- Have you already tried?
- What stopped you on that occasion?

What help is available for women with mental health problems in pregnancy?

- Health professionals: Primary care doctors, midwife, obstetrician, specialist perinatal teams
- Psychological therapies: CBT, counselling
- Pharmacology: Antidepressants, anxiolytics, antipsychotics
- Charitable organisations: For example, Tommy's

What is a Mother and Baby Unit (MBU)?

- A specialist unit available for women who have mental health needs in pregnancy, where they can get specialist input from psychiatrists, mental health nurses and many allied health professionals

 A Case to Learn From

A woman committed suicide a few months after giving birth. She had disclosed her previous history of mental health disorder in late pregnancy and presented postnatally with low mood and anxiety. A referral was made to mental health services. Shortly afterwards she attempted suicide and reported seeing intrusive violent images. She was referred by the midwifery team to the crisis team but was still managed at home. She contacted the crisis team before her death to express suicidal intent but had died by the time services arrived.

The focus of this woman's treatment was on cognitive approaches to deal with her intrusive thoughts, despite evidence of psychotic symptoms. Cognitive therapies will not work in isolation for psychosis and medication will be required. As she had clear intent of suicide and psychotic symptoms, this woman should have been admitted to an MBU ideally, or an inpatient mental health hospital, to have intensive treatment.

 Top Tip

Women often hide anxiety or domestic violence. If you actively look for it routinely, you'll pick up the hidden cases.

STATION 7.4: HISTORY: ANTEPARTUM HAEMORRHAGE

SCENARIO

You are a junior doctor on the labour ward and have been asked to see Priya Patel, a 28-year-old woman, who has presented with vaginal bleeding. She is 30 weeks pregnant. Please take a history from Mrs Patel and establish a differential diagnosis.

 Cardinal Symptoms

Abdominal pain

Vaginal bleeding

Reduced fetal movements

May be a history of trauma

Rupture of membranes

HISTORY OF PRESENTING COMPLAINT

- Quantity: For example, number of soaked pads, egg cups, spoonful
- Any clots passed: May signify very heavy bleeding or old blood loss
- Precipitating factors: Trauma, local or systemic infection, sexual intercourse

ASSOCIATED SYMPTOMS

Other symptoms to enquire about include:

- Pain: Abdominal or back pain may suggest abruption or labour
- Fetal movements: Whether they are as per normal
- Rupture of membranes: May suggest labour

CURRENT OBSTETRIC HISTORY

- Scans to date: Dating scan, anomaly scan, placental site, any additional scans and why
- Complications: Admissions to hospital, previous bleeding
- Rhesus status: Important in case the patient needs anti-D; may have had free fetal deoxyribonucleic acid (DNA) testing

PAST OBSTETRIC HISTORY

- Pregnancies to date: Year, livebirth, miscarriage, termination, mode of birth, birth weight
- Complications: Pre-eclampsia, haemorrhage, infections

PAST MEDICAL, SURGICAL AND GYNAECOLOGICAL HISTORY

- General: Ask about known medical conditions, relevant treatments and any hospital admissions
- Uterine surgery: Caesarean section and myomectomy increase the risk of uterine rupture
- Abdominal surgery: If planning an emergency surgery, you will have to anticipate adhesions if there has been any previous surgery
- Cervical smears: Up to date, any abnormal tests before

MEDICATION HISTORY

Enquire about prescribed and over-the-counter medications, including any recent changes. Allergies should also be included with the specific reaction noted. In this scenario be aware of medications that:

- Increase bleeding risk: For example, aspirin, LMWH

SOCIAL HISTORY

Social history includes enquiring about occupation, residence, lifestyle (diet, exercise, smoking, alcohol, substance abuse) and recent travel. Additionally in this scenario, consider:

- Drug use: Cocaine can increase the risk of placental abruption
- Smoking: Risk factor for placental abruption
- Domestic violence: One-third of domestic violence starts in pregnancy

FAMILY HISTORY

Enquire about significant family history, including:

- Conditions associated with bleeding; for example, haemophilia. However, these are unlikely to present for the first time in pregnancy

SYSTEMS REVIEW

On systems review, particularly pertinent questions to the above case may include questions regarding symptoms of hypovolaemic shock. These include:

- Dizziness
- Palpitations
- Shortness of breath
- Clamminess

Risk Factors for Placental Abruption

- Smoking
- Hypertension
- Increasing parity
- Increasing maternal age
- Trauma
- Cocaine use
- External cephalic version (ECV)

Differential Diagnosis

CONDITION	CLINICAL PRESENTATION	INVESTIGATIONS	MANAGEMENT
Placental abruption	• Pain and bleeding • May have reduced fetal movements • May have 'woody' uterus to palpate • Can present with stillbirth	• FBCs • Clotting and fibrinogen • CTG • Cross-match	• Intravenous (IV) access • Most likely emergency caesarean section if not in labour and suspected large abruption
Placenta praevia	• Painless bleeding, may be very heavy	• FBCs • Clotting and fibrinogen • CTG • Cross-match	• IV access • Emergency caesarean section if heavy bleeding
Vasa praevia	• Painless bleeding – small amount • Extreme fetal distress • Stillbirth	• FBCs • Group and save • CTG	• IV access • Emergency caesarean section if fetus is alive
Marginal placental bleed	• Predominantly bleeding • May have some period-type pain	• FBCs • Group and save • CTG	• IV access • Can normally manage conservatively • Consider steroids for fetal lung maturity
Cervical ectropion	• Painless bleeding	• Speculum • CTG	• Can reassure the patient that there is no risk to her or baby

MANAGEMENT OF AN ANTEPARTUM HAEMORRHAGE

- Manage like any other bleeding scenario using ABCDE
- The risk to the mother's life takes priority over that of the fetus at all times
- Remember anti-D for Rhesus-negative women
- Only the most serious and common causes are listed above, but don't forget non-obstetric causes; for example, vaginal trauma, cervical cancer or polyps, coagulopathy

 Present Your Findings

Mrs Patel is a 28-year-old woman who presents with an antepartum haemorrhage. She is 30 weeks pregnant in her first pregnancy. Her pregnancy has been uneventful so far and she is Rhesus-positive. She describes passing around 500 mL of blood over the last 3 h and she has not felt any fetal movements during this time. This is on a background of being normally fit and well.

I feel the most likely diagnosis is placental abruption, with the differentials being placenta praevia or vasa praevia. I would like to examine Mrs Patel fully, establish IV access and check her observations. I would like to send FBCs, clotting screen and fibrinogen and cross-match her for 4 units of blood. I would like a CTG to assess fetal well-being and to involve senior obstetricians and anaesthetists in case of an emergency caesarean section.

❓ QUESTIONS AND ANSWERS FOR CANDIDATE

Are there any tests for placental abruption?
- No, placental abruption is a clinical diagnosis and you would not wait for ultrasound scans or blood tests to confirm it

How would you assess fetal well-being?
- Ask about fetal movements
- Listen for the fetal heart with a Doppler or Pinard stethoscope
- If a fetal heart was present, you would perform a CTG

What is the difference between placenta praevia and vasa praevia?
- Placenta praevia is where the placenta covers the internal os of the cervix
- Vasa praevia is when placental vessels carrying fetal blood across the cervix

 A Case to Learn From

A woman presented from home at 35 weeks pregnant with a small antepartum haemorrhage. She was haemodynamically stable and around 100 mL of blood was on her pad. On arrival, her CTG was very abnormal, indicating fetal distress.

Due to the CTG and bleeding, an emergency caesarean section took place 20 min after she presented. There was a blood clot of 1000 mL in the uterus and placental abruption was diagnosed. Mothers can have concealed bleeds, and be much more unwell than the amount of reported bleeding suggests

 Top Tip

Young people can maintain their blood pressure despite significant blood loss. Don't let this mislead you in the context of signs of significant fetal distress or placental pathology.

STATION 7.5: HISTORY: VAGINAL DISCHARGE

SCENARIO

You are a junior doctor in the gynaecology outpatient clinic and have been asked to see Diane Bruce, a 39-year-old woman, who is complaining of vaginal discharge. Please take a history from Ms Bruce, present your findings and formulate an appropriate management plan.

 Cardinal Symptoms

Purulent discharge

Abdominal or pelvic pain

New sexual partner

Postcoital bleeding

HISTORY OF PRESENTING COMPLAINT

- Onset: Sudden or gradual
- Character:
  - Colour: Clear, yellow, green, blood-stained
  - Odour: Odourless, fishy, foul-smelling
  - Consistency: Watery, thick, sticky
- Duration: Days or weeks
- Exacerbating or relieving factors: For example, sexual intercourse, tampon use
- Previous episodes: Previous diagnoses or treatment

ASSOCIATED SYMPTOMS

Other symptoms to enquire about include:
- Itch or vulval pain: Intermittent or constant
- Abdominal or pelvic pain: Radiation
- Constitutional symptoms: Malaise or fever

SEXUAL HISTORY

- Sexual partners: Most recent sexual contacts in the last 3–6 months
- Type of intercourse: Oral, vaginal, anal
- Contraception used: Barrier and/or hormonal
- Previous sexually transmitted infections: For example, chlamydia or gonorrhoea
- Does the partner(s) have any symptoms? Discharge, itching

PAST GYNAECOLOGICAL HISTORY

- Last menstrual period: Note if it was different to normal; for example, heavier or lighter, bled for a longer or shorter period of time
- Menstruation history: Regularity of cycles, intermenstrual bleeding

- Contraception history: Used in the past or currently using, particularly intrauterine device (IUD)
- Cervical smear status: If up to date and any abnormalities diagnosed
- Gynaecological surgeries: Laparoscopies, sterilisation surgery
- Previous pregnancies:
  - Livebirths and mode of birth, as well as any pregnancy complications
  - Miscarriages and their management, any investigations
  - Terminations of pregnancy and their management (medical or surgical)
  - Ectopic pregnancies and their management (medical or surgical)
- Fertility treatment: For example, in vitro fertilisation (IVF)

PAST MEDICAL AND SURGICAL HISTORY

- General: Ask about known medical conditions, relevant treatments and any hospital admissions
- Uterine surgery: Any recent instrumentation of the uterus; for example, coil insertion, termination of pregnancy

MEDICATION HISTORY

Enquire about prescribed and over-the-counter medications, including any recent changes. Allergies should also be included with the specific reaction noted. In this scenario be aware of medications that:

- Affect vaginal flora: For example, antibiotics or immunosuppressants

- Changes to contraceptives: Which may affect vaginal discharge

SOCIAL HISTORY

Social history includes enquiring about occupation, residence, lifestyle (diet, exercise, smoking, alcohol, substance abuse) and recent travel. Additionally in this scenario, consider:

- Risk assessment for HIV and other blood-borne viruses: Ask about sexual history, IV drug use, tattoos, piercings, blood transfusions and episodes in prison

FAMILY HISTORY

Enquire about any significant family history.

SYSTEMS REVIEW

On systems review, particularly pertinent questions to the above case may include questions regarding systemic diseases. These include:

- Fever: Relating to infection
- Right upper-quadrant pain: Relating to perihepatic adhesions or Fitz-Hugh–Curtis syndrome
- Increased thirst or polyuria: New diagnosis of diabetes

Risk Factors for Pelvic Inflammatory Disease (PID)

- Recent IUD insertion (within 4 weeks)
- Multiple sexual partners
- Immunodeficiency

Differential Diagnosis

DISEASE	CLINICAL PRESENTATION	INVESTIGATIONS	MANAGEMENT
Candida albicans	• Curdy, thick discharge • Vulval itching and soreness • Vulval oedema • Superficial dyspareunia	• High vaginal swab (HVS) culture • Vaginal pH; normal reference range is 4.0–4.5	• Topical or oral antifungal treatment; for example, clotrimazole • Cotton underwear • Avoid irritants
Bacterial vaginosis	• Fishy white or grey discharge • Worse after sex	Amsel criteria (three of the four): • Characteristic discharge • Clue cells on microscopy • pH >4.5 • Fishy odour when adding alkali to slide	• Metronidazole • Clindamycin • Avoid douching and strongly perfumed products
Trichomonas	• Frothy, yellow, offensive discharge • Strawberry cervix • Itching • Abdominal pain and dysuria	• Wet smear slide • Polymerase chain reaction-based swab	• Metronidazole • Avoid sexual intercourse until both partners have been treated
Gonorrhoea	• Mucopurulent vaginal discharge • Abdominal pain • Dysuria • Postcoital and intermenstrual bleeding	• Endocervical swabs – nucleic acid amplification tests (NAATs)	• Full sexual health screen • Ceftriaxone 500 mg intramuscular (IM)
Chlamydia	• Purulent discharge • Abdominal pain • Dysuria • Postcoital and intermenstrual bleeding	• Endocervical swabs – NAATs	• Full sexual health screen • Azithromycin 1 g orally (PO) statum (stat) • Doxycycline 100 mg PO twice daily (BD) for 7days

PELVIC INFLAMMATORY DISEASE AND SUBFERTILITY

If untreated, PID can lead to irreversible tubal damage. The most likely causative organisms are chlamydia or gonorrhoea, which lead to salpingitis (inflammation of the fallopian tubes). Twenty per cent of women with a chlamydial infection will have a degree of PID and 3% will develop subfertility. The likelihood of tubal damage is increased with the number of episodes of PID and the time taken for treatment.

Tubal damage from PID may be diagnosed during investigations for subfertility, either at laparoscopy or hysterosalpingogram, where blocked fallopian tubes will be demonstrated. It is important that women have swabs taken before these investigations, as active infection should be treated before further intervention.

If the tubes are blocked, treatment options may be:

- Unilateral or bilateral salpingectomy, followed by IVF
- Tubal surgery

Women with blocked fallopian tubes from PID should be warned that they have an increased risk of an ectopic pregnancy if they do conceive and the relevant signs and symptoms to look for.

 Present Your Findings

Ms Bruce is a 39-year-old woman who has been referred to the gynaecology clinic with vaginal discharge. This has been present for around 3 months and she has never had it before. She describes the discharge as grey, with a fishy smell that is worse after sexual intercourse. Ms Bruce is fit and well, with no other health problems. She is up to date with her smear tests. She has had a regular sexual partner for 1 year and they use condoms for contraception.

I think the most likely diagnosis is bacterial vaginosis; however, I would like to examine Ms Bruce, perform an abdominal, speculum and bimanual examination, and perform a HVS and NAATs swab to exclude other infections.

❓ QUESTIONS AND ANSWERS FOR CANDIDATE

What is the link between vaginal douching and bacterial vaginosis?

- The pH of the vagina should be less than 4.5
- Feminine washes and douches can affect this balance, allowing lactobacilli to be replaced by other bacteria; for example, *Gardnerella vaginalis*, an anaerobic organism

What would make you more suspicious that the patient may have a sexually transmitted infection?

- A history of multiple sexual partners
- No barrier contraception being used
- New onset of purulent discharge and pelvic pain

How would you approach the issue of informing the patient's partner about the diagnosis?

- You cannot tell them, but you would encourage her to do so if treatment is going to be required
- Health advisors at the local sexual health clinic can help with this, as they are experienced at contact tracing in these situations

 A Case to Learn From

A young woman was admitted with symptoms of dyspareunia and pelvic pain. An ultrasound was unremarkable and so a diagnostic laparoscopy was carried out, showing dense pelvic and perihepatic adhesions. Her NAAT swab confirmed a chlamydia infection. Remember, women with pelvic infections may not present with discharge as their main symptom. In fact, chlamydia can be completely asymptomatic.

 Top Tip

Ask the doctors on your placement to show you the different types of swab so that you are familiar with them if you are given them in an OSCE station. There are different swabs for bacterial, viral and specific sexually transmitted infections.

STATION 7.6: HISTORY: POSTMENOPAUSAL BLEEDING

SCENARIO

You are a junior doctor in the gynaecology clinic and have been asked to see Bethany Bates, a 68-year-old woman, who has come in with postmenopausal bleeding. Please take a history from Mrs Bates, present your findings and formulate an appropriate management plan.

🚶 **Cardinal Symptoms**

Blood loss
Weight loss
Bloating
Vulval soreness/itching
Pain exacerbated on moving

HISTORY OF PRESENTING COMPLAINT

- Volume: Spotting, like a period, flooding
- Frequency: Single episode, regular occurrence
- Consistency: Fresh red blood, clots
- Precipitating factors: Sexual intercourse, physical activity, starting medication (tamoxifen, anticoagulants)

ASSOCIATED SYMPTOMS

Other symptoms to enquire about include:
- Weight loss: Unintentional, loss of appetite
- Bloating: Clothes getting gradually tighter, feeling full
- Vulval soreness or itching: May be related to dermatological conditions, e.g. lichen sclerosus

PAST GYNAECOLOGICAL HISTORY

- Menstruation: Age of menarche, age of menopause, problems with periods in the past
- Cervical smears: If up to date, any abnormalities diagnosed
- Parity: Total pregnancies as well as livebirths, mode of birth
- Gynaecological surgery: Hysteroscopies, endometrial ablations, hysterectomy
- Polycystic ovarian syndrome: What kind of treatment the patient is on
- Sexually transmitted infections (STIs): For example, chlamydia, gonorrhoea

PAST MEDICAL AND SURGICAL HISTORY

- General: Ask about known medical conditions, relevant treatments and any hospital admissions
- Malignancy: Any malignancy may cause the above presentation, but gynaecological malignancies, breast cancer and bowel cancer are important to enquire about both here, and in the family history
- Obesity: Ask about current weight, calculate the body mass index (BMI), and ask about any history of previous obesity
- Liver disease: Cirrhosis leads to decreased degradation of circulating oestrogen, therefore increases the risk of endometrial cancer

MEDICATION HISTORY

Enquire about prescribed and over-the-counter medications, including any recent changes. Allergies should also be included with the specific reaction noted. In this scenario be aware of medications that:
- Increase bleeding risk: Warfarin, aspirin, clopidogrel, rivaroxaban
- Increase risk of endometrial cancer: Hormone replacement therapy (HRT) – oestrogen only, tamoxifen
- Decrease risk of endometrial cancer: Combined oral contraceptive pill (COCP), continuous combined HRT

SOCIAL HISTORY

Social history includes enquiring about occupation, residence, lifestyle (diet, exercise, smoking, alcohol, substance abuse) and recent travel. Additionally in this scenario, consider:
- Smoking: Cigarette smoking is protective for endometrial cancer due to its antioestrogenic effect
- Change in sexual partner: Increased risk of new STI

FAMILY HISTORY

Enquire about any significant family history, including:
- History of bowel cancer: Hereditary non-polyposis colorectal cancer (HNPCC or Lynch syndrome) carries a 40–60% risk of endometrial cancer

SYSTEMS REVIEW

On systems review, particularly pertinent questions to the above case may include questions regarding other possible gynaecological causes (Fig. 7.1). These include:
- Night sweats: Relating to malignancy
- Jaundice or itching: Relating to liver disease
- Vulval itching or soreness: Relating to local vulval dermatoses
- Pelvic pain: relating to PID

Risk Factors for Endometrial Cancer

Risk factor	Further information
Age	Peak incidence is 65–75 years old
Early menarche or late menopause	Increased exposure to oestrogen
Parity	Pregnancy reduces the risk by 30% after the first birth, then 25% for each subsequent birth
Obesity	36% of endometrial cancer is related to obesity
HRT	If oestrogen only
Liver cirrhosis	Decreased oestrogen breakdown
Polycystic ovarian syndrome	Increased anovulatory cycles, therefore more unopposed oestrogen
Hereditary nonpolyposis colorectal cancer (HNPCC)	40–60% risk
Tamoxifen	Oestrogen modulator

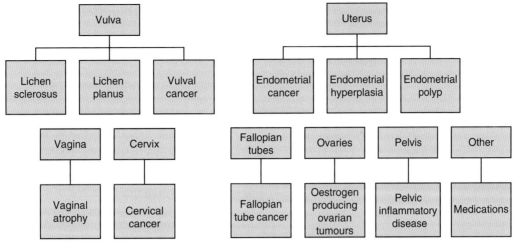

Fig. 7.1 Causes of postmenopausal bleeding.

Differential Diagnosis

DISEASE	CLINICAL PRESENTATION	INVESTIGATIONS	MANAGEMENT
Endometrial cancer	• Painless bleeding; may be a small amount only	• Transvaginal ultrasound scan • Endometrial biopsy	• Hysterectomy and bilateral salpingo-oophorectomy (BSO) • May need radiotherapy
Endometrial hyperplasia	• Painless bleeding, may be a small amount only	• Transvaginal ultrasound scan • Endometrial biopsy	• Consider local progesterone (Mirena coil) • Can consider hysterectomy and BSO
Endometrial polyp	• Painless bleeding, may be a small amount only	• Transvaginal ultrasound scan • Endometrial biopsy • Hysteroscopy	• Polypectomy at the time of hysteroscopy
Vaginal atrophy	• Bleeding can occur after sexual intercourse • Dryness • Soreness	• Speculum examination	• Topical oestrogen cream
Vulval skin conditions, e.g. lichen sclerosus or planus	• Vulval sores • Vulval itching • Bleeding after scratching or sexual intercourse	• Vulval examination (may be too sore to pass a speculum)	• Vulval hygiene advice • Topical steroid ointment

Present Your Findings

Mrs Bates is a 68-year-old woman who presents with a single episode of postmenopausal bleeding which occurred 3 weeks ago. She describes no intentional weight loss or history of malignancy. She has a BMI of 42 and was previously diagnosed with polycystic ovarian syndrome. She has had no children. She is otherwise fit and well.

I feel the most likely diagnosis is endometrial cancer, with other differentials being endometrial hyperplasia or vaginal atrophy. I would like to examine Mrs Bates fully, arrange an urgent transvaginal ultrasound scan and perform an endometrial biopsy.

❓ QUESTIONS AND ANSWERS FOR CANDIDATE

How is an endometrial biopsy performed?
• In the outpatient clinic, while performing a speculum examination, using a small Pipelle sampler

• A hysteroscopy can be carried out to visualise the endometrium directly and a biopsy can be taken at this time (a curettage)

What thickness of endometrium on transvaginal ultrasound would be associated with pathology?
• The accepted thickness at which a biopsy would need to be taken is 4 mm

What is the risk of endometrial hyperplasia progressing to an endometrial cancer?
• If there is no atypia, the chance of progression is less than 5% over 20 years; however, treatment with progesterone (Mirena coil or oral) would be recommended with 6-monthly follow-up
• If atypia is present, the risk is much higher and cancer is diagnosed in up to 43% of these women, who end up having a hysterectomy

A Case to Learn From

An elderly woman was admitted to the gynaecology ward from home with heavy vaginal bleeding. Her transvaginal scan showed that she had a thin normal endometrium. The nurses looking after her reported that her overnight pads were often blood-soaked. On further investigation, she had frank haematuria and had a bladder cancer. It is important to think outside the box in patients when no obvious cause can be found, particularly in those who may not be able to give a thorough history.

 Top Tip

Remember, some women will feel uncomfortable discussing vaginal bleeding and may have had several episodes before they have visited a doctor. Listen to the patient describe the problem in their own words, rather than using overly medicalised terms such as 'vulva' or 'introitus'. Take your time and use appropriate language for the patient in front of you.

STATION 7.7: HISTORY: PAIN IN EARLY PREGNANCY

SCENARIO

You are a junior doctor on the gynaecology ward and have been asked to see Alice Arden, a 24-year-old woman who has presented with abdominal pain and is 6 weeks pregnant. Her primary care doctor has referred her to the hospital. Please take a history from Miss Arden, present your findings and formulate an appropriate management plan.

 Cardinal Symptoms

Severe unilateral pain
Shoulder tip pain
Pain exacerbated on moving

HISTORY OF PRESENTING COMPLAINT

- Site: Unilateral, generalised
- Onset: Sudden, insidious
- Character: Throbbing, aching, stabbing
- Radiation: Shoulder tip, into the back, to the tops of thighs or hip
- Associations: Vaginal bleeding, fever, malaise, change in bladder or bowel function
- Timing: First occurrence, constant, intermittent
- Exacerbating or relieving factors: Analgesia, movement
- Severity: 1–10 pain scale, analgesia use

ASSOCIATED SYMPTOMS

Other symptoms to enquire about include:
- Bleeding: Any bleeding since the positive pregnancy test
- Changes in bowel habit: Any constipation or diarrhoea, pain opening bowels (dyschezia)
- Nausea or vomiting: Duration and frequency
- Urinary symptoms: Dysuria, increased frequency

CURRENT OBSTETRIC HISTORY

- Date of positive pregnancy test
- Planned or unplanned

PAST GYNAECOLOGICAL HISTORY

- Last menstrual period: Important to know the current cycle
- Menstruation history: Regularity of cycles, intermenstrual bleeding
- Contraception history: Used in the past or currently using, particularly IUD
- Cervical smear status: If up to date, and any abnormalities diagnosed
- Gynaecological surgeries: Laparoscopies, sterilisation surgery
- Previous pregnancies:
  - Livebirths, mode of birth, any pregnancy complications
  - Miscarriages and their management, any investigations
  - Terminations of pregnancy and their management (medical or surgical)
  - Ectopic pregnancies and their management (medical or surgical)
- STIs: Infections can impact on fertility
- Fertility treatment: Patients may have already had scans

PAST MEDICAL AND SURGICAL HISTORY

- General: Ask about known medical conditions, relevant treatments and any hospital admissions
- Surgical: For example, appendectomy and laparoscopies

MEDICATION HISTORY

Enquire about prescribed and over-the-counter medications, including any recent changes. Allergies should also be included with the specific reaction noted. In this scenario be aware of medications:
- Contraindicated in pregnancy: For example, ibuprofen

SOCIAL HISTORY

Social history includes enquiring about occupation, residence, lifestyle (diet, exercise, smoking, alcohol, substance abuse) and recent travel. Additionally in this scenario, consider:
- Living arrangements: Who does the patient have for support?
- Domestic violence: Important to ask about in any woman presenting with abdominal pain
- Smoking: Increased risk of miscarriage

FAMILY HISTORY

Enquire about any significant family history, including:
- History of pregnancy complications in first-degree relatives

SYSTEMS REVIEW

On systems review, particularly pertinent questions to the above case may include questions regarding possible intra-abdominal bleeding secondary to an ectopic pregnancy, infection secondary to urinary tract infection or appendicitis. These include:

- Fever: Relating to infection
- Loss of appetite: Decreased or increased appetite
- Shoulder tip pain: Associated with diaphragmatic irritation due to intra-abdominal blood

Risk Factors for Ectopic Pregnancy

- Previous ectopic pregnancy
- Tubal damage from infection or surgery
- Intrauterine contraceptive devices
- Smoking
- Infertility treatment
- Extremes of reproductive age

HCG MONITORING

It is usually not possible to see an intrauterine pregnancy until the blood level of hCG reaches 1500 IU. Therefore, in very early pregnancies, the ultrasound report may say, 'An ectopic pregnancy cannot be excluded'.

If the index of suspicion remains high, then hCG monitoring must take place. This involves a blood hCG level on the day of presentation and a repeat level 48 h later.

- An ongoing intrauterine pregnancy will usually result in a doubling of hCG level over 48 h
- A falling pregnancy will usually see a fall in hCG levels

- An ectopic pregnancy will usually result in a rise of less than 60%

In any case, if the hCG level is above 1500 IU and no intrauterine pregnancy has been seen, an ectopic should be highly suspected.

Present Your Findings

Miss Arden is a 24-year-old woman who is 6 weeks pregnant. She has had left iliac fossa pain for 24 h and it is increasing in severity. She has had no symptoms of fever or loss of appetite. She does not have any shoulder tip pain. She is fit and well at present but has previously been treated for chlamydia.

I feel the most likely diagnosis is an ectopic pregnancy, with the possible differential diagnosis of an ovarian cyst accident. I would like to examine Miss Arden and send bloods for an FBC and hCG. I would also like to perform a urine dipstick and arrange a transvaginal ultrasound scan.

QUESTIONS AND ANSWERS FOR CANDIDATE

Name three potential sites for ectopic pregnancy.

- Fallopian tube: 98% of ectopic pregnancies
- Interstitial tubal area (where the tube meets the myometrium): 1–2%
- Cornual: within a rudimentary horn of a bicornuate uterus
- Ovary
- Previous uterine surgery scar: For example, caesarean section
- Abdominal: Can be anywhere within the peritoneum
- Cervix
- Heterotopic: When an intrauterine pregnancy is present at the same time as an ectopic pregnancy

Differential Diagnosis

CONDITION	CLINICAL PRESENTATION	INVESTIGATIONS	MANAGEMENT
Ectopic pregnancy	• Unilateral, sharp pain • May have shoulder tip pain	• FBCs • Human chorionic gonadotrophin (hCG) • Transvaginal ultrasound scan	Surgical management: • Salpingectomy or salpingotomy Medical management: • Methotrexate
Ovarian cyst accident	• Usually unilateral • Character of pain can vary	• Transvaginal ultrasound scan	If it is a cyst rupture: • Analgesia onlyIf it is ovarian torsion: • Laparoscopy
Urinary tract infection	• Pain may be generalised or unilateral • Often accompanied by dysuria or frequency	• Urine dipstick • Midstream specimen of urine	• Oral antibiotics
Appendicitis	• Centralised pain, settling to right iliac fossa • Loss of appetite • Pyrexia	• FBC • CRP • Ultrasound scan	• Laparoscopic appendicectomy

What are the management options for an ectopic pregnancy?

- Conservative: Women must be asymptomatic and be willing to have regular close follow-up
- Medical: Methotrexate
- Surgical: Salpingectomy (removal of affected fallopian tube) or salpingotomy (incision of tube and removal of ectopic pregnancy)

What antibiotics should be used if a urinary tract infection is diagnosed?

- Be guided by microbiology results but avoid trimethoprim, as this is a folate antagonist and should not be used in the first trimester

 A Case to Learn From

A woman was admitted with pelvic pain in pregnancy but had a very low hCG result. The on-call doctor thought this risk of an ectopic pregnancy was low. While waiting for an ultrasound scan to confirm this, the patient became haemodynamically unstable and was transferred to theatre where a ruptured tubal ectopic pregnancy was diagnosed. It is important not to be falsely reassured by blood results and to act on the clinical presentation.

Top Tip

Remember that there is more in the pelvis and abdomen than a pregnancy. When confronted with a pregnant woman with abdominal pain, do not forget all other 'usual' pathologies like a urinary tract infection, appendicitis and PID.

STATION 7.8: EXAMINATION: OBSTETRIC EXAMINATION

SCENARIO

You are a junior doctor in the antenatal clinic and have been asked to see Clare Pfannenstiel, a 28-year-old woman, who is 30 weeks pregnant. Please perform an obstetric examination on Mrs Pfannenstiel and present your findings.

PREPARATION

- WIPER:
  - *Wash* your hands
  - *Introduce* yourself
  - Ask about *pain*
  - Appropriately *expose*
  - *Reposition*
- Explain the examination to the patient and your reasons for performing it
- Gain verbal consent
- Give the patient privacy to expose herself as required

- Start in a comfortable position (usually lying on the bed, positioned at 45°)
- Ensure that a female chaperone is present

OBSTETRIC EXAMINATION

GENERAL INSPECTION

- Environment: Vomit bowls, medication, walking aids (pelvic girdle pain)
- Patient: General appearance, oedema (possible sign of pre-eclampsia) and conjunctival pallor of anaemia

EXAMINATION OF THE ABODOMEN

Inspection

- Size: Estimate the size of the uterus
- Scars: For example, Pfannenstiel from previous caesarean section
- Skin changes of pregnancy: Linea nigra, striae gravidarum

Palpation

- First check that the patient does not have any pain
- Measure the SFH:
  - Feel for the fundus, starting at the xiphisternum with the left hand (if examining from the right side of the bed)
  - Feel for the symphysis pubis with the right hand
  - Measure between the two landmarks with a tape measure. Turn it over so that numbers are hidden to avoid operator bias
  - The length in centimetres should equate to the number of weeks' gestation with 2 cm either way; for example, a 30-week pregnancy may measure between 28 and 32 cm
  - Plot to check consistent growth with previous measurements
- Assess fetal lie:
  - With both hands, feel for the spine
  - It will be longitudinal, oblique or transverse (Fig. 7.2)
- Assess fetal presentation:
  - Assess which part of the fetus is closest to the maternal pelvis

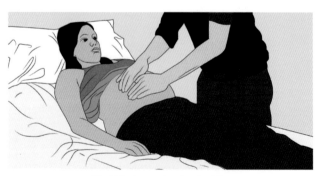

Fig. 7.2 Assessing the fetal lie.

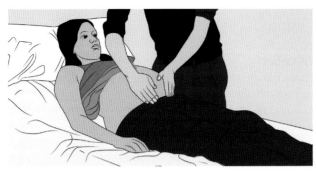

Fig. 7.3 Assessing the presenting part.

- Warn the patient that this may be slightly uncomfortable
- With one hand (thumbs and first two fingers) or two hands, palpate the presenting part to assess what part is presenting (Fig. 7.3)
  - If unsure, try to assess the non-presenting part
- Assess fetal engagement:
  - How much of the presenting part is within the maternal pelvis?
  - It is measured in finger breadths and assessed in fifths (i.e. one finger is a fifth)
  - If the whole head or bottom is palpable, this is five-fifths palpable
- Assess liquor volume:
  - This is tricky to assess, but in general if the fetal parts are easily palpable there may be reduced liquor, and if it is difficult to feel fetal parts there may be increased liquor

Auscultation
- Place the Doppler or Pinard stethoscope over the anterior shoulder of the fetus
- Normal rate is 110–160 bpm
- If you cannot find the fetal heart, then try the other end of the fetus, as presentation may have been assessed wrongly
- If you still cannot find the fetal heart, it is important to arrange an ultrasound scan immediately to exclude stillbirth

Finishing
- Offer to:
  - Assess for bleeding or labour progress: Perform a vaginal and/or speculum examination
  - Assess for venous thromboembolism: Examine the calves and chest
  - Assess for pre-eclampsia: Check reflexes and clonus
- Thank the patient
- Check she is comfortable and offer to help reposition her
- Wash your hands
- Leave the patient in privacy to get dressed

Important examination findings in pregnancy

General	• Whether she looks well • Weight • Oedema • Blood pressure and urine dip
Face	• Pale conjunctiva • Dry mucous membranes
Hands	• Pulse • Blood pressure • Palmar erythema
Chest	• Systolic murmur • Increased tidal volume • Spider naevi

Present Your Findings

Mrs Pfannenstiel is a 28-year-old woman who is 30 weeks pregnant. She has a normal blood pressure and pulse today. She was referred for reduced fetal movements. On examination, she has an SFH of 31 cm, which is in keeping with her previous SFH measurements by her community midwife. The fetal lie is longitudinal with a cephalic presentation. The fetal head is not engaged, with five-fifths palpable. The fetal heart rate is normal at 124 bpm. Fetal movements are regular again. She has had a normal growth scan.

She has been discharged from the consultant-led antenatal clinic today and will continue to see her community midwife for the rest of her antenatal care. To complete my examination, I would take a history and assess for pre-eclampsia and venous thromboembolism.

❓ QUESTIONS AND ANSWERS FOR CANDIDATE

Why would you not want a pregnant woman to lie flat on an examination couch?
- There is a risk of aortocaval compression from the pregnant uterus and this can result in maternal hypotension and fetal hypoperfusion

Why does a systolic murmur develop in pregnancy?
- Due to a hyperdynamic circulation
- It usually does not require investigation, unless it is loud, pansystolic or diastolic, or associated with symptoms

Why does determining the presentation of the fetus matter at each visit?
- The fetus should be in a fixed position by 36 weeks. If not, this is called an unstable lie
- If the fetus has an unstable or transverse lie after 36 weeks, then there is a risk of cord prolapse if the woman ruptures her membranes. Most hospitals would admit such a patient to hospital until delivery

A Case to Learn From

A woman presented in advanced labour with her first baby. Throughout her pregnancy the fetus had been thought to be cephalic; however when she was 9 cm dilated the fetal buttocks were found to be presenting and the baby was breech. Nobody had checked the presentation on arrival. Determining the fetal position at each visit is important, as is it may change affecting management.

Top Tip

Remember that obstetric pathology is not limited to the abdomen. Clues to other pathology may be found with general examination.

STATION 7.9: EXAMINATION: GYNAECOLOGY EXAMINATION (BIMANUAL AND SPECULUM)

SCENARIO

You are a junior doctor in gynaecology and have been asked to see Josephine Sapphire, a 28-year-old woman, who has presented with severe pelvic pain and vaginal discharge. She suddenly became unwell last night and has been referred by her primary care doctor. Please perform a relevant gynaecological examination on Miss Sapphire and present your findings.

PREPARATION

- WIPER:
  - *Wash* your hands
  - *Introduce* yourself
  - Ask about *pain*
  - Appropriately *expose*
  - *Reposition*
- Explain the examination to the patient and your reasons for performing it
- Gain verbal consent
- Give the patient privacy to expose herself as required. A sheet or blanket should be provided to cover the patient's genitalia
- Ensure that a female chaperone is present

GYNAECOLOGICAL EXAMINATION

GENERAL INSPECTION

- Environment: Swabs, medications
- Patient: General appearance, height, weight, pallor, ascites, peripheral oedema or jaundice

EXAMINATION OF THE ABDOMEN

Inspection
- Size
- Scars (from previous laparoscopy or caesarean section)
- Masses
- Distension

Palpation
First enquire regarding the patient's pain and where it is. Then, feel for:
- Superficial palpation: Tenderness, guarding, obvious masses
- Deep palpation: Determine nature and location of any masses; for example, whether the mass arises from the pelvis

Percussion
- Determine if the abdomen is tympanic, dull or there is shifting dullness

Auscultation
- Important to check, especially in postoperative patients

EXAMINATION OF THE PELVIS

Preparation
- Make sure that you are wearing non-sterile gloves
- Have the equipment you may need ready (speculum, swabs and lubricating jelly) before exposing the patient
- Ensure that the patient is comfortable and explain that you will move the sheet covering her in order to continue with the pelvic examination
- Position the patient in the dorsal position

Inspection
- Swelling
- Erythema
- Skin changes
- Lesions or bleeding should be looked for on the vulva, vagina and cervix

Speculum Examination
- Ensure that the speculum is lubricated
- Part the labia minora with your non-dominant hand
- Insert the speculum fully along the direction of the vagina with the blades closed using your dominant hand. It is usually more comfortable for the patient if the speculum is inserted 90° and rotated once in the vagina
- Open the blades to visualise the cervix
- This would be the time to take swabs if necessary
- Inform the patient you are about to withdraw the speculum
- Once you have inspected the cervix gradually, withdraw the speculum with the blades still open to examine the vaginal walls
- As you withdraw, slowly close the blades so they are closed at the introitus as to not cause pain to the patient

Bimanual Examination

- Ensure that the gloved index and middle fingers of your dominant hand are lubricated
- Insert these two fingers of your dominant hand into the vagina
- Place your non-dominant hand on the lower abdomen
- Palpate the uterus by keeping your fingers central on the cervix and your non-dominant hand just above the pubic symphysis (bimanual palpation)
- Palpate the adnexae by placing your fingers lateral to the cervix and your hand in the left and right pelvic region (bimanual palpation)
- Check for cervical motion tenderness by pushing one finger against the cervix
- Inform the patient when you are withdrawing your fingers

Finishing

- Offer to:
  - Perform a urine dipstick
  - Swab the discharge
- Thank the patient
- Check she is comfortable and offer to help reposition her
- Wash your hands
- Leave the patient in privacy to get dressed

🏃 Common diagnoses from pelvic examination

VULVA	VAGINA	CERVIX
• Female genital mutilation (FGM)	• Genital herpes	• Cervical ectropion
• Lichen sclerosus	• Genital infection	• Cervical polyps
• Lichen planus	• Vaginal cancer	• Nabothian cysts
• Bartholin's gland cyst/abscess		• Cervical cancer
• Candidiasis (thrush)		
• Genital warts		
• Genital herpes		
• Vulval cancer		

🔍 Present Your Findings

Miss Sapphire is a 28-year-old woman who presented with severe abdominal pain and vaginal discharge. On examination, she looked uncomfortable at rest with generalised lower abdominal pain with some guarding to deep palpation. External genitalia were normal, with profuse discharge seen on speculum examination. On bimanual examination, she was generally tender, but no masses were felt.

I feel the most likely diagnosis is PID, with the differentials being ovarian cyst accident. I would like to examine Miss Sapphire fully. To complete my examination, I would like to take a history and bloods to check her FBCs, U&Es and CRP. I would also organise an ultrasound scan of her pelvis and send off the vaginal swabs I have taken. It is likely that we will start her on antibiotics.

❓ QUESTIONS AND ANSWERS FOR CANDIDATE

What are the common swabs that can be taken during a gynaecological examination?

- Endocervical swab: For chlamydia ± gonorrhoea (depending on local policy)
- HVS: For vaginal flora and pathogens; for example, bacterial vaginosis

How is FGM classified?

- Type 1: Clitoridectomy (partial or total removal of the clitoris)
- Type 2: Excision (partial or total removal of the clitoris and labia minora; can also involve labia majora)
- Type 3: Infibulation (narrowing of the vaginal opening through the creation of a covering seal either by cutting or stitching the labia)
- Type 4: All other harmful procedures to the female genitalia (pricking, piercing, incising)

In the UK, if FGM is confirmed in a woman under the age of 18, then it is mandatory to report this to the police within 1 month of confirmation.

What should I do if the woman declines a chaperone?

- If the woman declines and you are happy to go ahead without a chaperone, then this discussion must be clearly documented in the patient's notes

---

A Case to Learn From

We had a patient who presented with pelvic pain but denied any other symptoms. It was not until she had a full gynaecological examination that it was noted that she had profuse offensive discharge. Swabs were taken and she was successfully treated for PID. If left untreated, this could have had implications for future fertility. It is important to remember that not all symptoms will be reported by patients, as they may not have noticed, or may be too embarrassed to say.

Top Tip

When performing a speculum examination, ensure that you are always watching the blades. Inadequate opening will make your examination difficult and keeping them fully open whilst withdrawing will be very uncomfortable for your patient.

STATION 7.10: COMMUNICATION: CONSENT FOR CAESAREAN SECTION

SCENARIO

You are a junior doctor in the antenatal clinic and have been asked to see Joanne Taylor, a 22-year-old woman, who is 39 weeks pregnant. This is her first pregnancy and the baby is in a frank breech presentation. She is considering an elective caesarean section. Please explain the risks and benefits of the procedure to her. She has already had counselling about ECV and vaginal breech birth.

CORE CONCEPT

- Although a common procedure, a caesarean section is a major operation with significant risk
- Women must be aware of the risks and benefits of any operation in order to make the best decision for them and their baby

Common Concerns

How long will the operation take?	Typically, an uncomplicated caesarean section takes around 30–45 min, but the patient may be in the operating theatre for up to 2 h
How long is the recovery?	Most women stay in hospital for 2 nights before going home. Full recovery from the operation takes 6 weeks and you will not be allowed to drive before this time
Will I be awake?	Yes. Most caesarean sections are carried out under spinal anaesthetic, as this is safer for women and their babies

GATHERING INFORMATION AND COMMUNICATIONS

- Ask Mrs Taylor what she has been told before she came to see you in antenatal clinic
- Ask what information she has found for herself already
- Ask whether there are any specific concerns that she would like you to address

This case has two parts:
1. Explaining what occurs during a caesarean section
2. Explaining the risks and benefits of the operation in order for her to make a decision

EXPLAINING THE PROCEDURE

Timing
- Elective caesarean sections are planned on or after 39 weeks' gestation. This is to decrease the rate of admission to the neonatal intensive care unit with transient tachypnoea of the newborn
- Most hospitals will give a date at the time when you decide to have a caesarean section
- If you go into labour before your caesarean section date, it is important to attend the hospital and the on-call obstetrician will discuss your options with you depending on the stage of labour

On the Day
- You will be expected to have had nothing to eat or drink for 6 h before your surgery
- You will meet the obstetrician performing the surgery, and they will confirm the consent form with you

- If the caesarean section is for breech position, you will have an ultrasound to confirm that this is still the case

What to Expect
- The anaesthetist will insert a drip into your hand or arm and then inject some anaesthetic to make you numb – usually a spinal block
- The midwife will insert a tube, called a catheter, into your bladder. This is because you will not be able to walk for several hours following the spinal block and it makes the surgery safer by emptying your bladder
- When the anaesthetic is working adequately and you are numb enough for the operation, your tummy will be cleaned with an antiseptic solution and you will be covered in sterile drapes. The obstetrician will ensure that you cannot see the operation
- You will hear the theatre team performing a safety check. This is called the World Health Organization safety checklist and it is mandatory before any operation
- When the operation starts, you are likely to feel some pushing and pulling until the baby is delivered. If it is your first caesarean section this part usually takes around 5 minutes
- After the baby is delivered, the baby can come to you and your birth partner while the obstetrician closes your womb and tummy wall. This part usually takes around 30 minutes

After the Operation
- You will initially be looked after in a recovery bay, before being transferred to a postnatal ward
- When full sensation returns to your legs, the tube emptying your bladder can be removed
- You will have compression stockings on your legs and you may need injections to thin the blood

COUNSELLING ON THE RISKS AND BENEFITS OF A CAESAREAN SECTION

Risks to the Mother
- Infection: Common
- Haemorrhage: Common
- Readmission: Common
- Venous thromboembolism: Uncommon
- Emergency hysterectomy: Uncommon
- Further surgery at a later date (for example, because of retained products): Uncommon
- Admission to intensive care unit: Uncommon
- Damage to internal structures: Uncommon

Risks to the Baby
- Laceration: Common
- Respiratory distress: Uncommon

Benefits to the Mother
- Timing of birth known

Benefits to the Baby

These will depend upon the reason for caesarean section, but include:

- Rapid delivery to relieve any source of distress
- Reduced likelihood of some birth complications; for example, getting stuck, especially when there is already evidence of foetal distress

INDICATIONS FOR A PLANNED CAESAREAN SECTION

- Breech position
- Placenta praevia
- Pre-eclampsia
- Previous caesarean section
- Fetal macrosomia
- Multiple pregnancy

VAGINAL BIRTH AFTER CAESAREAN (VBAC)

Women who have had a caesarean section before may be able to consider a vaginal birth in future pregnancies, depending on the reason and consequences of their surgery. This is known as VBAC. If you have had a previous vaginal birth, then the chances of a successful VBAC is higher. Individual risks and benefits will need to be weighed out through a detailed consultation. There are some circumstances in which a VBAC is advised against for example, three or more previous caesarean deliveries.

 Present Your Findings

Mrs Taylor is 39 weeks pregnant and this is her first pregnancy. She has been diagnosed with a baby in the breech presentation and is considering a caesarean section.

I have discussed what to expect during and after a caesarean section, as well as the risks and benefits to both Mrs Taylor and her baby. I have also given her a leaflet on caesarean sections and she will be given time to come to a decision.

❓ QUESTIONS AND ANSWERS FOR CANDIDATE

If there were no medical indications and a woman requested a caesarean section, what would you say to her?

- It is important to explore her reasons for requesting a caesarean section to assess if she has any misconceptions
- If she understands the risks fully and is willing to take those risks, many obstetricians would perform that caesarean section

Is a paediatrician present at all caesarean sections?

- No. If it is an uncomplicated elective caesarean section, a paediatrician will not be present. However, if the baby is likely to be born unwell; for example, after an abruption or with a poor CTG, neonatal presence is mandatory

Give an example of when a caesarean section may need to be performed under general anaesthetic.

- If there are fetal concerns and a general anaesthetic is deemed faster than a spinal
- If there are low maternal platelets, contraindicating a spinal anaesthetic

 A Case to Learn From

A woman came to antenatal clinic requesting a caesarean section for her first birth. She told the obstetrician that she was aware of all of the risks and wished to go ahead. When the obstetrician asked the woman to list the risks and benefits of a caesarean section, the only risks she said were bleeding and infection. During a frank and open discussion, the woman and obstetrician covered all of the risks and benefits of the surgery and a plan was made to see the patient again in 2 weeks after she had had time to do some reading and have a think. The woman returned and decided to opt for a vaginal birth, having been appraised of all of the information. If you don't provide all the information to the woman, she cannot make an informed decision.

 Top Tip

Ensure that the information you give parents is in a language that is digestible for them. For example, 'In this hospital we do 2000 caesarean sections a year and will see 30 babies born with transient tachypnoea of the newborn'.

STATION 7.11: COMMUNICATION: GROUP B STREPTOCOCCUS

SCENARIO

You are a junior doctor in the antenatal clinic and have been asked to see Victoria Jones, a 28-year-old woman, who has been diagnosed with GBS infection in pregnancy. She is worried about what this means for her and her baby and would like to know more. Please explore her concerns and explain the diagnosis to her.

CORE CONCEPT

- GBS (*Streptococcus agalactiae*) is present in the bowel flora of 20–40% of adults
- GBS is the most common cause of severe early-onset infection in neonates, less than 7 days of age
- If women are found to be carrying GBS, either in urine or on a vaginal swab, they should be offered antibiotics in labour to prevent this neonatal infection
- Current guidance in the UK does not support universal screening for GBS; however, in the USA, all women are recommended to have screening at 35–37 weeks
- When explaining this diagnosis to women and their partners, it is important to be clear and not use jargon at any time

Common Concerns

How did I get this infection?	20–40% of women carry GBS in their bowel flora (normal gut bacteria), but it does not affect them in any way
Can I have treatment now to treat it?	If the GBS has been diagnosed in a urine test, then you should have antibiotics to treat it as soon as possible, as this has been shown to decrease the chance of infection to the baby. You should also have antibiotics in labour
	If the GBS has been diagnosed on vaginal swab, then you should have antibiotics in labour to protect your baby
What are the risks to my baby if they get GBS?	GBS is a serious condition in babies, causing some form of disability in 7.5% of cases and death in 5%. However, the risk of infection being transmitted dramatically reduces with antibiotics in labour

GATHERING INFORMATION AND COMMUNICATIONS

- Ask Miss Jones what she has been told so far about her results
- Ask what she has heard about this before coming to see you. Most women will have done their own research before coming to clinic
- Explore her concerns about the GBS and find out what she is most worried about; for example, the infection, how it will affect her labour, or both

This case has two parts:
1. Explaining the diagnosis
2. Addressing her concerns

EXPLAINING THE DIAGNOSIS

Describe what GBS is:
- GBS, commonly referred to as 'group B strep', is a bacteria found in 20–40% of people in their bowel flora, as part of their normal gut bacteria
- It usually causes no harm to adults
- When you have it in your bowel, you are called a carrier.

Explain why it is important:
- GBS is the biggest cause of early-onset infection in babies
- Although rare, about 7 in 100 babies who get the infection will end up with a degree of disability, and 5–6 babies in 100 will die as a result of the infection

Explain why it is not screened for in pregnancy:
- Currently no test is accurate enough to use for screening
- Because so many women carry GBS and the infection is very rare, if we screened everyone many women and babies would end up with antibiotics that they did not need

ADDRESSING CONCERNS

Risks to mum and baby:
- There is a theoretical risk of anaphylaxis in woman from antibiotics, so it is important to check allergy status carefully
- There is also a risk of alteration of neonatal gut flora

How this will affect labour and hospital stay:
- The recommendation is to deliver in a hospital setting
- IV antibiotics would be offered in labour
- If these antibiotics are given 4 h before delivery, your baby may not need additional monitoring, compared to babies born without antibiotics
- If these antibiotics are not given before this time, the baby will need at least 12 h of monitoring
- There are no contraindications to water birth, as long as there are no other risks in the labour or pregnancy

What this will mean for future pregnancies:
- 50% chance of carrying GBS again
- Can choose either to have antibiotics in labour or to test at 35–37 weeks pregnant with a vaginal swab
- If the previous baby was affected by GBS infection, antibiotics would be offered in labour

REFUSAL OF TREATMENT

If a patient refuses to have antibiotics, we need to ensure that she has the capacity to make this decision and that she has been fully informed of the risks and benefits regarding this decision.

If the woman still refuses, and has the capacity to do so, we must respect her decision and document this clearly in the notes.

Then the baby must have at least 12 h of observations after birth to watch closely for signs of infection. The neonatologists at birth must also be informed and they may consider starting the newborn on a course of antibiotics.

Present Your Findings

Miss Jones is a 28-year-old woman in her first pregnancy. She has been found to be carrying GBS on a vaginal swab. She has had time to ask questions about this diagnosis.

I have explained this diagnosis to her and addressed her concerns. She is planning to deliver in the hospital unit and will be having antibiotics in labour to reduce the risk of passing the infection on to her baby.

QUESTIONS AND ANSWERS FOR CANDIDATE

Can you force Miss Jones to have antibiotics during her labour if she refuses?
- No. Women have the right to refuse treatment during pregnancy. You can, however, ensure that the neonatologists are aware at birth and insist on her baby having adequate levels of observations

What are the signs of GBS infection in a neonate?
- GBS sepsis has no specific signs; however, important signs of sepsis in a neonate include: Respiratory

distress, abnormal heart rate, temperature, floppy episodes, increased sleepiness, poor feeding and low blood sugar levels

Do women have symptoms of GBS?

- GBS is usually an asymptomatic infection in adults and is diagnosed on a vaginal swab or urine culture

A Case to Learn From

A woman insisting on a home birth was diagnosed with GBS in her urine at 28 weeks pregnant. After being told the risks, she felt that a home birth was the safest way for her baby to be born. Her consultant obstetrician and the supervisor of midwives reviewed her and discussed the plan at length. It was agreed that she could deliver at home, but then attend hospital for her immediate postpartum care in order for her baby to have the correct observations. By working closely with the woman, a plan was made that was as safe as possible for her baby and ensured that she did not disengage with the service or feel bullied or undermined.

Top Tip

When performing a speculum examination on a pregnant woman during antenatal care, it is good practice to take an opportunistic vaginal swab at the time. This is how many GBS carriers are identified.

STATION 7.12: COMMUNICATION: PLACENTA PRAEVIA

SCENARIO

You are a junior doctor in the antenatal clinic and have been asked to see Clare Smith, a 26-year-old woman, who has been diagnosed with placenta praevia on her anomaly scan. She is currently 20 weeks pregnant. She is worried about what this means for her and her baby and would like to know more. Please explain the diagnosis to her as well as the plan for the rest of her pregnancy.

CORE CONCEPT

- Placenta praevia exists when the placenta is sited in the lower segment of the uterus (Fig. 7.4)
- It can be either major or minor:
  - Major placenta praevia: Covers the internal os of the cervix
  - Minor placenta praevia: Within the lower segment of the uterus, but not covering the internal os
- When explaining this diagnosis to women and their partners it is important to be clear. Do not use jargon at any time

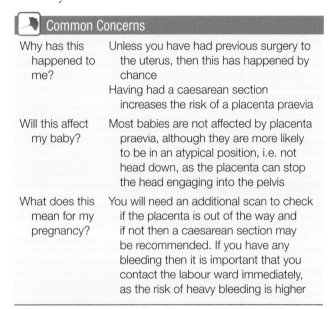
Common Concerns

Why has this happened to me?	Unless you have had previous surgery to the uterus, then this has happened by chance Having had a caesarean section increases the risk of a placenta praevia
Will this affect my baby?	Most babies are not affected by placenta praevia, although they are more likely to be in an atypical position, i.e. not head down, as the placenta can stop the head engaging into the pelvis
What does this mean for my pregnancy?	You will need an additional scan to check if the placenta is out of the way and if not then a caesarean section may be recommended. If you have any bleeding then it is important that you contact the labour ward immediately, as the risk of heavy bleeding is higher

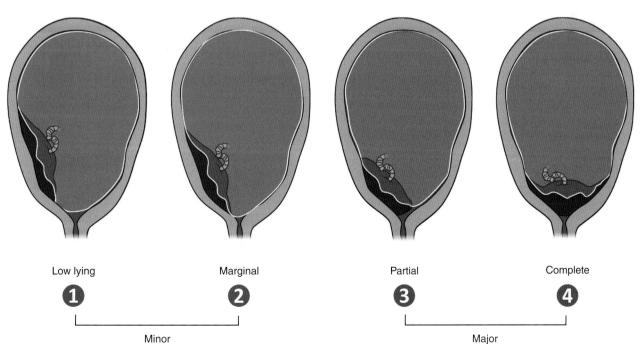

Fig. 7.4 Location of placenta.

GATHERING INFORMATION AND COMMUNICATIONS

- Ask the patient what she has been told so far about her scan
- Ask what she has found out about before coming to see you. Most women will have done their own research before coming to clinic
- Ask if she has had any uterine surgery before, increasing her risk of placenta accreta
- Explore her concerns about placenta praevia and find out what she is most worried about

This case has two parts:
1. Explaining the diagnosis
2. Making an ongoing plan for her pregnancy

EXPLAINING THE DIAGNOSIS

Describe what placenta praevia is:
- Major placenta praevia covers the internal os of the cervix
- Minor placenta praevia is within the lower segment of the uterus, but not covering the internal os

Explain why it is important:
- If the placenta is covering the cervix, then a vaginal birth will not be possible
- There is a risk of significant bleeding to the mother if labour were to start

MAKE A MANAGEMENT PLAN

Risks to mum and baby:
- The baby is unlikely to have any risks
- The mother is at risk of significant bleeding, either spontaneously or if labour starts

How to minimise these risks:
- Avoid sexual intercourse from the time of diagnosis
- If there is any bleeding, ask the mother to contact the labour ward immediately, as a small bleed can quickly progress to heavy bleeding

What this will mean for mode of birth:
- Women with a minor placenta praevia and no bleeding should have a scan at 36 weeks to check the placental site
- Women with a major placenta praevia, or previous uterine surgery, should have a scan at 32 weeks
- If the placenta has moved at least 20 mm from the internal os, a vaginal birth can be planned
- If not, an elective caesarean section should be carried out no earlier than 38 weeks
- If she were to have heavy bleeding, an emergency caesarean section might be needed sooner
- There is a high risk of heavy bleeding at this caesarean section and a significant risk of hysterectomy

What this will mean for future pregnancies:
- If the placenta has moved away and a vaginal birth is possible, the risk of another placenta praevia is low
- If a caesarean section is necessary, there is an increased risk of a further placenta praevia and an increased chance that this will become a placenta accreta

 Risk Factors for Placenta Praevia

- Increasing age
- Previous caesarean section
- Previous uterine surgery
- Increasing parity
- Smoking
- Multiple pregnancy
  Previous placenta praevia

TYPES OF ABNORMAL PLACENTA

 Abnormally adherent placenta

TYPE	DESCRIPTION
Placenta accreta	Placenta is adherent to the uterine wall
Placenta increta	Placenta invades the myometrium
Placenta percreta	Placenta invades the uterine serosa, that can extend into surrounding structures

Present Your Findings

Miss Smith is a 26-year-old woman in her first pregnancy. She is 20 weeks pregnant. She has been diagnosed with major placenta praevia at her anomaly scan.

I have explained this diagnosis to her and advised her to avoid sexual intercourse during the pregnancy. She is aware to contact the labour ward if she has any vaginal bleeding. She will have another scan at 32 weeks' gestation to assess if the placenta has moved, and if not, her mode of birth will be planned and will most likely be a caesarean section.

❓ QUESTIONS AND ANSWERS FOR CANDIDATE

How can the placenta move?
- The placenta does not migrate upwards on the uterus
- During the pregnancy the lower segment of the uterus develops and becomes larger, thus taking the placenta with it

What are the additional risks at caesarean section, compared to women without a placenta praevia?
- Increased risk of emergency hysterectomy
- Increased risk of massive obstetric haemorrhage
- Increased risk of a return to theatre during recovery

Do all women have symptoms of placenta praevia?
- Most women are asymptomatic and have no bleeding in pregnancy
- This is why it is important to check the placental site at the anomaly scan

A woman presented to the local delivery suite bleeding heavily in the early stages of labour. She did not have her antenatal notes with her. There was no sign of fetal distress but she continued to bleed. The obstetrician scanned her and she had a placenta praevia. An emergency caesarean section was carried out. Remember that blood loss from a placenta praevia may not affect the fetus, as it is maternal blood being lost.

 Top Tip

Visual aids can be really useful for patients when trying to explain diagnoses in parts of the body that most people will not have seen. You can either draw or find pictures online to explain a diagnosis like placenta praevia to patients.

STATION 7.13: COMMUNICATION: BREECH PRESENTATION

SCENARIO

You are a junior doctor in the antenatal assessment unit and have been asked to see Rachel Rae, a 26-year-old woman, who is 37 weeks pregnant and has been diagnosed as having a frank breech presentation during her first pregnancy. Please explain the diagnosis, then discuss the possibility of ECV as well as other options if this fails to turn her baby.

CORE CONCEPT

- Breech presentation occurs when the baby's bottom or feet are the presenting part at the maternal pelvis.
- 3–4% of babies at term are breech
- Vaginal breech deliveries are associated with a higher risk of perinatal mortality than cephalic deliveries
- To try to avoid a vaginal breech birth, women are offered an ECV to attempt to turn the fetus
- If this is unsuccessful or they decline, women are offered either a planned vaginal breech birth or an elective caesarean section
- All of these carry risks and it is important to explain these in as straightforward a manner as possible to allow women to make their decision based upon evidence

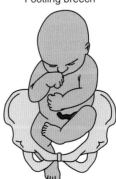 Common Concerns

What are the risks of an ECV?	Complications with an ECV are very rare. The risk of emergency caesarean section within 24 h is 0.5%. If you are Rhesus-negative, you will be offered anti-D to avoid a sensitising event
Will my baby turn back to breech after an ECV?	The chances of your baby turning back into the breech position are small
What are the risks with a vaginal breech birth?	The risks for the mother are very low and a successful vaginal breech birth is safer for the mother than a caesarean section. The risk of perinatal mortality in a vaginal breech is higher than a planned cephalic birth via caesarean section

GATHERING INFORMATION AND COMMUNICATIONS

- Ask Mrs Rae what she has been told so far about her baby's presentation
- Ask Mrs Rae if she has had any thoughts herself or done any research before seeing you on the management of babies in the breech position
- Explore her concerns

This case has two parts:
1. Explaining the diagnosis of frank breech presentation
2. Explaining the management options

EXPLAINING THE DIAGNOSIS

What a breech presentation is:
- Breech presentation is the term used to describe a baby that is presenting with its bottom or feet first
- There are three different types of breech (Fig. 7.5). This is a frank breech, i.e. the bottom is coming first into the pelvis, with the legs pointing straight upwards

Frank breech / extended breech   Complete breech / flexed breech   Footling breech

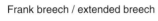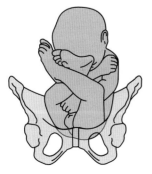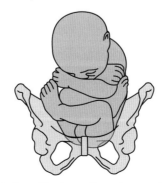

Fig. 7.5 Illustration of the type of breech presentations.

Why it has happened:

- 3–4% of babies are breech at term and in most of these cases, no cause is found
- Babies are more likely to be breech when there is something stopping them rotating in the uterus; for example, a bicornuate uterus or multiple pregnancies

EXPLAINING THE MANAGEMENT OPTIONS

External Cephalic Version

- ECV is done from 36 weeks' gestation to try to turn the baby
- The ECV success rate is around 50%
- It is performed in hospital, usually on the labour ward
- An ultrasound scan will confirm position before and after the procedure, and the baby's heart will be monitored
- An injection is given to relax the womb muscles to make it easier to turn the baby
- The obstetrician will press quite firmly on the tummy to try and turn the baby, while the mother is lying down on a bed
- Patients who are Rhesus-negative are recommended a dose of anti-D
- There is a small risk that an emergency caesarean section will be required within 24 h. The majority of these are for vaginal bleeding or abnormalities of the baby's heart beat

Vaginal Breech

- Vaginal breech carries a higher risk than a planned cephalic birth
- There are factors that are likely to make a vaginal breech birth riskier; for example, footling breech presentation or a baby that is large for gestational age
- The patient should deliver on a labour ward in case of deterioration
- There is a low threshold for converting to caesarean section and the baby's heart rate will be closely monitored

Caesarean Section

- Caesarean section is outinely offered at 39 weeks' gestation, but may be done earlier if other concerns

CONDITIONS THAT INCREASE THE CHANCE OF BREECH PRESENTATION

- Twins
- Polyhydramnios
- Oligohydramnios
- Prematurity
- Uterine fibroids
- Uterine malformations
- Placenta praevia
- Pelvic tumour

🔍 Present Your Findings

Mrs Rae is a 26-year-old woman in her first pregnancy. She is at 37 weeks' gestation and has attended today because she has been diagnosed with a breech presentation. The baby was in a frank breech position today.

I have explained the diagnosis to her and that we would recommend an ECV to turn her baby. I have explained the procedure and risks to her. I have also given her information on other options and time to decide what she wishes to do.

❓ QUESTIONS AND ANSWERS FOR CANDIDATE

Do any tests have to be done on a baby that is born breech?

- Normally, these babies will have their hips checked by the paediatrician for hip dysplasia before being discharged home and will need an ultrasound scan as an outpatient

Can women have a breech birth at home?

- Women can choose where they wish to have their babies, but it would not be recommended to have a breech birth at home, due to the potential complications and the absence of paediatric support if needed

If an ECV is successful, but the baby turns back again, what are the options?

- Most obstetricians will offer another ECV if the woman wishes, or discuss vaginal breech birth or caesarean section

🗨 A Case to Learn From

A woman was admitted in advanced labour with a breech presentation. She had an elective caesarean section booked for the next day, but the obstetrician felt that labour had progressed too far to do a caesarean section safely. The woman was frightened, having been told nothing about vaginal births, apart from that they were risky. If the patient chooses a caesarean section for a baby in the breech position, it is important to explain what could happen if she goes into labour before the planned caesarean section to reduce maternal anxiety from lack of information.

💡 Top Tip

If in any doubt regarding a change in the presentation of a baby, confirm it on an ultrasound scan. It is much better to have an extra scan than a surprise breech baby!

STATION 7.14: COMMUNICATION: MISCARRIAGE

SCENARIO

You are a junior doctor working in the early pregnancy unit (EPU) and have been asked to see Emma Parker, a 32-year-old woman, who has had an ultrasound scan today and has been informed that she has had a miscarriage. She was referred to the clinic by her primary care doctor after some vaginal bleeding 2 days ago. Please explain the diagnosis and discuss her options with her.

CORE CONCEPT

- 20% of pregnancies end in miscarriage and early pregnancy loss accounts for 50,000 admissions to hospital in the UK each year
- Most pregnancy losses are unexplained, and this can be difficult for women and their partners to come to terms with
- There are three options for management of a miscarriage: Conservative, medical and surgical. It is important to discuss these options clearly and with empathy with women and allow them time to make a decision

Common Concerns

Has this happened because I did something wrong?	You have not done anything wrong, but many women do feel this way. One in five pregnancies end in miscarriage and the vast majority of these are unexplained
What does this mean for future pregnancies?	Most women go on to have straightforward pregnancies in the future. A very small proportion of women are at risk for recurrent miscarriages but there is nothing to suggest that you will be one of these women
When can I try again for another pregnancy?	It is a good idea to wait until after your next period but apart from that, you can try when it feels right for you and your partner

GATHERING INFORMATION AND COMMUNICATIONS

- Ask the patient if she has anyone with her today, or anyone she would like you to call for her
- Ask what she has been told so far following her ultrasound scan
- Enquire about her last menstrual period
- Ask if this was a planned or unplanned pregnancy

This case has two parts:
1. Explaining the diagnosis
2. Discussing her ongoing options for management

EXPLAINING THE DIAGNOSIS

- One in five pregnancies ends in miscarriage, so sadly, it is very common
- Most of these are unexplained; however, miscarriage often happens with embryos that have a chromosomal abnormality and would not have grown into a healthy baby

- The bleeding that she had 2 days ago was likely a sign of this miscarriage; however, even if she had come to hospital sooner, it would not have stopped the miscarriage

MANAGEMENT OF MISCARRIAGE

There are three options for ongoing management in miscarriage: Conservative, medical or surgical.

Conservative

- This would normally be offered as the first option to women who have been diagnosed with a miscarriage
- Most miscarriages will take place without medical intervention, over the following 1–2 weeks
- The main risk is of retained products needing further intervention, but for most women this does not happen
- It is normal to expect bleeding, as heavy as or slightly heavier than a period
- It is also normal to have some crampy abdominal pain and you may need to take painkillers for this
- If the pain and bleeding settle down, it is likely that the miscarriage is complete
- A routine review should occur after 2 weeks
- A pregnancy test should be taken after 3 weeks. If this is positive, there may be some retained products of conception, requiring a different treatment. This should be discussed with the EPU

Medical

- This involves taking a medication called misoprostol (600–800 mcg), which will make the cervix open, and there will be a bleed like a heavy period, signifying that the treatment has worked
- This tablet is normally given vaginally (on the end of a tampon) but can also be swallowed
- The risks involved include:
  - Excessive bleeding
  - Retained products of conception
  - Fever
  - Nausea
  - Diarrhoea
  - Abdominal cramps (usually manageable with painkillers)
- If there is no bleeding, the EPU should be contacted, as it is likely the medication has not worked
- A pregnancy test should be taken after 3 weeks. If this is positive there may be some retained products of conception, requiring a different treatment. This should be discussed with the EPU

Surgical

- This involves opening up the cervix and passing a tube through to the womb to remove the pregnancy tissue

- It can either be done awake (manual vacuum aspiration) or under a general anaesthetic
- The risks involved include:
  - Bleeding
  - Infection
  - Damage to the cervix
  - Perforation of the womb
  - Development of intrauterine adhesions that can affect future fertility

! Presentations of different types of miscarriages

TYPE OF MISCARRIAGE	SYMPTOMS	SCAN FINDINGS	MANAGEMENT
Threatened	• Pain and/or bleeding	• Live pregnancy	• Return to EPU after 14 days if symptoms persist
Incomplete	• Pain and/or bleeding	• Evidence of pregnancy tissue (products of conception)	• Conservative • Medical (offer 600 mcg misoprostol) • Surgical
Missed	• None, often diagnosed at dating scan	• Fetus with no heart beat	• Conservative • Medical (offer 800 mcg misoprostol) • Surgical
Complete	• Pain • Bleeding	• Empty uterus; may see some blood clots only	• No further treatment needed

RECURRENT FIRST-TRIMESTER MISCARRIAGES

- Defined as three or more consecutive pregnancy losses
- Affect 1% of couples trying for a pregnancy
- Causes:
  - Maternal age:
  - 12–19 years: 13%
  - Over 45 years: 93%
  - Paternal age
  - Previous miscarriages: Risk is 40% if three previous miscarriages
  - Antiphospholipid syndrome
  - Parental chromosome rearrangements
  - Embryonic chromosomal abnormalities
  - Uterine malformations
- Investigations:
  - Antiphospholipid antibodies
  - Karyotyping of parents and products of conception

- Pelvic ultrasound scan
- Treatment:
  - Recurrent miscarriage clinic
  - If the patient has antiphospholipid syndrome, aspirin and LMWH should be started upon realising that the patient is pregnant
  - Referral to clinical genetics team if abnormal karyotyping result

🔍 Present Your Findings

Miss Parker is a 32-year-old woman who has been diagnosed with a first-trimester miscarriage today. Her primary care doctor referred her to the clinic after some vaginal bleeding 2 days ago. This was her first pregnancy and she was approximately 11 weeks pregnant. It was a planned pregnancy.

I reviewed her with her partner today and offered my condolences. I explained the diagnosis to them. We have discussed management options and she is going to go home and think about what she would like to do. I have given her written information as well as an emergency contact telephone number for the ward if she has any issues in the meantime.

❓ QUESTIONS AND ANSWERS FOR CANDIDATE

When should women be offered further investigations for miscarriages?
- Recurrent miscarriage investigations should take place when women have had three or more consecutive pregnancy losses

How long can conservative management be offered for?
- Normally women would perform a pregnancy test after 3 weeks and if this was positive, another ultrasound scan would be arranged and the patient would be offered medical or surgical management

What would you do if the woman was still bleeding heavily when she attended the EPU?
- In the case of heavy bleeding, the safest option is to carry out surgical management of miscarriage, usually under general anaesthetic, as the womb must be emptied to stop the bleeding. This can be a lifesaving intervention

📖 A Case to Learn From

A woman presented to the emergency department (ED) with heavy vaginal bleeding at 10 weeks' gestation. She was transferred to the gynaecology ward without being examined or having IV access established. When the woman was seen she had lost at least 1500 mL of blood and had to be transferred straight to theatre for emergency surgical management. Patients bleeding from a miscarriage can lose a very large amount of blood and should be treated no differently than any other bleeding patient. If you do not feel confident to do a speculum examination in such a setting, then at least look at pads to assess blood loss before transferring patients to another speciality.

Top Tip

Try to spend some time with the specialist staff in the EPU. They are excellent at breaking bad news and dealing with patients at a very emotive time.

STATION 7.15: COMMUNICATION: COMBINED ORAL CONTRACEPTIVE PILL

SCENARIO

You are a junior doctor in primary care and your next patient is Lauren Field, a 28-year-old woman, who wishes to start the COCP. She has a regular sexual partner and they have been using condoms up to this point. Please explain how the COCP works, how to take it, as well as the risks and benefits of this form of contraception.

CORE CONCEPT

- The COCP is a commonly used form of contraception that is well tolerated by most women
- It is important that women know how to take it correctly to prevent unwanted pregnancies and side effects
- It is important that women understand the risks and benefits of this type of contraception
- There are contraindications to taking the COCP and it is imperative to ensure that the patient does not have any of these contraindications

Common Concerns

Will the COCP affect my periods?	It should mean that your periods are regular, falling in your pill-free week and some women find them lighter and less painful
How effective is the COCP?	With perfect use, the failure rate is 0.3%. Studies have shown that with typical patient use the failure rate is 9%
Do I have to pay for the COCP?	This depends on where you live. In the UK, access to all contraception is free and this is the case in many European countries; for example, France and Germany. In many other countries, access to the COCP is subsidised
Will the COCP make me gain weight?	Some women do report this, but the evidence does not support a link between weight gain and COCP use

GATHERING INFORMATION AND COMMUNICATIONS

- Ask if she has taken the COCP before and if so, which one and how she got on with it

- Ask what contraceptive methods she has tried in the past
- Ask what has made her want the COCP and what she knows about it already
- Ask a full medical, drug and family history
- Measure her weight and blood pressure

This case has one part:
1. Counselling on the use of COCP

COUNSELLING ON THE USE OF COCP

How Does the COCP Work?
- The pill packet has 21 pills, which are a combination of oestrogen and progestogen
- In most packets, the first pills prevent ovulation, and the next 14 maintain anovulation
- In the 7-day pill break, there is a withdrawal of hormones, which causes the endometrium to shed and this is called the withdrawal bleed

When?
- Women who have regular cycles can start the COCP any time between days 1 and 5 of their cycle (days 1–5 of their period)
- Women who do not have periods can start at any time if it has been deemed reasonably certain that the woman is not pregnant

Missed Doses
- If a pill is missed, then there is a risk of pregnancy:
  - If one pill has been missed, or if a new packet has been started less than 48 h late, then the missed pill should be taken immediately and the remaining pills should be continued at the regular time
  - If two or more pills have been missed, or if the new packet is over 48 h late, then the missed pill should be taken immediately and the remaining pills should be taken at the regular time. Condoms should be used or sexual intercourse avoided until seven consecutive pills have been taken

Risks and Side Effects
- 20% of women get irregular bleeding
- It can be associated with mood changes
- The risk of VTE is twice that of women not on the COCP
- The COCP may also increase the risk of cardiovascular disease, with a very small increase in the risk of ischaemic stroke
- Studies show that there is a 24% increased risk in breast cancer compared to background risk, which is not associated with length of use and disappears within 10 years of stopping
- There is an increased risk of cervical cancer, which appears to be linked to duration of use and declines to normal levels 10 years after stopping

Benefits
- Able to control own fertility
- Easy to transport
- Generally well tolerated
- Reduced risk of ovarian, endometrial and colorectal cancers
- May help to improve acne
- Can lighten periods and improve period pain

UK MEDICAL ELIGIBILITY CRITERIA FOR CONTRACEPTIVE USE (UKMEC)

The UKMEC guide staff who provide contraception on restrictions in place for contraceptives for women. There are four categories, as shown in Table 7.1.

It is important to be familiar with the category 4 restrictions, as the COCP should not be prescribed to women who meet these criteria:
- Less than 6 weeks postpartum
- Age over 35, smoking more than 15 cigarettes per day
- Systolic blood pressure 160 mmHg or higher
- Diastolic blood pressure 100 mmHg or higher
- Vascular disease
- Current or history of ischaemic heart disease
- Stroke
- History of VTE
- Surgery with prolonged immobilisation
- Known thrombogenic mutations; for example, factor V Leiden
- Complicated valvular or congenital heart disease
- Cardiomyopathy with impaired cardiac function
- Atrial fibrillation
- Migraine with aura
- Current breast cancer
- Severe cirrhosis, hepatocellular adenoma or liver cancer
- Antiphospholipid antibodies

🔍 Present Your Findings

Miss Field is a 28-year-old woman who has presented today asking to start the COCP.

I have discussed the risks and benefits with her and explained how to take the pill effectively and safely. She has no contraindications to taking it. I have checked her blood pressure and weight today and given her a prescription for 3 months, when she will return to the practice for a review.

❓ QUESTIONS AND ANSWERS FOR CANDIDATE

Does the patient have to tell her partner that she is starting the COCP?
- No, and this remains confidential and will not be shared by any of her healthcare team

What should the patient do if she develops irregular bleeding?
- Up to one in five women will have this while on the COCP
- It is worth asking if her cervical smear tests are up to date, if she has any other symptoms and if she has had a sexual health screen, in case there is another cause

What if the patient develops hypertension while taking the COCP?
- Rechecking the blood pressure a week or so later would be sensible, as well as reviewing a full medical history. If her blood pressure remains raised, then another contraception method should be started

🗨 A Case to Learn From

A woman did not disclose to her doctor that she had a history of migraines with aura and developed a stroke after starting the COCP. It is important that women are made aware that none of their healthcare team are trying to hold them back from contraceptives and that there are lots of other effective and safe options to choose from.

💡 Top Tip

Always give patients written information on their contraception choices, as the breadth of choice can be confusing. Most obstetrics and gynaecology units and family care practices will have leaflets to hand out.

STATION 7.16: COMMUNICATION: EMERGENCY CONTRACEPTION

SCENARIO

You are a junior doctor in the sexual health clinic and have been asked to see Chloe Martin, a 16-year-old woman, who has presented to request emergency contraception. Please discuss her options with her and discuss the risks and benefits of each.

Table 7.1 Four categories of restrictions for contraception provided by the UKMEC

CATEGORY	DESCRIPTION
Category 1	A condition for which there is no restriction for the use of the method
Category 2	A condition where the advantages of using the method generally outweigh the theoretical or proven risks
Category 3	A condition where the theoretical or proven risks usually outweigh the benefits of using the method. Expert clinical judgement will be needed if it is going to be used
Category 4	A condition which represents an unacceptable health risk if the method is used

CORE CONCEPT

- Women have three options for emergency contraception: Two oral methods (ulipristal acetate and levonorgestrel) and the copper coil
- The options are limited by time from the episode of unprotected sexual intercourse (UPSI)
- It is important to ensure that patients fully understand the risks and benefits of each option
- Sexual health screening and ongoing contraception should be offered at the same visit

Common Concerns

Does emergency contraception cause an abortion?	No, it can work in different ways, but does not cause an abortion. Abortion only occurs after implantation. Emergency contraception can stop ovulation, prevent an egg from becoming fertilised or stop a fertilised egg from implanting
Where can I access emergency contraception?	Many places, including: Primary care practices, sexual health clinics, walk-in centres, minor injury units and some EDs. You can buy the tablets over the counter in most pharmacies
How will I know if it has worked?	If your period comes within 3 weeks of taking the medication, then it has worked. If not, then you should take a pregnancy test and contact your primary care doctor

GATHERING INFORMATION

- Check with the patient that the sexual intercourse was consensual, details about her partner and if she feels safe in the relationship
- Check whether she was using contraception that failed or not using any
- Ask whether she is on any medications (particularly enzyme-inducing medications which can interact with oral emergency contraception)
- Ask how many hours since the UPSI occurred
- Ask about her last menstrual period and cycle details in order to work out an ovulation date
- Ask whether she would like a sexual health screen and discuss ongoing contraception

This case has two parts:
1. Explaining the emergency contraception options
2. Explaining the risks and benefits for each emergency contraception option

HOW DO YOU DECIDE WHICH EMERGENCY CONTRACEPTION IS BEST?

The Faculty of Sexual and Reproductive Health (FSRH) has really useful guidelines with algorithms (Fig. 7.6).

Present Your Findings

Miss Martin is a 16-year-old woman who presents having had a single episode of UPSI 48 h ago. We have discussed her emergency contraception choices and I have given her some leaflets with more information. She is going to return to the clinic this afternoon once she has decided which option to go for.

Her partner is a regular sexual partner of the same age and she feels safe in the relationship. She has had swabs and blood tests taken for a full sexual health screen and if she decides to have oral medication for emergency contraception, then she is going to have a contraceptive implant fitted for ongoing contraception.

Details on the different types of emergency contraception

METHOD	MECHANISM OF ACTION	USAGE	RISKS	BENEFITS
Copper coil	• Stops implantation • Toxic to sperm	• Inserted within 5 days of first UPSI or 5 days of ovulation, whichever is later	• Discomfort on insertion • Risk of uterine perforation • Increased risk of PID • Risk of coil expulsion	• Most effective form of emergency contraception • Can be used as ongoing contraception • Can stay in for 5–10 years (depending on make) • Very few contraindications
Levonorgestrel	• Progestogen drug • Delays ovulation	• Can be given within 72 h of UPSI	• Not as effective as the other two methods • Affected by enzyme-inducing drugs and patient weight • Can cause vomiting	• Can be used more than once per cycle if another episode of UPSI occurs
Ulipristal acetate	• Progesterone receptor modulator • Delays ovulation	• Can be used within 120 h of UPSI	• Not as effective as the coil • Can cause vomiting	• Can be used more than once per cycle if another episode of UPSI occurs

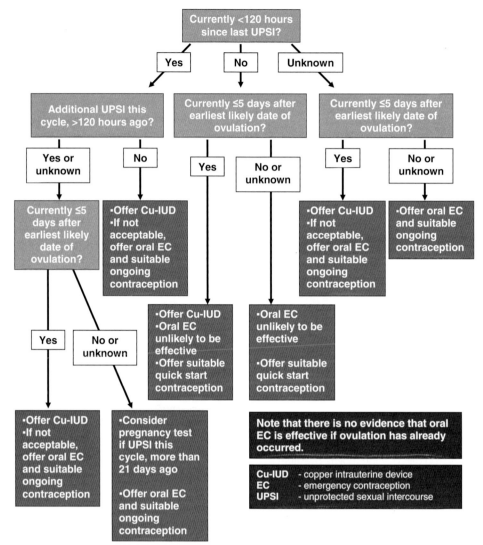

Fig. 7.6 FSRH guidance on emergency contraception types.

 QUESTIONS AND ANSWERS FOR CANDIDATE

What drugs are enzyme inducers and may affect the effectiveness of levonorgestrel?

- Antiepileptics: For example, carbamazepine, phenytoin
- Antibiotics: For example, rifabutin, rifampicin
- Antidepressants: For example, St John's wort
- Antiretrovirals

What if the woman vomits after taking oral emergency contraception?

- If this happens within 3 h of taking the medication, another dose should be given

If the patient was 15, would you need to tell her parent or guardian?

Contraception advice can be given to women under the age of 16, providing they meet the criteria of the Fraser Guidelines:

- They understand the advice
- They cannot be persuaded to tell their parents
- They are likely to begin or continue having sexual intercourse with or without contraception
- Unless they receive contraception, they will suffer physically or mentally
- It is in their best interest

A Case to Learn From

A young woman attended multiple times to the primary care practice requesting emergency contraception and staff became frustrated. Eventually the practice nurse managed to find out that she was in an abusive relationship and her partner abused both her and her child and would not allow her to take contraception.

Recurrent use of emergency contraception should be concerning. Without the practice nurse taking the time to gain the woman's trust, the situation would have continued.

Top Tip

When providing contraception to a young person it is important to check for any safety or safeguarding concerns.

STATION 7.17: COMMUNICATION: CERVICAL SMEAR COUNSELLING

SCENARIO

You are a junior doctor in a primary care practice and have been asked to see Miss Kerr, a 26-year-old woman who is worried about her first cervical smear result. It has shown mild dyskaryosis and human papillomavirus (HPV) and she has an appointment for colposcopy. Please explain the diagnosis to her and what will happen at her colposcopy appointment.

CORE CONCEPT

- Cervical screening is offered to all women aged between 25 and 64 in England
  - 3-yearly screening aged between 25 and 49
  - 5-yearly screening aged 50–64
- The aim of screening is to diagnose women with precancerous changes called cervical intraepithelial neoplasia (CIN) and treat these in order to reduce the number of cervical cancers
- HPV is strongly associated with cervical cancer
  - The highest risk subtypes are 16 and 18
- The smear test will test for changes in the cervical cells. If these are found, then the sample will also be tested for HPV
- Around five million women are invited to screening each year
- Cervical screening saves approximately 5000 lives per year in the UK

Common Concerns

Does this result mean I have cervical cancer?	This result does not mean that you have cancer, but it does mean that more investigations have to be done on your cervix. The most likely thing is that you have some precancerous changes which can be treated
Is HPV a sexually transmitted disease?	HPV is transmitted during sexual contact, and four out of five people in the world will become exposed to at least one strain of the virus during their life. It can lie dormant in the body for a long time and it is impossible to tell when you were exposed to this strain
Will I still be able to have children?	Yes. Most women who are found to have this will need minimal treatment

GATHERING INFORMATION AND COMMUNICATIONS

- Ask what the patient understands so far about her test results and what she has managed to find out for herself
- Ask what her main concerns are and what she would like to know today
- Do not use any jargon and be clear in explanations

This case has two parts:
1. Explaining the diagnosis
2. Explaining the colposcopy

EXPLAINING THE DIAGNOSIS

The cervical smear programme is designed to diagnose precancerous changes and there are seven possible results:
- Normal: Routine recall in 3 or 5 years
- Inadequate: Repeat in 3 months
- Borderline changes
- Mild dyskaryosis (CIN 1)
- Moderate dyskaryosis (CIN 2)
- Severe dyskaryosis (CIN 3)
- Glandular changes (CGIN)

How each abnormal result is treated depends on the area of the UK:
- In England, if there is borderline or mild dyskaryosis, then HPV testing will be carried out
- If this shows high-risk HPV, then you will be invited to colposcopy for further tests
- If the HPV test is negative, then you will return to routine screening, as at least 50% of these will return to normal without treatment

If there are moderate, severe or glandular changes, then you would be invited to colposcopy for further tests.

EXPLAINING THE COLPOSCOPY

- You will be seen by either a doctor or a specialist nurse
- There will also be a nursing assistant present, who will act as a chaperone
- When you attend, they will ask questions about your general health, as well as about your periods and history of any bleeding
- The colposcopist will look down a microscope (called a colposcope) at your cervix, in order to see in much closer detail. They may apply some fluid to your cervix to allow cells to show up better
- You may need a small biopsy, or a slightly larger area to remove, called a large loop excision of the transformation zone (LLETZ)
- The LLETZ aims to diagnose and help to clear any areas of precancerous changes
- Any biopsies are done under local anaesthetic
  You will normally receive your results in the post. This letter will tell you the result of your biopsy, any other treatment you may need and when your next smear or colposcopy visit will be.

CERVICAL INTRAEPITHELIAL NEOPLASIA

Many women become exposed to high-risk HPV, but not all women go on to develop cervical cancer, even without the cervical smear programme. This is because it is possible to clear HPV from the body.

There are different types of CIN that each have their own features (Table 7.2 and Fig. 7.7).

LLETZ AND PRETERM LABOUR

Most women who have a cervical smear abnormality will be of childbearing age, and many will not yet have completed their potential families and so will be concerned about the risk of damaging their fertility. While a LLETZ is unlikely to affect fertility, it can be associated with preterm labour. This is normally when women have had to have a LLETZ deeper than 10 mm, or when they have had to have repeated treatments. This will be discussed with them at their visit to colposcopy, and in future pregnancies they may need extra surveillance depending on their previous treatment.

 Present Your Findings

Miss Kerr is a 26-year-old woman who has attended to discuss her smear results, which have reported mild dyskaryosis and HPV.

I have explored her concerns about HPV and her smear result. She will attend colposcopy for further investigation and I have explained what is likely to happen at this appointment.

❓ QUESTIONS AND ANSWERS FOR CANDIDATE

Do all CIN have to be treated?

- No. Often CIN 1 does not need to be treated with a LLETZ because of the high chance of regression and the minimal chance of progression to an invasive cancer. These women will, however, need close follow-up in colposcopy

What is CGIN?

- Cervical glandular intraepithelial neoplasia
- This is a premalignant change in the glandular cells of the cervix, located within the cervical canal

What are the principles of an effective screening test?

- The condition must have the following features:
  - Be serious enough to affect life
  - Have a precancerous or early stage that can be treated
  - Have a high prevalence
- The programme itself should be:
  - Valid and reliable
  - Inexpensive
  - Acceptable to patients and easy to administer

 A Case to Learn From

A woman was referred to the EPU several times with bleeding starting at 8 weeks' gestation. Her last smear was over 5 years ago but had been normal. She was seen by multiple people during her admissions and had ultrasound scans which showed a viable intrauterine pregnancy. At 20 weeks, after further bleeding, a senior house officer did a speculum examination, which showed a cervical mass, found to be a cervical cancer. Remember, cervical abnormalities can be picked up for the first time in pregnancy.

💡 **Top Tip**

Take the time to explore the woman's concerns properly in these situations. Patients may be worried that the result means that they have cancer or that they will not be able to have children.

〰️ Table **7.2** The types of CIN and the likelihood of their progression

CERVICAL ABNORMALITY	HISTOLOGY	CHANCE OF REGRESSION	RISK OF PROGRESSION TO INVASIVE CANCER
CIN 1	Changes in basal third of epithelium	57%	1%
CIN 2	Changes in basal two-thirds of epithelium, with more nuclear atypia	43%	5%
CIN 3	Affecting entire epithelium; more severe changes	32%	>12%

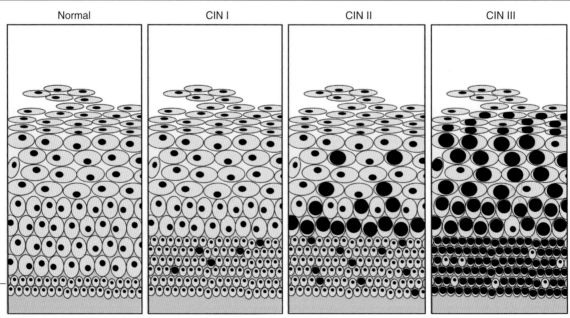

Fig. **7.7** Pictorial representation of cervical histology.

Psychiatry

8

Content Outline

Psychiatry can be perceived as a daunting and even difficult placement. It involves contact with patients who have often gone through extremely challenging life circumstances and having to communicate sensitively, whilst also coming up with an appropriate management plan.

New skills are required, not taught in other areas of medicine, like assessing thought form and content. There are also broader opportunities to develop generic skills, like assessing capacity, dealing with distressed patients and understanding psychiatric manifestations of medical illnesses.

Study Action Plan

- Speak to the staff on your ward to determine the most suitable patients for you regarding obtaining histories and performing mental state examinations (MSEs). Some patients may be unsafe to approach, others may not be able to provide a useful history for your stage of training and some may just be physically/emotionally exhausted
- Discuss your findings with ward staff afterwards to consolidate your learning, presenting them in the appropriate format
- Interviewing a patient in pairs can be helpful. It makes the process less intimidating and gives you an opportunity to get direct feedback from your colleagues
- Practise the routine for a Mini Mental State Examination (MMSE) on friends as well as patients to ensure that you are familiar with it. This is a common OSCE station
- Sharing the experiences of psychiatry patients can often be quite a difficult and emotional task, often more so than with other medical patients. This is common. If you think it might help, speak to psychiatry doctors, your colleagues, your educational supervisor, your pastoral tutor or whoever else might be helpful to 'debrief' from such experiences

STATION 8.1: HISTORY: ALCOHOL

SCENARIO

You are a junior doctor in primary care and have been asked to see Mr Chang, a 58-year-old man, who has presented with an elevated gamma-glutamyl transpeptidase (GGT). His wife is concerned about how much he is drinking. Please take a detailed alcohol history from Mr Chang, present your findings and formulate an appropriate management plan.

Cardinal Symptoms of Alcohol Dependence
Compulsion to drink with lack of control
Withdrawal
Tolerance
Neglect of other activities

HISTORY OF PRESENTING COMPLAINT

ALCOHOL INTAKE

- Amount: In a typical week, the recommended maximum weekly alcohol intake is 14 units for both men and women
- Frequency: Number of times in a day and total quantity
- Pattern: Binge drinking or regular drinking
- Timings: Drinking in the morning, during the work day and/or during the evening
- Triggers and/or motivation to drink: This may include stress or social situations
- Location of drinking: Alone or with company
- Type of alcohol: Beer, wine or spirits
- Describe a typical week of drinking: This should be like a diary

- Explore maintaining factors: What results in their continued drinking; for example, poor support

ALCOHOL DEPENDENCE SYNDROME

According to the *International Classification of Diseases*, 10th revision (ICD-10), three of the six criteria below must be met (over a 12-month period) to diagnose dependence:
- Strong desire or compulsion to drink
- Difficulty controlling intake of substance: Onset, termination or levels
- Physiological withdrawal symptoms or use of substances to prevent withdrawal symptoms
- Development of tolerance: A higher quantity required to achieve the same effect
- Neglect of other responsibilities in life
- Persistence despite evidence of harmful consequences

SCREENING METHOD

CAGE is a widely used screening method for alcohol abuse or dependence. The recommended cut-off for CAGE is ≥2 to screen for alcohol abuse or dependence:
C: 'Have you ever felt that you should *cut* down on your drinking?'
A: 'Have other people *annoyed* you by criticising the amount you drink?'
G: 'Have you ever felt *guilty* about your drinking?'
E: 'Do you ever need a drink first thing in the morning – an *eye-opener*?'

ASSOCIATED SYMPTOMS

Other symptoms to enquire about include:
- Mood or mental health problems
- Withdrawal symptoms; for example, anxiety, tremor, nausea and vomiting
- Weight loss or loss of appetite

PAST MEDICAL AND SURGICAL HISTORY

- General: Ask about known medical conditions, relevant treatments and any hospital admissions
- Alcohol history: Age of first alcoholic drink, pattern of alcohol use up until current situation, periods of abstinence, help in the past; for example,

detoxification programmes or counselling services like Alcoholics Anonymous
- Known physical complications of alcohol abuse: The complications of poorly managed alcohol withdrawal can be life threatening. These include seizures, Wernicke's encephalopathy, Korsakoff's syndrome and delirium tremens (Table 8.1)

MEDICATION HISTORY

Enquire about prescribed medications (including any recent changes) and over-the-counter medications. Allergies should be included with the specific reaction noted. In this scenario it is also important to note whether:
- Alcohol has ever caused disruption to regular medications
- Any over-the-counter medication has been used for withdrawal symptoms or 'hangovers'
- Any medications have been prescribed as aversion therapy; for example, disulfiram
- The patient has been prescribed any nutritional support

SOCIAL HISTORY

Social history includes enquiring about occupation, residence, lifestyle (diet, exercise, smoking, alcohol, substance abuse) and recent travel. Additionally, in this scenario, consider:
- Occupation: Explore any difficulties at work, including absenteeism, loss of job or decreased productivity
- Relationships: Differentiate between alcohol intake affecting relationships and relationship breakdown leading to increased alcohol intake
- Forensic: Explore any difficulties with the police, including driving convictions
- Illicit drug use: Ensure that there is no other risk-taking behaviour
- Impact of drinking on daily life: This may include shopping, eating, cooking, looking after dependants

FAMILY HISTORY

Enquire about any significant family history, including:

Table 8.1   Physical complications of alcohol abuse

BLOOD ABNORMALITIES	GASTROINTESTINAL	NEUROLOGICAL	PSYCHIATRIC	CARDIOVASCULAR
• Anaemia	• Cirrhosis • Pancreatitis • Gastro-oesophageal reflux disease (GORD) • Peptic ulcer disease • Hepatic encephalopathy	• Epilepsy • Ataxia • Peripheral neuropathy • Amnesia	• Depression • Psychosis • Wernicke's encephalopathy • Korsakoff's syndrome	• Ischaemic heart disease (IHD) • Cardiomyopathy • Hypertension

- Family history of alcoholism, noting which relatives
- Mental health problems

SYSTEMS REVIEW

On systems review, particularly pertinent questions to the above case may include questions regarding sequelae of alcohol abuse. These include:
- Jaundice: Liver disease
- Peripheral neuropathy: A neurological complication
- Memory concerns: Alcohol-related brain damage or memory blanks whilst drinking

- Sexual dysfunction: Impact of alcohol on reproductive organs

 Risk Factors for Chronic Liver Disease
- Alcohol
- Hepatitis B and C
- Obesity
- Autoimmune (autoimmune hepatitis, primary biliary cirrhosis or primary sclerosing cholangitis)

 Differential Diagnosis

DISEASE	CLINICAL PRESENTATION	INVESTIGATIONS	MANAGEMENT
Alcohol dependence	Withdrawal symptoms, including: • Tremor • Agitation • Confusion • Physical complications; for example, anaemia and signs of liver disease	• Full blood count (FBCs) • Liver function tests (LFTs) • Liver ultrasound scan (USS)	• Alcohol detoxification regime • Thiamine • Aversive medication; for example, disulfiram • Psychosocial support
Gallstones	• Biliary colic • Ascending Cholangitis (fever, jaundice, confusion)	• FBCs • LFTs • C-reactive protein (CRP) • Abdominal USS	• Analgesia • Cholecystectomy • Antibiotics • Endoscopic retrograde cholangiopancreatography (ERCP)/magnetic resonance cholangiopancreatography (MRCP)
Cholangiocarcinoma	• Jaundice • Abdominal pain • Pyrexia • Weight loss	• FBCs • LFTs • Computed tomography (CT) scan • Further detailed imaging of the biliary tree	• Chemotherapy and radiotherapy • Surgery

ASSESS MOTIVATION TO CHANGE

This can be illustrated by the Stages of Change model (Fig. 8.1). An individual progresses through all five stages before successfully achieving a new behaviour; for example becoming sober. This does not necessarily occur in a strictly linear manner and the patient may return to earlier stages on the path to achieving abstinence.

ALCOHOL WITHDRAWAL

The standard benzodiazepine-reducing regime is 20 mg chlordiazepoxide four times a day (QDS) orally, decreasing gradually over 6 days. However, administration of benzodiazepines should be titrated according to need, on the basis of objective symptoms (high blood pressure, tachycardia, tremor, agitation, sweating, confusion). Patients with severe alcohol dependence generally require doses of benzodiazepines that are substantially greater than those outlined in a standard protocol.

 Present Your Findings

Mr Chang is a 58-year-old man who presented with a raised GGT and a history of consuming 50 units of alcohol a week with tolerance. He described no symptoms of liver disease but has experienced withdrawal symptoms on previous attempts to stop drinking. This is on a background of being normally fit and well.

I feel the most likely diagnosis is alcohol dependence syndrome.

I would like to examine Mr Chang fully and take a collateral history. I would like to take further bloods tests to check his FBCs and LFTs and organise a liver USS. I would also refer him to drug and alcohol services so his alcohol detoxification can be appropriately managed.

❓ QUESTIONS AND ANSWERS FOR CANDIDATE

What is delirium tremens?
- Delirium tremens is an acute confusional state associated with tremor and autonomic dysfunction and is usually caused by the withdrawal of alcohol. It is a medical emergency

What is Wernicke's encephalopathy?

- Wernicke's encephalopathy is a condition associated with alcohol abuse and results from thiamine deficiency. It classically presents with a triad of acute confusion, ophthalmoplegia and ataxia. However, the triad may not be present in up to 90% of patients and magnetic resonance imaging (MRI) is a powerful tool to help prompt diagnosis

What is Korsakoff's syndrome?

- Korsakoff's syndrome is a preventable chronic memory disorder which can occur after Wernicke's encephalopathy and results from a severe deficiency of thiamine. It presents with impaired recent and anterograde memory, lack of insight, apathy and confabulation in an alert and responsive patient

 A Case to Learn From

A 65-year-old thin and unkempt man, of no fixed abode, presented to the emergency department (ED) with an acute confusional state. No clear history was obtained and he was admitted for a presumed delirium. It was not until a late ward round that an ataxic gait was noticed and parenteral thiamine was prescribed. The man then made a quick recovery and fortunately he was not left with any cognitive impairment.

People with alcohol dependence syndrome often have poor nutrition. The consequences of thiamine deficiency can be disastrous and therefore it should be thought about early, with immediate thiamine replacement being transformative.

 PRECONTEMPLATION: No intention to take action in the next six months

 CONTEMPLATION: Intends to take action in the next six months

 PREPARATION: Intends to take action in the next 30 days: has taken some steps in the direction

ACTION: Has changed behaviour for less than 6 months

 MAINTENANCE: Has changed behaviour for greater than 6 months

Fig. 8.1 Stages of Change model.

 Top Tip

CAGE is a widely used tool but remember it does not include important aspects like the frequency and pattern of drinking. All patients you are concerned about or those who score positive will need a full alcohol history.

 Top Tip

The experience of withdrawal is not a prerequisite for the diagnosis of dependence. An individual can be dependent on a substance even if they do not experience a clear withdrawal syndrome on ceasing use.

STATION 8.2: HISTORY: DEPRESSION

SCENARIO

You are a junior doctor in primary care and have been asked to see Mr Wood, a 50-year-old man, who has presented with difficulties sleeping. He has recently been made redundant and his wife has noticed that he is not enjoying things like he used to. She is worried about his mood. Please take a history from Mr Wood, present your findings and formulate an appropriate management plan.

Cardinal Symptoms of Depression

Reduced appetite
Sleep disturbance
Anhedonia
Dysphoria
Fatigue
Agitation and/or retardation
Diminished concentration
Low self-esteem and/or guilt
Suicide and/or thoughts of death

HISTORY OF PRESENTING COMPLAINT

CORE DEPRESSIVE SYMPTOMS

- Low mood: Present most of the day, nearly every day, with little variation
- Anhedonia: Loss of interest in things that used to be enjoyed
- Decreased energy: Less motivation and excess fatigue causing them to be slowed down

BIOLOGICAL SYMPTOMS

- Sleep disturbance: Insomnia with early-morning wakening or hypersomnia (atypical)
- Reduced appetite: Leading to weight gain when not dieting
- Loss of libido: Loss of sexual desire

COGNITIVE SYMPTOMS

- Worthlessness or excessive guilt: Marked reduction in self-esteem, not just self-reproach or guilt about being ill
- Poor concentration: Inability to think or concentrate, or indecisiveness
- Suicidal ideation: Recurrent thoughts of death or suicide, even if not acted on

SUICIDE RISK

It is not possible to take a full suicide history in a depression OSCE station, but a brief enquiry is necessary. If you run out of time, tell the examiner that you would go on to ask about it. Ask about:
- Feelings about their current situation
- Feelings about the future
- Thoughts that life is not worth living
- Thoughts of ending their life
- Thoughts about how they would do this
- Any plans made
- Past suicidal attempts
  Other risk factors for suicide should be assessed; for example:
- Unemployment
- Relationship status
- Chronic pain or disability
- Family history of deliberate self-harm or completed suicide
- Male > female

ASSOCIATED SYMPTOMS

Other symptoms to enquire about include:
- Psychotic symptoms: Delusional beliefs or perceptual abnormalities. Disturbances in the form of thoughts
- Premorbid personality: Personality before the episode of illness, as described by patient and friends/ family
- Insight: Find out what the patient subjectively thinks is happening to him

PAST PSYCHIATRIC, MEDICAL AND SURGICAL HISTORY

- General: Ask about known medical conditions, relevant treatments and any hospital admissions
- Chronic illness: Chronic pain, mobility issues or chronic illnesses
- Psychiatric illness:
  - Previous mental health diagnosis; for example, anxiety, self-harm
  - Previous psychological treatment; for example, cognitive behavioural therapy (CBT), previous medications for mental health problems

(including over the counter) and alternative therapies; for example, music therapy

MEDICATION HISTORY

Enquire about prescribed and over-the-counter medications, including any recent changes. Allergies should be included with the specific reaction noted. In this scenario, be aware of any medication that:
- Has been prescribed for mental health conditions; for example, selective serotonin reuptake inhibitors (SSRIs), anxiolytics and over-the-counter medications; for example, St John's wort
- Note any overdoses, including the amount taken

SOCIAL HISTORY

Social history includes enquiring about occupation, residence, lifestyle (diet, exercise, smoking, alcohol, substance abuse) and recent travel. Additionally, in this scenario, consider:
- Occupation: Any current employment, any difficulties at work, sick leave
- Home life: Where the patient currently lives and with whom, difficulties with relationships, impact of illness on home life
- Alcohol and illicit substance use: Any recent changes and why drugs and/or alcohol are used

FAMILY HISTORY

Enquire about any significant family history, including:
- Depression
- Other mental health illnesses

SYSTEMS REVIEW

On systems review, particularly pertinent questions to the above case may include questions regarding low mood. These include:
- Weight loss: Due to reduced appetite and self-neglect
- Insomnia: A biological symptom of depression
- Self-neglect: Evidence of malnutrition, not washing or looking after themselves, i.e. poor dental hygiene

Risk Factors for Depression

- Genetic
- Childhood experiences; for example, loss of parent, abuse
- Single and/or no confiding relationship
- Adverse life event(s)
- Physical illness
- Personality traits; for example, neuroticism, anxiety, impulsivity, obsessional

🏠 Differential Diagnosis

DISEASE	PRESENTATION	MANAGEMENT
Bipolar affective disorder	• Periods of elevated mood • Depression	• Antipsychotics • Mood stabilisers
Bereavement/grief reaction	• Low mood • Tearful • Poor sleep	• Bereavement counselling
Hypothyroidism	• Weight gain • Constipation	• Thyroxine
Stroke	• Visual and speech changes • Hemiparesis	• Anticoagulation/antiplatelet therapy (ischemic) • Rehabilitation
Malignancy (hypercalcaemia)	• Abdominal pain • Renal calculi	• Fluids • Diuretics • Treatment of primary malignancy
Parkinson's disease	• Bradykinesia • Tremor • Rigidity	• Levodopa
Drugs: • Alcohol • Withdrawal from stimulants • Oral contraceptives • Some antihypertensive drugs	• Variable presentation; for example, intoxication, low mood, weight gain, sun sensitivity	• Alcohol and drug support, including detoxification • Talking therapy • Medication review

AETIOLOGY OF DEPRESSION

🏃 Aetiological factors for depression

PREDISPOSING	PRECIPITATING	PERPETUATING
• Long-term adversity; for example, employment or marital difficulties • Poor support network; for example, lack of close-confiding relationships • Female gender	• Acute stressful life events • Poor compliance with medication	• Inability to solve precipitating or predisposing adversity • Poor insight • Alcohol or substance misuse

SELECTIVE SEROTONIN REUPTAKE INHIBITORS

The mnemonic: EFSPC (effective for sadness, panic and compulsion) is helpful:
- *Escitalopram*
- *Fluoxetine, fluvoxamine*
- *Sertraline*
- *Paroxetine*
- *Citalopram*

CONCERNING FEATURES OF DEPRESSION

- Psychotic features: Persecutory delusions, auditory hallucinations
- Self-neglect: Poor oral intake with weight loss
- Potential for harm: To self or others
- Suicide risk: Assess this thoroughly, including previous attempts

DIAGNOSING DEPRESSION

Key Symptoms
- Persistent sadness or low mood and/or
- Marked loss of interest or pleasure
  At least one of these, most days, most of the time for at least 2 weeks.

If any of above is present, ask about associated symptoms:
- Disturbed sleep (decreased or increased compared to usual)
- Decreased or increased appetite and/or weight
- Fatigue or loss of energy
- Agitation or slowing of movements
- Poor concentration or indecisiveness
- Feelings of worthlessness or excessive or inappropriate guilt
- Suicidal thoughts or acts

Depression Definitions (taken from DSM-IV)

- Subthreshold depressive symptoms: Fewer than five symptoms of depression
- Mild depression: Few, if any, symptoms in excess of the five required to make the diagnosis, and symptoms result in only minor functional impairment The ICD-10 threshold is lower, at four symptoms
- Moderate depression: Symptoms or functional impairment are between 'mild' and 'severe'
- Severe depression: Most symptoms, and the symptoms markedly interfere with functioning. Can occur with or without psychotic symptoms

🔍 Present Your Findings

Mr Wood is a 50-year-old man who presented with a 2-month history of low mood, with low energy and poor appetite associated with a 5-kg weight loss. Mr Wood displays no evidence of psychosis or mania and denies thoughts of self-harm or suicide. This is on a background of being normally fit and well with no psychiatric history.

I feel the most likely diagnosis is a moderate depressive episode.

I would like to take a collateral history and discuss psychological and medication management with Mr Wood. I will ensure he is followed up during this difficult time.

❓ QUESTIONS AND ANSWERS FOR CANDIDATE

Name three symptoms of atypical depression.
- Reactive affect
- Increased appetite and weight gain
- Hypersomnia
- Leaden paralysis; for example, heavy, leaden feelings in arms or legs
- Interpersonal rejection sensitivity that results in significant impairment

What is catatonia?
- Catatonic symptoms are abnormal movements and behaviours that can be caused by mental illnesses such as mania, depression or schizophrenia. In depression you might see a patient staying in one position for a long period of time, mutism, resistance to passive movements or stupor

What is a nihilistic delusion?
- This is a delusional belief that everything, including the person, does not exist and is not real. This type of delusional belief is most commonly seen in severe depression

A Case to Learn From

A 46-year-old patient was admitted to a psychiatric ward with severe depression and psychomotor retardation (slowing of physical and emotional responses). This meant that it took him a few minutes to answer questions. Initially he was seen during ward round but due to the schedule only a few questions could be asked at the time. The team, therefore, changed the day he was seen so that more time could be spent with him and he was not rushed, and a full history could be taken. This allowed him to ask questions and be involved in his care.

💡 Top Tip

There are often hints that a patient has severe depression before they even start speaking. Be aware of eye contact, body language, facial expressions and the feeling in the room as you enter.

STATION 8.3: HISTORY: MANIA

SCENARIO

You are a junior doctor in primary care and have been asked to see Mrs Jones, a 28-year-old woman, who has presented with her husband. He reports that she has been acting strangely and has been on huge shopping sprees, resulting in considerable debt. She has previously suffered from depression. Please take a history from Mrs Jones, present your findings and formulate an appropriate management plan.

Cardinal Symptoms of Mania

Elated, excited and enthusiastic mood

Increased activity

'Naughty' behaviour; for example, spending sprees, use of alcohol and drugs, increased sexual activity

Insomnia

Increased confidence

HISTORY OF PRESENTING COMPLAINT

MANIC SYMPTOMS

- Elevated mood: Distinct period of persistent high mood
- Increased activity: Reduced sleep, increased libido, racing thoughts, pressured speech
- Increased self-esteem: Grandiosity, overoptimistic, overfamiliarity, reduced social disinhibition

- Reduced attention: Distractible
- Risky behaviours: Overspending, increased sexual activity, preoccupation with extravagant schemes

ASSOCIATED SYMPTOMS

Other symptoms to enquire about include:
- Psychotic symptoms: Including hallucinations, pseudohallucinations and illusions
- Premorbid personality: Personality before the episode of illness, as described by patient and friends/family
- Insight: Find out what the patient subjectively thinks is happening to her

PAST PSYCHIATRIC, MEDICAL AND SURGICAL HISTORY

- General: Ask about known medical conditions, relevant treatments and any hospital admissions
- Psychiatric illness: Ask about previous depression, manic, psychotic or hypomanic episodes

MEDICATION HISTORY

Enquire about prescribed and over-the-counter medications, including any recent changes. Allergies should also be included with the specific reaction noted. In this scenario it is also important to note:
- Previous antipsychotics: For example, olanzapine, risperidone, haloperidol
- Previous antidepressants: For example, citalopram, sertraline, mirtazapine
- Previous mood stabilisers: For example, lithium, carbamazepine, sodium valproate

SOCIAL HISTORY

Social history includes enquiring about occupation, residence, lifestyle (diet, exercise, smoking, alcohol, substance abuse) and recent travel. Additionally in this scenario, consider:
- Home life: Where the patient currently lives and with whom
- Relationships: Any recent difficulties or arguments
- Occupation: Difficulties at work, concerns from colleagues
- Financial concerns: Including overspending and debt
- Substance abuse: Changes in substance use, check for risky behaviours

FAMILY HISTORY

Enquire about any significant family history, including:
- Mental health illnesses

SYSTEMS REVIEW

On systems review, particularly pertinent questions to the above case may include questions regarding mania. These include:
- Insomnia: Whether she is managing to sleep and if not, why
- Self-neglect: Whether she is managing to look after herself, washing and cleaning clothes, eating properly
- Sexually transmitted Infections: Pain, itching, discharge

Differential Diagnosis

DISEASE	PRESENTATION	MANAGEMENT
Psychotic disorders, including: • Schizophrenia • Schizoaffective disorder • Delusional disorder	• Hallucinations • Delusional thoughts • Disorganised speech • Negative symptoms	• Antipsychotics • Mood stabilisers • Talking therapy • Multidisciplinary team (MDT) support
Anxiety, posttraumatic stress disorder (PTSD)	• Palpitations • Sweating • Flashbacks • Hyperarousal	• Anxiolytics • Talking therapy
Brain tumour	• Personality changes • Headache • Vomiting	• Radiotherapy • Chemotherapy • Surgery
Hyperthyroidism	• Anxiety • Sweatiness • Weight loss • Tremor • Diarrhoea • Neck swelling	• Radioactive iodine • Beta-blockers • Carbimazole

Differential Diagnosis—cont'd

DISEASE	PRESENTATION	MANAGEMENT
Cushing's syndrome	• Weight gain (particularly centrally, between shoulders and on face) • Acne • Easy bruising • Skin thinning • Striae on skin	• Cortisol-inhibiting medications • Surgery
Head injury	• Headache • Vomiting • Seizures • Loss of power and/or sensation • Visual disturbances • Disorientation • Amnesia	• Conservative management or surgery depending on the injury
Drugs; for example: • Alcohol • Stimulants • Opiates • Hallucinogens • (Withdrawal from) antidepressants • Steroids	• Variable presentation; for example, intoxication, hallucinations, unkemptness, increased energy, disorientation	• Alcohol and drug support, including detoxification • Talking therapy • Medication review

Risk Factors for Mania

- Family history
- Substance misuse
- Stress
- Antidepressant use in bipolar affective disorder

SYMPTOMS OF A MANIC EPISODE MNEMONIC

A manic episode is a distinct period of persistently elevated, expansive and irritable mood. It must last for at least 1 week and features include:

- *Grandiosity*: Or inflated self-esteem
- *Sleep*: Decreased need
- *Talkative*: Pressure of speech
- *Pleasure*: Will engage in high-risk and irrational activities for pleasure; for example, sex, spending, drugs
- *Activity*: Goal-directed and psychomotor agitation increased
- *Ideas*: Flight of ideas
- *Distractibility*: Difficulty concentrating

The above features can be remembered using the mnemonic GST PAID.

HYPOMANIA

Although many of the same symptoms are experienced in hypomania as in mania, these are usually less severe.

Hypomanic periods must last for several days and should not necessitate hospitalisation or have psychotic features. With hypomania, an individual's ability to function in everyday life is not significantly impaired.

Present Your Findings

Mrs Jones is a 28-year-old woman who presented with a 2-week history of elevated mood, increased energy, reduced sleep and overspending. She describes no thoughts of self-harm or harm to others and displays no features of psychosis. This is on a background of depression.

I feel that the most likely diagnosis is a manic episode in the context of bipolar affective disorder because of her history, with differentials being hyperthyroidism and substance misuse.

I would like to examine Mrs Jones fully and take bloods to check her FBCs and TFTs. I will refer her urgently for a psychiatric assessment and discuss medication options with her today.

QUESTIONS AND ANSWERS FOR CANDIDATE

What is 'flight of ideas'?

- 'Flight of ideas' is a type of thought disorder in which there is a rapid shifting of ideas with minimal connections between the ideas. It is typically seen during manic episodes

What is the difference between bipolar type I and II?

The ICD-10 recognises bipolar I and bipolar II:

- Bipolar I: Episodes of mania and depression
- Bipolar II: Episodes of hypomania and depression

Name three examples of physical health medications that can precipitate mania.

- Antiparkinsonian medication: For example, levodopa, bromocriptine, amantadine
- Respiratory drugs: For example, aminophylline, salbutamol
- Benzodiazepines: For example, diazepam, lorazepam
- Cardiovascular medication: For example, captopril, digoxin, diltiazem

A Case to Learn From

A 62-year-old man with a new diagnosis of chronic obstructive pulmonary disease (COPD) presented to his primary care doctor with increased shortness of breath and a productive cough. He was prescribed a course of antibiotics and oral prednisolone for an infective exacerbation of COPD. A few days later he presented to the ED with his wife, who complained that he had irritable outbursts. She reported that he had hardly been sleeping and wouldn't rest like the primary care doctor had advised. The ED doctor identified that the steroids might have precipitated manic symptoms and stopped them, which resulted in a quick improvement in the patient's mental state.

Top Tip

Ask about a history of overactivity or irritability in recurrent depression, as prescribing antidepressants to someone with unrecognised bipolar affective disorder can be dangerous. Antidepressants can trigger a hypomanic or manic episode, cause rapid cycling and increase the risk of suicide, and this is why follow-up after starting a medication is so important.

STATION 8.4: HISTORY: POSTNATAL DEPRESSION (PND)

SCENARIO

You are a junior doctor in primary care and have been asked to see Mrs Roberts, a 24-year-old woman, who has presented after giving birth to her first child. Her partner is concerned because she does not appear to be coping well. Her mood has been persistently low and she has been very tearful. Please take a history from Mrs Roberts, present your findings and formulate an appropriate management plan.

Cardinal Symptoms of Postnatal Depression

Depressive symptoms

Anxiety

Concerns about the baby's health

Feelings of inadequacy and inability to cope

Lack of bonding with the baby

HISTORY OF PRESENTING COMPLAINT

SYMPTOMS OF PND

- Low mood: Sustained low mood with tearfulness and anhedonia
- Guilt or inadequacy: Parent may feel they are not able to cope or look after their baby properly
- Overwhelmed: Women can feel stressed and like they cannot manage
- Anxiety: Women may be very worried with no clear explanation
- Thoughts of harming the baby: These thoughts are rarely acted on and are very distressing to the parent Features of PND are similar to those of depression (low mood, tearfulness, anhedonia, self-harm), but

suicidal thoughts are less common and anxiety is particularly marked.

ASSOCIATED SYMPTOMS

Other symptoms to enquire about include:
- Low self-esteem
- Worthlessness
- Psychotic symptoms

PAST PSYCHIATRIC, MEDICAL AND SURGICAL HISTORY

- General: Ask about known medical conditions, relevant treatments and any hospital admissions
- Pregnancy history: Any problems such as pre-eclampsia or prolonged hospital admission
- Psychiatric illness: Previous mental health diagnosis; for example, depression or manic episodes, and previous talking therapies

MEDICATION HISTORY

Enquire about prescribed and over-the-counter medications, including any recent changes. Allergies should also be included with the specific reaction noted. In this scenario it is also important to note:
- Previous medication for a mental health condition; for example, antidepressants, antipsychotics or mood stabilisers
- Previous medication overdose(s)
- Medication prescribed during pregnancy

SOCIAL HISTORY

Social history includes enquiring about occupation, residence, lifestyle (diet, exercise, smoking, alcohol, substance abuse) and recent travel. Additionally, in this scenario, consider:
- Home life: Where the patient currently lives and with whom
- Relationships: Explore her support network and who helps with childcare

FAMILY HISTORY

Enquire about any significant family history, including:
- Depression
- Other mental health illnesses

SYSTEMS REVIEW

On systems review, particularly pertinent questions to the above case may include questions regarding low mood. These include:
- Weight loss: Due to reduced appetite and self-neglect
- Insomnia: A biological symptom of depression
- Self-neglect: Evidence of malnutrition, not washing or looking after herself, i.e. poor dental hygiene

Risk Factors for PND

- Family and/or personal history of PND or depression
- Adverse life events; for example, family death, loss of income
- Difficulties with breastfeeding
- Unplanned or unwanted pregnancy
- Poor social support or difficult home environment
- The risk factors outlined above can be remembered using the mnemonic FA BUS.

Differential Diagnosis

DISEASE	PRESENTATION	MANAGEMENT
Baby blues More than 50% of mothers will experience this type of low mood within the first week after childbirth	• Labile mood • Tearful • Feeling overwhelmed	• This generally resolves and requires reassurance as management
PND Depression experienced by a parent following childbirth	• Low mood • Anxiety • Guilt • Feelings of inadequacy	• Education • Support • Talking therapies; for example, CBT or interpersonal therapy • Antidepressant therapy • Mother and baby unit may be required
Puerperal psychosis The most severe form of mental illness following childbirth	• Psychotic symptoms • Thoughts of harming the baby	• Hospitalisation is usually required in a mother and baby unit • Antipsychotic and antidepressant therapy

INFORMATION ON PND

- Approximately 10–15 in 100 women suffer PND in the year after birth
- Usually gradual in onset
- 50% onset by 6 months
- It is typically a non-psychotic depression, with no loss of contact with reality

ADVICE FOR THE PARENT

- PND is common

- The Edinburgh PND scale can be a useful screening tool. It is a self-reported 10-item questionnaire that can be completed at 6–8 weeks postpartum
- PND will usually improve with treatment; for example, psychological interventions (CBT or interpersonal therapy)
- Antidepressants can play a role. It is important to discuss the risks and benefits of antidepressants in a breastfeeding mother as some psychotropic drugs are secreted in breast milk. At higher doses, one may advise against breastfeeding
- Tell the mother that it is helpful to discuss any concerns and her feelings

MANAGEMENT OF PND

- In cases of mild PND, antidepressants should be avoided. At this stage, guided self-help, exercise or watchful waiting should be attempted
- However, if severity warrants it, offer referral to psychiatry and antidepressants
- Adequately assess and monitor the safety of the mother and child:
  - Increase visits by health visitors and regularly see the mother yourself
  - If serious concerns arise regarding child and/or mother safety, urgent assessment by mother and baby psychiatry is required
  - It may be advisable to admit the patient to a mother and baby unit to allow treatment (generally with the baby being present in the unit)
  - Child protection issues may arise and need to be addressed

Present Your Findings

Mrs Roberts is a 24-year-old woman who presented 5 days postnatally with low mood and tearfulness. She reports no thoughts of harm to herself or others (including her baby) but describes finding it difficult coping as a mother. This is on a background of being normally fit and well, with no previous background of psychiatric illness. I feel the most likely diagnosis is 'baby blues'.

I would like to provide reassurance and organise support to be provided in the community, with involvement of the health visitor or primary care team.

QUESTIONS AND ANSWERS FOR CANDIDATE

When is the most likely time to develop PND?
- The peak onset is 3–4 weeks postpartum

What should you discuss with a new mother trying to decide whether to start antidepressants?
- Past history
- Severity of illness and the possible impact on the baby
- Past treatments and side effects
- Up-to-date information about the safety of medication in breastfeeding
- The benefits of breastfeeding

Name three investigations that you would ask for to rule out an organic cause of low mood.
- FBCs to look for infection
- Haematinics to look for folic acid deficiency
- TFTs to look for hypothyroidism

 A Case to Learn From

A 30-year-old woman with a history of moderate episodes of depression stopped her antidepressants during pregnancy as she was concerned about the possible damage it could do to her baby. The midwife picked up on this and alerted the primary care doctor who was able to monitor the woman regularly after she had given birth and pick up on the early signs of PND. This is an example of an MDT approach working well to support a patient.

 Top Tip

Keep PND in your mind when seeing parents. It can present up to 2 years after birth. Even when a paediatrician is seeing a child, symptoms in the parents may become apparent when taking the history.

STATION 8.5: HISTORY: SUICIDE RISK ASSESSMENT

SCENARIO

You are a junior doctor in the ED and have been asked to see Mr Smith, a 45-year-old man, who has presented after attempting to hang himself. He has recently separated from his wife and has been struggling with low mood. He is now medically fit. Please take a history from Mr Smith, present your findings and formulate an appropriate management plan.

HISTORY OF PRESENTING COMPLAINT

When assessing risk, try to conduct your questioning in a structured manner whilst simultaneously showing sensitivity by being flexible and exploring what the patient wants to talk about in greater detail.

A good approach to assessing suicide risk is to invite the patient to take you through an autobiographical timeline (starting at least 24 h before the act of self-harm).

The suicide attempt:
- Method: Identify how
  - Medication overdose: Note the drug(s) taken, how much and the time scale it was taken over
- Plans: Identify how long a plan existed for and the level of detail; for example, getting finances in order, preparing a suicide note
- Triggers: Relationship breakdown, job loss
- Avoiding detection: For example, not telling anyone or doing it where the individual might not be discovered
- Suicidal fantasy: Patient perception of lethality or likely consequence of their actions

- Event: Identify how they were found
- Current thoughts: Identify how patient is feeling now; for example, would they rather not be alive?
- Assessing future risk: Thoughts, intentions or plans for self-harm in the future
- Protective factors: Family, relationships and friends, hobbies, future plans
- Insight: Establish whether the patient subjectively understands that he may require help to deal with this and how he will keep himself safe

PAST PSYCHIATRIC, MEDICAL AND SURGICAL HISTORY

- General: Ask about known medical conditions, relevant treatments and any hospital admissions
- Chronic illnesses: Chronic pain or mobility issues
- Psychiatric illnesses:
  - Depression
  - Bipolar affective disorder
  - Personality disorders
  - Previous self-harm or suicidal attempts

MEDICATION HISTORY

Enquire about prescribed and over-the-counter medications, including any recent changes. Allergies should also be included with the specific reaction noted. In this scenario be aware of medications that:
- Have been previously prescribed e.g. antidepressants or anxiolytics
- Have been taken as an overdose

Check the amount of medication prescribed at a time, as some patients with a risk of overdose will be given weekly prescriptions

SOCIAL HISTORY

Social history includes enquiring about occupation, residence, lifestyle (diet, exercise, smoking, alcohol, substance abuse) and recent travel. Additionally, in this scenario, consider:
- Occupation: Any current employment, difficulties at work, financial concerns, including debt
- Home life: Where the patient currently lives and with whom
- Relationships: Any recent difficulties or arguments, whether the patient has any children and if so, who is looking after them
- Alcohol and illicit substance use: Any recent changes and past history

FAMILY HISTORY

Enquire about any significant family history, including:
- Depression
- Other mental health illnesses

SYSTEMS REVIEW

On systems review, particularly pertinent questions to the above case may include questions regarding low mood. These include:

- Weight loss: Due to reduced appetite and self-neglect
- Insomnia: A biological symptom of depression
- Self-neglect: Evidence of malnutrition, not washing or looking after themselves, i.e. poor dental hygiene

Risk Factors for Suicide

- *Sex*: Male
- *Age*: Over 40 or under 19 years old
- *Depression*
- *Previous* attempts or *plans* to retry
- *Ethanol* or drug abuse
- Loss of *rational* thinking; for example, psychosis
- *Social* isolation; for example, single, separated, widowed
- *Organised* plan; for example, leaving a suicide note, getting affairs in order
- *No* hobbies
- Physical illness
- Social problems; for example, unemployment, recent change in life circumstances

The risk factors outlined above can be remembered using the mnemonic SAD PERSON.

HOW MIGHT THE PATIENT BE HELPED?

- Any underlying disease could be treated, including depression. The patient could be counselled to deal with underlying emotions
- Specialist groups such as Relate could more specifically deal with relationship problems
- Methods to reduce work stresses; for example, reducing hours and avoiding tight deadlines, and financial aids could also be explored if this was a problem
- Beliefs could be challenged using CBT
- Charities and organisations to help support with financial debt, housing and coping with suicidal thoughts
- Referral to community mental health teams for ongoing support

Present Your Findings

Mr Smith is a 45-year-old man who presented after attempting to hang himself. He believed and intended the suicide attempt to take his life and made efforts to avoid detection. He describes no evidence of psychosis, but the attempt was preplanned and the stresses that led to it are still present. This is on a background of being normally fit and well. I feel the most likely diagnosis is untreated depression.

Mr Smith has a high risk of successfully completing suicide with multiple significant risk factors, including, sex, age and social isolation. I would like to keep Mr Smith in hospital for further psychiatric assessment.

❓ QUESTIONS AND ANSWERS FOR CANDIDATE

What are the three typical differences between features of completed suicide and non-fatal deliberate self-harm?

FEATURES	COMPLETED SUICIDE	NON-FATAL DELIBERATE SELF-HARM
Sex	More males	More females
Age	Late middle age	Late teens or early 20s
Setting	Concealed setting	Others are normally present

How many deaths in England and Wales are due to suicide, expressed as a percentage?

- 1%

Name three examples of mental illnesses that increase the risk of suicide.

- Depression
- Psychosis
- Anorexia nervosa
- Alcohol and drug misuse
- Personality disorders
- Organic mental illness

A Case to Learn From

A patient was settled on the medical assessment unit after being admitted for intentional overdose of paracetamol. After lunchtime, the emergency call bell was activated and it was found that the patient had a metal knife and was trying to harm himself with it. He had kept his knife after lunchtime and hid it under his pillow. It's important that patients at risk of harm to themselves or others are carefully taken care of in the correct facilities and with protective measures in place to avoid a dangerous situation for everyone.

Top Tip

Always ask the patient what they thought would happen after the attempt, as serious suicidal intent can be associated with medically trivial overdoses.

Top Tip

If a patient has written a suicide note you should read it, as it may provide insight into their motivation. A note that reads like an emotionally charged rant suggests a writer who desperately wants to be heard – the self-harm may be a 'cry for help'. In contrast, a note that reads like the instructions someone with a terminal illness would leave for surviving relatives is highly suggestive of suicidal intent – the writer expected to die.

STATION 8.6: HISTORY: SCHIZOPHRENIA

SCENARIO

You are a junior doctor in primary care and have been asked to see Mr Brown, a 19-year-old student, who has presented after hearing voices. He believes that his friends are out to get him and his parents are worried that he has been acting strangely. Please take a history from Mr Brown, present your findings and formulate an appropriate management plan.

 Cardinal Symptoms of Schizophrenia

Delusions

Hallucinations

Disorganised speech

Disorganised or catatonic behaviour

Negative symptoms, i.e. flattening of affect

HISTORY OF PRESENTING COMPLAINT

DELUSIONS

- Persecutory: Concern about harm or people being out to get them; for example, secret services
- Delusions of reference: Connecting strong personal significance to normal experiences; for example, believing that newspaper headlines are written for him
- Delusions of perception: Attributing false meanings to normal perceptions; for example, a red traffic light causing the belief that he has special powers
- Grandeur: Increased importance; for example, the belief he is very important and wealthy
- Nihilistic: Self/body/others/the world has ceased to exist; for example, he has the thought that his own internal organs are rotting
- Passivity: Lack of control of thoughts or actions; for example, feeling that others are controlling his movements
- Test conviction: It is important to clarify how strongly he holds this belief

HALLUCINATIONS

- Auditory: Hearing a running commentary of his actions, hearing his own thoughts being spoken or hearing voices
- Visual: Seeing figures; for example, Lilliputian hallucinations is where intricate small figures are seen
- Olfactory: Noticing smells that are not present
- Gustatory: Tasting something, typically unpleasant, when nothing is there
- Tactile: Feeling sensations when nothing is there

THOUGHT INTERFERENCE AND DISORGANISATION

- Thought insertion: Thoughts being placed into the mind
- Thought withdrawal: Thoughts being taken out of the mind
- Thought broadcast: People being able to hear thoughts like they are being broadcast without them being said
- Disorganised thought: Shown by disorganised speech; for example, speech that is difficult to follow and does not make sense. This includes thought blocking, when speech suddenly stops and tangential speech, where the speech diverts from its previous course and does not return

ASSOCIATED SYMPTOMS

- Disorganised or catatonic behaviour: Unusual movements which may be held for a long time; for example, waxy flexibility, a decreased response to stimuli and tendency to remain in an immobile position
- Premorbid personality: A schizoid personality, including symptoms such as detachment, lack of interest in others and excessive introspection, sometimes predates a diagnosis of schizophrenia
- Insight: Establish what the patient thinks is happening, whether they think they are unwell and require treatment

PAST PSYCHIATRIC, MEDICAL AND SURGICAL HISTORY

- General: Ask about known medical conditions, relevant treatments and any hospital admissions
- Psychiatric illness:
  - Depression
  - Anxiety
  - Previous self-harm or suicide attempts
  - Previous psychotic symptoms
  - Previous hospital admissions and if so, whether the patient was detained under the Mental Health Act

MEDICATION HISTORY

Enquire about prescribed medications, typical and atypical antipsychotics (including any recent changes) and over-the-counter medications. Allergies should be included with the specific reaction noted. In this scenario, be aware of medications that:

- Induce psychosis; for example, corticosteroids, ketamine, antihistamines and recreational drugs; for example, cannabis

SOCIAL HISTORY

Social history includes enquiring about occupation, residence, lifestyle (diet, exercise, smoking, alcohol, substance abuse) and recent travel. Additionally, in this scenario, consider:

- Smoking: Document pack years, calculated as the number of packets per day multiplied by the number of years smoked
- Alcohol and illicit substance use: For example, cannabis use
- Occupation: Any current employment and financial support
- Home life: Where he currently lives and with whom, any stressors, how the patient manages with activities of daily living

- Relationships: Any recent arguments or difficulties, support network

FAMILY HISTORY

Enquire about any significant family history, including:
- Mental health illnesses
- Physical health; for example, epilepsy, systemic lupus erythematosus, Cushing's syndrome

SYSTEMS REVIEW

On systems review, particularly pertinent questions to the above case may include questions regarding psychotic symptoms. These include:

Differential Diagnosis

DISEASE	PRESENTATION	INVESTIGATIONS	MANAGEMENT
Organic syndromes (for example, dementia, brain tumour, temporal-lobe epilepsy)	• Poor memory • Personality changes • Seizures	• FBCs • Vitamin B_{12} and folate • Calcium • LFTs • Thyroid function tests (TFTs) • Urea and electrolytes (U&Es) • Glucose • Erythrocyte sedimentation rate (ESR) • CRP • CT scan • Electroencephalogram (EEG)	• Dependent on the cause
Drug-induced (for example, by amphetamines, lysergic acid diethylamide (LSD), cocaine)	• Disorientated • Increased energy • Hallucinations	• Urine drug screen	• Drug management with detoxification
Mood disorder (for example, depression or mania with psychotic features)	• Mood changes • Delusional beliefs • Hallucinations	• FBCs • Vitamin B_{12} and folate • Calcium • LFTs • TFTs • U&Es • Glucose • ESR • CRP • Baseline ECG prior to treatment	• Antipsychotics
Schizoaffective disorder	• Affective and psychotic symptoms	• FBCs • Vitamin B_{12} and folate • Calcium • LFTs • TFTs • U&Es • Glucose • ESR • CRP • Baseline ECG prior to treatment	• As for schizophrenia, but treat mania and depressive episodes as per bipolar affective disorder

Continued

Differential Diagnosis—cont'd

DISEASE	PRESENTATION	INVESTIGATIONS	MANAGEMENT
Schizoid personality disorder	• Lack of interest in relationships • Solitary lifestyle • Emotional detachment	• FBCs • Vitamin B_{12} and folate • Calcium • LFTs • TFTs • U&Es • Glucose • ESR • CRP • Baseline ECG prior to treatment	• Psychological therapies • Medication
Acute psychotic reaction	• Hallucinations • Delusional beliefs • Disorganised speech	• FBCs • Vitamin B_{12} and folate • Calcium • LFTs • TFTs • U&Es • Glucose • ESR • CRP • Baseline ECG prior to treatment	• Antipsychotics

- Neurological: Headache, confusion, fits
- Genitourinary: Urinary retention secondary to psychotropic anticholinergic medications
- Gastrointestinal: Constipation secondary to psychotropic anticholinergic medications

Risk Factors for Psychosis

- Family history
- Perinatal complications
- Substance misuse
- Urbanisation at birth
- Stress

DEFINITION OF SCHIZOPHRENIA

ICD-10 states there must be at least one very clear symptom from group A or two or more from group B lasting longer than 1 month:

- Group A:
  - Thought echo, insertion, withdrawal or broadcasting
  - Delusions of control, influence or passivity
  - Hallucinatory voices, third-person or running commentary
  - Persistent bizarre delusions
- Group B:
  - Persistent hallucinations in any modality
  - Thought disorder: A disorder of cognitive organisation in which thoughts lack expected sequencing and it can be difficult to follow the train of thought
  - Catatonic behaviour
  - 'Negative' symptoms such as marked apathy, paucity of speech, and blunting or incongruity of emotional responses
  - Behavioural change

SYMPTOMS OF SCHIZOPHRENIA

The positive and negative symptoms of schizophrenia outlined above can be remembered using the mnemonic THREAD LESS (Table 8.2).

Table 8.2   Positive and negative symptoms of schizophrenia

POSITIVE SYMPTOMS	NEGATIVE SYMPTOMS
Thinking disturbed	*Loss* of volition, underactivity, social withdrawal
Hallucinations, typically auditory	*Emotionally* flat
Reduced contact with reality	*Speech* reduced, monosyllabic
Emotional control affected – incongruous effect	*Slowness* in movement, thought and psychomotor retardation
Arousal may lead to worsening of symptoms	
Difficulty concentrating	

Present Your Findings

Mr Brown is a 19-year-old student who presented with a persecutory delusion of his classmates wishing to harm him with associated auditory hallucinations and thought insertion. He describes no thoughts of harm to himself or others. This is on the background of being normally fit and well but misusing cannabis. I feel the most likely diagnosis is drug-induced psychosis, with the differentials being the onset of schizophrenia or schizoaffective disorder.

I would like to get a collateral history to further my assessment, examine Mr Brown fully and organise a urine drug screen.

❓ QUESTIONS AND ANSWERS FOR CANDIDATE

Define a 'delusion', 'hallucination' and 'psychosis'.

- Delusion: A fixed false belief which is not congruent with cultural norms
- Hallucination: A perception in the absence of a stimulus
- Psychosis: An umbrella term for a loss of contact with reality. There are many causes of psychosis, one of which is schizophrenia

Name three subtypes of schizophrenia recognised in ICD-10.

- Paranoid: Key symptoms include delusions and hallucinations
- Catatonic: Key symptoms include psychomotor disturbance
- Hebephrenic: Key symptoms include disorganised speech and flat or inappropriate affect
- Residual: This is when previous positive symptoms are less marked, but prominent negative symptoms remain
- Undifferentiated: This meets general criteria, but no specific subtype predominates
- Simple: There are no delusions or hallucinations; negative symptoms gradually arise without an acute episode

What is schizoaffective disorder?

- This is a disorder when schizophrenic and mood symptoms are present in approximately equal proportions. There needs to be at least one typical schizophrenic symptom present for a diagnosis

 A Case to Learn From

A 20-year-old patient presented to the ED and reported that he needed to hide as he was being followed by MI5. He was agitated, would not cooperate with staff and said he only felt safe if he lay under the bed. The ED doctor allowed him to remain under the bed and sat down next to him calmly. With open questions and observing his behaviour, the doctor was able to gather a lot of information about his current presentation without increasing his agitation. This case shows the value of observing patients and the importance of being flexible when completing assessments.

 Top Tip

Not all voices are psychotic in nature. Patients with emotionally unstable personality disorder or complex PTSD describe voices internally which are derogatory and distressing in nature. They may be aware that these voices are not real and do not respond to them. These can sometimes be called pseudohallucinations.

 Top Tip

The majority of patients with schizophrenia lack insight that their symptoms are caused by a mental illness. It is therefore very important to get a collateral history as soon as possible.

STATION 8.7: EXAMINATION: MENTAL STATE

SCENARIO

You are a junior doctor in a primary care practice and have been asked to see Mrs Bradley, a 58-year-old female, who has recently separated from her husband and lost her job. There is a concern that she is very depressed. Please perform an MSE, present your findings and formulate an appropriate management plan.

MENTAL STATE EXAMINATION

- Appearance
  - Loosely dressed: may occur with anorexia
  - Dishevelled: may occur with psychosis or dementia
  - Brightly coloured: may occur with mania (Fig. 8.2)
  - Evidence of self-harm: Cuts, bruising
  - Evidence of physical neglect: Personal hygiene
  - Evidence of physical illness: Hyperthyroidism (Fig. 8.3) or hypothyroidism, Cushing's disease
- Behaviour
  - Rapport: Quality, including consistency
  - Eye contact: Fleeting, normal or intense
  - Behaviour: Distracted, agitated, tearful, anxious or suspicious
- Mood
  - This is an assessment of the patient's sustained state of inner feelings; for example, low, anxious, angry, elated
  - Subjective: The patient's own impression, and it can be helpful to ask them to rate it numerically
  - Objective: Your impression of the patient's mood
- Affect
  - Observable expression of the patient's feelings from witnessing expressions and demeanour
  - It can be normal (reactive), blunted or labile (changes easily)
- Speech
  - Tone: Monotonous or tremulous

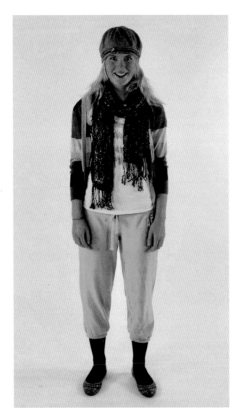

Fig. 8.2 Brightly coloured clothes, in the context of other features, may be consistent with possible mania.

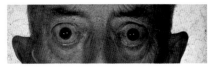

Fig. 8.3 Medical disorder that might be noted in 'appearance'; for example, lid retraction is suggestive of hyperthyroidism.

- Fluency and rhythm of speech: Articulate, clear or slurred
- Rate: Slow or pressure of speech
- Volume: Loud or quiet
- Content: Inappropriate or appropriate
- Thoughts
  - Thoughts are probably best considered as 'the how' (the 'mechanics' or the form of your thinking) and 'the what' (the content or the beliefs you hold) of thinking. Form is rarely disturbed but is highly significant when it is
    - Thought form
  - Thought content
    - Ask the patient to describe present worries, preoccupations, obsessional ruminations
    - Ask about thoughts of self-harm and/or suicide
    - Ask the patient about abnormal thoughts; for example, in psychosis
- Perceptions
  - Hallucinations: Ask whether the patient has ever seen, tasted, felt or heard anything, but there was nothing to explain it. Then ask whether they thought this was real
- Cognition

- Orientation: Assess whether the patient is orientated in time, place and person
  - Concentration: Ask the patient to list the months in reverse order
  - Other cognitive function tests: For example, MMSE
- Insight
  - Assess the level of insight into illness, including whether the patient thinks that she is ill, how severely and whether treatment is required

MNEMONIC FOR MSE

Each section of the MSE can be remembered using the mnemonic ASEPTIC:

- *Appearance* and behaviour
- *Speech*
- *Emotion*: Mood and affect
- *Perception*: Hallucination and illusion
- *Thought*: content and form
- *Insight* and judgement
- *Cognition*

Present Your Findings

Mrs Bradley is a 58-year-old female who presented with low mood. She was wearing appropriate clothes and was well kempt. She displayed good eye contact throughout the interview and was tearful at times. Her mood was subjectively and objectively low, with a reactive affect. Her appetite is reduced and her sleep is disturbed. Her thought form is normal and her content centres around the recent separation from her husband. She denies thoughts of harm to herself or others. She displays no evidence of abnormal perceptions. I assess Mrs Bradley to be of reasonable intelligence and she is orientated to time, place and person. She has good insight into her condition and is aware that she may need treatment.

I feel the most likely diagnosis is a moderate depressive episode.

To complete my examination, I would like to consider Mrs Bradley for talking therapy and discuss the possibility of pharmacotherapy with her, depending on the severity of her condition.

? QUESTIONS AND ANSWERS FOR CANDIDATE

What is an illusion?
- Illusions are altered perceptions in which a real external object is present, but an it is incorrectly percieved or interpreted

What are hypnagogic and hypnopompic hallucinations?
- These are transient false perceptions which occur when falling asleep (hypnagogic) or when waking (hypnopompic). They have the characteristics of hallucinations and are mostly visual or auditory

How are congruent and incongruent used to describe mood and affect?
- Congruent affect is used to describe when the mood and affect are in line with each other, such as smiling when happy. Incongruence is seen when this is not the case, such as laughing when anxious

A Case to Learn From

I was once in a psychiatric unit taking a history from a patient who was being treated for schizophrenia. When I asked her if she was having any hallucinations, she told me no. However, later when another senior doctor came to see the patient with me and asked if she had been seeing, hearing, smelling or tasting things that are not really there, she then revealed that she had been seeing bugs crawling all over her skin for the past 2 days. From this I learnt that it is essential to avoid the use of jargon and to enquire about each sensation in depth as the patient may not always reveal something until asked directly.

 Top Tip

During difficult assessments, remember that you can get a lot of the information in an MSE by just observing and listening to a patient.

 Top Tip

The single most important symptom predictor of suicide is hopelessness.

STATION 8.8: EXAMINATION: COGNITIVE

SCENARIO

You are a junior doctor in primary care and have been asked to see Mr Ahmed, a 68-year-old man, who has been referred because his son has noticed his increasing forgetfulness. The son is worried that his father may have some memory problems. Please perform a cognitive assessment on Mr Ahmed, present your findings and formulate an appropriate management plan.

THE MINI MENTAL STATE EXAMINATION

The MMSE gives us a standardised assessment of orientation, memory, concentration and performance. It is a screening tool, so if there are further concerns, we need to test specific cerebral-lobe function or do further general cognitive assessments. It is really important to gain collateral information from family or neighbours when assessing cognitive function.

GAIN CONSENT AND PREPARE THE PATIENT

- Explain that you would like to perform a memory test and that this will include some questions and tasks (Table 8.3)
- Explain that some of the questions may be easy, some difficult and some are strange, but that it is all part of a routine test we use and that they should just try their best. This helps to alleviate some concerns
- It is important to be patient and encouraging during cognitive assessments as patients can become upset or agitated

- emember you can also take a break and ask general questions or come back to repeat the test at another time

SCORES FOR THE MMSE

The MMSE is assessed out of a total of 30 points (Table 8.4). It is not a diagnostic test. Instead, it is helpful in monitoring progress over time; for example, response to treatment.

The MMSE does not provide information on executive function and ideally this should be supplemented with further tests such as the Frontal Assessment Battery (FAB) and/or the Addenbrooke's Cognitive Examination-Revised (ACE-R).

ASSESSING MEMORY

There is no clear consensus on which is the best cognitive assessment to use and it is therefore useful to have an awareness of which questions are testing which parts of the brain and memory. This can help you to adapt your assessment to the patient. There are particular questions that can be used to assess immediate, short-term and long-term memory which are completed by specialists.

The questions in the MMSE do not adequately cover frontal-lobe function and we therefore use the frontal assessment battery (FAB) to cover this. The frontal lobe is important in executive functioning, personality and memory.

FRONTAL ASSESSMENT BATTERY

The FAB consists of six tasks, each scoring up to 3 points, maximum 18 points (Table 8.5).

 Present Your Findings

Mr Ahmed is a 68-year-old man presenting with forgetfulness. He scores 15/30 on his MMSE, with a poor performance across all domains of the test.

This global impairment may be consistent with a diagnosis of dementia of moderate severity.

I would like to obtain a collateral history, particularly with respect to long-term cognitive impairment.

❓ QUESTIONS AND ANSWERS FOR CANDIDATE

Name three causes of dementia.
- Alzheimer's disease
- Vascular dementia
- Lewy body dementia
- Frontotemporal dementia
- Huntington's disease

Name three potentially reversible causes of dementia.
- Normal-pressure hydrocephalus
- Subdural haematoma
- Alcoholism

Name three risk factors for Alzheimer's disease.
- Age
- Down's syndrome
- Apolipoprotein ε4 allele/family history

Table 8.3 An example of tasks and questions for the MMSE

	AREA OF COGNITION	TESTS	ADDITIONAL INFORMATION	SCORE
1	Orientation	Time: 'What is the date?', 'The day?', 'The month?', 'The year?', 'The season?' (/5) Place: 'What country are we in?', 'What county?', 'What town/city?', 'What is the name of the building?', 'On what floor are we?' (/5)	It is important not to ask 'Do you know what…' for these questions, as the patient will commonly say yes, and then become frustrated, as the questions can appear very simple	(/10)
2	Registration	Say three common objects to the patient; for example, lemon, key and ball. 'Can you repeat the words I said?' (/1 point per word)	Check that the words are remembered, as that is important for the recall step. You can repeat the objects up to six times until all three are remembered (though no additional points are given if the answers arent given at the first attempt)	(/3)
3	Attention and calculation	Either spell the word 'WORLD' backwards (D-L-R-O-W) or keep subtracting from 100 and stop after five answers (93, 86, 79, 72, 65)	You can give the patient a choice with these options by asking them if they prefer doing tasks with numbers or letters	(/5)
4	Recall	'What were the three objects I told you earlier?' For example, lemon, key and ball (/1 point per word)	There is no need to tell the patient whether their responses are right and wrong. Try to be encouraging and use the same phrase regardless, such as 'Thank you'. Do not repeat the objects again here	(/3)
5	Language	Naming: 'Can you tell me the name of the following?' Point to your watch, then point to a pencil (Fig. 8.4) (/2). Repeating: Repeat the following after me: 'No ifs, ands or buts' (/ 1)	It is important to continue on even if the patient gets things wrong or can't complete a task	(/3)
6	Reading and writing	Reading: Show a card that says, 'Close your eyes' (Fig. 8.5). 'Can you read what is written and do what it says?' (/1) Writing: 'Can you write down a short sentence for me? It can be about anything' (/ 1)	Don't close your own eyes as well, to try and help the patient	(/2)
7	Three-stage command	'Take this paper in your right hand, fold it in half and place it on the floor' (Fig. 8.6)	Do not help the patient by miming or demonstrating during the task. The patient needs to complete the actions in the correct order	(/3)
8	Construction of interlocking pentagons	'Try to copy this drawing for me' (Fig. 8.7)	Score 1: Pentagon has five sides and there is a diamond shape in the middle Score 0: Any errors	(/1)

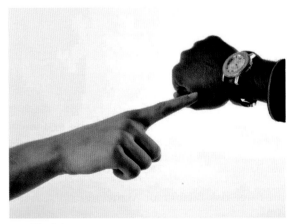

Fig. 8.4 'Can you tell me the name of the following?'

A Case to Learn From

Once I was assessing a patient's cognitive function and was asking her a lot of questions, but I got no response to anything. I thought that she couldn't perform any of the tasks or answer any of the questions, and had very severe cognitive impairment. It was only when I spoke to the nurse looking after her that I learnt that she was extremely hard of hearing and didn't have her hearing aids in. We inserted them into her ears for her and she was able to understand everything that I was asking her and scored 30/30 on her MMSE! From this I learnt always to think about other factors that may be limiting your communication with a patient before putting it down to cognitive impairment.

STATION 8.9: COMMUNICATION: ASSESSING CAPACITY

SCENARIO

You are a doctor in the later-life liaison psychiatry team and have been asked to see Mr Webber, an 80-year-old man with vascular dementia, who was admitted

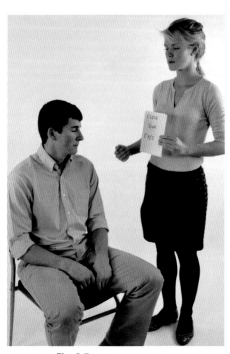

Fig. 8.5 'Close your eyes.'

following a fall. There is concern about how Mr Webber is coping at home, but he is refusing a package of care at discharge. Please assess his capacity to make the decision to refuse care at home and present your findings.

? CORE CONCEPT

- Assessment of capacity involves making a decision about whether the patient's mental state allows them to consent to or refuse treatment or care
- Consent is an informed, freely given decision from a patient with capacity to do so
- There are specific incapacity legislations that can be referred to for England and Wales (Mental Capacity Act 2005), Scotland (Adults with Incapacity Act 2000), Northern Ireland (Mental Capacity Act 2016) and Ireland (Assisted Decision-Making Capacity Act 2015). In Australia, there is no uniform standard for capacity and variation exists between the different territories
- Fundamental principles related to capacity are:
  - A patient aged 16 years or over has capacity unless proven otherwise
  - A patient must not be assumed to lack capacity until all steps have been taken to enhance it
  - Capacity is decision- and time-specific
  - Patients can have capacity but still make an unwise decision
  - If a patient does not have capacity, they are treated in their best interests and this should be the least restrictive option

INTRODUCTION

- Read the medical notes to understand Mr Webber's diagnosis, current support and physical state
- Always consider whether delirium could be affecting decision making
- Consider inviting a family member or friend to the review for further information
- Introduce yourself to Mr Webber and have a colleague with you to document and witness the interaction if needed

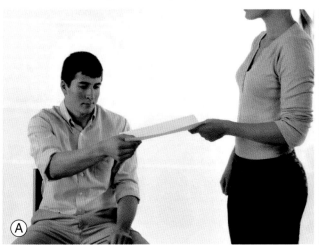
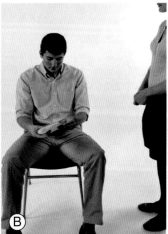
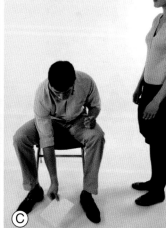

Fig. 8.6 (A–C) Three-stage command.

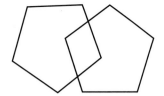

Fig. 8.7 Construction.

Table 8.4 Interpretation of MMSE score

SCORE	RESULTS SUGGEST...
27+	No significant cognitive impairment
24–27	Possible mild cognitive impairment
21–23	Possible early dementia
10–20	Possible moderate dementia
<10	Possible severe dementia

- Explain the fact that there are concerns about how he will manage at home at discharge and that this is what you are here to explore with him
- Ask Mr Webber to explain in his own words what's led to him coming into hospital and how he is feeling now to establish his current awareness level

ASSESSING CAPACITY

This follows the two-stage test of capacity and provides a useful framework (Figs 8.8 and 8.9).

ENHANCING CAPACITY

If the patient lacks capacity, several techniques can be used to try and enhance it:
- Using plain language
- Allowing the patient to have relatives and friends present
- Allowing time to pass or seeing them at the best time of day for them
- Enhancing the environment, such as finding a quiet side room

Table 8.5 Tasks and questions for the FAB

	AREA OF FRONTAL FUNCTION	TESTS	ADDITIONAL INFORMATION	SCORE / POINTS
1	Assessment of programming ability (fist–palm–edge test)	Demonstrate a series of hand movements (fist, palm, edge of your hand placed on a surface) three times. Ask the patient to repeat as many times as they can, the first two with the examiner	Do not provide any verbal prompts to help the patient, and don't do it with the patient	3: Six consecutive series 2: Three consecutive series 1: Requires assistance to perform three series
2	Assessment of conceptualisation	Ask how some objects are similar. For example, table and chair, or daisy and tulip	Make sure you use words from clear categories like flowers or fruit	1 point each (three categories)
3	Verbal fluency	Ask the patient to say as many words (excluding proper nouns) in one minute that begin with 'S'	If no response for 5 s, start them off with a word, 'For example, snake'	1: 3–5 words 2: 6–9 words 3: 9+ words
4	Sensitivity to interference (Go-No Go test)	Ask the patient to tap twice when you tap once, and to tap once when you tap twice. Perform a series of 10 single and/or double taps (randomised) to assess the patient's ability to follow both commands	Make sure the patient understands before starting by doing three trials of 1-1-1 taps and 2-2-2 taps	3: No errors 2: 1–2 errors 1: 3+ errors 0: 4 consecutive errors
5	Inhibitory control	Ask the patient to tap once when you tap once, and not to tap at all when you tap twice. Perform a series of 10 random single and double taps	Remember to perform examples of both instructions before starting to check that the patient understands	3: No errors 2: 1–2 errors 1: 3+ errors 0: 4 consecutive errors
6	Prehension test (read and grasp)	Ask the patient not to touch your hand and then reach out to touch the patient's hand. Repeat again	Make this a quick and natural movement like you are reaching for a handshake	3: Doesn't take hand 2: Hesitates but doesn't take hand 1: Takes hand without hesitation (but not on repeat) 0: Takes hand on both attempts

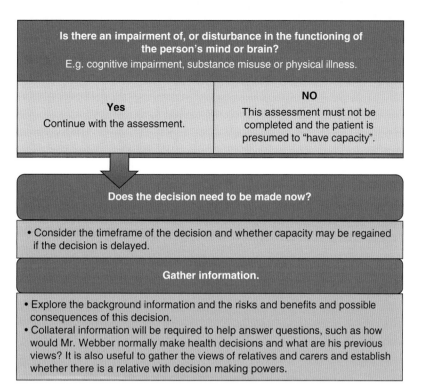

Fig. 8.8 Two-stage process to assessing capacity – stage 1.

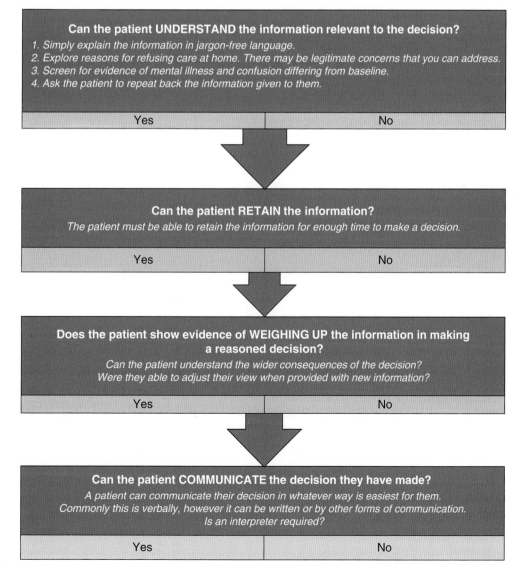

Fig. 8.9 Two-stage process to assessing capacity – stage 2. If the answer to all of the questions 1–4 is yes, the person 'has capacity' at this time for this decision only. Any 'no' means capacity is not present.

The capacity assessment must be clearly documented in the notes and communicated with the treating team.

LACK OF CAPACITY

- If the patient does not have capacity, it may be necessary to treat them under the relevant incapacity legislation
- If you are stopping a patient without capacity from doing things that they want to, for example, leaving the hospital, then you are depriving them of their liberties and you must put a Deprivation of Liberty Safeguards (DOLS) in place

ASSESSING CAPACITY

A useful mnemonic to use when assessing capacity is CURVES:

- *Choose* and *communicate*: Can the patient make a choice and communicate their decision?
- *Understand*: Can the patient understand the information?
- *Reason*: Can the patient make a logical, rational choice?
- *Value*: Is the choice the patient makes consistent with their values?
- *Emergency*: Is there an immediate risk to the patient?
- *Surrogate*: Is there a decision maker available?

Present Your Findings

Mr Webber is an 80-year-old man who presented following a fall. He has a diagnosis of vascular dementia and lives alone. He is refusing a package of care at discharge, despite concerns from his family and staff. Mr Webber's home situation has been explored with him and he feels that he is able to cope, despite two recent admissions following falls and evidence of self-neglect. I feel that Mr Webber was unable to understand fully the risks of him returning home without support and was not able to weigh up the information provided. This was despite relatives being present and clear, jargon-free language being used.

I do not feel that Mr Webber, therefore, has capacity to consent to care at home and he may require this to be organised in his best interests.

A social worker should be allocated and a best-interests meeting organised.

❓ QUESTIONS AND ANSWERS FOR CANDIDATE

What is a power of attorney?

- A power of attorney is when a person gives another person, or multiple people, power to make decisions relating to their personal welfare and/or property

What is an advance statement?

- An advance statement is a written statement which confirms a person's preferences, wishes and values regarding their future care
- It is not legally binding

- The aim is to provide a guide for anyone who may have to make decisions in someone's best interests in the future if they have lost the capacity to do so

What is an IMCA?

- IMCAs are Independent Mental Capacity Advocates. They are a legal safeguard for people who lack capacity and have no other person to represent them in decision making. The IMCA represents the patient and makes sure the Capacity Act is being followed

A Case to Learn From

Whilst on a ward round, we reviewed a patient admitted with a non-ST elevation myocardial infarction. The decision was made that an angiogram was required. However, the patient was partially deaf and verbal communication was difficult. To aid communication, we exchanged written messages to communicate both in terms of words and diagrams and were able to gain informed consent. The patient thanked us for explaining what we wanted to do and at the end had a clear understanding of the procedure. This case highlights how the method of communication can be adapted to the needs of the patient.

💡 Top Tip

Remember that if a patient lacks capacity for one decision, that does not mean that they lack capacity to make all decisions or that they will not be able to make similar decisions in the future. Capacity assessments are decision- and time-specific and capacity needs to be regularly assessed.

STATION 8.10: COMMUNICATION: COMMENCING LITHIUM TREATMENT

SCENARIO

You are a junior doctor working on a psychiatry ward and you have been asked to see Mr Wallace, a 36-year-old man, after his ward round where your consultant discussed the option of starting lithium. Please counsel Mr Wallace about starting lithium treatment for his bipolar affective disorder.

CORE CONCEPT

- Lithium is first-line treatment recommended by the National Institute for Health and Care Excellence (NICE) for long-term maintenance treatment in bipolar affective disorder
- It is known to be an effective medication and has been used for a number of years
- The exact mechanism of lithium is unknown, but it appears to modulate the neurotransmitter-induced modulation of second messengers

Common Concerns

Why do I need to have regular blood tests?	This is needed to ensure medication doses remain high enough to treat the underlying problem, but not too high to cause problems
Is there a risk of toxicity?	By monitoring blood tests, we try and spot toxic levels of lithium before it causes a significant problem
Will it cause weight gain?	This can be an issue with some people, but we will monitor your weight
Will I develop kidney problems?	We can adjust medication doses if there is any sign of the kidneys being affected
Will it cause change in personality or an inability to feel emotion in the same way as before?	Lithium may cause changes in personality that are unintended, but the overall effect is likely to be positive

GATHERING INFORMATION

- Before the review, read the patient's background, including previous treatments
- Introduce yourself and check the patient's name and date of birth
- Explain that you plan to talk to them about the possibility of starting lithium therapy and that this will involve discussing side effects, monitoring and lithium toxicity
- Be empathetic and maintain open body language so the patient feels able to ask questions
- Use appropriate language and avoid medical jargon, regularly check the patient's understanding and summarise back to them

COUNSELLING ABOUT LITHIUM THERAPY

INFORMATION ON LITHIUM

Provide the patient with some background information on what lithium is:
- Inform the patient that lithium is a mood stabiliser and therefore its aim is to maintain the patient's mood at a constant level
- Discuss that poor compliance or rapid reduction in dose can result in relapse

SIDE EFFECTS OF LITHIUM

Lithium can cause side effects but these are mostly dose-related and therefore can be improved by adjusting the dose.

Side effects include:
- Polyuria
- Polydipsia
- Weight gain
- Cognitive problems: Dulling, impaired memory, poor concentration, confusion
- Fine tremor
- Sedation or lethargy
- Impaired coordination
- Gastrointestinal disturbance: Nausea, vomiting, dyspepsia, diarrhoea
- Hair loss
- Acne
- Peripheral oedema

LONG-TERM EFFECTS OF LITHIUM

Lithium can affect the kidneys and thyroid glands in the longer term:
- After long-term treatment (>15 years) with lithium, the nephrogenic diabetes insipidus that causes polydipsia and polyuria may become irreversible
- Lithium can cause a reduction in glomerular filtration rate
- A very small number of people can also develop interstitial nephritis
- Lithium increases the risk of hypothyroidism in middle-aged women

LITHIUM TOXICITY

Lithium is a potentially toxic substance and it is important that this is understood:
- Lithium has a narrow therapeutic index, i.e. patients can easily become toxic
- The optimal range for plasma levels is 0.6–0.75 mmol/L. If the lithium level exceeds 1.5 mmol/L, most patients will experience some symptoms of toxicity. In levels > 2.0 mmol/L, life-threatening toxic effects occur
- Early signs of lithium toxicity include:
  - Marked coarse tremor
  - Poor appetite
  - Nausea and vomiting
  - Diarrhoea
  - Lethargy
- As the plasma levels rise, central nervous system effects can occur; for example, muscle weakness, drowsiness, ataxia, coarse tremor and muscle twitching
- Above 2.0 mmol/L, disorientation and seizures can occur, leading to coma and potentially death
- Patients on lithium need to be aware of these symptoms and ensure adequate hydration (especially in hot climates) and manage their salt intake, as the plasma lithium levels rise when the patient is dehydrated

- Advise patients to tell their doctor that they are taking lithium as it can interact with many drugs, and not to use non-steroidal anti-inflammatory drugs (NSAIDs) over the counter as they interact with lithium

LITHIUM MONITORING

- Lithium is a long-term treatment, which requires reviews with a psychiatrist for dose and blood monitoring. This process is initially quite frequent but becomes less frequent as the patient's mood is stabilised on the lithium treatment
- Prior to starting treatment, the following tests are required:
  - FBCs
  - Renal function
  - U&Es
  - TFTs
  - Baseline ECG
  - Baseline weight
- A plasma level is required after 7 days, and then 7 days after every dose change until the desirable level is reached. Blood tests are taken 12 h after the last dose
- When the dose is stable, a plasma level should be taken every 3 months for the first year. It can then be measured every 6 months, but should remain at 3 months in the following groups:
  - The elderly >65 years
  - People taking drugs that interact with lithium; for example, NSAIDs, diuretics
  - People with impaired renal or thyroid function
  - People whose symptoms are not managed well
  - Those who have poor compliance
  - People whose last plasma lithium level was 0.8 mmol/L or higher
- U&Es and TFTs will be needed every 6 months
- Weight should also be monitored, as weight gain can be a side effect

FEMALE CONSIDERATIONS

- If the patient you were interviewing was female, you would also warn her of the adverse effects of becoming pregnant whilst taking lithium
- Lithium has been shown to cause up to an eightfold increase in the risk of the fetus developing Ebstein's anomaly (a congenital malformation of the tricuspid valve in the heart) during the first trimester of pregnancy
- Other reported second- and third-trimester problems include: Polyhydramnios, premature delivery, thyroid abnormalities, nephrogenic diabetes insipidus and floppy-baby syndrome

Present Your Findings

Mr Wallace is a 36-year-old man who has struggled with a diagnosis of bipolar affective disorder type I for a number of years. He has recently recovered from an episode of mania and would like to try a mood stabiliser. Today I have discussed the side effects, longer-term complications, toxicity risks and monitoring with Mr Wallace. He was able to understand the information discussed and repeat it back to me. I have given him some written information so that he can discuss this with his wife.

If Mr Wallace would like to start lithium, we will complete FBCs, renal function, U&Es, TFTs and a baseline ECG and baseline weight.

QUESTIONS AND ANSWERS FOR CANDIDATE

Name two drugs that interact with lithium.
- Calcium channel blockers: Increase plasma lithium concentration
- Angiotensin-converting enzyme inhibitors (ACEi): Increase plasma lithium concentration

Name three risk factors for lithium toxicity.
- Infections: Viral or gastrointestinal infections causing diarrhoea and vomiting
- Decreased oral intake of water
- Medications altering renal function: NSAIDs, diuretics and ACEi
- Nephrogenic diabetes insipidus

Name three other uses of lithium.
- Augmentation of antidepressants in unipolar depression to increase mood
- To manage aggression and self-mutilating behaviour
- Treatment of steroid-induced psychosis
- To increase the white cell count in people taking clozapine

A Case to Learn From

A 50-year-old woman with bipolar affective disorder had been stable on lithium for 10 years. Her primary care doctor did some routine blood tests, which showed poor renal function. He therefore decided to stop the lithium. The patient quickly relapsed and required hospital admission. The doctor reflected that in the future, she would be more cautious about stopping lithium, as it can so easily precipitate a relapse. In this situation, the risks and benefits need to be carefully considered and the decision should be discussed with a specialist. Perhaps simply lowering the dose would have been sufficient.

Top Tip

As lithium is a complex drug, all patients on lithium should be given an information booklet so they have a reminder of the main issues when taking lithium.

Paediatrics

Content Outline

The small people of the world have the ability to terrify medical students and doctors alike, particularly during exams. Our aim is to give you a broad framework for paediatric history taking, illustrated through clinically relevant and commonly examined areas. Teaching and demonstration of practical procedures are other important skills we will explore. This applies not only to teaching colleagues, but also to educating patients or parents about conditions, treatments and side effects.

In real practice, vital information can be obtained from asking a verbal child about their presenting problem. If a child is present in your exam, remember to include them, using a 'three-way' consultation. You may need to deviate from the generally more structured approach used for adults to develop a rapport and gain the child's trust.

The paediatric OSCE at medical student level is not a test of your ability to be a paediatrician.

It is a test of three things:

1. Do you know how to take a paediatric history? This is an important skill because there are elements to the history that differ from an adult history, namely:
   (a) The history is indirect and you have to ask the carer for information, about which they may already have formed an opinion.
   (b) The perinatal, immunisation, nutrition and growth, and neurodevelopmental histories are unique to paediatrics.
   (c) The family and social history is more particular, given the utter dependence of the child upon these circumstances, the possible importance of congenital factors and the possibility of child protection issues.

2. Do you know how to conduct a paediatric examination? This means conducting a thorough physical assessment as you would do in any human being, but doing so in a child-friendly, age-appropriate, opportunistic but thorough way. Knowledge of what is normal, as regards physiology and development in particular, is crucial.

3. Do you know some basic facts about paediatric illness, loosely defined as facts that any non-paediatric doctor should know?

If you think about these three things, you will realise that, just like in trigonometry, showing your work is as important as, if not more important than, the answer. The diagnosis often only accounts for a small percentage of the mark compared to how you got there and leaping to a diagnosis is a great way of selling yourself short, even if it is correct, but particularly if is not.

Remember that it is impossible to know every detail about everything, so when in doubt, do not make something up or guess. Explain that you will find out the answer to the question or you will get someone who knows more about the subject to come back and speak to them. Being aware of your own limitations is one of the most important skills to acquire before your first day as a junior doctor. If you are ever in doubt or unsure, the slight dent to your pride from asking for help will always outweigh the deep water you might find yourself in by giving the wrong information or competent in or familiar with.

STATION 9.1: HISTORY: PAEDIATRIC HISTORY TAKING

INTRODUCTION

- Introduce yourself to the parents and child (if present)
- Establish the name and age of the patient
- Ask the child whom they have brought with them. Assumptions can lead to some embarrassing interactions; for example, 'grandmothers' might be mothers!
- Adapt the history taking to the child's developmental age (pregnancy and birth history are more pertinent for a neonate than a 15-year-old adolescent)
- Talk to the child as able, both to establish rapport and get initial information
- Speak to the parents, and the child alone if appropriate
  Note: Much of the adult history-taking structure can be adapted and used for paediatric history taking.

HISTORY OF PRESENTING COMPLAINT

- Start with broad open questions, giving the child space to talk about their agenda.
- Obtain a chronological description of the:
  - Mode of presentation
  - Sequence and duration of symptoms
  - Hospital admissions
  - Management of problem so far, including compliance
- Remember your job as a junior doctor is to get the story and by asking the right questions in the right way, turn that story into a coherent concise medical story
- The mnemonic used for describing pain, SOCRATES, can be used for other symptoms too

PAST MEDICAL HISTORY

- Previous illnesses and hospital admissions in chronological order
- Medical conditions, particularly those linked to the presentation; for example, for an asthmatic patient, ask about atopic conditions such as eczema and allergic rhinitis

BIRTH HISTORY

Especially in those less than 2 years old, check
- Pregnancy: Gestation at birth and any antenatal concerns (including anomalies on scans)
- Birth: Mode of birth and indications, need for resuscitation and initial Apgar scores (if known), birth weight
- Postnatal: Ask about neonatal intensive care unit (NICU) admission, any diagnoses made a diagnoses made, length of stay or antibiotics given length of stay

FEEDING HISTORY

- All ages: Ask about vomiting with feeds or concerns about weight gain
- Babies: Breast or bottlefed, volume, frequency and wet nappies
- Older children: Eating and drinking regularly and compare it with normal for them

DEVELOPMENTAL HISTORY

- Always ask screening questions around any developmental concerns or problems in school
- If the presentation is more relevant to developmental problems; for example, walking difficulty, ask more detailed questions covering all four developmental domains (gross motor, fine motor, vision/hearing and social/self-care) appropriate to age. (See Station 9.3: Developmental Delay)

MEDICATION HISTORY AND IMMUNISATIONS

- Enquire about prescribed and over-the-counter medications, including any recent changes
- Allergies should also be included with the specific reaction noted
- Immunisation status and, if relevant, reasons for not being immunised

FAMILY HISTORY

- Anything that runs in the family; for example, atopy, inflammatory bowel disease, migraines
- History of childhood death or recurrent miscarriage
- Parental consanguinity. Particularly relevant if unexplained constellation of symptoms and possible genetic diagnosis

SOCIAL AND TRAVEL HISTORY

- People around the child: Clarify who is at home; for example, parents/siblings/pets and any unwell contacts or smokers
- Housing situation: Housing issues; for example, mould
- Recent travel abroad: Travel in the last 3 months (particularly relevant for infective symptoms)

- Social issues: Clarify if there is any social worker involvement and if so, the reasons

SYSTEMS REVIEW

With experience these questions can be more focused, guided by the presenting complaint:
- General: Activity levels, behaviour, fever, rashes, unintentional weight loss
- Neurological: Headaches, drowsiness, fits
- Respiratory: Wheeze, breathlessness limiting activity, cough
- Cardiac: Chest pain, palpitations
- Gastrointestinal: Vomiting, bowel movements, abdominal pain, weight gain
- Musculoskeletal: Joint pain/swelling
- Genitourinary: Dysuria, urinary frequency and wetting episodes
- Haematology: Abnormal bruising or bleeding
- Ears, nose and throat (ENT): Snoring, noisy breathing, ear pain or discharge

ADOLESCENTS AND SOCIAL HISTORY

It is important to tailor the questions that you ask the patient (or parent) to the appropriate age group. For example, in young people, information on certain aspects of their social life can help to build a better picture of their general well-being. The acronym HEEADSSS can be used to structure some of the key points:
- *Home* and relationships
- *Education* and employment
- *Eating*
- *Activities* and hobbies
- *Drugs*, alcohol and tobacco
- *Sex* and relationships
- *Self-harm*, depression and self-image
- *Safety* and abuse

Note that some of the questions are very personal to the patient and therefore, it would be imperative for the clinician to ask them in a professional, non-judgemental manner.

ADOLESCENTS AND CONFIDENTIALITY

Confidentiality is one of the four pillars of medical ethics and is vital for building and maintaining a good relationship between the patient and the healthcare professional. For young people in particular, there may be sensitive topics that they want to discuss, for example, contraception, that they do not want to disclose to their carer(s)/parent(s). In these situations, it is important that the content of the conversation does remain confidential, as we need to respect the patient's right to confidentiality. However, if you have reasons to believe that there is a possible risk of harm to the patient or to others, then it is your duty to protect the patient/others and, in these circumstances, you may need to break confidentiality. If you were to do so, you should inform the patient of your plans and explain your reasoning.

❓ QUESTIONS AND ANSWERS FOR CANDIDATE

What tests can aid the diagnosis of coeliac disease?
- To screen for coeliac disease, you can test for specific immunoglobulin A (IgA) antigliadin or antiendomysial antibodies
- To make a definitive diagnosis of coeliac disease, you would need a jejunal biopsy

Name the three most common causative organisms of meningitis in neonates.
- *Escherichia coli*
- Group B streptococcus
- *Listeria*

Name three risk factors for cerebral palsy.
- Prematurity
- Factors during pregnancy; for example, multiple pregnancy, pre-eclampsia
- Low birth weight
- Complications during labour; for example, maternal sepsis, fetal distress, neonatal sepsis

 A Case to Learn From

I once reviewed a baby who had a new diagnosis of Down syndrome. I spoke to the family to update them, having been told the family had been updated by the consultant. When I asked whether dad had any further questions about Down syndrome, he asked, 'What's Down syndrome?'. It was actually the mum who had been updated, and dad inadvertently had the news broken to him quite harshly. Always note who is present, and who had been told what in a paediatric consultation.

 Top Tip

Remember some children have learning disabilities and their developmental age may be lower than their chronological age – in this case establish their level of understanding.

 Top Tip

Remember the assessment of neurodevelopment, growth and puberty is all about asking three questions for any parameter – is this within normal range, did they get there at a normal rate and is it consistent with other parameters I am assessing?

 Top Tip

Always think carefully about how to make the child as comfortable as possible. There are often toys and books available for them. Parents can be really helpful too. Simple things like sitting the child in mum's lap can really put them at ease, especially during parts of an examination.

STATION 9.2: HISTORY: A CRYING BABY

SCENARIO

You are a junior doctor in primary care and have been asked to see Mabel, a 4-month-old girl. Mabel's mother, Mrs Jackson, has brought her in because she will not stop crying. Please take a history from Mrs Jackson regarding Mabel, present your findings and formulate an appropriate management plan.

 Cardinal Symptoms

High-pitched cry

Fever

Vomiting/poor feeding

Respiratory distress

Lethargy

Floppy episodes

HISTORY OF PRESENTING COMPLAINT

CRYING

- Onset: Sudden onset; for example, trauma, post-illness, or gradual; for example, worsening reflux
- Character: High-pitched; for example, meningeal irritation, or distinctive cry; for example, cat-like cry (cri du chat)
- Time course: Intermittent (for example, infantile colic, gastro-oesophageal reflux, cow's milk protein intolerance) or constant (for example, trauma)
  - A normal baby's crying increases in frequency from birth to an average peak of 2.5 h/day by 2 months
- Exacerbating and relieving factors:
  - Feeds (colic, reflux)
  - Immunisations
  - Dietary change; for example, introduction of cow's milk
  - Paracetamol
  - Environment
  - Time of day; for example, infantile colic is worse in the evenings
  - Posture; for example, reflux is better in the upright position
- Severity: Whether it affects the baby's general well-being; for example, unable or unwilling to eat

ASSOCIATED SYMPTOMS

Other symptoms to enquire about include:
- Reflux; for example, drawing up of knees, back arching, vomiting
- Gastrointestinal upset; for example, blood/mucus in the stools, diarrhoea, constipation, rashes (cow's milk protein allergy)
- Head injury; for example, vomiting, seizures, floppy episodes

- Sepsis; for example, temperature, poor feeding, floppy episodes

Associated symptoms are vast, but two important differentials are sepsis and non-accidental injury (NAI).

PAST MEDICAL AND SURGICAL HISTORY

In this scenario, it is also important to enquire about:
- Pregnancy: Gestation, antenatal scans, maternal blood group, infections
- Risk factors for neonatal infection
  - Prolonged rupture of membranes
  - Maternal sepsis
  - Group B streptococcus colonisation
  - Third-trimester urinary tract infection
- Birth: Method, resuscitation, birth trauma

MEDICATION HISTORY

Inquire about prescribed and over-the-counter medications, including any recent changes. Allergies should also be included with the specific reaction noted. In this scenario, also ask about:
- Regular medications: Reflux medication, analgesia
- Immunisation status: Vaccine-preventable infections

SOCIAL HISTORY

- People around the child: Clarify who is at home; for example, parents, siblings, pets and any unwell contacts, smokers
- Housing situation: Housing issues; for example, mould
- Recent travel abroad: Travel in the last 3 months (particularly relevant for infective symptoms)
- Social issues: Clarify if there is any social worker involvement and if so, the reasons

FAMILY HISTORY

- Ask about any conditions that run in the family and if anyone experienced similar symptoms in the past or currently

SYSTEMS REVIEW (FIG. 9.1)

Crying is a non-specific symptom and so requires a full systems review, including the following (some have already been mentioned above):
- Gastrointestinal: Eating or drinking, vomiting and/or diarrhoea, masses, stool changes
- Genitourinary: Change in urinary frequency or smell of urine
- Respiratory: Cough, coryza, difficulty in breathing
- Neurological: Seizures, floppiness, vomiting, swelling
- General: Fevers, sleep, tiredness, irritable, rash, unwell contacts
- Pain: Drawing up of the legs or arching of the back, tugging at ear

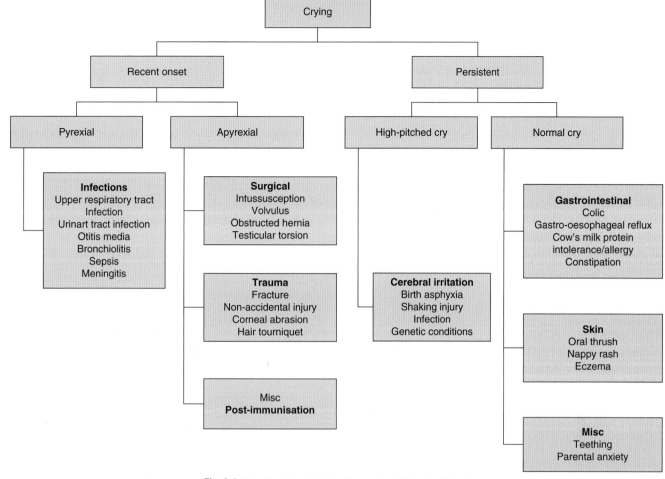

Fig. 9.1 Flowchart to aid in the diagnosis of 'A crying baby'.

Differential Diagnosis			
CONDITION	**CLINICAL PRESENTATION**	**INVESTIGATIONS**	**MANAGEMENT**
Cow's milk protein Intolerance	• Usually presents in the first few months of life • Discomfort during/after feeds • Vomiting • Diarrhoea or constipation • Blood/mucus in stool • Allergic-type rash (in IgE-mediated)	• Allergy testing/ radioallergosorbent test (RAST) often negative (not all IgE-mediated) • Trial of exclusion	• Hydrolysed or amino acid formula • Dairy-free diet
Gastro-oesophageal reflux	• Usually presents in first few months of life • Discomfort during feeds • Vomiting during/after feeds • Faltered growth in severe cases	• Barium study • pH study	• Reduce feed volumes • Feed thickeners • Antacids; for example, proton pump inhibitors (PPIs)/H_2 receptor blocker
Infection	• May be high-pitched/irritable cry • Fever is sometimes present • Poor feeding • Localising symptoms	• SPartial septic screen: FBCs, C-reactive proteins (CRP), blood, urine, CSF culture	• Broad-spectrum intravenous (IV) antibiotics
Intussusception	• Predominantly aged 3–18 months • Intermittent crying • Draws legs up • Vomiting • 'Redcurrant jelly' stools	• Abdominal X-ray (may have absence of gas in the right colon) • Ultrasound (target sign)	• Air enema can reduce the lesion • Surgery
Colic	• Usually presents at 6 weeks old and settles by 4 months old • Crying for greater than 3 h, for more than 3 night per week • Symptoms are often more evident in the evening • Otherwise well, thriving baby	• Diagnosis of exclusion, mainly from history	• Reassurance • Ensure that the parents are well supported

Present Your Findings

Mabel is a 4-month-old girl who presents with a 2-month history of crying associated with feeds, vomiting and an eczematous rash to her face and torso.

Mrs Jackson feels the symptoms have worsened since she changed from breast to formula feeding 6 weeks ago. Mabel has also dropped from the 25th to the ninth centile on her growth chart.

I feel the most likely diagnosis is cow's milk protein intolerance. I would like to perform a full examination of Mabel before starting her on a hydrolysed formula trial for at least 2 weeks and following up in clinic.

NON-ORGANIC CAUSES OF CRYING

- Organic causes should never be overlooked and the first priority is to exclude serious organic illness
- However, babies are sensitive to their environment and the emotional climate (if parents are stressed, anxious or irritable)
- This can be easily transmitted to the baby and manifest as persistent crying
- Persistent crying can also be a sign of neglect or NAI
- Parents can also complain of incessant crying when in fact the baby is crying a normal amount. In these cases, it is important to screen the mother for postnatal depression, which can present up to 2 years from the time of birth

QUESTIONS AND ANSWERS FOR CANDIDATE

How much should a baby feed?
Formula feeding:
- Day 1 of life: 60 mL/kg/day
- Day 2 of life: 90 mL/kg/day
- Day 3 of life: 120 mL/kg/day
- Day 4 of life until solids introduced: 150 mL/kg/day

Breastfeeding:
- Should be 'responsive' feeding (as often and for as long as they want)
- Often very frequent, even hourly, in the first weeks of life
- Generally, it settles to 2–4-hourly but will be more often in hot weather or during growth spurts
  Remember that this is a guide and the best way to know a baby is feeding enough is to see them growing along a centile line

What is intussusception?
- Part of the intestine (usually small) folds or 'telescopes' in on itself
- This causes bowel obstruction, ischaemia and, if not treated, perforation
- The blood and mucus produced mix with intestinal contents, which can sometimes produce stool that is classically like redcurrant jelly

When should you worry about infection in a crying infant?
- Presence of a fever
- Sudden or recent worsening of symptoms
- High-pitched, irritable cry
- Lethargy or behavioural changes

However, infants, particularly those < 3 months old, can have significant infections with minimal clinical signs or a fever. Therefore, a high degree of suspicion should be maintained when assessing children of this age group

 A Case to Learn From

A 3-month-old presented to the emergency department (ED) with vomiting and a high-pitched cry. There was nothing obvious from the history or examination until the vest was removed and four small round bruises, the size of a fingertip, were seen. Trauma was suspected, and it led us to do a computed tomography (CT) head. A large subdural haemorrhage was seen. This case of NAI reminded me always to undress the baby fully.

Top Tip

Crying is a non-specific symptom so be sure to do a full systems review to try and reveal the cause.

STATION 9.3: HISTORY: FEBRILE CONVULSIONS

SCENARIO

You are a junior doctor in the ED and have been asked to see Fred, a 2-year-old boy who has been brought in by his mother. He has presented with a temperature and a fit. You examined the patient and found signs consistent with acute otitis media. Take a history from the mother and arrive at a likely diagnosis.

Cardinal Symptoms

Length of seizure

Number of seizures within same illness

Neurological deficit

Focal seizures

HISTORY OF PRESENTING COMPLAINT

CONVULSIONS

- Before the convulsion:
  - Signs of infection: Fever, ear pain, coryza, respiratory distress
  - Other causes of seizure: Head injury, pain, temper tantrum or breath-holding event
- During the convulsion:
  - Body parts involved

- Change in colour or tone
- Loss of consciousness
- Eye rolling
- Incontinence (if toilet-trained)
- Injuries
- Duration (febrile convulsions generally last less than 5 min)
- Interventions (recovery position, medication)
- After the convulsion:
  - Weakness or lethargy
  - Reduced consciousness
  - Behavioural change
  - Time to complete recovery

ASSOCIATED SYMPTOMS

Other symptoms to enquire about include:
- Unable to eat and drink as normal
- Recent infections

PAST MEDICAL AND SURGICAL HISTORY

In this scenario, it is also important to enquire about:
- Known medical conditions, relevant treatments and any hospital admissions
- Previous seizures, known epilepsy/febrile convulsions

BIRTH HISTORY

- Gestation at birth
- Perinatal infections
- Resuscitation at birth
- Admission to NICU, duration and treatment
- Neonatal seizures

DEVELOPMENTAL HISTORY

- Any concerns voiced by parents, healthcare professionals or carers
- Loss of milestones (developmental regression)
- Most children at this age can:
  - Jump and kick a ball (gross motor)
  - Hold a pencil and scribble (fine motor)
- Speak more than 50 words (language/hearing)
- Feed themselves with spoon and fork (social)

MEDICATION HISTORY

Enquire about prescribed medications (including any recent changes) and over-the-counter medications. Allergies should be included with the specific reaction noted. In this scenario it is also important to note:
- Use of antipyretics; for example, paracetamol and ibuprofen
- Antiepileptics (uncommon in this age group)
- Recent immunisation (can trigger febrile seizure)

SOCIAL HISTORY

- People around the child: Clarify who is at home, for example, parents/siblings/pets and any unwell contacts, smokers
- Housing situation: Housing issues; for example, mould
- Recent travel abroad: Travel in the last 3 months, particularly relevant for infective symptoms
- Social issues: Clarify if there is any social worker involvement and if so, the reasons

FAMILY HISTORY

Ask about any significant family history, including:
- Febrile seizures (genetic link)
- Epilepsy

SYSTEMS REVIEW

On systems review, particularly pertinent questions to the above case include questions to help identify a focus for infection:
- Respiratory: Cough, wheeze
- ENT: Pulling at ears, ear discharge, food refusal (tonsillitis)
- Gastrointestinal: Poor appetite, diarrhoea, vomiting
- Genitourinary: Crying with urination, offensive smelling urine

🏠 Differential Diagnosis

CONDITION	CLINICAL PRESENTATION	INVESTIGATIONS	MANAGEMENT
Simple febrile seizure	• Age 6 months old to 6 years old • With febrile illness • Duration less than 5 min • Generalised tonic-clonic seizure • May be sleepy afterwards, for up to a few hours • No neurological deficit after	• Examination to find source of the fever • Bloods for septic screen (FBCs, CRP, blood culture) if unwell • Urine culture • Blood glucose	• Treat febrile illness • Advice for future episodes (see below) • Antipyretics as required; for example, paracetamol and ibuprofen

Continued

Differential Diagnosis—cont'd

CONDITION	CLINICAL PRESENTATION	INVESTIGATIONS	MANAGEMENT
Rigor	• All ages • With febrile illness • Duration of seconds to minutes • Exaggerated shivering • Does not feel sleepy after	• Examination to find source of the fever • Bloods for septic screen (FBCs, CRP, blood culture) if unwell • Urine culture • Lumbar puncture (LP) if suspected meningitis	• May be associated with bacterial infections • Treat underlying infection
Epilepsy	• All ages • Recurrent seizures with or without a fever • Focal or generalised • Feels sleepy after the seizure, for up to a few hours	• EEG • Imaging; for example, magnetic resonance imaging (MRI) or CT if focal seizures	• Dependent on the type of seizure and EEG findings • For a seizure of greater than 5 min, give benzodiazepines; for example, diazepam • For recurrent seizures, give antiepileptics; for example, sodium valproate
Reflex anoxic seizure	• Age under 4 years old • Without a fever • Triggered by pain or fear • Gasping/crying, followed by stiffening • Becomes pale/grey and loses consciousness • The body may jerk a few times • Lasts for less than 1 min • Feels sleepy afterwards, for up to a few hours	• None needed if clear history	• Reassurance • Caused by overstimulation of the vagus nerve • Causes no long-term damage • They generally stop by the time the child starts school
Breath-holding attack	• Age less than 4 years old • Without a fever • Prolonged cry without taking a breath in • Becomes blue • May lose consciousness • May be tired afterwards	• None needed if clear history	• Reassurance • Cause no long-term damage • They generally stop by the time the child starts school

FIRST AID IN SEIZURES

- Parents should not restrain the child/put things in their mouth
- Harmful objects should be moved away
- The child should be put in the recovery position, with chin lifted to open the airway (Fig. 9.2)
- Seizures should be timed. Call an ambulance if they last longer than 5 min

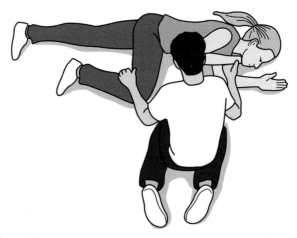

Fig. 9.2 Recovery position. (From St. John's Ambulance: www.sja.org.uk/sja/first-aid-advice/first-aid-techniques/the-recovery-position.aspx)

🔍 Present Your Findings

Fred is a 2-year-old boy who presented to the hospital with a 'fit' lasting 3 min. Fred became pale and began to shake all four limbs. He was less responsive after the seizure, but was back to his normal self after a few minutes. He has been suffering from an ear infection for the last 2 days, with a temperature of 38.5°C. His older brother and father both suffered from febrile convulsions.

Given that the examination findings are consistent with acute otitis media, this is consistent with a diagnosis of febrile convulsions, but I would check a urine dipstick and the blood glucose. I would reassure Fred's parents and also give them advice about how to prevent and manage any further febrile convulsions along with a written information sheet.

❓ QUESTIONS AND ANSWERS FOR CANDIDATE

What advice should be given to a parent after a first febrile seizure?

- There is no long-term damage and most children grow out of them

- This is not epilepsy, although the risk of developing it in the future is slightly increased
- Seizures can happen again with future feverish illnesses
- The parents can give paracetamol or ibuprofen during a febrile illness (although there is no evidence that this will prevent seizures)
- For future seizures:
  - Put the child into the recovery position (as above)
  - If the seizure lasts for less than 5 min and there is a known cause of infection/feverish illness, the child does not have to go to hospital
  - If it lasts for longer than 5 min or there is parental concern, call for an ambulance

What is an infantile spasm?
- An uncommon but significant seizure in children under 1 year old
- 'Spasms' most often manifest as sudden bending forward (flexor) with stiffening, but can be with arms and legs stretching out like a startle (extensor)
- Each spasm lasts for seconds
- Infrequent spasms are spasms that over time increase in frequency and happen in clusters
- It is associated with developmental delay and even loss of milestones
- It is associated with epilepsy syndromes; for example, Lennox–Gastaut syndrome

What is West syndrome?
A combination of:
- Infantile spasms
- Characteristic EEG (hypsarrhythmia – chaotic pattern)

 A Case to Learn From

We saw an 8-month-old child who presented with seizures. It would have been easy to diagnose febrile convulsions as the child had been suffering from acute otitis media. However, on further questioning of the mother, it was clear that there were multiple, short seizures, with head bending forwards, and limbs going stiff, characteristic of infantile spasms. The key was asking about the duration of the incidents, their frequency and the exact movements that the child made during them.

 Top Tip

In a febrile child, it is important to have a thorough search for a focus of infection, including an ear and throat examination (which you may not necessarily do in every febrile adult).

 Top Tip

Seizures can be very difficult to describe and so much of the diagnosis depends on this description. One of the advantages of mobile phones is that we are never far away from a good-quality video recording. Asking parents to video episodes really helps with diagnosis. Some seizures like infantile spasms are instantly recognisable to the experienced professional.

STATION 9.4: HISTORY: WHEEZE

SCENARIO

You are a junior doctor in the ED and have been asked to see Tommy, a 3-year-old boy who has presented with a wheeze. Please take a history from Mrs Shire, his mother, present your findings and formulate an appropriate management plan.

 Cardinal Symptoms

Work of breathing/respiratory effort
Exhaustion or altered consciousness
Responsiveness to inhalers
Ability to speak

HISTORY OF PRESENTING COMPLAINT

WHEEZE
- Site: Lower airways/wheeze (expiratory) or upper airways/stridor (inspiratory). Ask the patient to demonstrate if possible
- Onset. Duration, sudden or gradual, intermittent or constant
- Timing: Worse at night
- Exacerbating factors: Exercise, infection, history of inhaled foreign body
- Relieving factors: Inhaler use, rest, change of environment
- Severity. Lethargy or unable to speak in sentences

ASSOCIATED SYMPTOMS

Other symptoms to enquire about include:
- Difficulty breathing, which may manifest as sucking in of chest or flaring of nostrils
- Fever
- Cough/runny nose/productive sputum

PAST MEDICAL AND SURGICAL HISTORY

In this scenario, it is also important to enquire about:
- General: Ask about known medical conditions, relevant treatments and any hospital admissions
- Atopic conditions: Asthma, eczema, hay fever/allergic rhinitis
- Known 'wheezers'
  - Frequency of exacerbations and course of steroids
  - Hospital admission, including level of care (ward vs. intensive care), length of admission, IV medications
  - Previous investigations; for example, imaging, sputum cultures, sweat test, skin prick testing and lung function tests
- Chronic lung disease: Any home oxygen

BIRTH HISTORY

- Oxygen/ventilatory support, use of continuous positive airway pressure or intubation
- Prematurity
- Chronic lung disease is associated with more frequent and severe respiratory infections/wheezy episodes

FEEDING HISTORY

- Eating and drinking
- Breathless when feeding
- Height and weight
- Growth can be affected by high-dose steroids

DEVELOPMENTAL HISTORY

- Any concerns voiced by parents, healthcare professionals or carers
- Loss of milestones (developmental regression)
- Most children at this age can:
  - Confidently go up and down stairs (gross motor)
  - Copy a circle (fine motor)
  - Speak in short sentences (language/hearing)
  - Play with other children (social)

MEDICATION HISTORY

Enquire about prescribed medications (including any recent changes) and over-the-counter medications. Allergies should be included with the specific reaction noted. In this scenario it is also important to note:

- Regular medications: Corticosteroids, long-acting β agonists, montelukast
- Exacerbating medication: Salbutamol

- Compliance and inhaler technique
- Known allergies
- Immunisation status: Recurrent vaccine-preventable infections

SOCIAL AND TRAVEL HISTORY

- Environmental triggers:
  - Housing: Damp, mould
  - Pets: Allergy
  - Smoking: Toxins
  - Recent travel: Tuberculosis (TB) exposure
  - People: Unwell contacts
- Recent travel abroad: Travel in the last 3 months (particularly relevant for infective symptoms)
- Social issues: Clarify if there is any social worker involvement and if so, the reasons

FAMILY HISTORY

- Ask about any significant family history, including atopic conditions; for example, asthma, eczema and hay fever

SYSTEMS REVIEW

On systems review, particularly pertinent questions to the above case may include questions regarding cardiac conditions, ENT, reflux and infection:

- Constitutional: Weight loss, appetite
- Cardiac: Sweating/breathlessness with feeds, palpitations
- ENT: Snoring/noisy breathing, ear pain/discharge, throat pain
- Reflux: Vomiting after feeds
- Infection: Fever, night sweats (think TB)

Differential Diagnosis

CONDITION	CLINICAL PRESENTATION	INVESTIGATIONS	MANAGEMENT
Viral-induced wheeze	• Younger children (under 5 years old) • Gradual onset • Cough/runny nose/fever	• Chest X-ray (CXR) for severe/non-responsive presentations	• Inhaled bronchodilators (salbutamol) • Ipratropium may work better in younger children • Nebulised if there is oxygen requirement • Limited evidence for oral steroids without atopic features
Asthma	• Gradual onset • Night cough • Interval symptoms • May be triggered by infection, allergen or exercise • Associated with atopy	• Peak flow if greater than 7 years old and compliant • CXR if severe to exclude pneumothorax or pneumonia	• Inhaled bronchodilators (salbutamol) • Nebulised if there is oxygen requirement • IV magnesium • Salbutamol/aminophylline infusions • Oral/IV corticosteroid
Inhaled foreign body	• Sudden onset • Stridor/wheeze • Monophonic wheeze	• CXR (radiopaque foreign body/lung collapse seen)	• Often surgical; for example, bronchoscopy to remove the foreign body

CONDITION	CLINICAL PRESENTATION	INVESTIGATIONS	MANAGEMENT
Bronchiolitis	• Age under 1–2 years old • Wet cough • Wheeze/crackles	• Nasopharyngeal aspirate	• Oxygen • Feeding support; for example, smaller, more frequent feeds, nasogastric tube feeds • Bronchodilators unlikely to be of benefit
Cardiac failure	• Sweating or breathlessness with feeds • Faltering growth	• Electrocardiogram (ECG) • CXR • Echocardiogram	• Diuretics
Gastro-oesophageal reflux	• Vomiting after feeds	• Barium study • pH study	• Reduce feed volumes • Feed thickeners • Antacids; for example, PPIs or H_2 receptor blocker

! Asthma Severity

	MODERATE	SEVERE	LIFE-THREATENING
Oxygen saturations	≥ 92%	< 92%	< 92%
Peak expiratory flow rate (PEFR) (vs. expected)	> 50%	33–50%	< 33%
Other features	• No clinical features of severe respiratory distress	• Tachypnoea (> 40 breaths/min in 2–5 year olds, > 30 breaths/min in over-5 years olds) • Tachycardia (>140 beats/min in 2–5 year olds, >125 beats/min in over-5 year olds) • Unable to complete sentences, talk or feed	• Poor respiratory effort • Altered consciousness • Hypotension/tachycardia • Exhaustion • Cyanosis • Silent chest on auscultation

Present Your Findings

Tommy is a 3-year-old boy who presented with his first episode of wheeze. He has had 2 days of coryzal symptoms, associated with wheeze and difficulty breathing, not responding to salbutamol inhalers. He is unable to speak in complete sentences. Both parents are smokers, and his brother has asthma. I feel the most likely diagnosis is a viral-induced wheeze, with differentials being asthma, reflux and cardiac failure.

I would like to examine Tommy fully, review a full set of observations and consider doing a blood gas and inserting a cannula. Initial management includes prescribing oxygen and inhaled or nebulised bronchodilator therapy, with consideration of IV medication if no improvement.

? QUESTIONS AND ANSWERS FOR CANDIDATE

What would make you suspect an inhaled foreign body rather than asthma?
• Sudden onset of difficulty breathing
• Monophonic wheeze
• Reduced air entry on one side
• No history of asthma

Which medications are used in the chronic treatment of asthma?
• Short-acting bronchodilators; for example, salbutamol

• Long-acting bronchodilators; for example, salmeterol
• Inhaled corticosteroid; for example, beclomethasone
• Oral leukotriene receptor antagonists; for example, montelukast
• Oral corticosteroids
• Oral theophylline

Aside from escalating medical treatment, what other methods would you do for someone presenting with repeat exacerbations of asthma?
• Check medicine compliance
• Review inhaler technique
• Encourage family members or the patient to stop smoking
• Review and avoid triggers; for example, pets, mould, dustmites

 A Case to Learn From

I saw a child who had been referred for wheeze and difficulty breathing. He had not responded to inhalers, and so as he looked like he was going to be admitted, I reviewed him. We checked his blood glucose and it was 30 mmol/L. This was actually Kussmaul breathing with diabetes. Don't assume all breathlessness in children is asthma, especially if the child does not respond to conventional treatment.

Top Tip

Parents will often say that because of the child, they now only smoke outside. It is important to tell the parents that this is still harmful for the child (due to smoke particles remaining on their clothes and on their breath) and that they should ideally stop smoking completely.

Top Tip

Don't get too obsessed with wheeze in and of itself. A patient who is really sick may have no wheeze, because quite simply there is no air moving. Similarly, as a child gets better, their wheeze may get louder because there is more air entry.

STATION 9.5: HISTORY: NEONATAL JAUNDICE

SCENARIO

You are a junior doctor seeing Mrs Jones and her daughter Sarah, a 1-week-old baby. Mrs Jones has noticed a yellow tinge to her daughter's skin and is quite concerned. Please take a history from Mrs Jones, present your findings and formulate an appropriate management plan.

Cardinal Symptoms

Onset of jaundice

Colour of urine

Colour of stools

Anaemia

Neurological deficit

HISTORY OF PRESENTING COMPLAINT

NEONATAL JAUNDICE

- Site: Sclera or skin
- Onset: Sudden or gradual, who noticed it and when
- Progression: Worsening or improving
- Severity:
  - Reduced wet nappies (dehydration)
  - Weight loss

ASSOCIATED SYMPTOMS

Other symptoms to enquire about include:
- Pale stool
- Dark urine
- Poor feeding (reduction in frequency or volume)

PAST MEDICAL AND SURGICAL HISTORY

In this scenario, it is also important to enquire about:
- Pregnancy: Gestation, antenatal scans, maternal blood group, infections, e.g. cytomegalovirus
- Risk factors for neonatal infection:
  - Prolonged rupture of membranes
  - Temperature during labour
  - Maternal sepsis
  - Group B streptococcus colonisation
  - Third-trimester urinary tract infection
- Birth: Method (especially assisted vaginal birth), resuscitation, birth trauma

MEDICATION HISTORY

Babies are not usually on any medication; however in this scenario it is also important to note:
- Certain drugs; for example, nitrofurantoin, can trigger haemolytic anaemia in glucose 6 phosphate dehydrogenase (G6PD) deficiency
- Children with known cholestatic jaundice may be on fat-soluble vitamin supplements (A, D, E and K)
- Any phototherapy for jaundice

SOCIAL HISTORY

- Recent travel abroad: Travel in the last 3 months (particularly relevant for infective symptoms)
- Social issues: Clarify if there is any social worker involvement and if so, the reasons

FAMILY HISTORY

Ask about any significant family history, including:
- Blood disorders; for example, hereditary spherocytosis
- Siblings/relatives with infantile jaundice

SYSTEMS REVIEW

On systems review, particularly pertinent questions to the above case may include questions regarding possible kernicterus, fluid loss or haematological issues:
- Neurological: Floppy episodes, abnormal movements or lethargy
- Gastrointestinal: Vomiting, particularly projectile (pyloric stenosis) or bilious (intestinal obstruction)
- Haematological: Pallor, bruising or bleeding noticed

Differential Diagnosis

CONDITION	CLINICAL PRESENTATION	INVESTIGATIONS	MANAGEMENT
Haemolytic causes (ABO and Rhesus incompatibility, spherocytosis)	• Onset < 24 h of life • Associated with drop in haemoglobin • There may be a positive family history • Increased severity with subsequent births	• Blood group (mother and infant) • Direct antiglobulin test (DAT)/ Coombs' test (will be positive) • Blood film	• Phototherapy • Immunoglobulin • Exchange transfusion in severe cases
Neonatal infection	• Onset < 24 h of life is more common but can be later • Risk factors for sepsis; for example, maternal group B streptococcus colonisation • Unwell	• 'Septic screen'- FBCs, CRP, blood and urine culture • Likely to include lumbar puncture and CXR if there is a fever or systemically unwell	• IV antibiotics
Physiological jaundice	• Onset 24–72 h of life • More common in prematurity	• Serum or transcutaneous bilirubin	• Phototherapy
Breast milk jaundice	• Onset 24–72 h of life • Breastfeeding • Can persist for up to 12 weeks	• Serum or transcutaneous bilirubin	• Phototherapy
Biliary atresia	• Onset > 72 h of life • Persists for weeks • Dark urine • Pale stools	• 'Split' bilirubin (conjugate/ unconjugated) • Liver/abdominal ultrasound	• Referral for surgical management (Kasai procedure)

Differential diagnoses for neonatal jaundice presenting in the first 24 h of life

Haemolytic causes

Rhesus incompatibility	• Mother Rhesus-negative • Baby Rhesus-positive
ABO incompatibility	• The baby is A+, B+ or AB+ and the mother is negative to those groups; for example, the mother is A+, baby is B+. Group O mothers are most at risk of this
G6PD deficiency	• X-linked recessive • Affects red cell function and predisposes to haemolysis
Hereditary spherocytosis	• Autosomal dominant • Affects red blood cell shape, therefore increasing the likelihood of haemolysis

Infection

Group B streptococcus	• Maternal carriage of group B streptococcus • Previous children with group B streptococcus
Other	• Always suspect if jaundice on day 1, particularly if no haemolysis set up • Baby may be clinically well

Differential diagnoses for neonatal jaundice presenting between 24 h and 2 weeks

Polycythaemia	• Babies have a higher number of red cells and therefore greater red cell breakdown and bilirubin production
Resolving cephalohaematoma	• As the bleed in the cephalohaematoma breaks down, there is a higher red cell turnover, leading to jaundice
Physiological jaundice	• Usually presents on day 2 or 3 of life • It is related to an immature liver function and high red cell turnover
Breastfeeding jaundice	• Related to the inhibition of the enzyme glucuronyl transferase, which is responsible for the conjugation of bilirubin

Differential diagnoses for prolonged jaundice presenting at 2 weeks or beyond

Biliary atresia	• Biliary ducts absent/blocked/narrow, causing biliary obstruction • Urgent surgical assessment required • There will be a conjugated hyperbilirubinaemia
Hypothyroidism	• If identified and treated early, significant reduction of complications

Present Your Findings

Sarah is a 1-week-old breastfed baby who presented with a 1-day history of jaundice that started on day 3.

There are no risk factors for infection and no family history of haemolytic disease. Sarah is otherwise well, with good feeding and has regained her birth weight. I feel the most likely diagnosis is physiological jaundice, with the differential being breastfeeding jaundice.

I would like to check her bilirubin level and plot it on a bilirubin chart to assess if phototherapy may be required.

QUESTIONS AND ANSWERS FOR CANDIDATE

How do you determine the management of jaundice in a well baby?
- Check and plot bilirubin on treatment threshold graph
- Depending on the level: Discharge, observe or give phototherapy
- Consider blood film, FBCs, CRP, blood cultures and DAT

What is kernicterus?
- A complication of severe unconjugated hyperbilirubinaemia
- Bilirubin crosses the blood–brain barrier, binding to the basal ganglia, causing irreversible brain damage
- This eventually results in parkinsonism and severe developmental delay

What is an exchange transfusion?
- Removal of patient's blood and replacement of equal volume with donor blood
- Used in severe haemolytic jaundice not responding to phototherapy and immunoglobulin to prevent kernicterus

A Case to Learn From

A baby I saw had been seen previously with jaundice. The jaundice was felt to be mild, so the baby was not tested and was sent home. The baby came back in several days later, and their jaundice levels were so high they needed an exchange transfusion. All babies with jaundice should have a formal bilirubin check, as the human eye is a poor judge of severity. In this baby, an exchange transfusion could have been avoided.

Top Tip

If you are really worried about jaundice in a baby, check it on a blood gas as well as formal bloods. This way you get an immediate bilirubin result and can start provisional treatment.

Top Tip

In neonates, infections are really difficult to pick up. They may have a normal CRP, normal observations and seemingly normal behaviour. Therefore, antibiotics are started just on the basis of a combination of risk factors, and jaundice within the first 24 h, even if the baby is well, is one of these.

STATION 9.6: HISTORY: FALTERING GROWTH

SCENARIO

You are a junior doctor attached to the paediatric team. The primary care physician has referred 9-month-old James because of poor weight gain. You are asked to take a history from his mother, Lucy, present your findings and formulate an appropriate management plan.

Cardinal Symptoms

Reduced input; for example, dysphagia, poor feeding

Increased metabolic demand; for example, fever, recurrent cough/wheeze

Increased output/losses; for example, vomiting, diarrhoea, polyuria

HISTORY OF PRESENTING COMPLAINT

FAILURE TO THRIVE
- Onset:
  - Chronology of weight concerns, i.e. recent vs. long-term
  - Weight vs. length vs. head circumference
- Intake or feeding history:
  - Breast milk vs. formula-fed
  - Date of weaning
  - Quantity and frequency of milk/solids
- Feeding difficulty:
  - Food being offered vs. food taken
  - Known issues; for example, tongue tie, dysphagia, vomiting, fussiness

ASSOCIATED SYMPTOMS

Other symptoms to enquire about include:
- Stool and bowel movements; for example, diarrhoea, blood or mucus
- Abdominal pain, colic
- Wet nappies reduced or polyuria

PAST MEDICAL AND SURGICAL HISTORY

In this scenario, it is also important to enquire about:
- General: Ask about known medical conditions, relevant treatments and any hospital admissions
- Genetic: Condition causing small stature; for example, Down's syndrome
- Jaundice: Consider hypothyroidism or chronic liver disease
- Recurrent infections: Consider CF
- Heart disease: Consider congenital heart defects; for example, aortic stenosis

BIRTH HISTORY

- Growth concerns in pregnancy
- Gestation at birth
- Birth weight, weight gain during the first week of life
- Guthrie test result or if known CF
- NICU admission: Details of stay, including issues with feeding/growth
- Home oxygen

DEVELOPMENTAL HISTORY

- Any concerns voiced by parents, healthcare professionals or carers
- Most children at this age can:
  - Sit unsupported (gross motor)
  - Use an early pincer grip (fine motor)
  - Babble (language/hearing)
  - Have stranger danger (social)

MEDICATION HISTORY

Enquire about prescribed and over-the-counter medications, including any recent changes. Allergies should also be included with the specific reaction noted. In this scenario, also ask about:

- Regular medications: Corticosteroids, multiple antibiotic courses
- Immunisation status: Recurrent infections

SOCIAL HISTORY

- Environmental triggers:
  - Housing: Damp, mould
  - Pets: Allergy
  - Smoking: Toxins
  - Recent travel: Tuberculosis exposure
  - People: Unwell contacts
- Recent travel abroad: Travel in the last 3 months (particularly relevant for infective symptoms)
- Social issues: Clarify if there is any social worker involvement and if so, the reasons

FAMILY HISTORY

Ask about any significant family history, including:
- Bowel disorders: Coeliac, inflammatory bowel disease
- CF

SYSTEMS REVIEW

In addition to symptoms explored in the history of the presenting complaint, pertinent questions in a systems review would explore possible underlying chronic conditions:

- General: Activity level, lethargy, rashes, pallor
- Cardiac: Sweating/breathlessness with feeds (cardiac failure)
- Respiratory: Recurrent chest infections, chronic cough
- Infective: Recurrent fevers, rashes
- Neurological: Headaches, drowsiness, fits
- Musculoskeletal: Joint pain/swelling
- Genitourinary: Dysuria, urinary frequency and wetting episodes
- Haematological: Abnormal bruising or bleeding
- ENT: Stridor/ snoring

Differential Diagnosis

CONDITION	CLINICAL PRESENTATION	INVESTIGATIONS	MANAGEMENT
Gastro-oesophageal reflux	• Usually presents in the first few months of life • Discomfort during feeds • Vomiting during/after feeds • Back arching/knee indrawing	• Barium study • pH study • Impedance study	• Reduce feed volumes • Feed thickeners • Antacids; for example, PPI/H$_2$ receptor blocker
Cow's milk protein intolerance	• Usually presents in the first few months of life • Discomfort during/after feeds • Vomiting • Diarrhoea or constipation • Blood/mucus in stools • Allergic-type rash (in IgE-mediated)	• Allergy testing/RAST is often negative (not all are IgE-mediated) • Trial of exclusion	• Hydrolysed or amino acid formula • Dairy-free diet
CF	• Fatty stools that do not flush (steatorrhoea) • Recurrent chest infections	• Screened for on Guthrie test (day 5 blood spot) • Sweat test	• MDT management • IV antibiotics for respiratory infections • Pancreatic enzymes

Continued

Differential Diagnosis—cont'd

CONDITION	CLINICAL PRESENTATION	INVESTIGATIONS	MANAGEMENT
Coeliac disease	• Presents after weaning (> 6 months old) • Bloating • Buttock wasting • Diarrhoea/fatty stools (steatorrhoea)	• Coeliac screening bloods (anti-tissue transglutaminase antibody (TTG), anti-gliadin antibody and anti-endomysial antibody, total IgA) • Endoscopic intestinal biopsy (shows villous atrophy) • Note that the tests must be carried out while the child is having gluten in his diet	• Lifelong gluten-free diet
Inflammatory bowel disease	• Usually older children • Diarrhoea • Blood/mucus in stools	• Bloods, including FBCs, CRP, ESR, LFTs (albumin) • Stool culture (to exclude infection) • Faecal calprotectin, which is raised in bowel inflammation • Colonoscopy and biopsy for histology	• Elemental diet • Corticosteroids • Immune-modulating drugs; for example, aminosalicylates • Surgical resection of affected areas
Non-organic causes, e.g. neglect	• Unkempt child • Signs of NAI; for example, bruising • Poor carer–child interaction	• Diagnosis of exclusion	• Requires MDT input, including social services • Ensure care and safety of siblings

MANAGEMENT OF GASTRO-OESOPHAGEAL REFLUX

Conservative
• Babies:
  • Raising the cot base (not mattress) at the head end by 30°
  • Smaller, more frequent feeds
  • Feed thickeners; for example, Carobel or Nestrogel
• Older children:
  • Weight loss
  • Avoiding chocolate, acidic food and drink, peppermint and coffee
  • Avoid eating within 3 h of bedtime
  • Avoid smoking

Medical
• Antacid: For example, Gaviscon
• PPIs: For example, omeprazole
• Prokinetics: For example, domperidone
• Histamine receptor antagonist: For example, ranitidine

Surgical
• Nissen's fundoplication

Present Your Findings

James is a 9-month-old boy presenting with faltering growth, dropping two centiles in the last 2 months for weight and length.

His symptoms of bloating, diarrhoea and pale stools coincide with him starting to wean on to solids, and he had previously been growing well. There is no other significant past medical history.

This history is suggestive of coeliac disease and as such I would suggest a gluten-free diet and do serological testing for IgA anti-TTG and a villous biopsy to confirm the diagnosis.

❓ QUESTIONS AND ANSWERS FOR CANDIDATE

What is the most common cause of failure to thrive in the UK?

Non-organic causes, which may be associated with:
• Poverty
• Inappropriate diet for age; for example, excessive consumption of fruit juice
• Coercive feeding
• Distraction at mealtimes
• Social isolation
• Life stresses
• Poor parenting skills
• Child abuse or neglect
• Parental mental health issues; for example, postpartum depression
• Parental eating disorders; for example, anorexia nervosa

What contraindications are there to breastfeeding?
• Active TB in the mother
• Mothers with breast cancer undergoing chemotherapy
• Syphilitic lesions on the breast or nipple
• Infant inborn errors of metabolism precluding tolerance of breast milk components

What advantages might breastfeeding have over formula feeding?
• Presence of antibodies to protect against infection
• Mother–baby bonding
• Demand-led
• Free and available on demand at optimal temperature
• Contents vary according to changing nutritional requirements of infant

A Case to Learn From

We admitted a baby to the children's ward with faltering growth. She had barely gained any weight in a month. The older sibling was in foster care because of maternal drug use and neglect. Mum insisted things were different this time. A couple of days after admission, we got a call saying the day 5 blood spot (Guthrie) had showed CF, which explained the poor weight gain. Things improved with treatment.

While your index of suspicion needs to be high to detect non-organic causes, they remain a diagnosis of exclusion. Ensure your medical investigations continue alongside your conversations with social services.

 Top Tip

When you have a condition with as many differentials as faltering growth, it helps to go back to basics. Split causes up into logical groups: Do they have insufficient intake? Do they have excessive loss? Or do they have a high energy demand?

 Top Tip

Faltering growth is not diagnosed from one timepoint. It is crucial to see the time trend of weight/length/head circumference and to see the centile lines being crossed over time. Otherwise, you cannot tell if someone is just small, or if they are dropping centiles.

STATION 9.7: HISTORY: NON-ACCIDENTAL INJURY

SCENARIO

You are a junior doctor in the ED and have been asked to see Fred, a 3-month-old boy. Fred was brought in by his mother, Mrs Williams, after he 'rolled off the sofa'. He has broken his right humerus, which has been confirmed on X-ray. Please take a history from Mrs Williams about Fred, present your findings and formulate an appropriate management plan.

 Cardinal Symptoms

Injuries not consistent with mechanism

Injuries in children who are not yet mobile

Delayed presentation

Vague, changing story

Multiple admissions: Different surgeries or hospitals with no medical explanation

GENERAL POINTS

- Ask questions in a calm, non-judgemental manner
- Avoid leading questions
- When age-appropriate, try to speak to the child separately, with an additional professional present who can document the child's account accurately. Never make promises of confidentiality to a child, as you may need to break such promises in order to notify the police or social services
- Speak to all third parties involved
- If interpreters are required, use one from outside the family
- Whilst taking a history of this nature, family members may become very defensive or angry in response to questioning. Leave if you feel threatened (ensuring that the child is safe)

Things to look out for include:
- The child's manner and behaviour while recounting the history. Do they look uneasy or worried? Are they looking around for confirmation of their story from their parents?
- Inconsistency between family members or accounts of the history over time
- Does the history match the injury sustained, as well as the child's developmental age?

HISTORY OF PRESENTING COMPLAINT

DESCRIPTION OF THE EVENTS SURROUNDING INJURY
- Before:
  - Abnormal behavior or signs of illness
  - Meals and sleep that day
  - List all the people at home and outside who had exposure to child
  - Snapshot of exactly what was happening and exactly where everyone was just before event
- During:
  - What happened to cause the injury? For a fall, document the mechanism, height, type of surface
  - Head injury
  - Time
- After:
  - Length of crying
  - Swelling
  - Bleeding
  - Bruising
  - Obvious limb deformity
  - Medication given or help sought

ASSOCIATED SYMPTOMS

Other symptoms to enquire about include:
- Symptoms of intracranial bleed: Loss of consciousness, vomiting, seizures, headache, change in behaviour, lethargy
- Symptoms of musculoskeletal injury: Pain, weakness, deformity

PAST MEDICAL AND SURGICAL HISTORY

In this scenario, it is also important to enquire about:
- Previous hospital admissions or injuries, noting if anything is suspicious

- Medical:
  - Metabolic bone disease: Complication of prematurity
  - Birth trauma: Bleeding disorders may be suspected in disproportionate injury after vaginal birth
  - Osteogenesis imperfecta
  - Haemophilia
- Surgical:
  - Prolonged bleeding after a procedure; for example, circumcision

FEEDING HISTORY

- Feeding difficulties: Can be a precipitant to NAI or associated with significant injury

DEVELOPMENTAL HISTORY

- Any concerns voiced by parents, healthcare professionals or carers
- Most children at this age can:
  - Smile responsively
  - Fix and follow with eyes
  - Turn head to sound
  - Respond to noise
- Some may be able to roll

MEDICATION HISTORY

Babies are not usually on any medication. In this scenario it is also important to note:
- Vitamin K at birth: Prevents hameolytic disease of newborn
- Immunisation history: If there is neglect, it may also mean immunisations have been missed

SOCIAL HISTORY

- Family situation:
  - Household residents
  - Parental relationship
  - Family tree, including siblings of new/old partners
  - Additional carers
  - Personal difficulties; for example, financial
  - Support from friend and family
- Social services:
  - Previous and current
  - May have named social worker
  - Child in need/child protection plan

FAMILY HISTORY

Ask about any significant family history, including:
- Bleeding disorders
- Osteogenesis imperfecta
- Chronic illness or mental health issues with either parent, which are risk factors for NAI

SYSTEMS REVIEW

On systems review, particularly pertinent questions to the above case may include questions regarding:
- Gastrointestinal: Vomiting, weight gain, difficulty feeding, unexplained crying
- Haematological: Easy bruising or bleeding
- Neurological: Headache, drowsiness, difficulty sleeping, fits

Differential Diagnosis

DISEASE	CLINICAL PRESENTATION	INVESTIGATIONS	MANAGEMENT
NAI	• Changing history • Injury inappropriate for mechanism or developmental age • Spiral fractures • May be signs of neglect; for example, unkempt	• Skeletal survey • CT head • Ophthalmological examination for retinal haemorrhages (age <1 year old)	• Multidisciplinary involvement, including social services and police • Ensure safety of siblings/other dependants
Accidental injury/ fracture	• Consistent history • Expected injury for age/ mechanism	• Localised X-ray	• Splinting or casting • Surgery for unstable fractures
Osteogenesis imperfecta	• Variable depending on subtype • Blue sclera • Hypermobile joints • Deafness • Dental problems	• Severe variants diagnosed prenatally • Postnatally, diagnosis is made clinically • X-ray shows multiple healed fractures, bowing of bones	• Physiotherapy • Bisphosphonates • Surgery, for fracture fixation or to correct deformities
Bleeding disorders; for example, haemophilia or von Willebrand disease (vWD)	• Excessive bleeding and bruising • Often suspected after excess bleeding post-circumcision or related to birth trauma	• Blood tests for coagulation studies	• Desmopressin (for vWD) • Infusion of missing factors (for haemophilia and vWD) • During severe bleeding episodes

MANAGEMENT OF NAI

- The child's safety and well-being are the most important things. Act to ensure that this principle is maintained at all times, which can include overriding confidentiality and consent, if necessary
- The role of the student/junior is not necessarily to diagnose child abuse, but to refer to somebody more experienced in the field
- Talk to a senior doctor, nurse or child protection lead as soon as possible
- Document your findings without conjecture (useful for assessing consistency of story following subsequent assessments)
- In the case of sexual abuse, to avoid further unnecessary trauma to the child, the examination should be performed only once by the most senior child protection doctor, often in a specialist centre

EXAMINATION

- Although an examination is unlikely as an OSCE station, it is still important to know about
- Gain consent from the child (if competent), carers with parental responsibility, or if parents refuse to cooperate, consult social care and police (police protection order or emergency protection order may be required)
- Examination can be done without explicit consent if it is considered an emergency and in the child's best interest
- Clearly mark examination findings on a body map, which should be counter-signed by a second doctor (always sign and date clearly)
- Do not do anything invasive that will need repeating soon or that you are not experienced in doing, in particular, genital examination

OBSERVATION

- Note the appearance of and behaviour of the child and their interaction with carers
- Look for any sign of anxiety or apprehension in the child. Is the child very reluctant to be touched/undressed? Is the child excessively clingy? Look for signs of neglect; for example, clothing and hygiene
- Some children may be inappropriately friendly and fail to show healthy attachment to carers
- 'Frozen watchfulness' is a sign of severe abuse. The child looks watchful, carefully tracking other people's movements. They may also have an expression of fear on their face
- Observe the relationship of the parent to the child. Do they stop the child from speaking to healthcare professionals alone? Are they hostile to the child?

ESTABLISHING WHETHER THE INJURY PATTERN IS SUSPICIOUS

- Remember that children are often hurt/marked in places that are thought to be less likely to be seen or found, so be thorough in your examination
- Be as objective as possible and describe your findings without making conclusions or judgements

Details on the four types of abuse

DOMAIN	DEFINITION	EXAMPLES
Physical	Causing physical harm	• Hitting • Shaking • Poisoning • Burning • Suffocation
Emotional	Constant neglect or ill treatment, adversely affecting emotional development	• Making a child feel worthless • Inducing fear in a child • Deprivation of social activity
Sexual	Enforcing/enticing sexual activity, including non-penetrative acts	• Encouraging sexual behaviour • Looking at pornographic material • Sexual contact
Neglect	Constant failure to meet basic needs of the child (physical or psychological)	• Insufficient food, clothing, shelter or medical care

Present Your Findings

Fred is a 3-month-old boy who has sustained a fracture to the right humerus after his mother reported him rolling off the sofa 4 days previously.

The history given by Mrs Williams seems inconsistent, changing throughout our discussion. This, combined with the delayed presentation and other risk factors, including a history of domestic abuse, leads me to be concerned that Fred may have sustained an NAI.

Fred needs to be examined by a senior doctor and a body map of any other injuries documented. I would recommend a full skeletal survey, CT head and ophthalmological examination for retinal haemorrhages. Prompt discussion with social services and the police should be made to ensure the safety of his 3-year-old sister, and Fred should be admitted to hospital as a place of safety in the meantime.

QUESTIONS AND ANSWERS FOR CANDIDATE

What investigations might be requested in cases of suspected NAI?

If child abuse is suspected in a non-ambulant infant, they will need the following four investigations:
- Bloods: FBCs and clotting screen to exclude bruising/bleeding disorders

- Skeletal survey: A series of X-rays, that can take up to 1 h to complete, to exclude occult fractures (if any are found, X-rays should be repeated 2 weeks later to exclude previous subtle fractures)
- CT brain: To exclude intracranial bleeds (may need a subsequent MRI if abnormal)
- Ophthalmological assessment: To exclude retinal haemorrhages (seen in shaken babies)

Further investigations are based on the site and nature of injuries and may include:
- Ultrasound: For soft-tissue injury, for example, muscle haematoma
- Sexually transmitted infection screening: If sexual abuse is suspected
- Dentist review: To interpret bite marks, even to identify the abuser
- Plastic surgery review: To interpret and also guide further management of burns

Name five potential risk factors for child abuse.
- Domestic abuse
- Drug or alcohol misuse
- Previous child abuse in the family
- Illness or disability in parents or carers, both physical and mental illness
- Illness or disability in the child or sibling
- Criminal record
- Single-parent families or social isolation

What is fabricated or induced illness?
Previously called Munchausen syndrome or Munchausen syndrome by proxy, this complex form of child abuse ranges from carers exaggerating or lying about symptoms, to inducing them; for example, giving drugs to cause diarrhoea.

There may be a history of mental health disorder in the carer or multiple medically unexplained symptoms. It can be very hard to detect and even harder to prove.

> **Top Tip**
>
> Remember, you are not a police officer or social worker and are not collecting forensic evidence or building a case. You are simply doing your job by taking a history, assessing red flags and risk factors, forming a differential diagnosis and making a management plan.

> **Top Tip**
>
> Once away from their carer, children may speak up about their concerns. Document their exact words without asking leading questions. You will want to establish their trust, but remember, you can't promise confidentiality.

> **Top Tip**
>
> I once spoke to two children on their own after having taken a history with their mother present. When I asked about what happens if they do something wrong, the younger child said 'Mum hits me'. His older brother reacted in shock, saying 'Shh, Mum told you not to say that!'. With parents absent, vital clues can be ascertained around not just what happened, but also the child's safety going back home.

STATION 9.8: EXAMINATION: NEWBORN BABY CHECK

SCENARIO
You are a junior doctor covering the postnatal ward. You routinely perform a baby check on baby Barton, who is 12 h old. He is the first child of a 36-year-old woman and was born by normal vaginal birth. Combined antenatal screening was not undertaken. Before you see the baby, the midwife has called your attention to the baby's facial features.

PREPARATION
- Explain the examination to the parents and your reasons for performing it
- Gain verbal consent from the parents
- Verify key points in the antenatal history, including hospital admissions and abnormal scans
- Identify any parental concerns
- Ask about feeding, passing of urine (normal within 24 h) and meconium (normal within 48 h)
- Family history of congenital hip dislocation, heart disease or deafness

EXAMINATION
The newborn baby check is a head-to-toe examination, but like all paediatric examinations, it is best performed opportunistically. You will need the baby fully undressed to assess them, but you may choose to do this in stages to keep them warm and reduce the chance of them crying. Do what you can while they are asleep; for example, auscultate the precordium. A systemic approach to the examination follows.

INSPECTION
- General features:
  - Assess the tone, posture and movements of the baby and note any abnormalities
  - If there is Erb's palsy (waiter's tip posture) after shoulder dystocia, the baby may not move one of the arms
- Skin
  - Area: Skin should be examined over the entire body
  - Birthmarks (naevi): Common birthmarks include haemangioma (Fig. 9.3) and congenital dermal melanocytosis
  - Rash: It is common for babies to have erythema toxicum (a benign rash characterised by erythematous macules with overlying white/yellow papules). Exclude more worrisome rashes; for example, petechiae
  - Colour: Look for pallor, cyanosis, jaundice
- Cry: Listen to the cry and assess whether it is strong and of a normal pitch

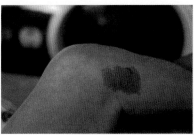
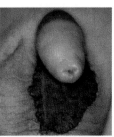
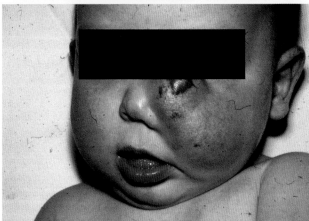

Fig. 9.3 Haemangiomas.

- Weight: Offer to weigh the baby and plot this on the growth chart

EXAMINATION OF THE HEAD

- Shape
  - Caput and chignon, which are swellings caused by pressure from the cervix or ventouse birth respectively
  - Bleeding can form under the scalp, known as cephalohaematoma
  - Examine sagittal and coronal suture lines. Check if any swelling crosses the suture lines
- Size
  - Measure and plot the head circumference. Do this by measuring the longest distance around the head from the occiput, and repeat twice, taking the longest measurement
- Fontanelles
  - Ensure normal size and shape of both anterior and posterior fontanelles
  - Check that they are not sunken or risen
- Face
  - Examine for abnormal facial features; for example, hypertelorism (widely spaced eyes) and micrognathia (undersized jaw), which may be consistent with an underlying syndrome
- Eyes:
  - Look through an ophthalmoscope to check for red reflexes from both pupils. Absence warrants further investigation to exclude cataracts or retinoblastoma
- Mouth:
  - Ensure normal shape with no cleft lip
  - Examine below the tongue to exclude tongue tie
  - Insert a gloved finger to assess suck reflex
  - Use a tongue depressor to visualise the palate all the way from the hard palate back to the uvula
- Ears:
  - Examine to ensure normal position (the superior aspect of the ear should be the same height as the eyes, or above) and exclude auricular skin tags and sinuses

EXAMINATION OF THE CHEST

Inspection

- Deformity; for example, pectus excavatum (caved-in appearance of chest), accessory nipples
- Effort of breathing by counting respiratory rate (normal is 40–60 breaths/min) and looking for recessions (sucking in between or under ribs)

Palpation

- Heaves and/or thrills

Auscultation

- Heart sounds and murmurs. Also, measure heart rate and rhythm (normal: 100–140 beats/min)
- Lung fields

EXAMINATION OF THE ABDOMEN

Inspection

- Masses
- Umbilical stump normally dries and separates over 5–10 days. Check for surrounding erythema, which could be a sign of infection
- Hernia, umbilical or inguinal
- Anus, checking patency and that it is in the normal position

Palpation

- Organomegaly or masses
- Femoral pulses (this takes practice!), by abducting the hips with the palms and using the forefingers to palpate the midinguinal point. Compare left and right. Weak or absent femoral pulses may be the only sign of coarctation of the aorta

Auscultation

- Bowel sounds

EXAMINATION OF THE GENITALIA

Inspection

- Ensure no ambiguity. If any doubt, do not assign a gender until the newborn has been reviewed by a senior colleague and relevant investigations are performed
- Female
  - A small amount of discharge or blood is normal (from residual maternal oestrogen)
- Male
  - Check that both testes have descended
  - Check for hypospadias (urethral opening on underside of penis)

EXAMINATION OF THE HIPS

- Barlow manoeuvre:
  - Adduct the hip and apply pressure posteriorly on the hip. If the hip moves posteriorly with a click, it is dislocatable
- Ortolani manoeuvre:
  - Stabilise the pelvis by firmly holding the symphysis pubis and coccyx between the thumb and middle finger of one hand. Then, with the baby's hips and knees flexed, and the index finger of your other hand on the greater trochanter, abduct the baby's hip. A palpable clunk signifies relocation of a posteriorly dislocated hip

EXAMINATIONM OF THE LIMBS

Inspection

- Digits for polydactyly (accessory digits) or syndactyly (fused digits)
- Hands for palmar creases (normally two, single or simian palmar creases are seen in Down's syndrome)
- Feet for talipes (in-turned or 'club' foot). If positive for this, determine if it is positional (can be moved to correct anatomical position) or fixed (cannot be moved)

EXAMINATION OF THE SPINE

Inspection

- Hold the baby in ventral suspension
- Tone
- Scoliosis or curvature of spine
- Sacral dimples or tufts of hair may indicate spinal fistulae or cord tethering

MOVEMENT AND REFLEXES

- Moro reflex
  - Hold the baby supine and allow the baby's head to drop backwards (warn the parents!). The baby will spread both arms. It may be asymmetrical in Erb's palsy
- Head lag
  - Support the shoulders and pull the baby to sit from the lying position. Assess tone
- Stepping reflex
  - While holding the baby in standing position, lower one foot to the underside of a flat surface; baby will slowly 'step' each foot
- Grasp
  - Place a finger in the palm of the baby's hand. A normal response is for the baby to grasp your finger with theirs

FINISHING

- Offer to redress the baby
- Thank the parents
- Wash your hands

Fig. 9.4 summarises the detailed explanation above to allow visualisation of the head-to-toe approach. This helps to ensure that no aspect of the examination is overlooked.

Present Your Findings

Baby Barton, born by spontaneous vaginal birth, with no antenatal or intrapartum concerns noted, is now 12 h old, I have performed a routine examination of the newborn on him.

On examination, there is evidence of hypertelorism, epicanthic folds, upslanting palpebral fissures and macroglossia. Reflexes are normal, there is a good cry, but tone is reduced throughout. Baby Barton also has single palmar creases with short broad hands. Cardiovascular and respiratory examination was normal.

In summary, this baby has features that may suggest trisomy 21 (Down syndrome).

To complete my examination, I would document the newborn baby check in the neonatal notes and, after appropriate counselling, genetic karyotyping will be required. He may require feeding support in the short term and if trisomy 21 is confirmed, will require multidisciplinary team (MDT) follow-up to monitor growth and development.

QUESTIONS AND ANSWERS FOR CANDIDATE

What is the management of suspected developmental dysplasia of the hip?
- Hip ultrasound
- If positive, this may require physiotherapy review and further treatment; for example, a Pavlik harness

What cardiac complications are associated with Down syndrome?
- Atrioventricular septal defect is the most common cardiac complication
- Ventral septal defect
- Patent ductus arteriosus
- Tetralogy of Fallot

What does the newborn blood spot (Guthrie card) test for?
This blood test is taken from a heel prick and screens for markers of diseases. The tests can vary depending on what has a higher prevalence in the geographical area, but generally include:
- Neonatal hypothyroidism
- CF
- Sickle cell disease
- Medium-chain acyl-CoA dehydrogenase deficiency
- Maple syrup urine disease
- Isovaleric acidaemia
- Glutaric aciduria type 1
- Homocystinuria

A Case to Learn From

Practical tip on the Moro. Be really careful performing this and do it over a bed. Years ago during an exam, a baby had a really exaggerated Moro reflex and 'leapt' out of the candidate's hands and fell to the floor. The candidate failed simply because the baby was not safe at all times. I tell my students this anecdote and then suggest in exams they ask, 'Would you like me to perform the Moro reflex?' It startles the child and can result in crying. Most examiners will decline your considerate offer.

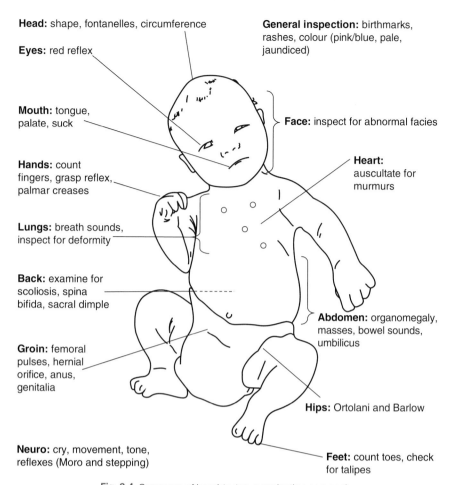

Head: shape, fontanelles, circumference

Eyes: red reflex

Mouth: tongue, palate, suck

Hands: count fingers, grasp reflex, palmar creases

Lungs: breath sounds, inspect for deformity

Back: examine for scoliosis, spina bifida, sacral dimple

Groin: femoral pulses, hernial orifice, anus, genitalia

Neuro: cry, movement, tone, reflexes (Moro and stepping)

General inspection: birthmarks, rashes, colour (pink/blue, pale, jaundiced)

Face: inspect for abnormal facies

Heart: auscultate for murmurs

Abdomen: organomegaly, masses, bowel sounds, umbilicus

Hips: Ortolani and Barlow

Feet: count toes, check for talipes

Fig. 9.4 Summary of head-to-toe examination approach.

 Top Tip

I prefer to undress a baby for myself when examining. It's a helpful way of understanding what their tone is like and how they respond to handling. However, it also reveals your experience handling infants so if you're not confident, ask the parents!

 Top Tip

Examining the hips can be extremely difficult to get right. Do one hip at a time, don't be afraid to repeat it if you're not sure and do it while the baby is settled, as if they are resisting, it makes a difficult procedure nearer impossible!

STATION 9.9: EXAMINATION: DEVELOPMENTAL DELAY

SCENARIO

You are a junior doctor in a neonatal outpatient clinic and have been asked to see Khalid, a 24-month-old boy who is attending with his mother Leila for routine developmental follow-up. He was born at 26 weeks' gestation and he left the NICU at 3 months of age, after overcoming numerous complications. Please examine Khalid and present your findings.

PREPARATION

- Introduce yourself, gain consent and wash your hands
- Explain the examination to Khalid's mother, stating that you are looking to assess his development and see if there are any ways that you can provide more help
- Remember to keep the child at ease; for example, you could try to make it like a game
- The appropriate equipment you will need may include:
  - Pencil, paper and scissors
  - Bricks
  - Toys, including dolls
  - Picture book
  - Beads and string
  - Cutlery or cup

THE EXAMINATION

A structured developmental examination incorporates finding the child's maximum ability in four key domains:
- Gross motor
- Fine motor and vision
- Language and hearing
- Social and self-care

INSPECTION

- Height, weight and head circumference
- Dysmorphic features; for example, in trisomy 21
- Developmental aids; for example, hearing aids
- Spontaneous demonstration of milestone; for example, walking/talking

GROSS MOTOR

Start at what appears to be the most appropriate stage (Table 9.1). If the child looks under 6 months old, start at the beginning. If they demonstrated walking with a steady gait on entering the room, there is no need to test for developmental milestones achieved before this landmark.

- Movements and position at rest:
  - Are they moving all four limbs, and are they moving them equally?
  - Can they roll over (5–6 months old)?
- Primitive reflexes (non-mobile child):
  - Moro: Sudden downward dropping of head (whilst supporting the bottom) results in both arms being flexed/abducted (under 3 months old)
  - Grasp: Place your finger in the baby's hand and the baby reacts by grasping it (under 3 months old)
  - Stepping: While you are holding the baby upright on a flat surface, the baby lifts one foot and then the other as if stepping/walking (under 4 months old and reappears at 12 months old)
  - Asymmetrical tonic neck reflex: With the baby lying on their back, when their head moves to one side, the arm and leg extend on the side the head is turned towards, and the opposite arm and leg flex (under 6 months old)
- Place the child in ventral suspension. Observe if the baby has:
  - Some head lag (6 weeks old)
  - No head lag. Also able to lift head above midline (3 months old)
- Place the child prone. Observe if the baby is able to:
  - Lift head and/or raise chest, resting on elbows (3 months old)
  - Raise chest with fully extended arms (5–6 months old)
- Place the child in a sitting position. Observe if the baby is able to:
  - Sit supported/unsupported with a curved back (5–6 months old)
  - Sit unsupported with a straight back (8–9 months old)
  - Crawl/bum shuffle (8–9 months old)
- Pull to a standing position. Observe if the baby is able to:
  - Stay in a standing position (10 months old)
- Moving on two legs. Observe if the baby is able to:
  - Cruise, walk while holding on to things (10 months old)

Table 9.1 Gross motor milestones

AGE	EXPECTATION
6 weeks	Good head control
3 months	Raising head and chest on forearms
6 months	Sitting up supported
8–9 months	Sitting up unsupported
9 months	Pulling to stand, crawling
12 months	Standing, walking unsteadily
18 months	Running, stooping down to pick things up
2 years	Jumping and kicking a ball, climbing stairs with two feet per step
3 years	Pedalling a tricycle, one foot per step going up
4 years	Hopping, climbing downstairs, one foot per step going down
5 years	Bouncing and catching a ball

- Walk with an unsteady gait (12 months old) or with a steady gait (15 months old)
- Run (18 months old)
- Stoop down to pick things up (18 months old)
- Jump and kick a ball (2 years old)
- Ride a tricycle (3 years old)
- Hop (4 years old)
- Stand on one foot for 10 s (5 years old)
- Walking up and down stairs. Observe if the baby is using:
  - Two feet per step (2 years old)
  - One foot per step going up, two feet per step going down (3 years old)
  - One foot per step going up, one foot per step going down (4 years old)
- Other:
  - Bounces and catches a ball (5 years old)
  - May be able to ride a bike without stabilisers (5 years old)

FINE MOTOR

- Start by generally observing the child playing and crudely assess what they can do
- Assess them whilst on the same level as they are, and make sure that there are no distractions around; for example, clear up building blocks when another test is being done
- Give them a crayon and see what they draw
- Use a piece of paper to assess grip
- Ask the child to copy your drawings of increasing complexity (from a line to a triangle, depending on the child's age). Remember to cover the image when drawing it so that the child cannot see how you have drawn it (Fig. 9.5)
- Watch the child for grasping, passing, mouthing and casting using a brick
- Demonstrate making shapes for the child using a brick (Fig. 9.6). For each shape with the bricks, produce it for the child first and then break the construction and ask them to make it again

- It is useful to separate into under 1 year old (Table 9.2) and over 1 year old (Table 9.3)

Additional tests include:
- Scissors
  - Using both hands (2 years old)
  - One-handed (3 years old)
- Page turning
  - Skimming pages (15–18 months old)
  - Turning pages singularly (2 years old)
- Threading beads
  - Large beads (3 years old)
  - Small beads (4 years old)

VISION

- Test the ability to fix and follow by holding up an interesting (silent) object and see if the child follows it with their eyes

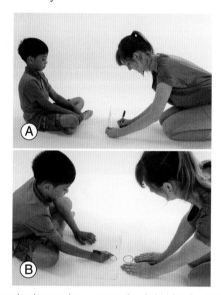

Fig. 9.5 Drawing images in a manner that is hidden from the child (A), and exposing each image individually for the child to copy (B).

- Children can follow to 90° by 6 weeks old, and 180° by 3 months old

SPEECH, LANGUAGE AND HEARING

- Ask what languages are spoken at home, and what is the child's preferred language
- Ask the parents if the child responds to their name, can say mum/dad or if they have any concerns about hearing
- Speak to the child, getting them to speak back. Note the landmarks described in Table 9.4
- Useful props include picture books and small objects, for example, bear, pencil and cup, to see whether the child can understand or say objects, adjectives and prepositions

Table 9.2	Fine motor landmarks in under-1-year-old
AGE	**ACTION**
6 weeks	• Holds hand in fist • Grasps anything put into palm • Tracks objects/faces
6 months	• Palmar grasp • Reaches out for objects • Brings object to midline • Hand-to-hand transfer (taking an object from one hand and putting it in the other) • Mouths objects (puts them in the mouth)
9 months	• Crude pincer grip
10 months	• Fine pincer grip
12 months	• Casts objects away • Bangs objects together • Object permanence (can be tested simply by dropping a toy and seeing if the child looks for the fallen object) • Points at things

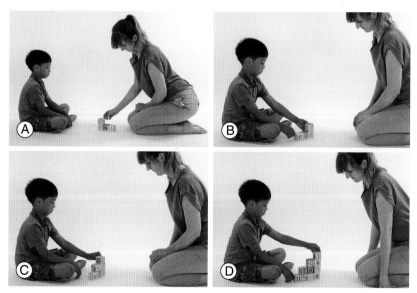

Fig. 9.6 Demonstrating building an L-shaped train (A), child replicating an L-shaped train (B), child replicating six-brick stairs (C), and child replicating 10-brick stairs (D).

Table 9.3 Fine motor landmarks for over-1-year-old

AGE	DRAWING		BUILDING BLOCKS	
15 months	Marks paper (cylindrical grasp)		Tower of two	
18 months	To-and-fro scribble		Tower of three	
2 years	Circular scribble		Tower of six	
2.5 years	Copies line		–	-
3 years	Copies circle (tripod grasp)		Tower of nine	
			Train with chimney (L-shaped)	
3.5 years	Copies cross		Three-brick bridge	
4 years	Copies square		Six-cube stairs	
5 years	Copies triangle (and can draw person, house with chimney/windows/door).		10-cube stairs	

Table 9.4 Language landmarks

AGE	UNDERSTANDING (RECEPTIVE LANGUAGE)	VOCALISING (EXPRESSIVE LANGUAGE)
Newborn	–	• Crying
6 weeks	–	• Startles to noise
3–4 months	• Turns to sound	• Cooing
5–6 months	• Turns to own name	• Babbling
8–9 months	–	• 'Mama' and 'dada' said indiscriminately
10 months	• Understands 'no'	–
12 months	• A few simple nouns; for example, 'mum' and first name	• A few individual words
15 months	• Follows simple commands • Points to body parts	–
18 months	• Lots of simple nouns; for example, leg. Knows 2–3 body parts	• 10–20 words
2 years	• Verbs and two-part commands	• 50 words and two-word phrases
2.5 years	• Prepositions; for example, put the doll under the table	• 3–4 words together
3 years	• Comparatives; for example, 'which circle is the biggest?' • Adjectives; for example, 'which one is red?' • Negatives; for example, 'which is not a fork?'	• What/where questions • Can give full name and sex
4 years	• Follows three-part/complex instructions; for example, 'first give me the pencil, then put the key in the cup'	• Why/when/how questions • Talks in narratives/sequences • 4–5-word sentences
5 years	• Enjoys jokes/riddles	• Talks about past/present/future

- Ask the child to use a sentence to describe what is happening
- Assess if the child can point to body parts
- Ask if the child knows their name, age, gender
- Ask the child to count

SOCIAL

- Assess if the child can smile or wave (Table 9.5)
- Ask the parents about how the baby eats and toilets (Table 9.6)

FINISHING

- Thank the parents
- Wash your hands

 Present Your Findings

Khalid is a 24-month-old boy (19 months corrected) who presented for routine developmental assessment in neonatal clinic with mum. On general examination Khalid looks well and has no obvious signs of dysmorphism or spasticity.

On gross motor assessment, Khalid is able to sit up and pull to stand and demonstrates walking but he is unable to demonstrate stooping to pick up toys or climb stairs.

On fine motor assessment, he has a good pincer grip and can hold a pen but is unable to scribble.

On language assessment, he is able to say 'mama' and 'dada' but is unable to point to body parts or say two-word phrases.

On social assessment, he is smiling and waving, and mum has told me he can finger feed but is unable to use a spoon well.

I feel that the most likely diagnosis is global developmental delay as Khalid is able to demonstrate features of a 12-month-old child but not a 24-month-old child, and this could be related to his prematurity, with the differentials being perinatal infection or a genetic disorder.

To complete my examination, I would like to do a general paediatric and neurological examination, an ophthalmology and audiology assessment, ask about perinatal history and plot his height, weight and head circumference on a growth chart. I would consider blood tests for liver function tests (LFTs), full blood count (FBC), urea and electrolytes (U&Es), thyroid function tests (TFTs) haematinics and genetic conditions and would want MDT input for ongoing management. I would also review the observation chart and ask the parents whether they have any concerns; for example, with toileting, dressing or feeding.

❓ QUESTIONS AND ANSWERS FOR CANDIDATE

What are the causes of developmental delay?

- Developmental delay can be idiopathic and self-resolving, or can be caused in the antenatal, intrapartum or postnatal period

- Examples include: Infection, prematurity and hypoxic ischaemic encephalopathy (Table 9.7)

What additional tests could be considered?

- Always ask for a growth chart, including head circumference, weight and height
- Consider full ophthalmology and audiology testing
- Consider FBCs, U&Es, haematinics, LFTs, metabolic and endocrine investigations, including thyroid function tests (TFTs)
- For suspected syndromic conditions, consider the need for genetics, creatine kinase, chromosomal tests
- Second-line investigations include neuroimaging and electroencephalogram (EEG)

How would you manage a child with developmental delay?

- You would require an MDT assessment (Table 9.8)
- Management planning may involve a paediatrician, a speech and language therapist, occupational therapist, physiotherapist, educational team, surgeons and health visitors

 A Case to Learn From

I had a child in clinic who was 24 months old but could only demonstrate skills at a 12-month level. I asked mum, who was adamant that her son was able to perform more than he was demonstrating. We gave the child a bit of a rest and came back later. He demonstrated all milestones and was discharged. Remember, developmental assessment only captures one timepoint and that it is very reliant on patient compliance.

 Top Tip

Remember that examiners are expecting you to demonstrate a structured approach to assessing development, rather than getting the developmental age spot on. You are trying to show what a child can and can't do, then make a rough estimate of developmental delay. In clinical practice, experienced paediatricians have an hour to do developmental assessments, so don't expect to get it right in a short OSCE!

Top Tip

Developmental assessment is actually easier to practise than most exams. Children often find it fun, and it can be practised on well children, including your own and those of friends. The more you practise, the more comfortable your routine will get, and you will become more used to establishing rapport with children.

Table 9.5 Social and self-care milestones. These can be observed, but this is best assessed by asking parents about toileting, dressing and eating

AGE	SOCIAL
6 weeks	• Social smile, i.e. child smiles back at you or when pleased
8–9 months	• Stranger anxiety (up until 2 years old) • Plays peekaboo • Holds/bites food
12 months	• Waves bye-bye • Claps • Points • Drinks from beaker
18 months	• Imitative play/domestic mimicry; for example, copying parents' actions at home • Symbolic play; for example, brushes doll's hair, may feed/put doll to bed • Removes socks/shoes
2 years	• Temper tantrums • Plays alongside other children (parallel play) • Eats with spoon • Starts toilet training • Loses stranger anxiety
3 years	• Plays with other children • Shares • Eats with fork and spoon
4 years	• Dresses and undresses • Concern/sympathy for others • Understands turn taking • Knife and fork
5 years	• Very definite likes and dislikes • Can amuse themselves for long periods of time • Can care for pets • Chooses best friends

Table 9.6 Average developmental milestones

	GROSS MOTOR	FINE MOTOR / VISION	LANGUAGE/HEARING	SOCIAL / SELF-CARE
6 weeks	• Holds head briefly in ventral suspension • Some head lag • Primitive reflexes • Symmetrical limb movement	• Holds fists closed • Turns to light • Fixes and follow 90°– especially faces	• Cries • Responds to mother's voice • Startles to noise	• Smiles
3–4 months	• No head lag • Raises chest (resting on elbows) when prone • More vigorous limb movements	• Holds object placed in hand • Reaches for objects; for example, mobile phone (later) • Fixes and follows through 180°	• Cooing • Quietens to mother's voice	• Laughs
5–6 months	• Sits supported/ unsupported with a curved back • Lifts chest on extended arms when prone • Rolls front to back, and later back to front	• Brings objects to midline • Transfers between hands • Consciously releases objects • Starts mouthing objects	• Early babbling (with consonants)	• Screams (happy) • No stranger anxiety yet
8–9 months	• Sits unsupported with a straight back • May crawl/ bum shuffle	• Early pincer grip (uses thumb with all fingers) • Looks for fallen objects	• Developed babbling – repetitive consonants • Says 'mama' and 'dada' non-specifically	• Stranger anxiety develops • Plays peekaboo

Table 9.6   **Average developmental milestones—cont'd**

	GROSS MOTOR	FINE MOTOR / VISION	LANGUAGE/HEARING	SOCIAL / SELF-CARE
10 months	• Pulls to stand • Cruising	• Developed pincer grip – picks grains of rice off the floor	• Understands 'no'	• Understands concept of 'bye-bye'
12 months	• Early walking – unsteady/broad-based gait	• Bangs objects together • Casts objects • Object permanence – looks for hidden toys • Points at things	• Few individual words • Imitates sounds and speaks jargon with conversational intonation • Understands name and simple objects	• Finger feeds • Can hold spoon and attempt use • Waves bye-bye/claps • Points to convey desire, shortly followed by pointing for excitement
15 months	• More confident walking	• Builds tower of two or three bricks • Turns thick cardboard pages	• Obeys simple commands • Can identify common objects	• Uses cup and spoon
18 months	• Squats to pick up object • Running	• Builds tower of four blocks • To-and-fro scribble • Points to pictures in books • Turns pages in book a few at a time	• 10–20 words, including common objects • Common two-word phrases; for example, 'all gone' • Points to body parts	• Removes socks/shoes • Imitative play/domestic mimicry; for example, copies parents' actions at home
2 years	• Jumps • Kicks ball • Climbs stairs with two feet per step/holding on	• Circular scribbles • Draws straight line (at 2.5 years old) • Builds tower of six blocks	• Has 50+ words • Links words. together to make two- or three-word sentences • Understands functions of objects; for example, 'which one do you eat with?', whilst pointing to a fork and a pencil, and verbs for example, 'who is running?' • Obeys two-part commands	• Feeds with fork and spoon • Starts toilet training • Temper tantrums • Plays alongside other children (parallel play) • Symbolic play
3 years	• Rides a tricycle • Goes upstairs with one foot per step, and downstairs with two feet per step	• Copies a circle • Builds a tower of nine bricks • Copies a bridge and stairs with six bricks	• Knows several nursery rhymes • Complex four- to five-word sentences • States first and last name • 'What' and 'who' questions • Understands prepositions; for example, under/behind • Understands sizes; for example, big or little, tall or small	• Washes hands • Plays with other children • Understands concept of sharing • Pretend play

Continued

Table 9.6   Average developmental milestones—cont'd

	GROSS MOTOR	FINE MOTOR / VISION	LANGUAGE/HEARING	SOCIAL / SELF-CARE
4 years	• Hops • Walks up and down steps like adult	• Copies a cross • Copies stairs with 10 bricks	• Can tell descriptive account of events • Uses 'why', 'when' and 'how' • Understands negatives; for example, 'which one is not a boy?'. • Understands three-part commands	• Undresses, but cannot dress independently • Understands turn-taking
5 years	• Skips • Catches ball	• Copies a triangle/square	• Tells a complex story using all tenses – future and past	• Dresses, including buttons and zips • Can eat with knife and fork • Chooses and names best friends • Imaginative play, including role playing and made-up stories

Table 9.7   Common diagnoses or problems from developmental delay

GENERALISED	MOTOR DELAY	LANGUAGE DELAY	SOCIAL DELAY
• Genetic • Perinatal infections • Hypoxic brain injury • Prematurity	• Cerebral palsy • Muscular dystrophies	• Deafness • Familial	• Autism • Attention deficit hyperactivity disorder (ADHD)

Table 9.8   Important situations where referral for further specialist paediatric assessment is indicated

AGE	FEATURE
6–8 weeks	• Asymmetrical Moro reflex • Unable to fix and follow • Not smiling • Excessive head lag • No startle to sound
12 weeks	• Persistent squint
8 months	• Persistent primitive reflexes • Not vocalising
1 year	• Hand preference • Not responding to their own name
18 months	• Not walking
2 years	• No or few words spoken by child
3 years	• Not speaking in sentences • Not interacting with other children • Not following simple commands • Unable to use the toilet • Unable to use a spoon

STATION 9.10: COMMUNICATION: TYPE 1 DIABETES MELLITUS

SCENARIO

Zac White is a 10-year-old boy who has recently been diagnosed with type 1 diabetes mellitus and is about to commence insulin therapy. Please explain the diagnosis and insulin treatment to him. Address any concerns that he or his parents might have.

CORE CONCEPT

• This station assesses your ability to explain a new diagnosis of a chronic condition and make a management plan with a patient
• You are most likely to be given a parent to talk to in an OSCE, but be prepared to talk to an older child as well
• Type 1 diabetes requires daily lifelong treatment. Involving the child in the management of their condition is vital to ensure compliance with treatment, particularly in the teenage years

Common Concerns

Why did I get diabetes?	• Type 1 diabetes is an autoimmune condition that occurs because the body attacks the cells that make insulin • Insulin is the hormone that allows the body to utilise glucose • It is not a result of poor diet or lifestyle choices
Will I have to inject myself for life?	• Lifelong insulin is required as the body cannot make its own
Can I keep playing sport?	• Yes. However, insulin levels need to be adjusted around activity, as there is an increased risk of hypoglycaemia

GATHERING INFORMATION AND COMMUNICATIONS

This case has two parts:
1. Establishing the patient's level of understanding and current concerns
2. Explaining the diagnosis

ESTABLISHING THE PATIENT'S LEVEL OF UNDERSTANDING AND CURRENT CONCERNS

• Ask about the experience of diabetes, via friends, family or other means
• Ask what they have already been told and a brief history of what has happened so far
• Identify any specific concerns to address

EXPLANATION OF THE DIAGNOSIS

Explain what type 1 diabetes mellitus is:

• Glucose (sugar) is a fuel required for cells to function
• Insulin is a hormone that allows glucose to be taken up and used by those cells
• People with type 1 diabetes stop producing their own insulin
• Without insulin, the sugar stays in the blood stream and can lead to people feeling unwell
• It can lead to things like weeing a lot, being very thirsty, losing weight and stomach aches
• Without insulin, people with type 1 diabetes get ill very quickly

Insulin treatment and monitoring:
• Insulin replacement is via daily injections
• The most common regime is an injection with each meal and again at bedtime, though there are many options
• To ensure the right amount of insulin is given, blood sugar levels have to be checked regularly with a finger prick blood. testor a continuous glucose monitoring device, which avoids the need for regular blood tests
• A specialist team of healthcare professionals, including doctors, nurses and dieticians, look after patients with type 1 diabetes, making it clear how to identify:
  • Low blood sugar ('hypos')
  • High blood sugar (hyperglycaemia)
  • Being unwell ('sick day rules')
  • Problems associated with diabetes in the long term

! Treatment of diabetes

INSULIN REGIME	ADVANTAGES	DISADVANTAGES
Twice dailyMixture of short- and long-acting insulin give twice daily	• Fewer injections	• Less physiological • Stricter mealtimes • Regular snacking needed to prevent hypoglycaemia
Basal bolusShort-acting insulin given with meal and long-acting insulin given once daily	• More physiological • Greater flexibility for mealtimes • Insulin doses can be adjusted depending on meal size/carbohydrate content	• More frequent injections • Children will need to inject during school hours
Insulin pumpContinuous infusion of short-acting insulin via a small pump worn by the patient	• More precise blood sugar control • Physiological	• Patient must be motivated (need to carbohydrate count, more frequent blood sugar checks) • Expensive • At higher risk of diabetic ketoacidosis (DKA) if there is a problem with the insulin pump (no background insulin)

Present Your Findings

Zac is a 10-year-old boy who has presented with his parents for a discussion about a new diagnosis of type 1 diabetes. Zac is generally well in himself otherwise.

This is the family's first encounter with type 1 diabetes. I have explained the cause of the disease, treatment with insulin and different options for how it might be given, and long-term prognosis. I clarified the distinction between type 1 and type 2 diabetes as the parents had concerns relating to type 2 diabetes in other family members.

I have given them an information leaflet and will follow them up with the rest of the MDT.

? QUESTIONS AND ANSWERS FOR CANDIDATE

What are the short-term complications of type 1 diabetes?
Hypoglycaemia:
• This occurs when blood sugar levels drop below 4 ('four is the floor')
• Some may be completely asymptomatic, hence the stress on the importance of regular monitoring
• Symptoms can be divided into
  • Neuroglycopenic; for example, headache, irritability, confusion, seizures, coma

- Adrenergic; for example, tremor, tachycardia, sweating, hunger, pallor, visual changes
- Treatment
  - Dextrose tablets or 50 mL sugary drink; for example, Lucozade
  - Followed by a longer-acting carbohydrate; for example, bread, banana
  - If the patient is drowsy, give Glucogel
  - If the patient is unconscious, give glucagon

Diabetic ketoacidosis:

- Occurs when insulin is low and therefore glucose cannot enter cells
- As a result, the body metabolises fatty acids which produce ketone bodies
- Symptoms include:
  - Kussmaul breathing
  - Pear drop breath
  - Vomiting
  - Dehydration
  - Confusion
  - Coma
- Treatment is with insulin and careful rehydration with IV fluids

What are the microvascular complications of diabetes?

- Retinopathy, which leads to blindness
- Nephropathy, which leads to renal failure
- Neuropathy, with leads to impotence and sensory/motor disturbances, particularly in the feet

What are the macrovascular complications of diabetes?

Macrovascular complications of diabetes include cardiovascular events (myocardial infarction and stroke) and peripheral arterial disease.

 A Case to Learn From

A 4-year-old boy was referred to the rapid-access (to be seen within 1 week of referral) paediatric clinic with suspected diabetes because of polydipsia and polyuria. However, he deteriorated before this, having to attend the ED 48 h later with vomiting and drowsiness in severe DKA.

Children with suspected diabetes need to be assessed by a paediatric doctor the same day. Almost all diabetes in children is type 1 and therefore, without insulin, they can rapidly progress to DKA.

 Top Tip

Use your time on placement to take advantage of speaking to children with chronic diseases like diabetes. These children and their parents become 'expert patients' and will often love explaining how they manage their condition, as well as showing you all the insulin pens and blood sugar-monitoring equipment.

 Top Tip

Remember that children with diabetes will need continuous re-education as they grow up and their level of understanding improves. New issues such as driving may then become important.

STATION 9.11: COMMUNICATION: MMR VACCINE

SCENARIO

You are a junior doctor working in primary care and have been asked to see Mr and Mrs Fletcher, who have come to see you with their daughter, Sandy. They are keen to get the MMR vaccine for her but have some concerns about what they have read on social media. Please discuss the risks and benefit of the vaccination and gain consent.

CORE CONCEPT

- There has been a significant decrease in the uptake of the MMR vaccine, which has been associated with an increased rate of measles
- Some children have legitimate contraindications to the MMR vaccine, but the vaccine is generally very safe and effective
- It is important to be aware of common concerns, for example, autism risk, so that they can be adequately addressed so parents can make an informed choice

 Common Concerns

Why should I give a vaccination to my child when they are perfectly well?	• Measles, mumps and rubella were very uncommon due to a high vaccination rate • Unfortunately, due to a decline in the number of children being vaccinated, these conditions have re-emerged • While sometimes self-limiting, these conditions can have severe complications, including: Meningitis, deafness and encephalitis (swelling of the brain) • Vaccination reduces the risk of these conditions for both your child and the children around them
What about single vaccinations as an alternative?	• There is no evidence of benefit • By spacing out the vaccinations further, there is more delay in children receiving this vital vaccination • There is a higher chance of missed doses due to need for repeat visits
Can my child get measles, mumps or rubella from the vaccination?	• The vaccine involves giving a small dose of a modified version of the three viruses • This is an effective way to induce immunity and prevent more severe infections • In a few cases, it can result in some of the features of the infection but this is mild and short-lived

GATHERING INFORMATION AND COMMUNICATIONS

This case has two parts:

1. Establishing the parents' level of understanding and current concerns
2. Explaining the MMR vaccine

ESTABLISHING THE PARENTS' LEVEL OF UNDERSTANDING AND CURRENT CONCERNS

- Establish what the parents already know about the MMR vaccination
- Ask about their previous experience of vaccinations, whether they are fully immunised and any complications
- Ask about the general health of their child, particularly looking for contraindications; for example, infection, immunocompromise, malignancy, neomycin/gelatin allergy, recent live vaccine
- Identify any specific concerns to address

EXPLANATION OF THE MMR VACCINE

- Injections will be given in the upper thigh at 12 months, in an identical manner to any previous vaccines
- The injection may cause local discomfort, which is short-lived and eased with oral paracetamol if needed
- It is given at the same time as other vaccinations (meningitis B/C, pneumococcal and *Haemophilus influenzae* type B (HiB) so no extra appointments are required
- A booster is then given at 3 years and 4 months to maintain immunity

Benefits

- A single dose gives 90% protection against MMR
- Herd immunity protects the community and potentially eradicates the disease if there is a greater than 95% vaccination rate

Risks

- Common: Fever, rash, malaise (feeling unwell), localised pain
- Uncommon or rare: Febrile seizures, parotid swelling

All usually manifest within 1 week of vaccination and are less common with the second dose.

Studies that suggested a causal link between MMR and autism have been discredited. Many subsequent research papers show no link between MMR and autism.

❗ Conditions protected against by MMR vaccine

	RUBELLA	MEASLES	MUMPS
Presentation	• Headaches • General body aches • Anorexia • Low-grade fever • Nausea • There may also be a discrete rose-pink maculopapular rash ranging from 1 to 4 mm • Eye pain on lateral and upward movement • Conjunctivitis • Tender lymphadenopathy (particularly posterior auricular and suboccipital lymph nodes)	• Fever • Coryza • Cough • Lymphadenopathy • Generalised maculopapular, erythematous rash • Koplik spots are pathognomonic	• Fever • Malaise • Rash • Swelling of parotid glands • Cervical lymph nodes
Complications	• The major risk of rubella occurs when it is acquired during pregnancy, resulting in congenital rubella • In childhood, it can cause arthritis and, rarely, thrombocytopenia and encephalitis	• Pneumonia • Otitis media • Haemorrhagic problems • Blindness • Subacute sclerosing panencephalitis • Potentially lethal in immunosuppressed patients	• Unilateral deafness • Meningitis • If infected after puberty, epididymo-orchitis and infertility may occur

CONTRAINDICATIONS

Some people cannot have the MMR vaccine. Contraindications include:

- Immunocompromised
- Malignancy
- Another live vaccination given in the previous 3 weeks
- Acute febrile illness (defer until recovered)
- Allergies to gelatine or neomycin. Egg allergy is not an official contraindication to MMR vaccine (due to miniscule amounts of egg protein)

TACKLING VACCINATION MYTHS

- There is no evidence of any link between the MMR vaccine and autism, leukaemia or inflammatory bowel disease

- Studies have shown that children can cope with having multiple vaccinations, and this will not 'overload' their immune system. Children constantly come into contact with bacteria and viruses on a daily basis, and this makes their immune system stronger.

 Present Your Findings

Mr and Mrs Fletcher have presented to clinic to discuss the MMR vaccine for their daughter Sandy, who is their first child. Sandy is fit and well, with no contraindications.

I have explained how the vaccine works. I discussed their initial concerns around autism with them and they are reassured. The parents are now happy to go ahead with the vaccination.

❓ QUESTIONS AND ANSWERS FOR CANDIDATE

What is herd immunity?
- \> 95% of the population have been vaccinated for MMR to confer herd immunity
- After reaching this threshold, the whole population becomes more protected, even those who are unvaccinated, because of the lower chance of spread
- A decreased uptake rate of MMR in the UK has been associated with a loss of herd immunity and increased cases of measles as a result

What are Koplik spots?
- These spots are pathognomonic of measles. They are small red spots with a white centre on the buccal mucosa

What is a notifiable disease?
- It is a disease that doctors are obligated to report nationally (to Public Health England)
- These include diseases such as MMR, but also other highly infectious conditions such as salmonella, TB and scarlet fever

 A Case to Learn From

I saw a girl, Millie, in clinic for follow-up of her asthma. Mum revealed that Millie was unvaccinated. However, after a short discussion mum elected to get the vaccinations done, as actually, she hadn't given much thought to vaccination as her family/friends didn't believe in it. Every consultation is an opportunity, if parents are willing, to re-discuss vaccination, and parents' views may change over time.

 Top Tip

Having trained in a time when vaccine uptake was high, many parents and even doctors haven't seen children with conditions such as measles. Set aside some time to look up cases of such conditions so you can fully inform parents and be prepared for the result of changing vaccination uptake rates.

STATION 9.12: COMMUNICATION: GENETIC COUNSELLING – CYSTIC FIBROSIS

SCENARIO

Mr and Mrs Taylor have been called to the rapid-access paediatric clinic as their 2-week-old baby, Matthew, has suspected CF from the newborn-screening blood (Guthrie) test.

CORE CONCEPT

- This station assesses your ability to explain a condition and make a plan with the patient to confirm diagnosis
- CF is a lifelong, multisystem disease that will require active management from an MDT
- How the disease is introduced is key to the family's perception of living with it. It is important to make the family aware not only of what CF is, but also the implications for different organ systems over a lifetime and the risk of recurrence in other children

 Common Concerns

Does the screening test mean my child definitely has CF?	• The screening test increases our suspicion of the disease, meaning it is highly likely, but not certain • Further tests will be done to confirm the diagnosis
Will my child die?	• Children with CF will generally have a shorter life than they would have done otherwise • New advances in CF treatment mean children are living well into adulthood • Childhood death is now uncommon. Average survival is to 41 years old
What gene causes CF?	• Thousands of gene mutations are known • p.Phe508del (previously known as ΔF508) accounts for 85% of cases in UK White Northern European patients

GATHERING INFORMATION AND COMMUNICATIONS

This case has two parts:
1. Establishing the parents' level of understanding and current concerns
2. Explanation of CF

ESTABLISHING THE PARENTS' LEVEL OF UNDERSTANDING AND CURRENT CONCERNS

- Ask about additional tests during pregnancy and any concerns (there may be delayed passage of meconium or poor weight gain)

- Ask about experience of CF via friends, family or other means
- Ask what they have already been told and a brief history of what has happened so far
- Identify any specific concerns to address

EXPLANATION OF CYSTIC FIBROSIS
What?
- A genetic condition causing some of the secretions produced by the body to thicken, due to a defect in a protein affecting the cell wall in the cells of the body
- Main organs affected:
  - Lungs (affecting breathing)
  - Pancreas (affecting digestion)
- There is an increased risk of chest infections and poor nutrition due to not being able to absorb food properly. It can also lead to blockages in the bowel, infertility and growths in the nose, polyps, that can cause obstruction

Testing
- A baby who has screened positive for CF on their Guthrie test is very likely to have CF; i.e. there is less than 1 in 100 chance that they do not have it
- Full confirmation is with a sweat test and genetic testing

Management
- For less than 5% of cases, there is a treatment for the defect in the cell wall, but all other cases rely on just helping the body adapt to having CF
- Life with CF is different for every child
- There will be specialist MDT input, with more tests looking at the lungs, liver, pancreas and bones
- Treatments such as physiotherapy, antibiotics and enzyme replacement prolong and improve the quality of life
- The child will need daily medication to support the absorption of nutrients
- Chest infections are more common and require more intensive treatment

Final Steps
Finish by checking understanding and offering written information and further time to meet and discuss.

ADDITIONAL INFORMATION

TESTING FOR CYSTIC FIBROSIS
1. Carrier testing: Simple mouthwash test can tell if you or your partner carries the gene
2. Antenatal testing: If both parents are carriers, the test can be carried out early in the pregnancy to tell whether the baby has CF:
   - Chorionic villous sampling: At 11–14 weeks' gestation (1% risk of miscarriage)
   - Amniocentesis: At 16–20 weeks' gestation (0.5% risk of miscarriage)
3. Newborn testing: The newborn screening programme (heel prick) includes testing for immune-reactive trypsinogen levels, which are markers of pancreatic function. If these levels are elevated, further tests are carried out, including a sweat test and genetics

Present Your Findings

Mr and Mrs Taylor have presented to clinic after Matthew's newborn screening test was suggestive of CF. Matthew is generally well, although he is still under the health visitor, as he has not regained his birth weight.

This is the family's first encounter with CF. I have explained the next stage of confirming the diagnosis with a sweat test and have explained some of the problems children with CF have, including chest infections and problems with absorption of nutrients. They have specific concerns around the amount of follow-up and the prognosis, which we have had an initial discussion about.

I have given them an information leaflet and, after confirmation of the diagnosis, I would refer the patient to the CF team.

QUESTIONS AND ANSWERS FOR CANDIDATE

What is the pathology of CF?
- The genetic defect causes a defective CF transmembrane conductance regulator
- This receptor is responsible for the transfer of chloride out of the cell and inhibition of the epithelial sodium channel
- Chloride does not leave the cell and sodium enters the cell uninhibited, creating a highly concentrated cell with a high osmolality
- Water follows salt and so water enters the cell from the outside and causes a thick mucus that builds up in various sites in the body

What happens during a sweat test?
- Sweat is stimulated by the application of a chemical (pilocarpine) to the skin and then a little electrical stimulation is applied
- The test is not painful; at most, tingling or warmth is felt
- Sweat is collected from a patch of gauze on either the arm or leg of the child, over approximately 30 min
- The aim is to measure the chloride content of sweat collected. If the sweat contains > 60 mmol chloride, then it is highly likely to be a positive diagnosis of CF

What is the inheritance pattern of CF?
- CF is generally inherited in an autosomal-recessive pattern
- For a baby to have CF, the baby needs to inherit two affected genes, one from each parent. Therefore both parents must be carriers
- If both parents are carriers there is a one in four chance of the baby having CF

A Case to Learn From

Premature twins were admitted to the special care baby unit for feeding support. On day 2 of life, twin B developed abdominal distension and bilious vomiting. He had not passed meconium and required surgery for obstruction due to meconium ileus (thick meconium causing small-bowel obstruction). Both twins tested positive for CF. CF can present with either no symptoms (twin A) or purely meconium ileus with no respiratory symptoms (twin B).

Top Tip

Be careful of using statistics when explaining the complications of a condition or treatment. Phrases like 1 in 100 may be better understood than risk or percentages. If pushed, maybe use phrases like 'common problems include...' or 'most children with this condition....'

Top Tip

When explaining CF to parents, remember that they are going to have a lifetime of conversations about it and you do not have to say everything in one go. The most important thing to do is ensure their initial concerns are addressed and that the very basic information (in this station) is conveyed in the first meeting.

STATION 9.13: COMMUNICATION: COUNSELLING FOR DOWN'S SYNDROME

SCENARIO

Mr and Mrs Bradley are pregnant with their fourth child. They are concerned about the possibility of Down's syndrome due to Mrs Bradley's age (35 years old). Please advise the couple as to what Down's syndrome is and what screening options are available.

CORE CONCEPT

- This station assesses your ability to explain a condition to patients in the context of screening and elevated risk
- Down's syndrome is a chromosomal disorder associated with characteristic physical features, a degree of learning disability and a higher chance of certain medical problems
- How the disease is introduced will be key to the parents' perception of the likelihood of it occurring, the support they might get and the impact on any child over their lifetime

Common Concerns

What will life be like for a child with Down's syndrome?	• Children with Down's syndrome have a degree of learning disability • There is a risk of some medical problems; for example, heart defects, hearing and visual problems and bowel problems • Many children with Down's syndrome are able to attend mainstream school, have relationships and work
Do the screening tests have any risks for my baby?	• The combined screening test involves an ultrasound scan and blood tests • There is no risk to the baby in performing these tests • People who are identified as having a higher chance of having a baby with Down's syndrome will be offered further testing that can be associated with a small chance of miscarriage
What does a higher-chance screening test mean?	• This value is calculated from a combination of maternal age, ultrasound and blood test results • A high-chance screening result is a greater than 1 in 150 chance of having Down's syndrome • This does not mean you will have a child with Down's syndrome, and 149 out of 150 with a positive screening test will be completely unaffected

GATHERING INFORMATION AND COMMUNICATIONS

This case has two parts:
1. Establishing the parents' level of understanding and current concerns
2. Explanation of Down's syndrome

ESTABLISHING THE PARENTS' LEVEL OF UNDERSTANDING AND CURRENT CONCERNS

- Ask about additional tests during pregnancy and any concerns
- Ask about the experience of Down's syndrome via friends, family or other means
- Ask what they have already been told and a brief history of what has happened so far in the pregnancy
- Identify any specific concerns to address

EXPLANATION OF DOWN'S SYNDROME

What?

- Genes that determine our characteristics are divided across units called chromosomes. Normally we have two copies of each chromosome, but in

Down's syndrome there is a third copy of chromosome 21
- Down's syndrome is the most common chromosomal abnormality in humans, but it is not inherited
- The probability of it occurring increases with maternal age (1 in 1500 when the mother is aged 20, 1 in 100 when the mother is aged 40)

Aetiology
- Down's syndrome is the result of an extra copy of genetic material, chromosome 21
- There is nothing you can do to change the chance of having a baby with Down's syndrome
- It is generally not inherited, but a result of a spontaneous change in the egg or sperm

Features of Down's Syndrome
- Physical features that are distinctive from other people, for example, the position of the ears, the position of the eyes and the creases in their hands (must not compare to 'normal')
- Slower to develop and grow
- Will have some degree of learning difficulty
- May develop or be born with heart and bowel problems
- Many adults with Down's syndrome are active, mobile and able to lead semi-independent lives
- The average life expectancy of someone with Down's syndrome is 50–60 years

Screening Tests
- These look to see if there is an increased risk of Down's syndrome, but they do not confirm the diagnosis
- 'Combined testing' (blood test and ultrasound) is offered to all pregnant women between 10 and 14 weeks
- Blood test for certain markers; for example, pregnancy-associated plasma protein A, human chorionic gonadotrophin, inhibin-A, oestriol, alpha-fetoprotein
- Ultrasound to measure fluid at the baby's neck (nuchal translucency) in utero
- The result is expressed as a higher-chance (>1 in 150) or lower-chance (<1 in 150) result and can also be a marker of other conditions (Edward's (trisomy 18) and Patau's (trisomy 13) syndrome)
- The severity of learning and behaviour difficulties, and in many cases the congenital defects; for example, cardiac abnormalities, cannot be predicted before birth

Diagnostic Tests
- These confirm the diagnosis before birth
- They are offered to women with higher-chance (>1 in 150) results

- Chorionic villous sampling is a sample of chorionic villi taken from the baby's placenta, between 11 and 13 weeks
- Amniocentesis is a sample taken from the fluid around the baby, between 16 and 20 weeks
- A diagnosis allows planning of the pregnancy/birth
- There are non-invasive prenatal testing (NIPT) maternal blood tests available for diagnosis. However, they are not available in all centres across the UK

🔍 Present Your Findings

Mr and Mrs Bradley presented to their primary care physician to discuss testing for Down's syndrome in pregnancy. They have had three previous children through uncomplicated pregnancies, and these children are fit and well.

They have no friends or family members with Down's syndrome but are familiar with the condition through the media, which also is how they knew that there was a correlation with increased maternal age.

I have explained the syndrome and the testing, and they are reassured about the screening tests. They expressed that they would not want diagnostic testing if recommended from the screening tests due to the risk of miscarriage and want to have a child regardless of any diagnosis.

I have directed them to the Down's Syndrome Association website for further reading but have reassured them that we have no suggestion of the baby having Down's syndrome at present.

❓ QUESTIONS AND ANSWERS FOR CANDIDATE

How is Down's syndrome diagnosed after birth?
- A clinical examination of the baby looks for characteristic features, including hypotonia (Fig. 9.7)
- A blood test is then sent for karyotyping (chromosome analysis)
- The result is normally available within 48 h

People with Down's syndrome have a higher risk of which conditions?
- Cardiac: Atrioventricular septal defect, tetralogy of Fallot
- Gastrointestinal: Duodenal atresia, coeliac disease
- Endocrine: Hypothyroidism, type 1 diabetes mellitus
- Immune: Leukaemia, autoimmune disorders
- Behavioural: Autistic spectrum disorder and ADHD
- Other: Hearing and visual impairment

What is the management of Down's syndrome?
- A multidisciplinary approach tailored to the needs of the child/family
- Teams include: Dieticians, community paediatricians, speech and language therapists
- Other specialists may get involved depending on medical complications; for example, cardiologists
- Children with Down's syndrome may require specialist support within school and assistance with behavioural difficulties

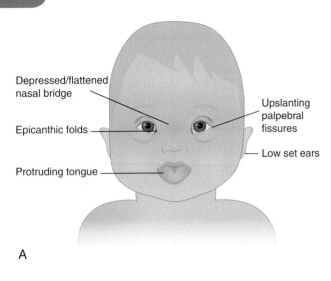

Depressed/flattened nasal bridge

Epicanthic folds

Protruding tongue

Upslanting palpebral fissures

Low set ears

A

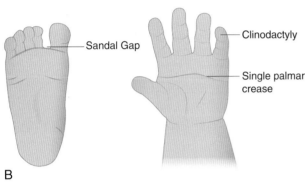

Sandal Gap

Clinodactyly

Single palmar crease

B

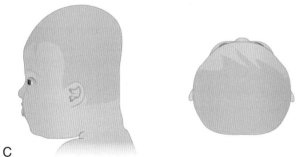

C

Fig. 9.7 (A–C) Clinical features of Down's syndrome.

A Case to Learn From

A term baby of a 21-year-old mother was admitted to the special care baby unit with poor feeding and hypotonia. She had many characteristic features of Down's syndrome. When this was explained, the mother was very confused how this could be the case as she was young and understood all her screening test to be 'negative'. Remember that although older mothers have a higher chance of having a baby with Down's syndrome, it can still occur in those with negative screening tests, and those with no risk factors.

Top Tip

Given the life expectancy of people with Down's syndrome, along with the fact that many can attend mainstream school and go on to work, we need to think carefully about the language we use with families. Avoid phrases such as 'risk of Down's' and try not to treat this as a 'breaking bad news' scenario. For many families, this is just not the case and can be highly offensive.

 ### Top Tip

Down's syndrome is a condition that we are very familiar with. This means we have the ability to anticipate problems and proactively manage them early. In many cases, it is diagnosed before birth, so it means from day 1, doctors will be doing extra tests and extra assessments to reduce the risk of anything being missed

STATION 9.14: PRACTICAL SKILLS: INHALER TECHNIQUE

SCENARIO

Mrs Andrews has come to your clinic with her son James, an 8-year-old boy. He has recently been diagnosed with asthma and has commenced using regular inhalers. Please teach him how to use an inhaler with a spacer, explaining the steps to the examiner.

GENERAL ADVICE

- Check the patient's identification and gain valid consent
- Check if they have used the inhalers before and if they have any concerns
- Ask them to demonstrate

BACKGROUND INFORMATION

- The blue inhaler is a reliever, for when the patient is symptomatic. If it is being used more than three times per week, or if greater than six puffs are required per day, asthma control should be reviewed
- The brown inhaler (steroid) is a preventer and it is used daily
- The inhalers have a use-by date printed on the side. If this expires, you will need to get another inhaler from your doctor. They usually last around 200 puffs
- Inhaled steroids produce fewer side effects than systemic steroids. Side effects are more likely to occur with higher doses and when the inhaler technique is poor. They include:
  - *Candida* infection of the mouth
  - Hoarseness
- In comparison with non-asthmatic children, children with asthma may have a later onset of puberty and growth retardation. Rarer side effects include:
  - Adrenal suppression: Non-specific symptoms; for example, anorexia, abdominal pain, weight loss, headache, nausea and vomiting
  - Skin: Easy bruising and thinning of skin
  - Weakened immunity: Instruct the patient that they should inform their doctor if they are ill
- Depending on the age, different systems are used for delivery of inhaled asthma medications:

- Older child or adult: metered-dose inhaler (MDI) with or without a spacer
- 2–10-year-olds: MDI with a spacer
- Over 2-year-olds: MDI with a spacer and mask.
- Spacers ensure better delivery of medication into the lungs and can be used around 200 times, and are highly preferred.. There are different types of spacer. For example:
  - Babyhaler: In under 2-year-olds (with a face mask). The patient does not have to be upright and remember to listen for five clicks
  - Volumatic: In over 2-year-olds (with or without a face mask). The patient should be seated upright
  - Aerochamber: Three different-sized masks for infants, children and adults (it is now the most commonly prescribed spacer in the UK)

Note: When starting patients on inhalers, it is important to highlight that they will feel immediate symptomatic relief after using the reliever inhaler (blue) but the effect of the brown inhaler is longer term. Emphasising this early on should improve adherence.

USING AN MDI WITHOUT A SPACER

Ask the patient to:
1. Check the expiration date of the inhaler.
2. Shake the inhaler.
3. Lift his chin and sit up straight.
4. Remove the inhaler cap.
5. Empty his lungs as fully as possible.
6. Put the inhaler in the mouth.
7. Ensure a good seal with his lips firmly around the mouthpiece (not biting).
8. Take a slow deep breath whilst pressing the canister simultaneously.
9. Once the lungs are full, take out the inhaler and hold the breath for 10 s, then breathe out.
10. Wait 30 s and repeat the above steps if further doses are required.
11. Replace the lid on the inhaler.
12. Rinse the mouth with water (or mouthwash) if the patient is taking a steroid inhaler, in order to prevent side effects.

USING AN MDI WITH A SPACER

Ask the patient to:
1. Check the expiration date of the inhaler.
2. Assemble the spacer as per manufacturer's instructions.
3. Shake the inhaler.
4. Remove the inhaler cap and slot the inhaler into the spacer.
5. Press the canister once to release a dose into the spacer.
6. Get the patient to take five normal tidal breaths. In the case of babies, leave it over their face for 10 s, ensuring that it clicks or the valve in the spacer moves.
7. Remove the device from the mouth.
8. Wait 30 s and repeat the above steps if further doses are required.
9. Replace the lid on the inhaler.
10. Rinse the mouth with water (or mouthwash) if the patient is taking a steroid inhaler in order to prevent side effects.

Wash the spacer once a week by taking it apart, washing it in warm, soapy water and leaving it to drip dry. It should be replaced every 3–6 months.

INHALED CORTICOSTEROIDS VS. BRONCHODILATOR

Reliever inhalers are usually blue and the medication itself is a bronchodilator. The medication works by relaxing the muscles in your airways, to open them up in order to relieve symptoms of wheeziness and chest tightness. Examples include salbutamol and terbutaline.

Inhaled corticosteroids are usually brown and the medication itself is a corticosteroid. They reduce inflammation in the airways, which reduces the likelihood of airways becoming narrow. Examples include beclomethasone and budesonide.

ESCALATION

If a patient is using their reliever inhaler at least two to three times per week, then the patient's medications should be reassessed as they may need to commence/increase the patient's steroid inhaler.

🔍 **Present Your Findings**

James Andrews, an 8-year-old boy, has recently been diagnosed with asthma and has commenced using regular inhalers. Today I have shown him how to use an MDI with a volumatic spacer. He has demonstrated good technique. I would follow this up by giving him a written asthma management plan, making it clear when his inhalers are to be used.

❓ QUESTIONS AND ANSWERS FOR CANDIDATE

Name three types of inhaler devices.
- MDIs; for example, Ventolin. Require good technique for coordination of pressing down on the inhaler and taking a breath at same time. Best used with spacers
- Breath-actuated inhalers; for example, Easi-Breathe can overcome hand–breath coordination problems. Spray is released as breath is initiated
- Dry-powder inhalers; for example, Accuhaler. Disc-shaped and require rapid, forceful intake of breath

Young children may not be able to generate the force of inhalation required for breath-actuated and dry-powder inhalers.

When should a spacer be used?

- Ideally for all children, but especially for those with an MDI who find it difficult to coordinate the hand–breath technique required
- *Routinely* for children less than 5 years of age with a:
  - Mask for children < 3 years
  - Mouthpiece for children >3 years

When is a nebuliser used?

- For delivery of short-acting beta agonist in acute asthma when respiratory effort is significantly reduced and there is an oxygen requirement
- Rarely used in chronic asthma management

 A Case to Learn From

We had a 12-year-old child who came to clinic with worsening asthma control. She was taking her salbutamol inhaler every day and was on both a daily steroid and a daily long-acting beta agonist. She was being referred to escalate her treatment, but when we reviewed her technique, it was apparent she had never used a spacer and didn't hold her breath after each inhaler dose. Once her technique was improved, her symptoms significantly improved and this stopped unnecessary escalation of treatment.

 Top Tip

Good technique should be reinforced on several occasions, not just once, especially if the asthma is worsening.

 Top Tip

An asthma review is not just a medication review. Look at other factors that may be contributing to worsening control, such as parental smoking, pollution and household mould. Improving these may improve control without having to escalate medication.

STATION 9.15: PRACTICAL SKILLS: PEAK FLOW

SCENARIO

You are the junior doctor in clinic. Mrs Patel has come to your clinic with her 7-year-old son, Sandeep. He has recently been diagnosed with asthma and has been advised to keep a peak flow diary. Please teach him how to perform a peak flow, explaining the steps to the examiner.

GENERAL ADVICE

- Check the patient's identification and gain valid consent
- Check if they have used the peak flow before and if they have any concerns
- Ask them to demonstrate

BACKGROUND INFORMATION

- Peak flow tracks lung function over time
- It helps assess the severity of asthma to inform management, both long-term and acutely
- Good technique and regular readings are critical to allow accurate interpretation
- The patient may be asked to keep a peak flow diary. This is important to establish diurnal variation in peak flow associated with asthma, and in establishing any environmental triggers associated with asthma. If so, show the child the peak flow diary and give them an example of how to record measurements

EQUIPMENT CHECKLIST

- Peak flow
- Cleansing wipe
- Mouthpiece
- Peak flow diary

PERFORMING PEAK FLOW

PREPARATION

1. Wash hands.
2. Clean the mouthpiece if it is being reused.
3. Assemble equipment, i.e. attach the mouthpiece to the peak flow meter, with a tight seal.
4. Set the dial to zero on the peak flow meter.

USING THE PEAK FLOW METER

Ask the patient to:
1. Stand up, holding the assembled peak flow meter in one hand.
2. Inhale as deeply as possible.
3. Put his lips around the mouthpiece.
4. Lift his chin and straighten his back.
5. Breathe out as hard and fast as possible.
6. Check dial, record, move back to zero.
7. Repeat three times, with a short recovery time in between.
8. Record the highest reading out of the three.

🔍 **Present Your Findings**

Sandeep Patel, a 7-year-old boy, has recently been diagnosed with asthma and has been advised to keep a peak flow diary. Today I have explained to him the importance of keeping an accurate peak flow diary and have shown him how to use the peak flow meter. He has demonstrated good understanding of both the equipment and the diary. I have also advised for him to use this alongside his asthma action plan and asked him and his mother to go to the family care physician if peak flow drops or he becomes symptomatic. To follow up I have asked to review his diary in 2 weeks' time.

QUESTIONS AND ANSWERS FOR CANDIDATE

Name three factors that are taken into account when calculating an individual's best/predicted peak flow score.
• Gender
• Age
• Height

Note that there is also diurnal variation in peak flow scores so, for the same individual, their peak flow readings may be lower in the morning.

When and how often should a patient measure peak flow?

Ideally a patient should check peak flow twice a day, once in the morning and once in the evening. This should also be done before taking any asthma medications, as this could alter the peak flow readings.

What are the four warning symptoms outlined on a peak flow diary?
• Used reliever inhaler
• Had asthma symptoms such as shortness of breath, tight chest, coughing or wheezing
• Waking at night with asthma symptoms
• Feeling like you can't keep up with your normal day-to-day activities

 A Case to Learn From

We had a 12-year-old child who seemed be very distressed with his asthma. He had come into hospital with worsening difficulty in breathing and mum wanted him admitted to hospital. He was objectively quite well. The peak flow meter proved helpful, as when the child focused on it, we demonstrated that his peak flow was similar to his baseline and we were able to reassure the family. Peak flow meters are a useful objective measure of the severity of an asthma exacerbation, as well as a marker of more long-term control.

 Top Tip

Make sure the patient can perform a peak flow independently. After talking them through it, watch them do it completely on their own and make sure they do it standing up!

Top Tip

Peak flow is reliant on patient compliance and therefore is not usually very helpful in those under 7. If a child isn't using it correctly, then a low reading is of no value.

Content Outline

Ophthalmology is a unique specialty which is often covered only briefly during undergraduate studies. Becoming proficient in the examination of the eye, especially fundoscopy, will equip the aspiring medic with the fundamental skills required to diagnose and classify systemic conditions affecting the eyes.

Overall, ophthalmology is a diverse and pioneering specialty based primarily in the outpatient setting. Day-to-day activity ranges from surgery, such as cataract extraction and retinal detachment repairs, to diagnosis, investigation and treatment in outpatient clinic. Often the ophthalmologist will work closely with other specialties; for example, general medicine, neurology and endocrinology.

Study Action Plan

- Outpatient clinic is abundant with opportunities to learn from patients with a variety of conditions. Medical retina clinic is especially useful for practising fundoscopy skills, particularly as all patients will have had their eyes dilated, so it will be much easier to examine the fundus with a direct ophthalmoscope and view retinal pathology
- Practise your fundoscopy skills on friends and family before heading off to clinic. This will give you an idea of the normal appearance of the fundus, so you are able to focus on the pathology seen in clinic
- Find out where theatre is and see if you can attend a list. This is a good opportunity to see and revise the anatomy of the eye

STATION 10.1: HISTORY: RED EYE

SCENARIO

You are a junior doctor in the ED and have been asked to see Aaron James, a 62-year-old man who has presented with a red right eye associated with pain and photophobia. He has a past medical history of ankylosing spondylitis. Please take a history from Mr James, present your findings and formulate an appropriate management plan.

Cardinal Symptoms

Red eye
Pain
Photophobia
Reduced vision

HISTORY OF PRESENTING COMPLAINT

RED EYE

- Site: Unilateral or bilateral. If bilateral, and one eye had started before the other, this would generally suggest conjunctivitis. Check which part of the eye is affected; for example, global, around the ciliary border, or segmental. Conjunctivitis usually causes a diffuse redness whereas segmental injection may suggest episcleritis or scleritis
- Onset: Sudden or gradual
- Timing: Associated with certain locations or exposures; for example, any recent contacts with new facial products or change in contact lens provider, etc
- Severity and progression: Small amount of redness, or intense redness. Establish if it is getting progressively redder or if the redness is beginning to settle; the latter would be less concerning

EYE PAIN

- Site: Bilateral or unilateral. Specify the location; for example, inside, around or behind the eye. Clarify the origin of the pain as it could be from the eye itself, or sinuses, orbit or intracranial space
- Onset: Sudden or gradual

- Character: Describe the pain. A gritty uncomfortable feeling could suggest dry-eye disease whereas a sharp deep, pushing sensation could be a migraine or scleritis
- Timing: Constant or intermittent. Dry-eye disease is usually intermittent
- Exacerbating or relieving factors: Analgesia and its effect. Whether anything in particular brings it on; for example, the eyes moving in a particular direction
- Severity: Rate the pain on a scale of 0–10

PHOTOPHOBIA

When presented with a patient complaining of photophobia (light sensitivity), it is important to enquire about the signs of meningism detailed below:
- Neck stiffness
- Fever
- Nausea and vomiting
- Headache

ASSOCIATED SYMPTOMS

Other symptoms to enquire about include:
- Watery eye but no sticky discharge tends to suggest viral conjunctivitis whereas purulent discharge suggests bacterial conjunctivitis
- Reduced vision: Would need to rule out AACG
- Headache
- Tender sinuses
- Inflammation of the periorbital skin; for example, signs of blepharitis or orbital cellulitis
- Trauma to the eyes

PAST MEDICAL AND SURGICAL HISTORY

- General: Ask about other diagnosed medical conditions, treatments and hospital admissions
- Recent eye surgery: An infection inside the eye (endophthalmitis) can rarely occur a few days after eye surgery or after injections into the eye. The vision will also be affected. This is an emergency!
- Contact lens wearer: Use of contact lenses is a risk factor for corneal ulcers
- Explore systemic diseases associated with anterior uveitis:
  - Joint diseases: Ankylosing spondylitis, juvenile chronic arthritis
  - Bowel diseases: Ulcerative colitis, Crohn's disease, Whipple's disease

- Sarcoidosis
- Herpes zoster ophthalmicus
- Behçet's syndrome

MEDICATION HISTORY

Enquire about prescribed medications (including any recent changes) and over-the-counter medications. Allergies should be included with the specific reaction noted. In this scenario it is also important to note:
- Use of any new eye drops

SOCIAL HISTORY

Social history includes enquiring about occupation, residence, lifestyle (diet, exercise, smoking, alcohol, substance abuse) and recent travel. Additionally in this scenario, consider:
- Smoking: Document pack years (calculated as the number of packs per day multiplied by the number of years smoked)
- Alcohol and illicit drug use
- Recent outdoor activities: Injury or trauma
- Impact of symptoms on daily life
- Sexual history: This is particularly important because chlamydial conjunctivitis can also be a cause of red eyes

FAMILY HISTORY

Enquire about any significant family history, including:
- Anterior uveitis can be related to the gene human leukocyte antigen (HLA) B27
- Allergies may run in families

SYSTEMS REVIEW

On systems review, particularly pertinent questions to the above case may relate to the anterior uveitis-associated systemic diseases:
- Joint: Including back pain
- Skin: Erythema nodosum
- Gastrointestinal: Diarrhoea, constipation, bloating
- Respiratory: Shortness of breath, reduced exercise tolerance

Risk Factors for Anterior Uveitis
- Previous anterior uveitis
- HLA B27-positive
- Any of the anterior uveitis-associated systemic diseases

Differential Diagnosis

DISEASE	CLINICAL PRESENTATION	INVESTIGATIONS	TREATMENT
Anterior uveitis	• Red eye • Eye pain • Photophobia • Reduced vision (usually mild)	• Measure IOP • Investigate for relevant systemic diseases based on clinical presentation	• Steroid eye drops • Dilating eye drops

AACG	• Unilateral, red eye
	• Painful eye
	• Significantly reduced vision (often counting fingers at presentation)
	• May be associated with nausea and vomiting
	• Periocular pain and headache
		• Pressure check: IOP >40 mmHg (reference range is 11–21 mmHg)	• Urgent referral to ophthalmologist for IOP-lowering treatment:
			  • Pressure-lowering topical drops; for example, apraclonidine 1% immediately
			  • Pressure-lowering acetazolamide oral or IV

Conjunctivitis	• Mild discomfort • Generalised inflammation of the conjunctivaBacterial • Purulent discharge that may stick the eyelids togetherViral: • Watery discharge • Photophobia • Vision can be affected mildlyChlamydial: • Persistent red eyeAllergic: • Watery discharge • Seasonal	• Conjunctival swabs (bacterial, viral, chlamydia)	Bacterial: • Chloramphenicol ointmentViral: • Supportive • Cool compresses • Artificial tearsChlamydial: • Chloramphenicol ointment • Referral to genitourinary medicine clinic for systemic treatment (oral azithromycin or doxycycline) Allergic: • Antihistamine eye drops
Orbital cellulitis	• Proptosed eye • Reduced eye movements • Swollen and erythematous eyelids	• Temperature • Blood culture • Computed tomography (CT) orbit and head, looking for abscesses that may need draining	• IV antibiotics • Ears, nose and throat specialist assessment to assess for sinus drainage
Subconjunctival haemorrhage	• Bright red haemorrhage on the sclera • May be spontaneous or due to trauma	• Blood pressure (high blood pressure can cause it) • Investigate blood clotting disorders, including anticoagulant therapy	• Self-resolving
Corneal abrasions	• Can be extremely painful and cause epiphora • Absence of a white opacity (infiltrate) on the cornea, which is usually associated with a corneal ulcer	• Fluorescein eye drops may help detect foreign bodies/abrasions	• Remove any foreign bodies • Chloramphenicol ointment • An ulcer will require referral to ophthalmology
Episcleritis or scleritis	• Sectoral or generalised inflammation of the episclera • Mild discomfort and normal vision • Scleritis is a more painful condition compared to episcleritis. It may be associated with connective tissue diseases	• None	• Self-resolving but the speed of recovery can be increased with oral non-steroidal anti-inflammatory drugs (NSAIDs) • Scleritis requires referral to ophthalmology

RED EYE

During the examination, look to see where the eye is red. This can give you clues as to the diagnosis. See Figs 10.1–10.3 for photographs of red eyes.

 Present Your Findings

Mr James is a 62-year-old man who presented with a 1-day history of right-eye pain, generalised redness and photophobia. He describes the pain as a sharp aching pain. It is gradual in onset, constant, radiates to the forehead and is made worse by bright light and accommodation. The vision is unaffected. This is on a background of having ankylosing spondylitis and taking ibuprofen.

I feel the most likely diagnosis is anterior uveitis, with the differentials being episcleritis and corneal abrasion.

I would like to perform a visual acuity test, IOP measurement and slit-lamp examination on Mr James, and then refer to ophthalmology.

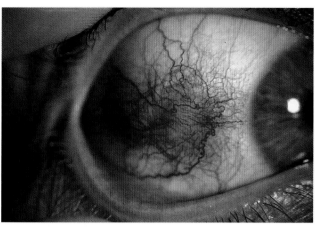

Fig. 10.1 Sectoral: This could be episcleritis or scleritis.

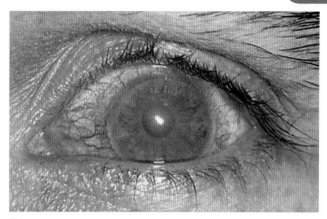

Fig. 10.2 Ciliary (around the limbus): This is the classic pattern of redness around the corneal border seen in iritis.

 QUESTIONS AND ANSWERS FOR CANDIDATE

What is ankylosing spondylitis?
- It is a seronegative (rheumatoid arthritis-negative) spondyloarthropathy
- There is inflammation of the joints, tendons and ligaments of the spine

Name three symptoms of ankylosing spondylitis.
- Pain and stiffness, worse in the morning and after periods of inactivity
- Most commonly affected areas are lower back, hips and shoulder joints
- Neck pain
- Fatigue

Name three potential complications of ankylosing spondylitis.
- Fusion of parts of the vertebrae, resulting in stiffness and inflexibility
- Uveitis
- Compression fractures
- Increased risk of cardiovascular disease

 A Case to Learn From

A patient who had recurrent anterior uveitis went to his primary care physician with a red eye and photophobia. His primary care physician did not have a slit lamp but gave him steroid eyedrops, thinking this was another anterior uveitis episode. Unfortunately, the patient had a corneal ulcer and the steroid drops made it a lot worse, meaning that the patient was left with permanent scarring. Steroid eye drops must only be prescribed after a full examination with an experienced practitioner.

Top Tip

Anterior uveitis and AACG can appear quite similar in their presentation to a non-ophthalmologist. To prevent permanent visual loss, always speak to the on-call ophthalmologist to discuss suspicious cases.

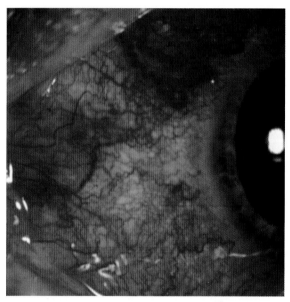

Fig. 10.3 Diffuse: This suggests a larger area of the eye is involved; for example, scleritis.

STATION 10.2: HISTORY: SUDDEN LOSS OF VISION

SCENARIO

You are a junior doctor in the ED and have been asked to see Monica Goodfellow, a 62-year-old woman, who has presented today with sudden visual loss in her left eye. She has also been having terrible headaches and generally feels unwell. Please take a history from Mrs Goodfellow, present your findings and formulate an appropriate management plan.

 Cardinal Symptoms

Visual disturbance
Headache
Jaw claudication
Scalp tenderness
Malaise

HISTORY OF PRESENTING COMPLAINT

VISUAL LOSS

- Character: Clarify the type of visual loss, whether it is blurring of the vision or complete visual loss. Specify if there is any double vision, which could suggest ophthalmic nerve palsy
- Site: Unilateral or bilateral. If both eyes are affected, consider whether this is a neurological event; for example, stroke, migraine, space-occupying lesion. Optic neuritis is typically unilateral
- Onset: Establish how long the symptoms have been present and if there were any significant events at the time of onset. If head trauma had occurred, this could indicate an intracranial bleed. Lifting a heavy weight may suggest a Valsalva-induced vitreous haemorrhage
- Timing: Is the visual loss transient or permanent?
- Progression: Gradual progressive blurred vision may be associated with infection or optic neuritis

HEADACHE

- Site: Location of the pain; for example, frontal, temporal or occipital. Unilateral headache is typical of migraine or sinusitis
- Onset: Of recent onset
- Character: A 'tight band around the head' is often used to describe tension headache, whereas with a 'thunderclap headache' or the 'worst pain ever to the back of the head', it is important to rule out a subarachnoid haemorrhage
- Radiation: Whether it radiates to the neck, jaw or ears
- Associated features: See below
- Timing: Headaches associated with GCA may be worse at night
- Exacerbating and relieving factors: Enquire about use of analgesia and its effectiveness
- Severity: Give a pain score on a scale of 0–10

ASSOCIATED SYMPTOMS

Other symptoms to enquire about include:
- Weight loss, fever, night sweats: Suggest vasculitis such as GCA
- Malaise and fatigue: These symptoms suggest systemic disease, which can range from lymphoma to hypothyroidism, a risk factor for CRVO
- Depression: Hypothyroidism, vasculitis, renal failure can result in a change of mood
- Symptoms associated with GCA:
  - Scalp tenderness:
Pain on brushing hair: The scalp can be extremely tender, making brushing the hair a real challenge
Pain on putting head on the pillow: Another question to explore how tender the scalp is
  - Jaw claudication:
Pain in the jaw when talking or chewing: It is important to clarify that the pain starts when using the jaw and gradually gets worse as the patient continues to use the jaw. You don't want to mistake toothache for jaw claudication!

- Polymyalgia rheumatica:
Muscle and joint pain, especially around the neck, shoulders, upper arms and hips
Stiffness located proximally

PAST MEDICAL AND SURGICAL HISTORY

- General: Enquire about other diagnosed medical conditions, treatments and hospital admissions
- Specific:
  - Whether there is already a diagnosis of polymyalgia rheumatica. This is a different manifestation of the same disease process as GCA
  - Whether there is a history of aortic aneurysm or dissection or large-artery stenosis. These are known complications of GCA

MEDICATION HISTORY

Enquire about prescribed medications (including any recent changes) and over-the-counter medications. Allergies should be included with the specific reaction noted. In this scenario it is also important to note:
- Steroids: These can mask symptoms of GCA

SOCIAL HISTORY

Social history includes enquiring about occupation, residence, lifestyle (diet, exercise, smoking, alcohol, substance abuse) and recent travel. Additionally in this scenario, consider:
- Smoking, alcohol and illicit drug use: This can cause visual loss due to nutritional deficiencies
- Occupation: Stress can trigger migraines or cause tension headaches
- Travel in the last 3 months: Abroad or within the country
- Impact of symptoms on daily life: Stress can trigger migraines with visual disturbances or cause tension headaches

FAMILY HISTORY

Enquire about any significant family history, including:
- Polymyalgica rheumatica
- GCA
- Migraines

SYSTEMS REVIEW

On systems review, particularly pertinent questions to the above case may include questions regarding other possible (although rare) systemic manifestations of GCA. These include:
- Neurological: Difficulty with speech and limb weakness or numbness
- Cardiac: Chest pain, breathlessness, palpitations
- Back/abdominal pain (thoracic aorta/aortic route involvement)

Differential Diagnosis

DISEASE	CLINICAL PRESENTATION	INVESTIGATIONS	MANAGEMENT
GCA	• Scalp tenderness • Jaw claudication • Temporal artery tenderness • Non-pulsatile temporal artery • Unilateral headache	• Full blood count (FBCs) • ESR • CRP • Temporal artery biopsy	• Steroids (oral or IV)

AACG	• Unilateral, red eye
	• Painful eye
	• Significantly reduced vision (often counting fingers at presentation)
	• May be associated with nausea and vomiting
	• Periocular pain and headache
		• Pressure check: IOP >40 (reference range is 11–21 mmHg)	• Urgent referral to ophthalmologist for IOP-lowering treatment:
			  • Pressure-lowering topical drops; for example, apraclonidine 1%
			  • Pressure-lowering acetazolamide oral or IV

Vitreous haemorrhage	• Floaters or decreased visual acuity in the affected eye • Usually unilateral • Poor fundal view (due to the blood)	• Ultrasound scan of the eye (B scan) if cannot see the retina, to check for retinal tear or detachment	• Mild: Can wait to clear • Severe: Surgical intervention; for example, vitrectomy
Retinal detachment	• Unilateral flashes and floaters • Has visual acuity or field loss	• Fundoscopy: Areas of raised retina and a retinal tear may be visible within this	• Urgent referral to ophthalmologist for surgical intervention to reattach the retina
CRAO	• Persistent painless loss of vision • White retina with a cherry-red spot	• Blood pressure • Serum glucose level • Serum cholesterol level	• If within 24 h: Decrease the IOP with acetazolamide
CRVO	• Painless loss of vision or blurring of vision, often on waking • Engorged veins • Retinal haemorrhages • Cotton-wool spots	• Blood pressure • Glucose • Cholesterol • Optical coherence tomography scan, to check for macular oedema	• Only treat complications; for example, macular oedema

COMPLICATIONS OF GCA

- Blindness: Due to reduced blood flow to the eyes, and often the loss of vision is permanent
- Aortic aneurysm: This may occur years after the diagnosis of GCA
- Stroke

 Present Your Findings

Mrs Goodfellow is a 62-year-old woman who presented with sudden vision loss in her left eye. She describes recent severe headaches, scalp tenderness and malaise but no jaw claudication. This is on a background of being normally fit and well. I feel the most likely diagnosis is GCA.

I would like to perform a visual acuity test, IOP measurement and dilated fundal examination on Mrs Goodfellow at the slit lamp, as well as examining her temporal arteries. I would like to take blood to check her FBCs, ESR and CRP, and organise an urgent temporal artery biopsy.

❓ QUESTIONS AND ANSWERS FOR CANDIDATE

What would you expect to find on examining the temporal arteries in a patient with GCA?
I would expect to find an abnormality; for example, an absent pulse, tenderness, feeling beaded or enlarged.

Name three possible complications from high-dose oral steroid treatment.
- Osteoporosis
- High blood pressure
- High blood sugar
- Risk of stomach ulcers
- Weight gain
- Thin skin, easy bruising
- Muscle weakness
- Mood and behavioural changes
- Risk of developing cataracts
- Increased risk of infections

Name three possible mechanisms of CRAO.
- Fibrinoplatelet clot
- Cholesterol embolus
- Calcific embolus

 A Case to Learn From

I met an elderly diabetic woman who went to her family care physician with diplopia (double vision). The family care physician thought it was an ocular cranial nerve palsy due to her diabetes so did a routine referral to the orthoptists (allied health professional specialising in eye movement disorders). She was given an appointment 2 weeks after the referral but came to the ED a week later with irreversible loss of her vision in both eyes due to GCA. Always consider GCA in patients presenting with diplopia, even if it is painless.

 Top Tip

Have a very low threshold for checking GCA bloods (FBCs, ESR, CRP). Some people only present with one symptom. Missing a presentation can have disastrous consequences for that patient, as the visual loss is quick and irreversible.

STATION 10.3: HISTORY: THE WATERY EYE

SCENARIO

You are a junior doctor in the ED and have been asked to see Phyllis Jones, a 43-year-old woman who has presented with constantly watery eyes, which have felt increasingly sore. She is very anxious and thinks that her vision is slightly blurred. Please take a history from Mrs Jones, present your findings and formulate an appropriate management plan.

 Cardinal Symptoms

Watering (epiphoria)

Soreness

Double vision (diplopia)

Proptosis

Blurred/lost vision

Red eyes

HISTORY OF PRESENTING COMPLAINT

WATERING EYES
- Onset: Sudden or gradual. Sudden suggests an acute change has occurred; for example, foreign body in the eye or exposure to chemical irritants
- Timing: Intermittent or constant. Variation with time of day. Dry-eye disease is often worse in the morning
- One eye or both eyes affected: Bilateral suggests dry-eye disease or environmental factors; for example, exposure to chemical fumes. Unilateral symptoms may be associated with lid laxity abnormalities and there may be signs and symptoms of a facial nerve palsy
- Trauma: Usually it will be sore and unilateral
- Occupational: Has there been exposure to alkaline fumes, which led to watering? Ask if eye protection is worn regularly
- What makes it worse? If reading or looking down, then it is likely to be an eyelid positional problem

SORENESS
- Nature of pain:
  - Gritty, foreign-body sensation: Typical of dry-eye disease
  - Sharp, constant, pain: May be a defect in the corneal surface
  - Deep, pushing sensation: Can range from migraine to scleritis
- Exacerbating and relieving factors: Driving or use of computers often exacerbates dry-eye disease. Ask whether lubricating drops or cool compresses have helped
- Timing: Constant or intermittent. Dry-eye disease is usually intermittent
- Quantify the pain: Dry-eye disease is usually (scoring 3–5/10), whilst corneal ulcers and epithelial defects are likely to give 8–10/10 pain scores

BLURRED VISION
- Describe the vision loss: 'Misty' (consider cataracts) or 'a black curtain' (consider retinal detachment or amaurosis fugax)
- Timing: Constant or intermittent. Quantify this using a frequency within a range of minutes, hours or days

ASSOCIATED SYMPTOMS

Other symptoms to enquire about include:
- Double vision
- Red eye
- Change in appearance to the eye(s)
- Facial nerve palsy on the affected side

PAST MEDICAL AND SURGICAL HISTORY
- General: Ask about other diagnosed medical conditions, treatments and hospital admissions
- Specific:
  - Autonomic disturbance; for example, Parkinson's disease, hyperthyroidism, eczema and/or rosacea
  - A history of recurrent eye infections; for example, herpes simplex virus keratitis and conjunctivitis. Both can lead to scarring, obstruction or eversion of the punctum, which drains tears

- Facial nerve palsy is associated with a reduced blink reflex. A unilateral watery eye would more commonly be seen in this context

MEDICATION HISTORY

Enquire about prescribed medications (including any recent changes) and over-the-counter medications. Allergies should be included with the specific reaction noted. In this scenario it is also important to note:
- Reflex watering: For example, lubrication drops with preservatives, eyelid skin creams which may have entered the eye inadvertently
- Increase parasympathetic drive: For example, pilocarpine

SOCIAL HISTORY

Social history includes enquiring about occupation, residence, lifestyle (diet, exercise, smoking, alcohol, substance abuse) and recent travel. Additionally, in this scenario, consider:
- Smoking: Relates to poor prognosis of thyroid eye disease and worsening severity
- Alcohol and illicit drug use: Recreationally and method of use; for example, IV injections
- Occupation: Metal grinding, cement use, close exposure to solvents
- Travel in the last 3 months: Abroad or within the country
- Impact of symptoms on daily life: Social and work life

FAMILY HISTORY

Enquire about any significant family history, including:
- Thyroid eye disease is autoimmune, and therefore, a family history of other autoimmune conditions, for example, diabetes mellitus type 1 or vitiligo, may increase suspicion

SYSTEMS REVIEW

On systems review, particularly pertinent questions to the above case may include:

- Respiratory: Chronic cough ± haemoptysis may indicate systemic disease; for example, sarcoidosis with lacrimal gland infiltration
- Joints: Autoimmune disease; for example, rheumatoid arthritis and Sjögren's syndrome are often associated with dry-eye disease
- Skin: A salmon-pink, scaly rash may indicate psoriasis and in Graves' disease, pretibial myxoedema is pathognomonic
- Endocrine: palpitations, diarrhoea, restlessness

Risk Factors for Thyroid Eye Disease

- Known diagnosis of hyperthyroidism
- Family history of hyperthyroidism
- Other concurrent autoimmune disease; for example, diabetes mellitus type 1, vitiligo

Present Your Findings

Mrs Jones is a 43-year-old woman who presented with bilateral continuously watery eyes (Fig. 10.4), which were associated with a 'gritty feeling' and intermittent blurred vision. She also reported a change to the appearance of her eyes, such that they appeared more protuberant. She is normally fit and well; however, recently she has become increasingly anxious, experiencing palpitations, recent unintentional weight loss and increased frequency of bowel movements.

The most likely diagnosis is thyroid eye disease associated with exposure keratopathy from untreated hyperthyroidism.

To complete the consultation, I would like to do a full examination, including a neck examination. I would also complete TFTs and organise a referral to ophthalmology to complete a full ophthalmic assessment, owing to the risk of optic neuropathy associated with thyroid eye disease.

QUESTIONS AND ANSWERS FOR CANDIDATE

Which parasympathetic pro-secretory drugs are you aware of?
- Donepezil
- Neostigmine
- Domperidone
- Metoclopramide

Differential Diagnosis

DISEASE	CLINICAL PRESENTATION	EXAMINATION FINDINGS AND INVESTIGATION	TREATMENT
Dysfunctional tear syndrome (imbalance of the three constituents of tears, leading to 'dry-eye disease' and increased lacrimation)	• Gritty, sore eyes with intermittent watering • Worse when reading or using computers	• Assessment of eyelid margins and lashes – may find debris and blocked glands	• If debris on eyelashes: Eyelid hygiene with Blephasol solution and cotton-tipped bud, once daily • If blockages to meibomian glands: Warm compress

Continued

Differential Diagnosis—cont'd

DISEASE	CLINICAL PRESENTATION	EXAMINATION FINDINGS AND INVESTIGATION	TREATMENT
Thyroid eye disease-related exposure keratopathy	• Bilateral red, sore eyes with increased watering • May present with altered appearance of eyes 'pushed out' • Intermittent double vision if posterior soft tissue is involved; for example, extraocular muscles	• Thyroid function tests (TFTs) • Thyroid autoantibodies • Orbital imaging: MRI for soft-tissue involvement	• Multidisciplinary team (MDT) input with endocrinologists for control of thyroid function • Ocular lubricants to relieve exposure of the corneal surface • Smoking cessation, as smoking worsens severity of thyroid eye disease and prognosis • Surgical: Orbital decompression if the optic nerve is compressed
Lacrimal pump failure associated with lid laxity	• Unilateral or bilateral watery eyes of gradual onset • Minimal soreness to the eyes	• Absence of fluorescein staining on slit-lamp biomicroscopy • Able to distract the lower eyelid from its usual position by more than 1.5 cm	• Supportive therapy • Surgical correction of any eyelid positional problems

Increased tear production	Lacrimal pump failure	Decreased tear drainage

• Increased parasympathetic drive from pro-secretory drugs leads to increase in basal secretion
• Reflex lacrimation e.g. ocular irritants, dysfunctional tear syndrome, systemic disease leading to exposure keratopathy in TED or inflammatory ocular surface disease e.g. rosacea
	• Lid laxity: age-related loss of tone of the eye lid and weakness of orbicularis oculi
	• Previous facial nerve palsy leading to weakness of orbicularis oculi and lacrimal pump
		• Lacrimal apparatus obstruction at :
		  • Punctum
		  • Canaliculus
		  • Nasolacrimal duct-can be associated with trauma, tumours, post-irradiation, vasculitis e.g. GPA or nasal pathology

Fig. 10.4 Aetiology of 'the watery eye'.

What are the systemic complications of untreated hyperthyroidism?
- Nervousness
- Anxiety
- Cardiac arrhythmia
- Palpitations
- Weight loss
- Change in bowel habit

How do you differentiate between a lower motor neurone facial nerve palsy and an upper motor neurone lesion causing facial weakness?
- Sparing of the forehead muscle: The frontalis indicates this is likely an upper motor neurone lesion
- A lower motor neurone lesion will involve the forehead

 A Case to Learn From

A 36-year-old woman presented to eye casualty with right worse than left gritty, sore eyes with blurred vision and intermittent watering of the eyes. Her past medical history includes Sjögren's syndrome. Examination revealed no evidence of swelling of the tissues around her eyes; however, she did have bilateral red eyes with conjunctival swelling and 'dots' on the cornea (punctate epithelial erosions). She was treated as keratoconjunctivitis sicca (aqueous-deficient dry-eye disease); however, after 3 weeks her eye continued to become increasingly red and sore. She was now developing diplopia. The diagnosis was thyroid eye disease. Never forget the risk factors for other concurrent autoimmune disease and systems review.

Top Tip

It is important to consider the systemic causes of ocular problems which, if missed, can result in a delayed diagnosis.

STATION 10.4: HISTORY: FLASHING LIGHTS AND FLOATERS

SCENARIO

You are a junior doctor in the ED and have been asked to see Sheila Jameson, a 67-year-old woman who has presented with flashes and floaters, with a small black curtain in her right-eye vision. Please take a history from Mrs Jameson, present your findings and formulate an appropriate management plan.

Cardinal Symptoms

Flashes
Floaters
Black curtain

HISTORY OF PRESENTING COMPLAINT

FLASHING LIGHTS (PHOTOPSIA)

- Site: Right, left or both eyes. Both eyes would generally suggest less sinister pathology; for example, migraine
- Onset: Sudden or gradual. If they came on intensely that should make you more suspicious for a sinister pathology; for example, retinal tear or detachment. If it was a gradual onset, it suggests a more benign pathology; for example, posterior vitreous detachment
- Character: Circles or zigzag lines suggest migraine, as do colourful lights. An arc of white light is associated with vitreous traction on the retina
- Exacerbating and relieving factors: If flashing lights are brought on with head or eye movement, this suggests vitreous traction on the retina
- Timing: Ask the patient if they notice a specific time of day when their symptoms are worse
- Severity: If the patient states that the flashes were present for a few days but have now resolved, this indicates that there is no more vitreous traction taking place on the retina

FLOATERS

These are opacities floating in the field of vision and are common, so a good history will enable you to decipher if these are sinister or not.
- Site: Right, left or both eyes
- Onset: Chronic or acute. Some people have had floaters for years; determine if there has been a sudden change in these floaters or if they are new

- Character: Spots, thread-like strands or squiggly lines
- Timing: Constant or intermittent. Constant new floaters suggest a more sinister pathology

BLACK CURTAIN

- Always ask if a patient can see a black curtain in their vision when presented with a 'flashes and floaters' history. This is the classic sign of a retinal detachment
- Site: The black curtain would be in the eye in which the patient is experiencing flashes and floaters
- Progression: Classically patients will describe the black curtain as slowly progressing over their field of vision in one eye
- Pain: Painless visual field loss suggests retinal detachment. Headache could suggest migraine

ASSOCIATED SYMPTOMS

Other symptoms to enquire about include:
- Reduced vision
- Red eye
- Eye pain

PAST MEDICAL AND SURGICAL HISTORY

- General: Ask about other diagnosed medical conditions, treatments and hospital admissions:
  - Any recent head injury or neck trauma
  - Recent illnesses; for example, sinusitis
- Ophthalmic history: Identify high-risk patients for retinal detachment:
  - Myopic: If they are short-sighted, they have a higher risk of getting a retinal tear or detachment
  - Previous retinal tear or detachment: If they have had them before, they are more likely to get them again
  - Amblyopia: Would account for poor vision in one eye
  - Previous trauma
  - Any previously diagnosed eye conditions
  - Recent ocular surgery increases risk of retinal detachment

MEDICATION HISTORY

Enquire about prescribed medications (including any recent changes) and over-the-counter medications. Allergies should be included with the specific reaction noted.

SOCIAL HISTORY

Social history includes enquiring about occupation, residence, lifestyle (diet, exercise, smoking, alcohol, substance abuse) and recent travel. Additionally in this scenario, consider:

- Smoking: Document pack years, calculated as the number of packs per day multiplied by the number of years smoked
- Alcohol and illicit drug use: Document alcohol units per week
- Recent travels abroad: Abroad or within the country
- Occupation: Enquire about any stresses at work

FAMILY HISTORY

Enquire about any significant family history, including:
- Any history of headaches, particularly migraines
- Family history of retinal detachment

SYSTEMS REVIEW

On systems review, particularly pertinent questions to the above case include neurological symptoms:
- Recent head trauma

- Symptoms of stroke:
  - Loss of sensation
  - Limb weakness
  - Speech impairment
  - Urinary incontinence
  - Personality change
- Symptoms of meningitis:
  - Neck pain or stiffness
  - Vomiting
  - Photophobia
  - Headache

Risk Factors for Retinal Detachment

- Myopic (short-sighted)
- Previous retinal detachment
- Trauma
- Recent eye surgery
- Family history

Differential Diagnosis

DISEASE	CLINICAL PRESENTATION	EXAMINATION FINDINGS AND INVESTIGATION	TREATMENT
Posterior vitreous detachment	• Unilateral flashes and floaters • No visual acuity or field loss	• Fundoscopy: Circular opacity in the vitreous, known as a Weiss ring, where the vitreous used to be attached to the optic nerve	• None
Retinal detachment	• Unilateral flashes and floaters • Reduced visual acuity or field loss	• Fundoscopy: Areas of raised retina and a retinal tear may be visible within this	• Urgent referral to ophthalmologists for surgical intervention to reattach the retina
Migraine	• Zigzag or circular patterns of flashing lights and floaters • Unilateral or bilateral • If associated with a unilateral headache, this is a normal migraine. If there is no headache it may be an ocular migraine	• Fundoscopy: Normal • No limb weakness, paraesthesia or slurred speech	• Acute treatment: • Combination of oral triptan and NSAIDs or paracetamol
Proliferative diabetic retinopathy	• Past medication history of poorly controlled diabetes • Lines or dots or floaters (bleeding inside the eye), causing reduced visual acuity • Flashing lights due to abnormal blood vessels pulling on the retina, which can rarely cause a retinal detachment	• Fundoscopy: Abnormal. Features of hard exudates, venous abnormalities, cotton-wool spots (small infarcts), new vessel formation, retinal haemorrhages	• Urgent referral to ophthalmologist

TYPES OF RETINAL DETACHMENT

- Rhegmatogenous: Most common. This can happen if there is a retinal tear, allowing vitreous to get behind the retina
- Tractional: This can happen if there is scar tissue on the retina, pulling the retina away from the back of the eye; commonly seen in proliferative diabetic retinopathy
- Exudative: This is when enough fluid builds up behind the retina to cause it to detach from the back of the eye, without the presence of any tears or breaks in the retina. It often results from an inflammatory cause or condition

Present Your Findings

Mrs Jameson is a myopic 67-year-old woman who presented with a 3-day history of flashes and floaters and a small black curtain in her right-eye vision. The floaters are lots of tiny dots and the flashes come in an arc. The black curtain is in her inferior right vision but is progressing in size. She is experiencing no pain. She is on no medication and has no other relevant medical history.

The most likely diagnosis is a retinal detachment in her right eye.

The differential diagnoses include posterior vitreous detachment and migraine. I would like to perform a slit-lamp examination on her and refer her to ophthalmology.

QUESTIONS AND ANSWERS FOR CANDIDATE

Why is a myope (short-sighted person) more susceptible to a retinal detachment than a hypermetrope (long-sighted person)?

- The more myopic a patient is, the bigger their eye is and the more susceptible they are to retinal detachments. As the eye becomes bigger, the layers of the eye stretch, making them weaker and more vulnerable to getting damaged. So, as the retina is stretched it becomes prone to separating from the other layers
- A hypermetrope has a small eye in comparison to a myope, so the layers are not stretched in the same way that myopic eyes are. Therefore, they are less susceptible to retinal detachments

What is the main prognostic indicator for good vision after treatment in a retinal detachment?

- If the macula is still attached when the retinal detachment is being treated, this is a good prognostic indicator. If the macula has detached, this is a poor prognostic indicator

What other conditions may cause an increase in floaters apart from degeneration of the vitreous (jelly)?

- Inflammation within the vitreous (vitritis), which may be caused by systemic diseases; for example, sarcoidosis
- Vitreous haemorrhage; for example, from proliferative diabetic retinopathy
- Asteroid hyalosis, which is described as 'a starry sky' in the back of the eye. This is largely asymptomatic, although in some cases it may lead to increased floaters

 A Case to Learn From

A young hypermetropic woman went to the ED on a Friday afternoon with flashes and floaters in her left eye and perfect vision. The on-call ophthalmologist booked the patient into clinic for Monday, thinking it couldn't be a retinal detachment as she was hypermetropic. On Monday the vision in her left eye was very poor, as she had had a retinal detachment and her macula had come off. She had surgery that day but the vision in her left eye remained poor the rest of her life. Myopes may be at a higher risk of retinal detachments than hypermetropes but hypermetropes can still get them!

Top Tip

Any patient who presents persistently with flashes and floaters needs to be seen by an ophthalmologist to rule out retinal detachment.

STATION 10.5: HISTORY: PERIOCULAR PAIN WITH HEADACHE

SCENARIO

You are a junior doctor in the ED and have been asked to see John Wright, a 77-year-old man who has presented with pain around his right eye, extending over his head. He also has a facial rash, which came up 2–3 days after the pain. Please take a history from Mr Wright, present your findings and formulate an appropriate management plan.

 Cardinal Symptoms

Periocular pain
Headache
Blurred vision
Red eye
Dermatomal rash

HISTORY OF PRESENTING COMPLAINT

HEADACHE

- Site: Right, left, frontal temporal, parietal or occipital
- Onset: Sudden or gradual. Sudden may suggest a more sinister pathology; for example, intracranial bleed, meningitis
- Character: Sharp, dull ache, deep-boring pain; the latter may suggest scleritis
- Radiation: Limited to one side or travels to another side. Migraines are normally unilateral, as are headaches associated with GCA
- Associated symptoms: See below
- Timing: Intermittent or constant
- Exacerbating factors: Worse when bearing down; for example, on the toilet or when lying flat. Worse on standing suggests a low-pressure headache; for example, from cerebrospinal fluid leak
- Relieving factors: Simple analgesia, sitting in a quiet and dark room, sleep
- Severity: Score out of 10

PERIOCULAR PAIN

- Description: Periocular pain includes pain in, around or behind the eye. It may originate from the eye, sinuses, orbit or intracranial space
- Onset: Before, after or at the same time as the headache
- Site: Bilateral or unilateral. Only around the eye or the eye itself feels sore
- Tender to touch: Pain on firm touch could indicate sinusitis
- Nature of the pain:
  - 'Sharp pressure behind the eye' is typically described in sinusitis. However, it can also be seen with migraines
  - 'Sharp burning sensation' indicates neuropathic pain from shingles or trigeminal nerve inflammation

RASH

- Distribution: Whether multiple areas are involved, and whether it is within a dermatomal distribution;

for example, trigeminal nerve ophthalmic division in herpes zoster reactivation
- Associated symptoms: Itching, erythema
- Fluid: Discharge or a golden crust can indicate infection with *Staphylococcus aureus* bacteria
- Size: Progression. A rapidly growing rash may suggest facial cellulitis or something more serious, such as necrotising fasciitis

BLURRED VISION

- Description: A brown spiral may suggest new bleeding at the back of the eye
- Timing: Constant or intermittent. Quantify this using a frequency, within a range of minutes, hours or days
- What the patient was doing at the time

ASSOCIATED SYMPTOMS

Other symptoms to enquire about include the following:
- Nausea, vomiting, neck stiffness and photophobia suggest meningism
- Slurred speech and limb weakness suggest a stroke
- Ocular features; for example, reduced vision, red eye and light sensitivity, are typical of iritis
- 'Zigzags in vision' are suggestive of migraines with aura

PAST MEDICAL AND SURGICAL HISTORY

- General: Ask about other diagnosed medical conditions, treatments and hospital admissions. Specifically, enquire about any recent illnesses or colds, diabetes mellitus or other cause for being immunocompromised
- Specific: A history of joint problems and rashes may be associated with iritis

MEDICATION HISTORY

Enquire about prescribed medications (including any recent changes) and over-the-counter medications.

Allergies should be included with the specific reaction noted.

SOCIAL HISTORY

Social history includes enquiring about occupation, residence, lifestyle (diet, exercise, smoking, alcohol, substance abuse) and recent travel. Additionally in this scenario, consider:
- Smoking: Document pack years, calculated as the number of packs per day multiplied by the number of years smoked. Smoking impairs the immune system, which may become vulnerable to reactivation of viruses like varicella zoster
- Alcohol and illicit drug use
- Recent travels: Insect bites, transmissible infectious disease
- Occupation: Exposure to solvents
- Impact of symptoms on daily life: Social and work life

FAMILY HISTORY

Enquire about any significant family history, including:
- Any history of headaches, particularly migraines

SYSTEMS REVIEW

On systems review, particularly pertinent questions to the above case may include:
- Respiratory symptoms: Recent upper respiratory tract infection or flu. If the immune system is compromised, then it is more likely that herpes zoster ophthalmicus (shingles with ocular involvement) can occur
- Constitutional features: Fatigue, stress
- Joints: Autoimmune disease; for example, ankylosing spondylitis is associated with iritis
- Skin: A blistering (vesicular) rash may indicate shingles

Risk Factors for Herpes Zoster Ophthalmicus
- Diabetes mellitus
- Human immunodeficiency virus (HIV) infection
- Recent hospitalisation for debilitating illness
- Stress (severe)

Differential Diagnosis

DISEASE	CLINICAL PRESENTATION	EXAMINATION FINDINGS AND INVESTIGATION	TREATMENT
Migraine ± aura	• 'Zigzag' or circular patterns of flashing lights and floaters • Unilateral or bilateral • If associated with a unilateral headache, this is a normal migraine. If there is no headache, it may be an ocular migraine	• Fundoscopy: Normal • No limb weakness, paraesthesia or slurred speech	• Acute treatment: • Combination of oral triptan and NSAID or paracetamol

Differential Diagnosis—cont'd

DISEASE	CLINICAL PRESENTATION	EXAMINATION FINDINGS AND INVESTIGATION	TREATMENT
AACG	• Unilateral red eye • Painful eye • Significantly reduced vision (often counting fingers at presentation) • May be associated with nausea and vomiting • Periocular pain and headache	• Pressure check: IOP >40 (normal is 11–21 mmHg)	• Urgent referral to ophthalmologist for IOP-lowering treatment • Pressure-lowering topical drops; for example, apraclonidine 1% • Pressure-lowering acetazolamide oral or IV
Herpes zoster ophthalmicus	• Unilateral dermatomal rash • Periocular pain • If eyes are involved, it may be only mildly sore despite severe redness and reduced vision • Eyelid oedema	• Examination may show fluorescein staining	• Start high-dose oral acyclovir 800 mg five times per day for 7–10 days • Neuropathic pain can be treated with gabapentin or amitriptyline

AETIOLOGY OF HERPES ZOSTER OPHTHALMICUS

Herpes zoster ophthalmicus is caused by the varicella zoster virus, which has reactivated from its dormant state and replicates in the nerve cells.

 Present Your Findings

Mr Wright is a 77-year-old man who presented with unilateral periocular pain around his right eye associated with a right-sided headache and a vesicular rash. The headache first appeared 5 days ago followed by a dermatomal rash. The eye itself appears red but is painless and the vision is reduced. He is on medication for diabetes mellitus type 2, hypertension and oesophageal reflux, and has recently recovered from an upper respiratory tract infection.

The most likely diagnosis is herpes zoster ophthalmicus. The differential diagnosis includes ocular surface disease or preseptal cellulitis.

I am going to refer him urgently to ophthalmology, give analgesia and start acyclovir treatment.

❓ QUESTIONS AND ANSWERS FOR CANDIDATE

What does the presence of blistering to the tip of the nose in shingles affecting the ophthalmic division of the trigeminal nerve (herpes zoster ophthalmicus) indicate, and what is the name of this eponymous sign?
• Involvement of the tip of the nose indicates that the nasociliary nerve has been affected by shingles, increasing the probability of corneal involvement. This is known as Hutchinson's sign

Define 'opportunistic infection' in the context of acquired immune deficiency syndrome (AIDS).
• Infections which occur when the CD4+ count is < 100 cells/µL

Name three opportunistic infectious agents affecting the eyes which may be present in people with AIDS.

• Cytomegalovirus: Often necrotising retinitis results
• Herpes zoster ophthalmicus
• Toxoplasmosis
• *Mycobacterium avium*

 A Case to Learn From

A 27-year-old man presented with a painful left eye associated with reduced vision, photophobia and a rash on his forehead that was unresponsive to oral antibiotic therapy. He noticed, after playing golf, that there was a spot on his forehead, which he presumed was an insect bite and was treated in the community for facial cellulitis. Ophthalmic examination revealed a hazy cornea with a fixed pupil and an IOP of 55 mmHg (raised). Treatment for AACG was started. Further examination revealed that the rash had a vesicular appearance. He was diagnosed and treated for herpes zoster ophthalmicus. The rash provided an important diagnostic clue that changed the management plan.

 Top Tip

When examining a skin rash, it is good to ensure that you cover the following: Size, shape, colour, contour and type. Patients presenting with eye symptoms may have systemic features too!

STATION 10.6: HISTORY: BLURRED VISION

SCENARIO

You are a junior doctor in the ED and have been asked to see Claire Reynolds, a 21-year-old woman, who has presented with blurred vision in the right eye. She thought the vision would resolve by itself, but unfortunately it has worsened and now her visual acuity is hand movements in that eye. Please take a history from Miss Reynolds, present your findings and formulate an appropriate management plan.

Cardinal Symptoms

Blurred vision

Painful eye movements.

Reduced colour intensity

Asymmetrical pupil

HISTORY OF PRESENTING COMPLAINT

BLURRED VISION

- Character: A gradual, constant 'fog' versus a temporary black curtain suddenly appearing across the vision represents two distinct eye problems. For example, corneal decompensation ('fog') and amaurosis fugax (temporary black curtain)
- Onset: Sudden blurred vision that is constant suggests an acute event. For example, vascular occlusion
- Timing: Whether the visual changes started at a specific time point or if they are worse at certain times of the day
- Progression: Gradual, progressive blurred vision may be associated with infection or optic neuritis
- Events preceding the blurred vision: If head trauma occurred at the time, this could indicate an intracranial bleed. Lifting a heavy weight may suggest a Valsalva-induced vitreous haemorrhage
- Unilateral or bilateral: If both eyes are affected, consider whether this is a neurological event; for example, stroke, migraine, space-occupying lesion. Optic neuritis is typically unilateral

ASSOCIATED SYMPTOMS

Other symptoms to enquire about include:
- Reduced colour vision: This usually suggests a problem with the optic nerve; for example, in optic neuritis, traumatic axonal neuropathy (damage to the optic nerve due to trauma to the eye) and orbital cellulitis
- Eye movements:
  - Pain: When looking in one particular direction or all directions. Optic neuritis may have pain in some or all directions, with a white eye that appears grossly 'normal'
  - Double vision: Whether it is double with one eye open, or only when both eyes are open. Clarify the direction in which there would be double vision
- Pupil asymmetry: A large pupil in bright and dark conditions suggests an afferent pathway defect. To test for this, use the swinging-torch test to look for an RAPD in the affected eye

PAST MEDICAL AND SURGICAL HISTORY

- General: Ask about other diagnosed medical conditions, treatments and hospital admissions

- Specific:
  - A history of eating disorders may suggest a nutritional cause for optic nerve problems
  - Previous anterior uveitis may suggest a masquerade syndrome; for example, systemic lupus erythematosus, lymphoma, vasculitis or sarcoidosis
  - A previous diagnosis of multiple sclerosis makes optic neuritis related to demyelination more likely

MEDICATION HISTORY

Enquire about prescribed medications (including any recent changes) and over-the-counter medications. Allergies should be included with the specific reaction noted. In this scenario it is also important to note:
- The following medications may cause optic nerve damage:
  - Amiodarone
  - Ethambutol
  - Cyanide
  - Isoniazid
  - Triethyltin

SOCIAL HISTORY

Social history includes enquiring about occupation, residence, lifestyle (diet, exercise, smoking, alcohol, substance abuse) and recent travel. Additionally, in this scenario, consider:
- Smoking: Document pack years, calculated as the number of packs per day multiplied by the number of years smoked. This may lead to optic neuropathy
- Alcohol and illicit drug use: Alcohol toxicity and methanol use are risk factors
- Recent travels abroad: Insect bites, transmissible infectious disease; for example, Lyme disease, syphilis, tuberculosis (TB)
- Diet: Vitamin B_1, B_2, B_6, B_{12} and folic acid deficiency

FAMILY HISTORY

Enquire about any family history of significantly reduced vision, this may suggest Leber's hereditary optic neuropathy, which affects males more often than females.

SYSTEMS REVIEW

On systems review, particularly pertinent questions to the above case may include:
- Respiratory: Cough or coryzal symptoms. If the immune system is compromised, the patient may acquire postviral or vaccination optic neuritis. Chronic cough may be associated with TB, sarcoidosis and vasculitis
- Neurological: Limb weakness (multiple sclerosis)

- Constitutional features: Fatigue and weight loss suggest systemic disease; for example, vasculitis or cardiac failure, which may lead to increased risk of anterior ischaemic optic neuropathy, due to reduced blood flow to the eye

Risk Factors for Optic Neuritis due to Demyelination
- Aged 20–30 years old
- Female:male ratio is 3:1
- Prior diagnosis of multiple sclerosis

Differential Diagnosis

DISEASE	CLINICAL PRESENTATION	EXAMINATION FINDINGS AND INVESTIGATION	TREATMENT
Optic neuritis	• Unilateral, blurred vision, which may rapidly progress to severe loss of vision over hours to days • Pain behind the eye and on eye movements	• General inspection: The affected eye is white externally with no swelling or proptosis • The swinging-torch test: demonstrates RAPD in the affected eye • Colour vision: Reduced in the affected eye • Visual fields: Increased size of blind spot • Fundoscopy: Disc may appear swollen or hyperaemic in comparison to the unaffected eye • Investigation: MRI head	• Monitor; spontaneously improves 2–3 weeks following onset • IV steroids may be recommended if the vision loss is severe; however there is conflicting evidence of benefit
Traumatic axonal injury	• Unilateral posttraumatic reduced vision • May be associated with double vision if there are orbital fractures present or periorbital bruising and swelling • Pupil asymmetry may be noted	• General inspection: Small conjunctival haemorrhages or bruising around the eye may be present • The swinging-torch test: Pupil may be dilated and sluggish. RAPD may be present • Colour vision: Reduced in the affected eye • Visual fields: Reduced globally • Fundoscopy: The optic disc may appear hyperaemic, swollen or normal • Examination: Reduced sensation in the maxillary (V2) distribution	• Urgent referral to ophthalmologist to check that the globe and structures are intact
Anterior ischaemic optic neuropathy	• Unilateral sudden reduction in vision • If associated with GCA, there may be symptoms of scalp tenderness, jaw claudication, temporal artery tenderness and non-pulsatile, unilateral headache	• The swinging-torch test: May demonstrate RAPD in affected eye • Visual fields: Horizontal visual field defect • Fundoscopy: Early stages may demonstrate swelling or hyperaemia of the optic disc • Bloods, including: FBCs, ESR, CRP: Need to rule out GCA • Haemoglobin A_{1c} (HbA$_{1c}$), lipid profile and glucose: Need to rule out microvascular disease	• Risk factor management; for example, antihypertensive medication, treatment of diabetes and hypercholesterolaemia • High-dose steroids are needed in cases of GCA • Smoking cessation advice • Lifestyle modification; for example, diet and exercise

CAUSES OF A PUPIL THAT IS DILATED OR SLUGGISH TO REACT

These include:
- Pharmacological dilating agents: For example, tropicamide
- Traumatic injury: To the iris sphincter muscle
- Third-nerve palsy: This requires urgent referral to ophthalmology
- Physiological Adie's pupil: A normal variant

Present Your Findings

Miss Reynolds is a 21-year-old woman who presented with unilateral blurred vision in the right eye for 1 week. This was gradual, but progressive, such that the vision is now limited to hand movements in the affected eye. This has been associated with a constant, dull ache behind the eye and pain on eye movements in all directions. She reports that the right pupil was much larger than the left in bright light and her colour intensity is significantly reduced. Otherwise, she feels fit and well and she is not on any medication.

I feel the most likely diagnosis is optic neuritis. The differential diagnosis includes demyelination and nutritional optic neuropathy.

I would complete my consultation with a focused neurological examination to look for signs associated with multiple sclerosis. I would also complete a set of bloods including FBCs, urea and electrolytes, CRP and ESR and order an MRI head.

QUESTIONS AND ANSWERS FOR CANDIDATE

What visual field defect would you expect to find in a case of early optic neuritis?
- Enlarged blind spot in the affected eye

Prolonged swelling of the optic nerve results in optic nerve atrophy. Describe the transition of the appearance of the optic nerve from the acute phase to the chronic phase of the disease.
- Acute phase:
  - Hyperaemia
  - Blurred disc margins
  - Indistinct blood vessels around the optic nerve
- Chronic phase:
  - Disc pallor
  - Enlarged cup-to-disc ratio
  - Clear, well-demarcated disc margins

What is an afferent pupillary defect?
- An afferent pupillary defect is caused by a complete lesion to the optic nerve, anterior to the optic chiasm

 A Case to Learn From

A 20-year-old woman presented with an 8-week history of bilateral temporal headaches, associated with worsening blurred vision in both eyes. She reported no nausea, vomiting, neck stiffness or photophobia. Examination confirmed bilateral swollen discs. She was investigated for intracranial causes of papilloedema through MRI and magnetic resonance venography head, but both were reported as unremarkable. Routine bloods tests revealed a significantly raised creatinine, suggesting renal failure. Her blood pressure measured 210/100 mmHg. The diagnosis was acute malignant hypertension. Blood pressure must be measured in all patients with disc swelling.

 Top Tip

When you are taking an ophthalmic history, always have in the back of your mind which extraocular muscles are involved in what action and its respective innervation. It is also important to think about the anatomy of the optic nerve, especially when a patient presents with a visual field defect.

STATION 10.7: EXAMINATION: OPHTHALMIC

SCENARIO

You are a junior doctor in the emergency department (ED) and have been asked to see Keri Whalen, a 67-year-old woman, who has presented with a constantly watery eye with mild irritation. She is otherwise fit and well. Please perform a relevant eye examination on Mrs Whalen and present your findings. You are not required to complete fundoscopy for this station.

PREPARATION

- WIPER:
  - *Wash* your hands.
  - *Introduce* yourself
  - Ask about *pain*

- Appropriately *expose*
- *Reposition*
- Explain the examination to the patient and your reasons for performing it
- Gain verbal consent
- Ensure that the patient is positioned so that you are able to use either your ophthalmoscope comfortably or, if required, the slit lamp
- Positioning on slit lamp: Place the slit lamp at a height comfortable for your back, then adjust the patient's position so that the eyes are level with the horizontal markers on each side of the microscope

EYE EXAMINATION

A complete ophthalmic assessment includes fundoscopy, which is especially important if the vision is blurred or reduced.

GENERAL INSPECTION

- Environment: Reading aids (glasses or magnifying glass)
- Patient: Facial asymmetry ± scars, jaundice, pallor, head tilt

EXTERNAL EYE EXAMINATION (UNDER SLIT-LAMP MICROSCOPE PREFERENTIALLY)

Inspection
Pupils
- Check that the light reflex is symmetrical in both eyes
- Check that the pupils are reactive to both light (direct and consensual) and accommodation. Note if constriction is normal on accommodation
- Check for a relative afferent pupillary defect (RAPD) using the swinging-torch test. If positive, this indicates optic nerve dysfunction to the afferent nerve pathway

Eyelids
- Look for:
  - Lumps on the periocular skin and lid margins
  - Scars (from previous surgery)
  - Hypo- or hyperpigmentation
  - Position of the eyelids to the globe
- Compare the right eye with the left eye for asymmetry between the eyes
- Note any abnormal movements; for example, blepharospasm
- Look from above and from the sides for any evidence of proptosis

Conjunctiva
- Look for:
  - The colour; for example, redness (erythema) or white areas (leukoplakia) and location or pattern

- Masses; for example, cysts, thickening or traction bands (symblepharon)
- If erythema is present, note whether it is diffuse or localised

Cornea
- Describe the appearance of the cornea
- If the cornea is hazy, note the location – central cornea, middle or on the outer aspect. Try to draw a picture and describe it
- Note whether there is anything stuck on the surface; for example, foreign bodies
- Note whether there are vessels growing on the surface
- Note if there is a defect on fluorescein staining. If so, note whether it is clear to look through or opaque. An abrasion is clear; an ulcer is white and opaque

Anterior chamber (space between the cornea and iris)
- Check that the anterior chamber is clear so that you can see the details of the iris without difficulty. Otherwise, describe what is obstructing your view; for example, blood (hyphaema), white cells moving around or stuck to the inner cornea (keratic precipitates)

Visual Acuity
- Locate the Snellen chart. This may be a chart for use at 6 m or commonly, 3 m. Ensure that the patient is assessed at the correct distance
- Cover one eye and ask them to read the smallest print possible
- Repeat with the other eye
- Check the vision with the pinhole for each eye separately. This tells you whether the macula is functioning well and is an indicator of visual potential; for example, if glasses are usually worn, but forgotten for the assessment, this is an indicator of central retinal function
- In documenting your findings, remember the top number is the distance the assessment was conducted at and the lower number refers to the line which was correctly read; for example, 6/9 indicates that at 6 m the line numbered 9 was read. If a letter from line 9 was missed, add –1 i.e. 6/9 – 1

Visual Fields
- Sit directly opposite the patient, 1 m away
- Close your left eye and ask the patient to close their right eye
- Ask the patient to focus on your uncovered eye and to keep that focus throughout this part of the examination
- Using a red-tipped object, for example, a pen or your finger, ask the patient to say 'yes' when she first sees the red-tipped object or finger appear in the outskirts of her vision

- There are eight meridians to test (two horizontals, four diagonals and two verticals) with your arm outstretched and the red-tipped object moving in slowly
- Repeat for the opposite eye

Eye Movements
- Remain sitting directly opposite the patient
- Note the position of the patient's eyes when facing straight ahead
- With both eyes open, ask the patient to follow the pen with her eyes only and without moving her head. Ask the patient to inform you if she sees two pens at any point
- Ensure to check horizontal and vertical meridians fully using the 'H' technique
- Note whether there is nystagmus (repetitive flickering movement sideways with a fast and slow component), the position of any double vision and what the eye is doing (drifting upwards and out on lateral gaze suggests a trochlear nerve palsy)

FINISHING
- Offer to:
  - Test for colour blindness using the Ishihara chart
  - Examine the eye using an ophthalmoscope
  - Test the other cranial nerves if relevant
- Thank the patient
- Check they're comfortable and offer to help reposition them
- Wash your hands

HORNER'S SYNDROME
- Defined as a triad of ptosis, mitosis (constriction) and anhidrosis on the same side
- Causes of Horner's syndrome include:
  - First-order neurone: Lesions of hypothalamus, brainstem and spinal cord. For example, stroke, demyelinating disease like multiple sclerosis, neoplasms
  - Second-order neurone: Lesions of the thoracic outlet such as pulmonary apex tumour. For example, Pancoast's tumour, thyroid malignancies, trauma to neck or thoracic spine
  - Third-order neurone: For example, base-of-skull tumours, trauma or iatrogenic from surgery, internal carotid artery dissection, thrombosis, pituitary malignancies

UNILATERAL LOSS OF VISION
Common causes of unilateral loss of vision (hand movement vision) include:
- Vascular, for example, central retinal vein occlusion (CRVO), central retinal artery occlusion (CRAO), giant cell arteritis (GCA)
- Retinal detachment
- Acute angle closure glaucoma (AACG)

Present Your Findings

Keri Whalen is a 67-year-old woman who presented with bilateral sore eyes associated with constant watering. On examination, visual acuity is 6/7.5 in both eyes. There is no facial asymmetry or scars on her eyelids. The conjunctiva is red diffusely and swollen. She has a palpable pre-auricular node on both sides of her face. There is eyelash debris present on close inspection of her eyelids, with an absence of purulent discharge. Pupils are round and reactive to light; there is no impairment to range of eye movements. The most likely diagnosis is viral conjunctivitis, with the differentials being allergic conjunctivitis.

To complete my examination I would like to take a swab for adenovirus polymerase chain reaction (PCR) testing. Her treatment involves cool compresses over both eyes. I would advise 1–2 weeks off work if working in close proximity with other individuals and good hand hygiene.

❓ QUESTIONS AND ANSWERS FOR CANDIDATE

A complete third cranial nerve palsy (oculomotor) may result in which features?
- Downward- and outward-positioned eye
- Enlarged pupil
- Complete eyelid lowering (ptosis)

A 55-year-old woman presents to the ED with double vision. She is unable to abduct her left eye. There is no history of head injury. She denies headache, jaw or tongue claudication, scalp tenderness or proximal muscle weakness. Bloods for C-reactive protein (CRP) and erythrocyte sedimentation rate (ESR) are normal. Which nerve is resulting in her diplopia and what is the most likely cause?
- Lateral rectus is paralysed, therefore it is the sixth cranial nerve, abducens nerve
- The most likely cause in this age group is microvascular, commonly due to diabetes or hypertension

A right-sided homonymous hemianopia indicates a lesion of the brain affecting which areas?
- Left optic tract
- Left occipital cortex

🗣️ **A Case to Learn From**

A 40-year-old man presented with headache and new-onset double vision. He denied any head injury and was otherwise fit and well. Blood pressure was normal on a one-off measurement. Examination revealed a sixth cranial nerve palsy, with an otherwise normal ophthalmic assessment. His risk factors for ischaemic-related sixth-nerve palsy were low, so a magnetic resonance imaging (MRI) head was completed and this revealed a large meningioma. It is important to note that a sixth-nerve palsy may indicate intracranial pathology, as it has the longest intracranial trajectory and may present as a false localising sign.

💡 **Top Tip**

When assessing eye movements, you can place one hand on the patient's chin or forehead gently. This will encourage the head to remain still and allow for accurate assessment of the eyes only.

STATION 10.8: PRACTICAL SKILL: FUNDOSCOPY TECHNIQUE

SCENARIO

You are a junior doctor in the ED. You have been asked to see Thomas Grey, a 72-year-old man who has presented with painless loss of vision in his right eye. Please complete fundoscopy on Mr Grey and present your findings.

PREPARATION

- WIPER:
  - *Wash* your hands
  - *Introduce* yourself
  - Ask about *pain*
  - Appropriately *expose*
  - *Reposition*
- Explain the examination to the patient and your reasons for performing it. Explain that you would like to assess the eyes by shining a bright light into them and warn the patient that you may get quite close
- Gain verbal consent
- Ensure the patient is sat down and you are in a position to reach their eye at close proximity without difficulty. You may prefer to stand

EQUIPMENT CHECKLIST

- Fundoscope
- Pupil-dilating eye drops; for example, tropicamide, cyclopentolate

FUNDOSCOPY

INITIAL SET-UP

- Dim the room lights
- Preferably dilate the patient's pupil for both ease of examination and increased peripheral view; for example, cyclopentolate 1% eye drops
- Ask the patient to focus on a distant target; for example, a large letter on the Snellen chart
- When examining the patient's right eye, use your right hand to hold the ophthalmoscope and look with your right eye, and vice versa for examining the patient's left eye
- Place your thumb or index finger on the focus dial located on the side, so that you can adjust the focus during the assessment

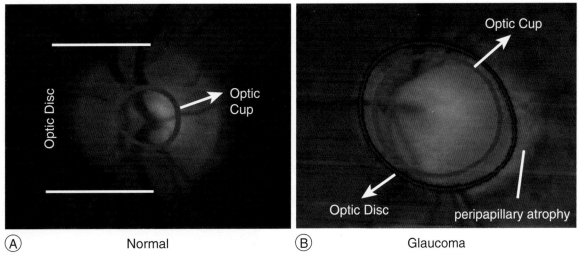

Fig. 10.5 Cup size relative to the optic disc.

- Ensure the dial is at zero, indicating that there is no adjustment for short-sightedness or long-sightedness

APPROACH TO FUNDOSCOPY

Red-Eye Reflex
- Look through the ophthalmoscope whilst shining it at the patient's eye from a distance of 30 cm
- Once the red-eye reflex (orange glow) has been identified, zoom in towards this reflex. Imagine a straight line towards the patient and follow this
- This orange glow may not be a perfect circle; it may have grey areas. These are likely to be cataract reflections

Retinal Structures
Optic Disc
- If the patient is looking straight ahead, aim the light from the ophthalmoscope towards the nose (at around 45°)
- Rotate the ophthalmoscope gently from side to side until you locate the disc, or you may find some vessels
- Use the focus dial: If the vessels appear out of focus, rotate it anticlockwise (red) to make it more negative and short-sighted (myopic), or clockwise (white) for long-sighted (hypermetropic), which is positive
- Once you have located the vessels, follow their trajectory until you reach the disc. If the vessels are getting smaller in diameter, you need to follow them the other way to find the disc
- Once you have located the disc, comment on the:
  - Colour: pale or hyperaemic (very red)
  - Contour: normal or blurred margins in optic nerve swelling
  - Size of the disc: normal, small, enlarged
  - Cup size (Fig. 10.5): For example, large cup suggests possible optic nerve atrophy

Vessels
- Follow the vessels from the optic disc towards the periphery
- There are four arcades to follow (each a pair of vein and artery). Veins appear wider and darker than arteries
- Comment on:
  - Narrowing: Arteriovenous nipping is narrowing at vein–artery crossing points, found in hypertensive retinopathy
  - Increased tortuosity: Found in hypertensive retinopathy

Macula
- This is located temporally to the optic disc
- Comment on any deposits; for example:
  - Drusen (subretinal deposits of waste products), macular haemorrhages and pigmentation are all indicators of age-related macular degeneration (ARMD)
  - Exudates (yellow deposits), haemorrhages or cotton-wool spots (white fluffy deposits) are present in hypertensive and diabetic retinopathy

Peripheral retina
Comment on:
- Retinal deposits
- Haemorrhages
- Chorioretinal atrophy (white patches with a pigmented edge)

Try to complete this when following the vessels into the periphery.

FINISHING
- Offer to:
  - Check the patient's blood pressure
  - Check the serum glucose and cholesterol levels
- Thank the patient
- Wash your hands

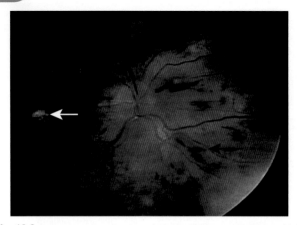

Fig. 10.6 Left-eye colour fundus photograph demonstrating multiple flame-shaped haemorrhages (black arrow), cotton-wool spots and central exudates at the macula (white arrow).

GRADES	CLASSIFICATION
I	• Mild retinal arteriolar narrowing
II	• Focal narrowing of arterioles and arteriovenous crossings • Silver wiring (retinal arterioles that have become white if there is an occlusion)
III	• Retinal haemorrhages (dot, blot or flame) • Exudates • Cotton-wool spots
IV (severe hypertensive retinopathy)	• Grade III + papilloedema.

Table **10.1** Grades of hypertensive retinopathy

HYPERTENSIVE RETINOPATHY

Accelerated hypertension occurs with severe hypertension, usually greater than 180 mmHg systolic and 110 mmHg diastolic, and evidence of end-organ disease, which may include severe hypertensive retinopathy (Fig. 10.6).

Table 10.1 outlines the grades of hypertensive retinopathy.

DIABETIC RETINOPATHY

Duration of diabetes is the most important risk factor. After 30 years of diabetes, 90% have diabetic retinopathy (Figs 10.7 and 10.8). This is more likely with poor control, especially in type 1 diabetes mellitus, and concurrent pregnancy and hypertension.

Table 10.2 outlines the grades of diabetic retinopathy.

AGE-RELATED MACULAR DEGENERATION

• ARMD is the leading cause of blindness in the over-50s population
• 26% of over 65-year-olds will be affected
• Signs are symptoms are detailed in Table 10.3
• Most cases are the slowly progressive dry form of ARMD

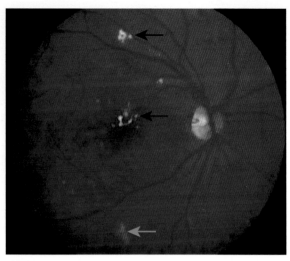

Fig. 10.7 Features of non-proliferative diabetic retinopathy: Dot and blot haemorrhages (black arrow), hard exudates (blue arrow) and cotton-wool spots (green arrow).

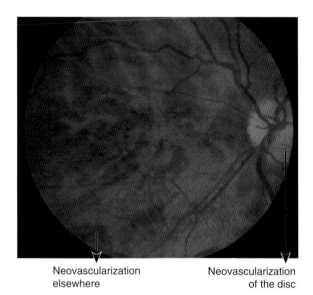

Neovascularization elsewhere   Neovascularization of the disc

Fig. 10.8 Colour fundus photograph showing proliferative diabetic retinopathy.

• The less common wet form of ARMD leads to rapid and severe vision loss
• Treatment with anti-VEGF (vascular endothelial growth factor) therapy exists for wet ARMD

OPTIC DISC SWELLING

• Disc margins appear fluffy or blurred, with obscured blood vessel entry and exit points (Fig. 10.9)
• There may also be haemorrhages at the disc, especially in severe hypertensive retinopathy with papilloedema
• If unilateral, it is termed optic neuritis. Causes include: Demyelination, infection, inflammation, drugs
• If bilateral, it is presumed to be papilloedema (optic disc swelling secondary to raised intracranial pressure) until other causes are excluded

Table 10.2 Categories of diabetic retinopathy

GRADES	CLASSIFICATION
Background	• Dot haemorrhages • Hard exudates • Minimal cotton-wool spots
Pre-proliferative	• Intraretinal microvascular abnormalities • Venous beading/loops • Blot haemorrhages • Multiple cotton-wool spots
Proliferative	• New fragile bleeding vessels; may be at the disc or elsewhere in periphery

Table 10.3 Symptoms and signs of ARMD

SYMPTOMS	SIGNS
• Distortion • Reduced vision: Gradual with dry ARMD, sudden with wet ARMD • Missing areas in vision (scotomas)	• Central visual field loss • Macular drusen spots on fundoscopy • Macular haemorrhages (wet form) • Geographic retinal atrophy (map-like areas of retinal degeneration) • Scarring (dark pigmented areas)

 Present Your Findings

Thomas Grey is a 72-year-old man who has presented with painless loss of vision in his right eye. He describes this as persistent with no other symptoms. He is known to be hypertensive and admits to omitting his medication on a regular basis. On fundoscopy, the retina appears white and a cherry-red spot is seen. I feel the most likely diagnosis is CRAO.

I would like to perform a visual acuity test and intraocular pressure (IOP) measurement and perform dilated fundal examination on Mr Grey at the slit lamp. I would like to take blood to check his serum glucose and cholesterol levels.

❓ QUESTIONS AND ANSWERS FOR CANDIDATE

Identify the differences in appearance of the retina on fundoscopy in dry ARMD compared to wet ARMD.

• Dry ARMD: Discrete yellow lesions at the macula, which may be accompanied by pigmentary changes and thinning of the retina
• Wet ARMD: Macular haemorrhages, which may be accompanied by discrete yellow lesions and hyperpigmented lesions at the macula

What is the treatment for wet ARMD and how does it work?

• Mainstay of treatment is anti-VEGF intravitreal injections (into the vitreous)
• Anti-VEGF injected into the eye has been shown to block VEGF, which promotes growth of abnormal vessels (neovascularisation). This results in a

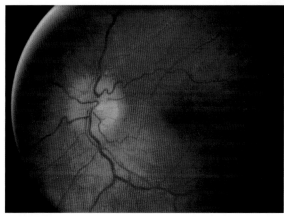

Fig. 10.9 Optic disc swelling. There is blurring of the vessels leaving the optic disc and loss of clarity of the disc margins.

reduction in the retinal fluid through regression of abnormal, leaky vessels in the choroid

How does the fundus appearance of a CRVO differ from a CRAO?

• The fundoscopic image seen in CRVO typically consists of multiple widespread retinal haemorrhages (flame-shaped, dot and blot haemorrhages), yellow soft-edged lesions (exudates) and white fluffy lesions (cotton-wool spots) due to ischaemia to the nerve layer. In severe cases, there may also be optic disc swelling
• The fundoscopic image seen in CRAO typically consists of widespread pallor to the retina, a cherry-red spot at the macula and a shiny embolus in the artery

 A Case to Learn From

A patient was seen in the ED after a 2-day history of progressive vision loss in the right eye. She described a curtain coming down over the right eye, starting superiorly, then progressing to obscure her vision completely. She was referred to eye casualty urgently. Her visual acuity in the right eye was perception to light and in the left eye 6/6 (Snellen chart), with a large superior visual defect in the left eye on confrontation field testing. Fundoscopy demonstrated an established CRAO in the right eye and a swollen disc in the left eye, indicating acute anterior ischaemic optic neuropathy. Detailed history taking revealed a 2-week history of temporal headache on the right side accompanied by neck pain, jaw claudication, increasing difficulty using her arms and intermittent double vision. The diagnosis was vision-involving GCA. In this case, she was treated with high-dose pulsed intravenous (IV) methylprednisolone (1 g/day for 3 days). An earlier diagnosis would have potentially saved the visual field in the left eye, and perhaps even the right eye, if she had presented when she first developed symptoms.

Top Tip

Practise fundoscopy on friends and family to become proficient in the technique for your exam and future clinical practice. This will also help you understand where the (hopefully) normal retina structures are located in relation to one another before identifying retinal changes.

Content Outline

Prescribing in emergencies can be a daunting experience for a junior doctor and scary stations for medical students. Below are some key points to help you establish a systematic and safe approach to prescribing.

- Write clearly with black ink and use capital letters
- The patient's name, date of birth (DOB) and hospital number should be clearly documented on every page of the drug chart and on all additional charts; for example, insulin and heparin prescription charts
- Allergies should be clearly documented on the front of the drug chart, detailing the reaction
- Acceptable dose abbreviations include mg (milligrams), g (grams), ml (millilitres). All other units must be written in full (micrograms NOT mcg)
- Never abbreviate ORAL or INTRATHECAL, other routes of administration may be abbreviated, e.g. IV (intravenous), IM (intramuscular), SC (subcutaneous), PR (per rectum), INH (inhaled), NEB (nebulised)
- Antibiotic prescriptions should detail the indication and the duration, stop date or review date
- Oxygen is a drug and should be prescribed on the drug chart, with the prescription detailing the device, starting flow rate and target saturations
- Consider prophylaxis for VTE in all patients on admission to hospital and regularly thereafter. Compression devices should be prescribed on the drug chart if indicated
- Consider whether any of a patient's usual medications should be stopped or withheld during admission
- Your signature must be accompanied by your name, clearly printed, and a contact number

Study Action Plan

- Practice, practice, practice is the key to prescribing
- Don't worry about remembering all the doses for common drugs; you can always check in the *British National Formulary* (BNF)

- Review the drug chart of every patient you see on the wards to observe which medications have been started, stopped or amended
- Try developing scenarios with friends – this chapter shows you some of the more common medical and surgical emergencies

STATION 11.1: ACUTE LEFT VENTRICULAR FAILURE

SCENARIO

You are the junior doctor covering a cardiology ward overnight. The nurses fast bleep you to see John Smith, an 85-year-old man, who has become acutely breathless and is coughing up frothy pink sputum. An echocardiogram performed on this admission showed severe left ventricular dysfunction. He had been written up for intravenous (IV) fluids overnight (1 L IV sodium chloride 0.9% over 8 h) since he was deemed to be dehydrated. Please review the patient, formulate an appropriate management plan and complete the drug chart provided.

Patient Details

Name	John Smith
DOB	12/02/1935
Hospital number	1202350034
Weight	75 kg
Height	1.82 m
Consultant	CAP
Hospital/ward	WGH/53
Current medications	Glyceryl trinitrate, ramipril, spironolactone, memantine, paracetamol, lansoprazole
Allergies	None
Admission date	11/05/2019

INITIAL ASSESSMENT

AIRWAY

- Patent

BREATHING

- Respiratory rate (RR) 30 breaths/min
- SpO_2 74% on 2 L/min oxygen via nasal cannulae
- Acutely dyspnoeic, panicked
- Loud crepitations bilaterally

CIRCULATION

- Heart rate (HR) 142 bpm
- Blood pressure (BP) 148/86 mmHg
- Peripheries warm with capillary refill time (CRT) < 2 s
- Jugular venous pressure (JVP) raised to the earlobes
- A third heart sound is present

DISABILITY

- Temperature 37.6°C
- Glasgow Coma Scale (GCS) 15/15
- Capillary glucose level 6.2 mmol/L

EXPOSURE

- Bilateral pitting oedema to the mid-shins

INITIAL INVESTIGATIONS

ELECTROCARDIOGRAM (ECG)

- Sinus rhythm at 150 bpm with anterolateral ST depression

Bloods

COMPONENTS	RESULTS	REFERENCE RANGES
Haemoglobin (Hb)	145	130–170 g/L
White cell count (WCC)	5.6	$3.7–11.1 \times 10^9$/L
Neutrophils	4.0	$1.5–7.4 \times 10^9$/L
Platelets	220	$150–400 \times 10^9$/L
C-reactive protein (CRP)	1	0–10 mg/L
Troponin	25↑	0–14 ng/L
Sodium	133↓	136–145 mmol/L
Potassium	3.8	3.5–5.1 mmol/L
Urea	4.0	2.1–7.1 mmol/L
Creatinine	78	62–106 µmol/L
Estimated glomerular filtration rate (eGFR)	>60	>60 mL/min/1.73 m²

Arterial blood gas (ABG)

COMPONENTS	RESULTS	REFERENCE RANGES
pH	7.31↓	7.35–7.45
PaO_2	6.3↓	>8 kPa
$PaCO_2$	5.7	4.7–6.0 kPa
HCO_3^-	19↓	22–26 mmol/L
Base excess	−3.2↑	−2.0–2.0 mEq
Lactate	2.1↑	0.5–1.0 mmol/L

CHEST X-RAY (CXR)

- Fluid in the horizontal fissures, upper-lobe diversion, 'bat's wing shadowing' and Kerley B lines

IMPRESSION

- Flash pulmonary oedema secondary to acute left ventricular failure, with rate-related ischaemic changes on ECG
- This patient is acutely unwell and requires immediate management to prevent deterioration
- Differential diagnoses include: Asthma, pneumonia, myocardial infarction (MI) and metabolic acidosis

INITIAL MANAGEMENT

- L, M, N, O, P:
  - *Loop* diuretic: Give furosemide. Higher doses may be required if currently on diuretics or in renal failure. Lower doses may be required if elderly or of low body weight. Consider a furosemide infusion
  - *Morphine*: Titrate to pain, 5–10 mg IV over 5–10 min. This has multiple effects: As an analgesic, anxiolytic (reducing hyperventilation) and weak venodilator, directly reducing pulmonary oedema. Prescribe with an appropriate antiemetic
  - *Nitrates*: Give glyceryl trinitrate (GTN) spray if systolic BP > 100 mmHg. If there is inadequate response to furosemide or sublingual nitrates, and BP is still holding, consider starting a GTN infusion (starting dose, depending on baseline BP, 0.3–1 mg/h)
  - *Oxygen*: Give high-flow oxygen (> 60% via Venturi mask). If the patient is in type 1 respiratory failure, consider continuous positive airway pressure (CPAP) early for refractory hypoxia
  - *Posture*: Sit the patient up

PLUS

- Consider early high dependency unit (HDU)/intensive therapy/ treatment unit (ITU) referral: Either for monitoring (central venous pressure, arterial BP) or for treatment (CPAP for type 1 respiratory failure or bilevel positive airway pressure (BiPAP) for type 2 respiratory failure). If the patient is deemed unsuitable for HDU/ITU, then an urgent resuscitation and ceiling of care decision needs to be made
- Thromboprophylaxis: Ensure that this is prescribed
- Monitor urine output: It is important to assess whether good diuresis has occurred. Insert a urinary catheter if not already in place

DRUG CHART

The important aspects to consider when prescribing for this patient are:
- Allergies: Should be considered in all cases

- Oxygen therapy: Should be considered in all cases. When prescribing oxygen therapy, indicate the device, desired oxygen flow and target saturations
- IV fluids: Always check all prescription charts. The patient may have a separate fluid chart and it is vital in these cases that it is stopped
- Regular medications: Regular medication should be reviewed every time the medication chart is looked at

COMPLICATIONS OF ACUTE LEFT VENTRICULAR FAILURE

- Respiratory failure
- Respiratory arrest
- Hypotension
- Cardiogenic shock
- Cardiac arrest

❓ QUESTIONS AND ANSWERS FOR CANDIDATE

Name three CXR findings associated with pulmonary oedema.
- Pleural effusions
- Cardiomegaly
- Kerley B lines
- Upper-lobe pulmonary venous congestion
- Interstitial oedema

 Prescription and Administration Record

Prescription and Administration Record

Name: JOHN SMITH	Weight: 75 KG	Known allergies:
DOB: 12./02./1935	Age: 85 YEARS	NO KNOWN DRUG ALLERGIES
Hospital number: 12.02.350034	Consultant: CAP	Signature: Date: C.Price 11/05/19 CATHERINE PRICE

Once-Only Medications

Date	Time	Medicine (approved name)	Dose	Route	Prescriber – sign and print	Time given	Given by
11/05/19	2.000	FUROSEMIDE	40 MG	IV	C.Price CATHERINE PRICE		
11/05/19	2.000	GTN SPRAY	2 PUFFS	SUBLINGUAL	C.Price CATHERINE PRICE		
11/05/19	2.000	MORPHINE (TITRATE TO PAIN)	1–10 MG	IV	C.Price CATHERINE PRICE		
11/05/19	2.000	METOCLOPRAMIDE	10 MG	IV	C.Price CATHERINE PRICE		
11/05/19	2.000	ENOXAPARIN	2.0 MG	SC	C.Price CATHERINE PRICE		

Start				Route		Stop	
Date	Time	Mask (%)	Prongs (L/min)	Prescriber – sign and print	Administered by	Date	Time
11/05/19	2.000	VENTURI (60)		C. Price CATHERINE PRICE			

Venous Thromboembolism (VTE) Prophylaxis

VTE risk assessment: Yes [X] Prophylaxis not required [ ] Contraindicated [ ]		Comment: Signature: **C. Price** CATHERINE PRICE Date: 12/09/19							
	Date: → Time: ↓	12/05							
Drug: ENOXAPARIN		1800							
Dose:	Freq:	Route:							
20 MG	OD	SC							
Start: 13/09	Stop/review:								
Signature: **C. Price** CATHERINE PRICE									

Regular medications

	Date: → Time: ↓	12/5							
Drug: RAMIPRIL		02							
Dose:	Freq:	Route:	06						
5 MG	BD	ORAL	⑩						
Start: 12/09/19	Stop/review:		14						
Signature: **C. Price** CATHERINE PRICE			⑱						
Indication: HYPERTENSION			22						

Drug: SPIRONOLACTONE		02							
Dose:	Freq:	Route:	06						
100 MG	OD	ORAL	⑩						
Start: 12/09/19	Stop/review:		14						
Signature: **C. Price** CATHERINE PRICE			18						
Indication: ASCITES			22						

Continued

Prescription and Administration Record—cont'd

Drug: MEMANTINE			02								
Dose: 5 MG	Freq: OD	Route: ORAL	06 ⑩								
Start: 12/09/19		Stop/review:	14								
Signature: C. Price CATHERINE PRICE			18								
Indication: DEMENTIA			22								

Drug: PARACETAMOL			02								
Dose: 1 G	Freq: QDS	Route: ORAL	⑥ ⑫								
Start: 12/09/19		Stop/review:	14								
Signature: C. Price CATHERINE PRICE			⑱								
Indication: BACK PAIN			㉔								

Drug: LANSOPRAZOLE			02								
Dose: 15 MG	Freq: OD	Route: ORAL	06 ⑩								
Start: 12/09/19		Stop/review:	14								
Signature: C. Price CATHERINE PRICE			18								
Indication: DUODENAL ULCER			22								

Prescription and Administration Record—cont'd

PRN Medications

		Date:	12								
		Time:									
Drug: GLYCERYL TRINITRATE											
Dose: 2 PUFFS	Freq: PRN	Route: SC									
Start: 11/05/19	Stop/review:										
Signature: **C. Price** CATHERINE PRICE											
Indication: ANGINA											

Fluid Prescriptions

Date	Fluid	Additive	Volume	Route	Rate	Signature	Given	Batch
12/09/19	0.9% SODIUM CHLORIDE	NONE	1 L	IV	OVER 8 H	C. Price CATHERINE PRICE		

Stopped due to fluid overload 12/09/19 C. Price (CATHERINE PRICE)

Which three groups of medications are known to improve mortality in patients with chronic heart failure?

- Beta-blockers
- Potassium-sparing diuretics
- Angiotensin-converting enzyme inhibitors (ACEi)

Note: Digoxin does not improve mortality!

Name three factors which might precipitate decompensation of heart failure.

- Sepsis
- Overhydration: Iatrogenic
- Acute kidney injury (AKI)
- Introduction of medications; for example, beta-blockers
- Stopping of medications, for example, diuretics

A Case to Learn From

At the end of a long night shift, I was bleeped to review a patient who was tachypnoeic and looking grey and unwell. He was an elderly man with lymphoma, atrial fibrillation (AF) and ischaemic heart disease. He had been admitted with a chest infection and was being treated with antibiotics and IV fluids. A–E assessment revealed coarse bi-basal crackles, a loud ejection systolic murmur and a jugular venous pulse visible by his ear, even with him sitting up at 90°. I was about to prescribe furosemide and GTN for his pulmonary oedema, but his BP was only 82/46 mmHg. I stopped his IV fluids and called my registrar for advice. We gave a very cautious bolus of furosemide and when it became apparent it was well tolerated, started an infusion. An hour later, he was looking much more comfortable. This was a lesson for me in ensuring that I have completed my A–E assessment before launching treatment, as my eagerness to treat his pulmonary oedema nearly resulted in me acting without checking the BP, which could have caused more harm than good.

Top Tip

Always ensure that you perform a thorough assessment of a patient with shortness of breath. There may be multiple pathologies. Acute ventricular failure may be exacerbated by infection, which would also need prompt treatment.

STATION 11.2: ACUTE MYOCARDIAL INFARCTION

SCENARIO

You are the junior doctor covering the acute receiving unit overnight. The nurses fast bleep you to see Perry Terrant, an 80-year-old man, who has been admitted with acute severe chest pain. Please review the patient, formulate an appropriate management plan and complete the drug chart provided.

Patient Details

Name:	Perry Terrant
DOB:	12/03/1940
Hospital number:	1203408558
Weight:	85 kg
Height:	1.75 m
Consultant:	CAP
Hospital/ward:	WGH/54
Current medications:	Allopurinol, amlodipine, esomeprazole, gliclazide, alendronic acid, citalopram, co-careldopa
Allergies:	Penicillin (rash)
Admission date:	03/10/2019

INITIAL ASSESSMENT

AIRWAY

- Patent

BREATHING

- RR 30 breaths/min
- SpO_2 90% on 2 L/min oxygen via nasal cannulae
- Chest clear on auscultation

CIRCULATION

- HR 128 bpm
- BP 152/94 mmHg
- Peripheries warm with CRT < 2 s
- Heart sounds are normal with no added sounds

DISABILITY

- Temperature 36.2°C
- GCS 15/15
- Capillary glucose level 6.8 mmol/L

EXPOSURE

- Appears sweaty and complaining of nausea

INITIAL INVESTIGATIONS

ECG

- Sinus rhythm at 122 bpm with 2 mm ST elevation throughout the anterior leads

Bloods

COMPONENTS	RESULTS	REFERENCE RANGES
Hb	152	130–170 g/L
WCC	7.4	3.7–11.1 × 10⁹/L
Neutrophils	5.6	1.5–7.4 × 10⁹/L
Platelets	315	150–400 × 10⁹/L
CRP	3	0–10 mg/L
Troponin	30,000↑	0–14 ng/L
Sodium	142	136–145 mmol/L
Potassium	4.6	3.5–5.1 mmol/L
Urea	6.2	2.1–7.1 mmol/L
Creatinine	113↑	62–106 µmol/L
eGFR	58↓	>60 mL/min/1.73 m2

ABG

COMPONENTS	RESULTS	REFERENCE RANGES
pH	7.25	7.35–7.45
PaO_2	7.8↓	> 8 kPa
$PaCO_2$	4.7	4.7–6.0 kPa
HCO_3^-	16↓	22–26 mmol/L
Base excess	−4.6↓	−2.0–2.0 mEq
Lactate	5.3↑	0.5–1.0 mmol/L

CXR

- Portable CXR is unremarkable

IMPRESSION

- This is an acute ST elevation MI (STEMI)
- Differential diagnoses include: Aortic dissection, pericarditis and pulmonary embolism (PE)

INITIAL MANAGEMENT

- ROMANCE:
  - *Reassure*
  - *Oxygen*: Keep saturations > 94%
  - *Morphine*: 2.5–10 mg IV initially, titrating to pain
  - *Aspirin*: 300 mg to chew

- *Nitroglycerine*: Sublingual spray. If chest pain continues, consider a nitrate infusion
- *Clopidogrel*: 300 mg oral tablet. Alternatively, prasugrel 60 mg oral tablet or 180 mg ticagrelor oral tablet may be used
- *Enoxaparin* (or fondaparinux): If the patient is already anticoagulated or the renal function is poor, this may be contraindicated

PLUS

- IV access
- Antiemetic: Metoclopramide 10 mg IV
- Contact: Cardiology and/or critical care areas (coronary care unit/HDU/ITU) for definitive management of STEMI and further support. Patients with ST elevation acute coronary syndrome (ACS) should be considered for primary percutaneous coronary intervention (PCI) as soon as the ECG is identified as an acute MI, even without a troponin level. When primary PCI cannot be provided within 90 min of diagnosis, patients with ST elevation ACS should be considered for immediate thrombolytic therapy. Consider whether there are any contraindications. Patients undergoing primary PCI, or those with other ACS presentations that are considered high-risk, may also be treated with a glycoprotein IIb/IIIa receptor antagonist
- Thromboprophylaxis: Be aware that patients who are receiving anticoagulant drugs as part of their treatment for an acute MI do not usually need VTE prophylaxis. However, this should be assessed on a case-by-case basis, with risks and benefits weighed up

DRUG CHART

The important aspects to consider when prescribing for this patient are:
- Allergies: Should be considered in all cases
- Oxygen therapy: Always prescribe oxygen therapy, indicating the device, desired oxygen flow and target saturations
- Antiemetics: Metoclopramide should be avoided in young women due to the risk of oculogyric crisis. Consider cyclizine 50 mg IV instead
- Regular medications: Regular medication should always be reviewed every time the medication chart is looked at

CONTRAINDICATIONS TO THROMBOLYSIS

- Known or suspected intracranial tumour
- Aortic dissection or pericarditis
- Stroke
- Gastrointestinal (GI) or genitourinary haemorrhage within the last 3 months
- Major surgery
- Trauma
- Biopsy or head injury within the last 6 weeks
- Puncture of a non-compressible vessel

- Bleeding diathesis
- Prolonged cardiopulmonary resuscitation (> 10 min)
- Impaired consciousness following cardiac arrest and pregnancy

COMPLICATIONS OF ACUTE MYOCARDIAL INFARCTION

- Left ventricular failure
- Valvular incompetence
- Conduction abnormalities and arrhythmias
- Rupture of the myocardial wall leading to tamponade
- Cardiac arrest

❓ QUESTIONS AND ANSWERS FOR CANDIDATE

Explain how patients with inferior STEMI may develop second- or third-degree heart block.
- In inferior MI, the right coronary artery is usually occluded
- The right coronary artery supplies the atrioventricular (AV) node (in about 80% of the population)
- Ischaemia of the AV node may then lead to heart block

Infarction of which area of the heart carries the worst prognosis, and why?
- Anterior MI carries the worst prognosis
- It is caused by occlusion of the left anterior descending artery, which supplies the largest area of the myocardium, hence carrying the worst prognosis

Name three causes of raised troponin, other than MI.
- Chronic kidney disease
- PE
- Sepsis
- Subarachnoid haemorrhage (SAH)
- Stroke
- Heart failure
- Tachyarrhythmia, for example, AF
- Myocarditis
- Cardiac contusion
- Aortic dissection

 Top Tip

Trust your instincts. If a patient looks unwell, they probably are. If someone with chest pain is grey and clammy, musculoskeletal chest pain is going to fall fairly low on your list of differentials.

STATION 11.3: EXACERBATION OF CHRONIC OBSTRUCTIVE PULMONARY DISEASE

SCENARIO

You are the junior doctor working in acute medical admissions and you are asked to see Mary Finn, a 78-year-old woman with a history of chronic obstructive pulmonary disease (COPD), who is currently breathless. She

Prescription and Administration Record

Prescription and Administration Record

Name: PERRY TERRANT	Weight: 75 KG	Known allergies:
DOB: 12/03/1940	Age: 80 YEARS	NO KNOWN DRUG ALLERGIES
Hospital number: 1203408558	Consultant: CAP	Signature: Date: C.Pratt 03/10/19 C.PRATT

Once-Only Medications

Date	Time	Medicine (approved name)	Dose	Route	Prescriber – sign and print	Time given	Given by
03/10/19	2200	ASPIRIN	300 MG	ORAL	C.Pratt C.PRATT		
03/10/19	2200	CLOPIDOGREL	300 MG	ORAL	C.Pratt C.PRATT		
03/10/19	2200	GTN SPRAY	2 PUFFS	SUBLINGUAL	C.Pratt C.PRATT		
03/10/19	2200	MORPHINE (TITRATE TO PAIN)	1–10 MG	IV	C.Pratt C.PRATT		
03/10/19	2200	ONDANSETRON	4 MG	IV	C.Pratt C.PRATT		

Oxygen Therapy

Start		Route				Stop	
Date	Time	Mask (%)	Prongs (L/min)	Prescriber – sign and print	Administered by	Date	Time
03/10/19	2200	VENTURI (60)		C.Pratt C.PRATT			

VTE Prophylaxis

VTE risk assessment: Yes [ ] Prophylaxis not required [ ] Contraindicated [X]	Comment: Signature: C.Pratt C.PRATT Date: 03/10/19

Prescription and Administration Record—cont'd

Regular Medications

	Date: →	3/10								
	Time: ↓									

Drug: ALLOPURINOL

Dose:	Freq:	Route:	02								
100 MG	OD	ORAL	06								
			(10)								
Start: 03/10/19		Stop/review:	14								
Signature: C.Pratt C.PRATT			18								
Indication: GOUT PROPHYLAXIS			22								

Drug: AMLODIPINE

Dose:	Freq:	Route:	02								
5 MG	OD	ORAL	06								
			(10)								
Start: 03/10/19		Stop/review:	14								
Signature: C.Pratt C.PRATT			18								
Indication: HYPERTENSION			22								

Drug: ESOMEPRAZOLE

Dose:	Freq:	Route:	02								
20 MG	OD	ORAL	06								
			(10)								
Start: 03/10/19		Stop/review:	14								
Signature: C.Pratt C.PRATT			18								
Indication: PEPTIC ULCER DISEASE			22								

Continued

Prescription and Administration Record—cont'd

			Date: →	3/10								
			Time: ↓									
Drug: GLICLAZIDE			02									
Dose:	Freq:	Route:	06									
30 MG	OD	ORAL	(10)									
Start: 03/10/19		Stop/review:	14									
Signature: C.Pratt C.PRATT			18									
Indication: DIABETES			22									

Drug: ALENDRONIC ACID			02									
Dose:	Freq:	Route:	06									
10 MG	OD	ORAL	(10)									
Start: 03/10/19		Stop/review:	14									
Signature: C.Pratt C.PRATT			18									
Indication: OSTEOPOROSIS			22									

Drug: CITALOPRAM			02									
Dose:	Freq:	Route:	06									
10 MG	OD	ORAL	(10)									
Start: 03/10/19		Stop/review:	14									
Signature: C.Pratt C.PRATT			18									
Indication: DEPRESSION			22									

Drug: CO-CARELDOPA			02									
Dose:	Freq:	Route:	(06)									
25/100 MG	TDS	ORAL	10									
Start: 03/10/19		Stop/review:	(14)									
Signature: **C.Pratt** C.PRATT			18									
Indication: PARKINSON'S DISEASE			(22)									

PRN Medications

			Date: → Time: ↓									
Drug: GLYCERYL TRINITRATE												
Dose: 2 PUFFS	Freq: PRN	Route: SC										
Start: 11/05/19	Stop/review:											
Signature: **C.Pratt** C.PRATT												
Indication: ANGINA												

Drug: MORPHINE												
Dose: 1-10 MG	Freq: PRN	Route: IV										
Start: 11/05/19	Stop/review:											
Signature: **C.Pratt** C.PRATT												
Indication: ANGINA												

A Case to Learn From

An elderly woman had been treated for non-ST elevation MI (NSTEMI) in the emergency department (ED) on the basis of a history of chest pain, with a raised troponin and an ECG showing T-wave inversion in the lateral leads. She divulged a history of intermittent central burning retrosternal pain, associated with nausea, on a background of several months of early satiety and weight loss. Her chronic kidney disease and AF could account for the mildly raised troponin. Old clinic letters mentioned lateral T-wave inversion on ECG. Bloods also showed iron-deficiency anaemia. These findings led to an endoscopy, revealing a malignant oesophageal stricture. Always start from scratch with your history taking and try to avoid leading and closed questions.

normally controls her COPD with inhalers alone and has no home nebulisers or long-term oxygen therapy. She also reports a worsening cough productive of green sputum. The patient is acutely dyspnoeic with an audible wheeze and some use of accessory muscles. The nurses are concerned about carbon dioxide (CO_2) retention so they have given her oxygen at 2 L/min via nasal cannulae. Please review the patient, formulate an appropriate management plan and complete the drug chart provided.

Patient Details

NAME:	MARY FINN
DOB:	12/05/1942
Hospital number:	1205427431
Weight:	65 kg
Height:	1.72 m
Consultant:	RE
Hospital/ward:	NGH/18
Current medications:	Seretide 250, salbutamol, levothyroxine, allopurinol, omeprazole
Allergies:	Ibuprofen (peptic ulcer)
Admission date:	12/09/2019

INITIAL ASSESSMENT

AIRWAY

- Patent

BREATHING

- RR 28 breaths/min
- SpO_2 83% on 2 L/min oxygen via nasal cannulae
- Widespread expiratory wheeze with inspiratory crepitations and increased vocal resonance in the right lower zone

CIRCULATION

- HR 98 bpm
- BP 120/82 mmHg
- Peripheries warm with CRT < 2 s
- JVP not raised
- Heart sounds are normal with no added sounds

DISABILITY

- Temperature 38.2°C
- GCS 15/15
- Capillary glucose level 5.4 mmol/L

EXPOSURE

- No other significant findings on examination

INITIAL INVESTIGATIONS

ECG

- Sinus rhythm at 100 bpm with no ischaemic changes

PEAK FLOW

- Not helpful in the acute management of COPD (in contrast to acute asthma)

Bloods

COMPONENTS	RESULTS	REFERENCE RANGES
Hb	159↑	120–150 g/L
WCC	17.1↑	3.7–11.1 × 10⁹/L
Neutrophils	15.3↑	1.5–7.4 × 10⁹/L
Platelets	401↑	150–400 × 10⁹/L
CRP	132↑	0–10 mg/L
Sodium	138	136–145 mmol/L
Potassium	4.2	3.5–5.1 mmol/L
Urea	5.4	2.1–7.1 mmol/L
Creatinine	112↑	44–80 µmol/L
eGFR	54↓	>60 mL/min/1.73 m²

ABG (on 2 L/min oxygen)

COMPONENTS	RESULTS	REFERENCE RANGES
pH	7.44	7.35–7.45
PaO_2	6.2↓	> 8 kPa
$PaCO_2$	4.7	4.7–6.0 kPa
HCO_3^-	26	22–26 mmol/L
Base excess	0.2	–2.0–2.0 mEq
Lactate	1.3↑	0.5–1.0 mmol/L

CXR

- Highly lucent lung fields in an otherwise appropriately penetrated film
- The diaphragm appears flat
- There is a well-circumscribed area of consolidation around the right base, with an air bronchogram. There is no pneumothorax

IMPRESSION

- Infective exacerbation of COPD and pneumonia
- Type 1 respiratory failure on ABG
- Differential diagnoses include: Pneumonia and PE

INITIAL MANAGEMENT

- Oxygen: Best delivered by Venturi mask as this allows controlled oxygen delivery. Oxygen is required to treat hypoxia, but must be used carefully in a certain cohort of COPD patients who rely on a hypoxic drive for respiration. However, in the acute setting, the patient will die faster from hypoxia than from hypercapnoea. Titrate oxygen therapy using ABG results as indicated above
- Bronchodilators: Give nebulised salbutamol 5 mg and ipratropium bromide 500 mcg immediately and then 4–6-hourly. Nebulisers can be driven with oxygen or air, depending on the result of ABGs. If the

patient is not responding, salbutamol can be given more frequently and the medical (or respiratory) registrar on call should be contacted
- Steroids: Prednisolone 40 mg oral OD (or hydrocortisone 200 mg IV if oral route is unavailable) should be given if there are no contraindications

PLUS

- Antibiotics: If indicated by fever or CXR findings. The choice depends on local policy. One option is amoxicillin 500 mg oral three times daily (TDS) or doxycycline 100 mg OD if the patient is allergic to penicillin
- IV fluids: Patients with an infection, particularly those who are septic, often require IV fluids. If the patient is shocked, use fluid challenges to assess the response to fluid resuscitation. It is important to exclude heart failure as the cause of dyspnoea before prescribing fluids. In addition, an acute exacerbation of COPD may tip a patient into right heart failure
- Consider early HDU/ITU referral: Also, contact the on-call medical (or respiratory) registrar if the patient is not responding to treatment. The patient may need some form of ventilation (CPAP if in type 1 respiratory failure or BiPAP if in type 2 respiratory failure)
- Thromboprophylaxis: Ensure that the patient is on appropriate thromboprophylaxis as per local protocol

DRUG CHART

The important aspects to consider when prescribing for this patient are:
- Allergies: Should be considered in all cases
- Oxygen therapy: If there is any known or suspected current or past CO_2 retention, for example in certain subgroups of COPD patients, then aim for target oxygen saturations 88–92%. Review regularly, titrating according to ABG results
- IV fluids: Always check all prescription charts; the patient may have a separate fluid chart and it is vital in these cases that these are cross-checked to ensure that we are not overprescribing fluids to the patient, to avoid iatrogenic fluid overload
- Regular medications: Regular inhalers should be withheld while the patient is on nebulisers

COMPLICATIONS OF COPD

- Infections, most commonly respiratory
- Pulmonary hypertension
- Depression

VACCINATION ADVICE FOR PATIENTS WITH COPD

It is advised that patients who suffer from COPD should take up an annual flu vaccination and regular vaccination against pneumococcal pneumonia. This should hopefully prevent them from getting infections as frequently.

? QUESTIONS AND ANSWERS FOR CANDIDATE

This patient has CXR changes consistent with pneumonia. What is the CURB-65 score used for and what does the acronym stand for?

CURB-65 predicts mortality in patients with pneumonia. It is used to aid decision making about inpatient versus outpatient treatment, single- versus double-agent antibiotic therapy and oral versus IV treatment. Patients are assigned 1 point for meeting each of the following criteria:
- *Confusion* (Abbreviated Mental Test Score < 8/10)
- Raised *urea* (acute and > 7 mmol/L)
- Raised *RR* (≥ 30 breaths/min)
- Low *BP* (systolic < 90 mmHg or diastolic ≤ 60 mmHg)
- *65* years or older

Score of 0–1: Indicates that outpatient treatment with oral antibiotics may be most appropriate. Score of 3–5: Indicates that the patient should be admitted and treated with IV antibiotics.

On which receptors does salbutamol act?
- Beta 2 receptors

Name three side effects of long-term prednisolone use.
- Immunosuppression
- Steroid-induced diabetes mellitus
- Central obesity, classic 'moon face' and 'buffalo hump' appearances
- Poor wound healing
- Hyperlipidaemia
- Osteopenia and osteoporosis
- Peptic ulceration
- Striae
- Muscle wasting
- Thinning of skin and hair

 A Case to Learn From

In the acute medical unit (AMU) I was clerking a young quadriplegic man with severe cerebral palsy and kyphosis who had been commenced on treatment for community-acquired pneumonia in the ED. On arrival into AMU, his oxygen saturations were 86% on air and the nurse started him on oxygen, 6 L/min by facemask. An hour later I came to clerk him and found him to be drowsy. The family were worried that this was not normal for him. Although I thought this was possibly a hypoactive delirium secondary to his infection, I thought it was worth checking an ABG, which revealed pH of 7.22 and $PaCO_2$ of 14 kPa, with PaO_2 of 16 kPa. We switched him to a Venturi mask with controlled oxygen at 24% and within 30 min he was alert and smiling. Repeat $PaCO_2$ was 8 kPa with PaO_2 11 kPa. This patient had a restrictive ventilatory defect due to his severe kyphosis which led to CO_2 retention when his oxygen saturations rose. Always be aware of CO_2 retention as a cause of drowsiness and perform an ABG early!

 Top Tip

Hypoxia will kill before hypercapnia will. In a severely hypoxic patient, start with high-flow oxygen and titrate down, rather than starting with 24% and titrating up.

Prescription and Administration Record

Name: MARY FINN	Weight: 65 KG	Known allergies:
DOB: 12/05/1942	Age: 78 YEARS	IBUPROFEN (RESPIRATORY DISTRESS)
Hospital number: 12.0542.7431	Consultant: RE	Signature: Date: R.Edmond 12/09/19 RICHARD EDMOND

Once-Only Medications

Date	Time	Medicine (approved name)	Dose	Route	Prescriber – sign and print	Time given	Given by
12/09/19	1600	SALBUTAMOL (DRIVEN WITH OXYGEN)	5 MG	NEB	R. Edmond RICHARD EDMOND		
12/09/19	1600	IPRATROPIUM BROMIDE (DRIVEN WITH OXYGEN)	500 MCG	NEB	R. Edmond RICHARD EDMOND		
12/09/19	1645	AMOXICILLIN	500 MG	ORAL	R. Edmond RICHARD EDMOND		
12/09/19	1645	PREDNISOLONE	30 MG	ORAL	R. Edmond RICHARD EDMOND		
12/09/19	1800	ENOXAPARIN	20 MG	SC	R. Edmond RICHARD EDMOND		

Oxygen therapy

Start		Route				Stop	
Date	Time	Mask (%)	Prongs (L/min)	Prescriber – sign and print	Administered by	Date	Time
12/09/19	1600	VENTURI (60)		R. Edmond RICHARD EDMOND			

VTE Prophylaxis

VTE risk assessment: Yes [X] Prophylaxis not required [ ] Contraindicated [ ]	Comment: Signature: R. Edmond RICHARD EDMOND Date: 12/09/19

		Date: → Time: ↓	13/09						
Drug: ENOXAPARIN			1800						
Dose: 20 MG	Freq: OD	Route: SC							
Start: 13/09/19	Stop/review:								
Signature: R. Edmond RICHARD EDMOND									

Regular Medications

			Date: →	12./9							
			Time: ↓								
Drug: SERETIDE 250 (SALMETEROL 25 MCG/FLUTICASONE 250 MCG)			02								
Dose:	Freq:	Route:	(06)								
2 PUFFS	BD	INH	10								
Start: 12/09/19		Stop/review:	(14)								
Signature: R. Edmond RICHARD EDMOND			18								
Indication: COPD			22								

Drug: LEVOTHYROXINE			02								
Dose:	Freq:	Route:	(06)								
50 MCG	OD	ORAL	10								
Start: 12/09/19		Stop/review:	14								
Signature: R. Edmond RICHARD EDMOND			18								
Indication: HYPOTHYROIDISM			22								

Drug: ALLOPURINOL			02								
Dose:	Freq:	Route:	06								
100 MG	OD	ORAL	(10)								
Start: 12/09/19		Stop/review:	14								
Signature: R. Edmond RICHARD EDMOND			18								
Indication: GOUT PROPHYLAXIS			22								

Continued

Prescription and Administration Record—cont'd

Drug: OMEPRAZOLE	02										
Dose: / Freq: / Route: / 06	06										
20 MG / OD / ORAL / (10)	(10)										
Start: 12/09/19 / Stop/review: / 14	14										
Signature: R. Edmond RICHARD EDMOND / 18	18										
Indication: GASTRO-OESOPHAGEAL REFLUX DISEASE / 22	22										

Drug: AMOXICILLIN	02										
Dose: / Freq: / Route: / (06)	(06)										
500 MG / TDS / ORAL / 10	10										
Start: 12/09/19 / Stop/review: / (14)	(14)										
Signature: R. Edmond RICHARD EDMOND / 18	18										
Indication: COPD EXACERBATION / (22)	(22)										

Drug: PREDNISOLONE	02										
Dose: / Freq: / Route: / 06	06										
30 MG / OD / ORAL / (10)	(10)										
Start: 12/09/19 / Stop/review: / 14	14										
Signature: R. Edmond RICHARD EDMOND / 18	18										
Indication: COPD EXACERBATION / 22	22										

Prescription and Administration Record—cont'd

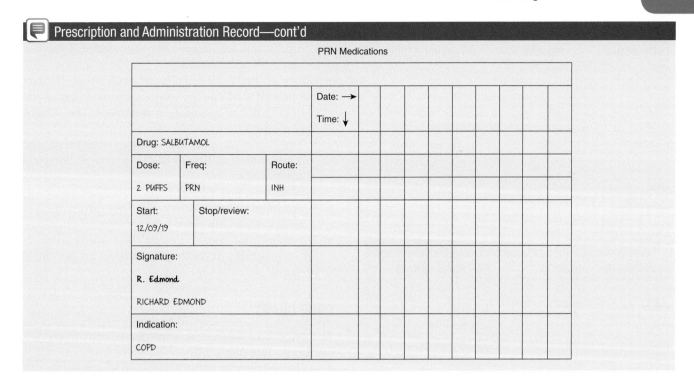

PRN Medications

			Date: →						
			Time: ↓						
Drug: SALBUTAMOL									
Dose:	Freq:		Route:						
2 PUFFS	PRN		INH						
Start:	Stop/review:								
12/09/19									
Signature:									
R. Edmond									
RICHARD EDMOND									
Indication:									
COPD									

STATION 11.4: EXACERBATION OF ASTHMA

SCENARIO

You are the junior doctor in the medical assessment unit. The nurse asks you to see Mark McDonald, a 28-year-old male, who has a background of asthma and has become breathless. Please review the patient, formulate an appropriate management plan and complete the drug chart provided.

Patient Details

NAME:	**MARK MCDONALD**
DOB:	25/03/1992
Hospital number:	2503920145
Weight:	83 kg
Height:	1.86 m
Consultant:	MJS
Hospital/ward:	RIE/45
Current medications:	Salbutamol
Allergies:	Penicillin (facial swelling, breathlessness)
Admission date:	15/09/2019

INITIAL ASSESSMENT

AIRWAY

- Patent

BREATHING

- RR 32 breaths/min
- SpO$_2$ 88% on 2 L/min oxygen via nasal cannulae
- Dyspnoeic and distressed, struggling to speak in sentences, using accessory muscles
- Audible expiratory wheeze throughout

CIRCULATION

- HR 128 bpm
- BP 148/86 mmHg
- Peripheries warm with CRT < 2 s
- JVP not raised
- Heart sounds are normal with no added sounds

DISABILITY

- Temperature 36.9°C
- GCS 15/15
- Capillary glucose level 6.0 mmol/L

EXPOSURE

- No other significant findings on examination

INITIAL INVESTIGATIONS

ECG

- Sinus tachycardia at 138 bpm with no ischaemic changes

Peak Flow

Peak expiratory flow rate (PEFR)	140	L/min
Predicted PEFR	530	L/min

Bloods

COMPONENTS	RESULTS	REFERENCE RANGES
Hb	153	130–170 g/L
WCC	11.6↑	3.7–11.1 × 10⁹/L
Neutrophils	9.8↑	1.5–7.4 × 10⁹/L
Platelets	475↑	150–400 × 10⁹/L
Sodium	136	136–145 mmol/L
Potassium	4.3	3.5–5.1 mmol/L
Urea	4.2	2.1–7.1 mmol/L
Creatinine	102	62–106 µmol/L

ABG (on 2 L/min Oxygen)

COMPONENTS	RESULTS	REFERENCE RANGES
pH	7.52↑	7.35–7.45
PaO_2	7.8↓	> 8 kPa
$PaCO_2$	2.1↓	4.7–6.0 kPa
HCO_3^-	30↑	22–26 mmol/L
Base excess	1.8	–2.0–2.0 mEq
Lactate	0.8	0.5–1.0 mmol/L

CXR

- Hyperexpanded lungs, clear lung fields
- No pneumothoraces

IMPRESSION

- Life-threatening asthma attack with SpO_2 88% on 2 L/min oxygen and PEFR < 33% of predicted
- Differential diagnoses include: Anaphylaxis, pneumonia and PE

INITIAL MANAGEMENT

- Senior input: Call for help early if the patient is unwell
- Oxygen: Via a non-rebreathe bag or Venturi mask, titrate according to ABG results. Aim for an oxygen saturation of 94–98%. In contrast to COPD patients, abolishing the hypoxic drive for respiration in asthmatic patients is not usually an issue. However, any severe type 1 respiratory failure can lead to tiring, and subsequent type 2 respiratory failure
- Bronchodilators: Give nebulised salbutamol 5 mg, repeated every 10 min if necessary (back to back). Consider nebulised ipratropium bromide 500 mcg 4–6-hourly in severe or life-threatening episodes
- Steroids: Give prednisolone 40 mg PO or hydrocortisone 200 mg IV if there are no contraindications. Remember that IV steroids do not work more quickly than oral steroids unless the patient has specific issues such as GI problems (impairing absorption)

PLUS

- IV fluids and antibiotics: May be needed if there is evidence of an infection
- Consider early HDU/ITU referral: Also, contact the on-call medical (or respiratory) registrar if the patient is not responding to treatment. The patient may require:
  - Ventilatory support: CPAP if the patient is in type 1 respiratory failure or BiPAP if in type 2 respiratory failure
  - Magnesium sulphate: 2 g IV over 20 min
  - Aminophylline infusion: Usually given in ITU with cardiac and renal function monitoring
- Thromboprophylaxis: Ensure that the patient is on appropriate thromboprophylaxis as per local protocol

DRUG CHART

The important aspects to consider when prescribing for this patient are:
- Allergies: Should be considered in all cases
- Oxygen therapy: Should be considered in all cases. When prescribing oxygen therapy, indicate the device, desired oxygen flow and target saturations
- IV fluids: Always check all prescription charts. The patient may have a separate fluid chart and it is vital in these cases that it is stopped
- Regular medications: Regular inhalers should be withheld while the patient is on nebulisers

Assessing severity of acute asthma

MODERATE	ACUTE SEVERE	LIFE-THREATENING
• Increasing symptoms • Peak expiratory flow > 50–75% of best or predicted • No features of acute severe asthma	Any one of: • Peak expiratory flow 33–50% of best or predicted • RR > 25 breaths/min • HR > 110 bpm • Unable to complete sentences in one breath	Acute severe asthma plus any one of: • Peak expiratory flow < 33% of best or predicted • Oxygen saturation < 92% • PaO_2 < 8 kPa • Normal $PaCO_2$ (4.6–6 kPa) • Silent chest • Cyanosis • Poor respiratory effort • Arrhythmia • Exhaustion, altered conscious level

INTERPRETING ABGS IN ASTHMA

All patients are likely to be hypoxic. Furthermore, as they are hyperventilating, their $PaCO_2$ should be low, giving a respiratory alkalosis (low H^+/high pH). As the patient tires, $PaCO_2$ rises. A normal $PaCO_2$ and normal

Prescription and Administration Record

Name: MARK MCDONALD	Weight: 83 KG	Known allergies: PENICILLIN (FACIAL SWELLING/ BREATHLESSNESS)
DOB: 25/03/1992	Age: 28 YEARS	
Hospital number: 2503920145	Consultant: MJS	Signature: Date: **M. Slack** 15/09/2019 MATT SLACK

Once-Only Medications

Date	Time	Medicine (approved name)	Dose	Route	Prescriber – sign and print	Time given	Given by
15/09/19	1100	SALBUTAMOL (DRIVEN WITH OXYGEN)	5 MG	NEB	**M. Slack** MATT SLACK		
15/09/19	1100	PREDNISOLONE	40 MG	ORAL	**M. Slack** MATT SLACK		
15/09/19	1115	IPRATROPIUM (DRIVEN WITH OXYGEN)	250 MCG	NEB	**M. Slack** MATT SLACK		

Oxygen Therapy

Start						Stop	
Date	Time	Mask (%)	Prongs (L/min)	Prescriber – sign and print	Administered by	Date	Time
15/09/19	1100	NON-REBREATHE MASK	15 L/MIN	**M. Slack** MATT SLACK			

VTE Prophylaxis

VTE risk assessment: Yes [X]	Comment:
Prophylaxis not required [ ]	Signature: **M. Slack** MATT SLACK
Contraindicated [ ]	Date: 15/09/19

	Date: → Time: ↓	15/9						
Drug: ENOXAPARIN	1800							
Dose: 20 MG	Freq: OD	Route: SC						
Start:	Stop/review:							
Signature:								

Continued

Regular Medications

			Date: →								
			Time: ↓								
Drug: PREDNISOLONE			02								
Dose:	Freq:	Route:	06								
40 MG	OD	ORAL	(10)								
Start: 15/09/19	Stop/review:		14								
Signature: **M. Slack** MATT SLACK			18								
Indication: ASTHMA			22								

Drug: IPRATROPIUM			02								
Dose:	Freq:	Route:	06								
250 MCG	TDS	NEB	10								
Start: 15/09/19	Stop/review:		14								
Signature: **M. Slack** MATT SLACK			18								
Indication: ASTHMA			22								

PRN Medications

			Date: →								
			Time: ↓								
Drug: SALBUTAMOL											
Dose:	Freq:	Route:									
2 PUFFS	PRN	INH									
Start: 12/09/19	Stop/review:										
Signature: **M. Slack** MATT SLACK											
Indication: ASTHMA											

H^+/pH can signify a severe episode, and high $PaCO_2$ and H^+/low pH signify a life-threatening episode. Note also that, as the patient improves, a low $PaCO_2$ will return to normal.

COMPLICATIONS OF ASTHMA

- Pneumothorax
- Respiratory failure
- Respiratory arrest
- Cardiac arrest

QUESTIONS AND ANSWERS FOR CANDIDATE

Name three drugs that may cause an exacerbation in sensitive asthmatics.
- Beta-blockers: For example, bisoprolol
- Non-steroidal anti-inflammatory drugs (NSAIDs): For example, ibuprofen
- ACEi: For example, ramipril
- Verapamil
- Adenosine
- Aspirin

Name three potential triggers of asthma exacerbation, other than drugs.
- Viral illness
- Allergens; for example, pollen, dust, animal hair, food allergens
- Sudden temperature change
- Exercise

Aspirin-induced asthma is characterised by a triad of which three characteristics?
- Asthma
- Aspirin intolerance
- Nasal polyposis

A Case to Learn From

A middle-aged woman had been admitted the previous day with an exacerbation of her asthma and had been transferred to the ward for regular salbutamol nebulisers. She told me that she felt that her breathing had deteriorated in the last couple of hours before she was transferred, and she was now unable to speak in full sentences. On reviewing her drug chart, I noticed that she had not received the steroids that she had been prescribed on admission. I repeated an ABG which showed a rising $PaCO_2$. I commenced steroid therapy, along with back-to-back salbutamol nebulisers. Do not assume drugs have been given just because they have been prescribed and remember that asthmatics can deteriorate even after they have been admitted and 'stabilised'. Adequate monitoring on an acute medical or respiratory unit is important in detecting this.

Top Tip

A quiet wheeze is not necessarily a sign of a mild exacerbation. Quiet wheeze may be due to poor air entry with severe bronchoconstriction.

STATION 11.5: HYPERKALAEMIA

SCENARIO

You are the junior doctor in the medical assessment unit and you have been asked to see Peter Jones, an 82-year-old patient, who has been admitted from the ED with a 3-day history of vomiting and dehydration. You are asked to chase his bloods and review him overnight. The patient's vomiting has settled with intramuscular (IM) cyclizine but he feels thirsty. His regular medications are aspirin, ramipril, bisoprolol, co-amilofruse, simvastatin and spironolactone. Please review the patient, formulate an appropriate management plan and complete the drug chart provided.

Patient Details

NAME:	PETER JONES
DOB:	22/06/1938
Hospital number:	2206381254
Weight:	65 kg
Height:	1.73 m
Consultant:	MJK
Hospital/ward:	RIE/14
Current medications:	Aspirin, ramipril, bisoprolol, co-amilofruse, simvastatin and spironolactone
Allergies:	Erythromycin (rash)
Admission date:	10/09/2019

INITIAL ASSESSMENT

AIRWAY
- Patent

BREATHING
- RR 20 breaths/min
- SpO_2 99% on air
- Chest is clear on auscultation

CIRCULATION
- HR 103 bpm
- BP 110/68 mmHg
- Peripheries cool with CRT 5 s
- JVP not visible, dry mucous membranes
- Heart sounds are normal with no added sounds

DISABILITY
- Temperature 36.9°C
- GCS 15/15
- Capillary glucose level 6.2 mmol/L

EXPOSURE
- No other significant findings on examination

INITIAL INVESTIGATIONS

ECG

Sinus rhythm, no prolongation of the PR interval or QRS complex.

Bloods

COMPONENTS	RESULTS	REFERENCE RANGES
Hb	130	130–170 g/L
WCC	11	3.7–11.1 × 10⁹/L
Neutrophils	8.4↑	1.5–7.4 × 10⁹/L
Platelets	240	150–400 × 10⁹/L
Sodium	135↓	136–145 mmol/L
Potassium	7.1↑	3.5–5.1 mmol/L
Urea	21↑	2.1–7.1 mmol/L
Creatinine	192↑	62–106 µmol/L

ABG

COMPONENTS	RESULTS	REFERENCE RANGES
pH	7.4	7.35–7.45
PaO$_2$	7.8↓	> 8 kPa
PaCO$_2$	5.0	4.7–6.0 kPa
HCO$_3^-$	30↑	22–26 mmol/L
Base excess	1.8	–2.0–2.0 mEq
Lactate	0.8	0.5–1.0 mmol/L
Sodium	134↓	136–145 mmol/L
Potassium	6.9↑	3.5–5.1 mmol/L

IMPRESSION

- This is hyperkalaemia secondary to dehydration, AKI, medications and/or metabolic acidosis
- Differential diagnosis includes: Spurious results; for example, sample taken from drip arm, long tourniquet time, raised WCC or platelet count

INITIAL MANAGEMENT

- Cardiac stabilisation:
  - Calcium chloride or gluconate: If there are ECG changes associated with myocardial instability, give IV 10% calcium chloride or calcium gluconate titrated in 1-mL aliquots to resolution of ECG changes. If no ECG monitoring is available, give 10 mL IV calcium chloride or gluconate slowly and repeat the ECG. This stabilises the myocardium but does not lower the serum potassium. Note that excessive calcium chloride or gluconate can cause cardiac arrest. Therefore, always titrate to the ECG if available
- Reduce serum potassium:

- Salbutamol: Nebulised salbutamol 5 mg is quick to administer and will drive some of the extracellular potassium into cells
- Insulin: Give 10 units Actrapid in 50 mL 50% dextrose (or equivalent) IV. This drives extracellular potassium into the cells. Blood glucose must be monitored closely. A slow infusion of 10% dextrose at 10–50 mL/h may be required to maintain the blood glucose
- Sodium bicarbonate: This may be required if the patient is acidotic
- Eliminate the potassium:
  - IV fluids: This patient has clinical signs of hypovolaemia. Give a fluid challenge, for example, 500 mL 0.9% sodium chloride over 15 min, and assess the response. Repeat if required. Once the deficit has been replaced, prescribe maintenance fluids, taking into account ongoing losses. Potassium is eliminated via diuresis

OTHER CONSIDERATIONS

- Catheter: This helps exclude a postrenal cause of renal impairment and allows accurate urine output measurement
- Withhold nephrotoxic drugs: Medications, for example, ramipril, co-amilofruse and spironolactone, may impair renal function and should be withheld. Spironolactone and ramipril will also increase serum potassium
- Haemodialysis or haemofiltration: May be required if the above measures are effective
- Prescribe appropriate thromboprophylaxis: Note that in patients with renal impairment, for example, eGFR<30 mL/min, heparin 5000 units twice daily (BD) is more appropriate than low-molecular-weight heparin

DRUG CHART

The important aspects to consider when prescribing for this patient are:
- Allergies: Should be considered in all cases
- Oxygen therapy: Should be considered in all cases. When prescribing oxygen therapy, indicate the device, desired oxygen flow and target saturations
- IV fluids: To treat the AKI and flush out the potassium. Plasmalyte is widely used as a resuscitation fluid but, as it contains potassium, it should not be used in this scenario
- Regular medications: Some of these may be contributing to hyperkalaemia and AKI, and should be withheld until these have normalised

Prescription and Administration Record

Prescription and Administration Record

Name: PETER JONES	Weight: 65 KG	Known allergies:
DOB: 22/06/1938	Age: 82 YEARS	ERYTHROMYCIN (RASH)
Hospital number: 2206381254	Consultant: MJK	Signature: Date: **M. Khan** 10/09/19 MO KHAN

Once-Only Medications

Date	Time	Medicine (approved name)	Dose	Route	Prescriber – sign and print	Time given	Given by
10/09/19	2040	CALCIUM GLUCONATE 10% (TITRATE TO ECG)	1–10 ML	IV	**M. Khan** MO KHAN		
10/09/19	2050	SALBUTAMOL (DRIVEN IN AIR)	5 MG	NEB	**M. Khan** MO KHAN		
10/09/19	2050	ENOXAPARIN	20 MG	SC	**M. Khan** MO KHAN		

Oxygen Therapy

Start		Route				Stop	
Date	Time	Mask (%)	Prongs (L/min)	Prescriber – sign and print	Administered by	Date	Time
10/09/19	2040		2 L/MIN	**M. Khan** MO KHAN			

VTE Prophylaxis

VTE risk assessment: Yes [X] Prophylaxis not required [ ] Contraindicated [ ]	Comment: Signature: **M. Khan** MO KHAN Date: 10/09/19

		Date: →	10/9						
		Time: ↓							
Drug: HEPARIN			1000						
Dose: 5000 UNITS	Freq: BD	Route: SC							
			22						
Start: 10/09	Stop/review:								
Signature: **M. Khan** MO KHAN									

Continued

Regular Medications

			Date: →	10/9							
			Time: ↓								
Drug: ASPIRIN			02								
Dose:	Freq:	Route:	06								
75 MG	OD	ORAL	(10)								
Start: 10/09/19		Stop/review:	14								
Signature: **M. Khan** MO KHAN			18								
Indication: SECONDARY PREVENTION OF ACS			22								

			Date:								
Drug: RAMIPRIL			02								
Dose:	Freq:	Route:	06								
5 MG	BD	ORAL	(10)			Stopped due to hyperkalaemia and acute kidney injury 20/11/19 **M. Khan** (MO KHAN)					
Start: 10/09/19		Stop/review:	14								
Signature: **M. Khan** MO KHAN			(18)								
Indication: SECONDARY PREVENTION OF ACS			22								

			Date:								
Drug: BISOPROLOL			02								
Dose:	Freq:	Route:	06								
10 MG	OD	ORAL	(10)								
Start: 10/09/19		Stop/review:	14			Stopped due to hypotension 20/11/19 **M. Khan** (MO KHAN)					
Signature: **M. Khan** MO KHAN			18								
Indication: SECONDARY PREVENTION OF ACS			22								

Prescription and Administration Record—cont'd

Drug:			02									
CO–AMILOFRUSE 5/40												

Dose:	Freq:	Route:	06									
1 SACHET	OD	ORAL	(10)									

Start: 10/09/19	Stop/review:	14							

Stopped due to hyperkalaemia and acute kidney injury 20/11/19 **M. Khan** (MO KHAN)

Signature:	18								
M. Khan									
MO KHAN									

Indication:	22								
SECONDARY PREVENTION OF ACS									

Drug: SIMVASTATIN			02									

Dose:	Freq:	Route:	06									
40 MG	ON	ORAL	10									

Start: 10/09/19	Stop/review:	14							

Signature:	18								
M. Khan									
MO KHAN									

Indication:	(22)								
SECONDARY PREVENTION OF ACS									

Drug: SPIRONOLACTONE			02									

Dose:	Freq:	Route:	06									
25 MG	OD	ORAL	(10)									

Start: 10/09/19	Stop/review:	14							

Stopped due to hyperkalaemia and acute kidney injury 20/11/19 **M. Khan** (M. KHAN)

Signature:	18								
M. Khan									
MO KHAN									

Indication:	22								
MODERATE HEART FAILURE									

Continued

Prescription and Administration Record—cont'd

Fluid Prescriptions

Date	Fluid	Additive	Volume	Route	Rate	Signature	Given	Batch
10/09/19	10% DEXTROSE	10 UNITS OF INSULIN (ACTRAPID)	250 ML	IV	OVER 30 MIN	M. Khan MO KHAN		
10/09/19	0.9% SODIUM CHLORIDE	NONE	500 ML	IV	OVER 20 MIN	M. Khan MO KHAN		

Further fluid prescriptions will be determined by the patient's response to this fluid challenge: Repeat observations are performed after the initial bag had gone through. There is a transient improvement with SpO₂ 99%, RR 18 breaths/min, HR 98 bpm, BP 116/72 mmHg, temperature is 36.9°C. His peripheries are cool and the JVP is not visible. He is improving but still hypovolaemic.

Date	Fluid	Additive	Volume	Route	Rate	Signature	Given	Batch
10/09/19	0.9% SODIUM CHLORIDE	NONE	1 L	IV	OVER 20 MIN	M. Khan MO KHAN		

Further fluid prescriptions will be determined by the patient's response to this fluid challenge: This patient needs reassessing before more fluids can be prescribed.

COMPLICATIONS OF HYPERKALAEMIA

- Cardiac arrhythmia
- Cardiac arrest

 QUESTIONS AND ANSWERS FOR CANDIDATE

Name three ECG changes that are associated with hyperkalaemia.
- Tall tented T waves
- Flattened P waves
- Loss of P waves
- Broad QRS complexes
- Sine-wave pattern

What is the role of calcium gluconate in the treatment of hyperkalaemia?
- Calcium gluconate stabilises the myocardium to prevent arrhythmia
- It does not have any role in reducing the serum potassium level

Name a metabolic condition that might be associated with hyperkalaemia.
- Any cause of metabolic acidosis; for example, type IV renal tubular acidosis, addisonian crisis or Addison's disease and adrenal insufficiency

 A Case to Learn From

A patient who was admitted with chronic myeloid leukaemia was obese with very difficult venous access. The potassium on admission was 9.3 mmol/L. There were no hyperkalaemic changes on the ECG but we treated with calcium gluconate and started insulin and dextrose infusion. The repeat potassium was 8.9 mmol/L. Were these spurious results due to a long tourniquet time or due to his lymphocytosis? An ABG showed potassium of 5.3 mmol/L and we were able to stop the treatment.

Top Tip

If hyperkalaemia is diagnosed on a venous blood gas or ABG sample, always take a serum blood potassium level to confirm, but do not necessarily delay treatment while awaiting the result.

STATION 11.6: BOWEL OBSTRUCTION

SCENARIO

You are the junior doctor working on a general surgical ward and are asked to see William McDonald, an 80-year-old man, who has presented with abdominal pain, severe nausea and vomiting. He is an average-sized man who is confused and looks dehydrated. On closer questioning, you discover that he has not had a bowel motion for the last 5 or 6 days. His past history is remarkable for ischaemic heart disease. He is on aspirin, simvastatin, ramipril and atenolol for a previous MI, and other medications. Please review the patient, formulate an appropriate management plan and complete the drug chart provided.

Patient Details

NAME:	WILLIAM MCDONALD
DOB:	07/06/1940
Hospital number:	0706401225
Weight:	70 kg
Height:	1.78 m
Consultant:	DNA
Hospital/ward:	WGH/27
Current medications:	Aspirin, ramipril, atenolol, atorvastatin, metformin, Movicol
Allergies:	Penicillin (rash)
Admission date:	10/09/2019

INITIAL ASSESSMENT

AIRWAY

- Patent

BREATHING

- RR 18 breaths/min
- SpO$_2$ 93% on air
- Chest is clear on auscultation

CIRCULATION

- HR 96 bpm
- BP 102/86 mmHg
- Pulse is weak
- Peripheries cool with prolonged CRT of 7 s
- Heart sounds are normal with no added sounds

DISABILITY

- Temperature 37.4°C
- GCS 15/15
- Capillary glucose level 6.0 mmol/L

EXPOSURE

- Abdomen distended, with generalised tenderness. No peritonism. Fullness in the right iliac fossa
- Loud, 'tinkling' bowel sounds
- Per rectum (PR) examination reveals no masses

INITIAL INVESTIGATIONS

ECG

- Sinus rhythm at 92 bpm

Urine Dipstick

Blood	++
Leukocytes	+
Nitrites	–
Protein	+
Bilirubin	–
Ketones	+++

Bloods

COMPONENTS	RESULTS	REFERENCE RANGES
Hb	123↓	130–170 g/L
WCC	9.1	3.7–11.1 × 10⁹/L
Neutrophils	6.8	1.5–7.4 × 10⁹/L
Platelets	324	150–400 × 10⁹/L
Bilirubin	16	0–21 µmol/L
Alanine aminotransferase (ALT)	43↑	0–41 IU/L
Alkaline phosphatase (ALP)	165↑	40–129 IU/L
Gamma-glutamyl transferase (GGT)	98↑	6–42 IU/L
Sodium	134↓	136–145 mmol/L
Potassium	3.0↓	3.5–5.1 mmol/L
Urea	8.1↑	2.1–7.1 mmol/L
Creatinine	129↑	62–106 µmol/L
CRP	8	0–10 mg/L
Amylase	49	28–100 IU/L
Lactate	1.0	0.5–2.2 mmol/L

ABG

COMPONENTS	RESULTS	REFERENCE RANGES
pH	7.28↓	7.35–7.45
PaO$_2$	9.7	> 8 kPa
PaCO$_2$	3.5↓	4.7–6.0 kPa
HCO$_3^-$	13↓	22–26 mmol/L
Base excess	–5.6↓	–2.0–2.0 mEq
Lactate	6.4↑	0.5–1.0 mmol/L

ABDOMINAL X-RAY (AXR)

- Dilated small bowel proximal to the caecum with no gas seen in the distal bowel

Table 11.1	Potential outcomes following a fluid challenge	
RAPID RESPONDER	**TRANSIENT RESPONDER**	**NON-RESPONDER**
• These patients respond fully to the challenge and become haemodynamically stable • Fluid deficit has been replaced • May still require maintenance IV fluids	• These patients have a brief response to the challenge but return to being haemodynamically unstable • They continue to have a fluid deficit which needs to be replaced	• In these cases, there is no response to the fluid challenge • This implies either the fluid deficit is so large that the fluid administered is not sufficient for any correction of haemodynamic instability, or the shock is not hypovolaemic

ERECT CXR

• Clear lung fields, no evidence of pneumoperitoneum

IMPRESSION

• This is small-bowel obstruction that has resulted in dehydration, metabolic acidosis, hypokalaemia and hypovolaemic shock
• The patient requires fluid resuscitation and intervention to decompress the distended bowel and prevent perforation

INITIAL MANAGEMENT

• Decompress the stomach: This patient should be made nil by mouth and a wide-bore nasogastric tube should be inserted
• Fluid resuscitation: This patient is peripherally shut down, has a relative tachycardia (on atenolol) and is hypotensive with a narrow pulse pressure. He needs aggressive fluid resuscitation to restore organ perfusion. Obtain IV access with two wide-bore cannulae and give 500 mL 0.9% sodium chloride into each cannula. IV potassium replacement may be required but should not be given in resuscitation fluid. Once the deficit has been replaced, maintenance fluids, including ongoing losses, can be prescribed. There are three potential outcomes following a fluid challenge (Table 11.1)
• Catheter: A urinary catheter should be inserted to monitor urine output and help assess fluid balance
• Analgesia: Use the World Health Organization (WHO) analgesic ladder (Fig. 11.1). Give paracetamol 1 g) IV four times daily (QDS). IV/SC/IM morphine should be titrated to pain
• Antiemetic: Cyclizine 50 mg IV/IM/SC 6–8-hourly is an appropriate choice. Ondansetron 4 mg IV/IM/SC 6–8-hourly can also be used. Metoclopramide should be avoided as it is a prokinetic and therefore may exacerbate the symptoms of bowel obstruction
• Thromboprophylaxis: Ensure that the patient is on appropriate thromboprophylaxis as per local protocol and consider any potential operation. Liaise

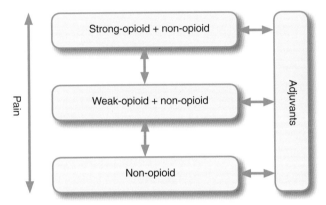

Fig. 11.1 WHO analgesic ladder.

with seniors before prescribing anticoagulants in emergency surgical patients
• Early senior review: Once stable the patient will need investigations to identify the cause of the obstruction and allow potential operative planning

DRUG CHART

The important aspects to consider when prescribing for this patient are:
• Allergies: Should be considered in all cases
• Oxygen therapy: Should be considered in all cases. When prescribing oxygen therapy, indicate the device, desired oxygen flow and target saturations
• IV fluids: To replace losses and then to maintain hydration status and to replace electrolytes
• Nil by mouth: The oral route is not available for this patient and an alternative route must therefore be considered
• Withhold regular medications: Ramipril should be withheld until the renal function has improved. Also withhold the atenolol, statin and metformin as these increase lactic acidosis and are contraindicated in AKI
• Impaired renal function: This will mean slower excretion of opiate metabolites, increasing the likelihood of opiate toxicity. Prescribe opiate analgesia with caution. Consider oxycodone instead of morphine sulphate (MST)

Prescription and Administration Record

Prescription and Administration Record

Name: WILLIAM MCDONALD	Weight: 70 KG	Known allergies:
DOB: 07/06/1940	Age: 80 YEARS	PENICILLIN (RASH)
		Signature: Date:
Hospital number: 0706401225	Consultant: DNA	**D. Akin** 10/09/2019
		DEBBIE AKIN

Once-Only Medications

Date	Time	Medicine (approved name)	Dose	Route	Prescriber – sign and print	Time given	Given by
10/09/19	1400	MORPHINE (TITRATE TO PAIN)	1–10 MG	IV	**D. Akin** DEBBIE AKIN		
10/09/19	1400	CYCLIZINE	50 MG	IV	**D. Akin** DEBBIE AKIN		
10/09/19	1400	PARACETAMOL	1 G	IV	**D. Akin** DEBBIE AKIN		

Oxygen Therapy

Start		Route				Stop	
Date	Time	Mask (%)	Prongs (L/min)	Prescriber – sign andprint	Administered by	Date	Time
10/09/19	1400	NASAL CANNULA	4 L/MIN	**D. Akin** DEBBIE AKIN			

VTE Prophylaxis

VTE risk assessment:	Comment: AWAITING POSSIBLE SURGERY
Yes [ ]	Signature: **D. Akin** DEBBIE AKIN
Prophylaxis not required [ ]	Date: 20/11/19
Contraindicated [X]	

			Date: →							
			Time: ↓							
Drug:										
Dose:	Freq:	Route:								
Start:	Stop/review:									
Signature:										

Continued

Regular Medications

		Date: →	10/09								
		Time: ↓									
Drug: ASPIRIN		02									
Dose:	Freq:	Route:	06								
75 MG	OD	ORAL	(10)								
Start: 20/11/19	Stop/review:	14									
Signature: D. Akin DEBBIE AKIN		18									
Indication: SECONDARY PREVENTION OF ACS		22									

Drug: RAMIPRIL		02									
Dose:	Freq:	Route:	06								
5 MG	BD	ORAL	(10)								
Start: 20/11/19	Stop/review:	14									
Signature: D. Akin DEBBIE AKIN		(18)									
Indication: SECONDARY PREVENTION OF ACS		22									

Drug: Atenolol		02									
Dose:	Freq:	Route:	06								
25 MG	OD	PO	(10)								
Start: 20/11/19	Stop/review:	14									
Signature: D. Akin DEBBIE AKIN		18									
Indication: SECONDARY PREVENTION OF ACS		22									

Prescription and Administration Record—cont'd

Drug: ATORVASTATIN		02								
Dose:	Freq:	Route:	06							
80 MG	OD	ORAL	(10)							
Start: 20/11/19	Stop/review:		14							
Signature: D. Akin DEBBIE AKIN			18							
Indication: SECONDARY PREVENTION OF ACS			22							

Drug: METFORMIN		02								
Dose:	Freq:	Route:	06							
500 MG	OD	ORAL	(10)							
Start: 20/11/19	Stop/review:		14							
Signature: D. Akin DEBBIE AKIN			18							
Indication: DIABETES			22							

Drug: MOVICOL		02								
Dose:	Freq:	Route:	06							
1 SACHET	BD	ORAL	(10)							
Start: 20/11/19	Stop/review:		14							
Signature: D. Akin DEBBIE AKIN			(18)							
Indication: CONSTIPATION			22							

Continued

Prescription and Administration Record—cont'd

Fluid Prescriptions

Date	Fluid	Additive	Volume	Route	Rate	Signature	Given	Batch
10/09/19	HARTMANN'S SOLUTION	NONE	500 ML	IV	OVER 20 MIN	D. Akin DEBBIE AKIN		
10/09/19	HARTMANN'S SOLUTION	NONE	500 ML	IV	O ver 20 MIN	D. Akin DEBBIE AKIN		
10/09/19	HARTMANN'S SOLUTION	NONE	1000 ML	IV	O ver 20 MIN	D. Akin DEBBIE AKIN		

FLUID OVERLOAD

Given his age and background of ischaemic heart disease, there may be some concern regarding fluid overload in this patient. However, the fluid deficit is likely to be large for two reasons:

- 1. The obstruction is likely to have been developing for several days
- 2. In addition to obvious fluid losses from vomiting, GI secretions collecting proximal to the obstruction (third-space losses) will be adding to the fluid deficit

These, combined with his clinical evidence of shock (reduced peripheral perfusion, confusion), mean that he is likely to be in a large negative fluid balance. To overload this patient, we would first have to replace the entire fluid deficit and then add enough further fluid to compromise his cardiac output. This would take a substantial amount of fluids in this scenario.

COMPLICATIONS OF SMALL-BOWEL OBSTRUCTION

- Aspiration of gastric content
- Dehydration and electrolyte disturbance, due to vomiting
- Bowel perforation
- Intra-abdominal sepsis

QUESTIONS AND ANSWERS FOR CANDIDATE

What is Rigler's sign?
This is seen on AXR when there is large pneumoperitoneum. When air is present both inside and outside the bowel wall, both the inner and outer edges of the bowel wall can be seen on the AXR.

Why is metoclopramide contraindicated in bowel obstruction?
Metoclopramide is prokinetic and could therefore cause severe pain and even perforation of obstructed bowel by stimulating peristalsis.

Name three potential causes of bowel obstruction.
- Previous abdominal surgery causing adhesions
- Inflammatory bowel disease, particularly Crohn's disease
- Other bowel pathology, including bowel cancer
- Intestinal malformation
- Hernias
- Constipation
- Volvulus

A Case to Learn From

While working in ITU, I cared for a 70-year-old woman who had been admitted to us postoperatively. She initially presented to the ED with severe abdominal pain. She had been taking oxycodone for back pain and had been suffering from constipation for several months. On initial examination, her abdomen was peritonitic and venous blood gas showed a metabolic acidosis. Her AXR showed dilated large-bowel loops and faecal loading and her erect CXR showed pneumoperitoneum. She required a laparotomy for sigmoid perforation which was secondary to constipation. The most important lesson from this case was always to consider a prescription of laxatives to accompany your opiate prescriptions.

Top Tip

Constant severe pain and peritonism are very concerning features, indicating that perforation may have already occurred.

STATION 11.7: ABDOMINAL SEPSIS

SCENARIO

You are the junior doctor working on a general surgical admissions unit. Your next patient is a 43-year-old woman, Miss Jennifer Williams, who has presented with a 3-day history of worsening left iliac fossa pain and vomiting. She has had some loose stools over the last couple of days. She has a background of diverticular disease and asthma. She is clearly in pain. Please review the patient, formulate an appropriate management plan and complete the drug chart provided.

Patient Details

NAME:	JENNIFER WILLIAMS
DOB:	12/05/1977
Hospital number:	0706401225
Weight:	70 kg
Height:	1.62 m
Consultant:	MHS
Hospital/ward:	WGH/27
Current medications:	Seretide 250, salbutamol, desogestrel, simvastatin
Allergies:	Erythromycin (rash)
Admission date:	20/11/2019

INITIAL ASSESSMENT

AIRWAY
- Patent

BREATHING
- RR 22 breaths/min
- SpO$_2$ 96% on air
- Chest is clear on auscultation

CIRCULATION
- HR 96 bpm
- BP 136/72 mmHg
- Good-volume pulse
- Warm peripheries with CRT of 2 s
- Heart sounds are normal with no added sounds

DISABILITY
- Temperature 38.3°C
- GCS 15/15
- Capillary glucose level 5.7 mmol/L

EXPOSURE
- The abdomen is tender in the left iliac fossa. No peritonism

- Bowel sounds are normal
- PR examination reveals no masses

INITIAL INVESTIGATIONS

Urine Dipstick

Blood	++
Leukocytes	+++
Nitrites	–
Protein	++
Bilirubin	+
Ketones	-

Beta-human chorionic gonadotrophin (hCG) negative.

Bloods

COMPONENTS	RESULTS	REFERENCE RANGES
Hb	143	120–150 g/L
WCC	18.9↑	3.7–11.1 × 10⁹/L
Neutrophils	16.0↑	1.5–7.4 × 10⁹/L
Platelets	532↑	150–400 × 10⁹/L
Bilirubin	8	0–21 µmol/L
ALT	43↑	0–33 IU/L
ALP	120↑	35–104 IU/L
GGT	65↑	6–42 IU/L
Sodium	135↓	136–145 mmol/L
Potassium	4.0	3.5–5.1 mmol/L
Urea	6.8	2.1–7.1 mmol/L
Creatinine	109↑	44–80 µmol/L
CRP	286↑	0–10 mg/L
Amylase	46	28–100 IU/L
Lactate	4.3↑	0.5–2.2 mmol/L

ABG

COMPONENTS	RESULTS	REFERENCE RANGES
pH	7.22	7.35–7.45
PaO$_2$	11.7	> 8 kPa
PaCO$_2$	4.1↓	4.7–6.0 kPa
HCO$_3^-$	15↓	22–26 mmol/L
Base excess	–4.5↓	–2.0––.0 mEq
Lactate	6.3↑	0.5–1.0 mmol/L

AXR
- Non-specific bowel gas pattern, no evidence of obstruction or perforation

ERECT CXR

- Clear lung fields, no evidence of pneumoperitoneum

IMPRESSION

- This is systemic inflammatory response syndrome (SIRS). Given the clear CXR and negative urinalysis, the most likely source is intra-abdominal infection, probably diverticulitis. This is therefore defined as sepsis (SIRS plus confirmed or suspected source of infection). There is an associated metabolic acidosis
- Differential diagnoses include: Pancreatitis, ruptured ectopic pregnancy and urosepsis

INITIAL MANAGEMENT

Sepsis is a serious condition with a high mortality rate. Successful outcomes require early recognition and treatment.

- Nil by mouth: This patient may require surgical intervention. She should be nil by mouth until senior review
- Antibiotics: The time between onset of sepsis and delivery of antibiotics is important for prognosis. Antibiotic choice depends on local antimicrobial policy. One option is 4.5 g piperacillin and tazobactam (Tazocin) IV TDS
- IV fluids: Septic patients are relatively hypovolaemic due to peripheral vasodilatation. Tachypnoea and pyrexia result in increased insensible losses. Fluid challenges should be used to correct shock, with regular reassessment. Patients with septic shock not responding to fluid resuscitation should be discussed with intensive care for consideration of vasopressor support. Note that while the patient is nil by mouth, they will require maintenance fluid following fluid resuscitation and replacement
- Analgesia: Analgesia prescribing should follow the WHO analgesic ladder, starting at the most appropriate level. An appropriate regimen would be regular paracetamol 1 g IV and as-required morphine 10 mg IV/IM/SC hourly

PLUS

- Catheter: Urinary catheter should be considered to monitor urine output
- Antiemetic: For example, cyclizine 50 mg IV/IM/SC TDS
- Thromboprophylaxis: Liaise with seniors before prescribing thromboprophylaxis in emergency surgical patients, especially if surgery is being planned
- Early senior review: This is to decide further investigations; for example, computed tomography (CT) abdomen and pelvis, and definitive management

DRUG CHART

The important aspects to consider when prescribing for this patient are:
- Allergies: Should be considered in all cases
- Antibiotics: Should be prescribed and given as soon as possible after the recognition of sepsis and certainly within 1 h
- Oxygen therapy: Should be considered in all cases. When prescribing oxygen therapy, indicate the device, desired oxygen flow and target saturations
- IV fluids: Resuscitate first and then remember to replace ongoing losses
- Nil by mouth: The oral route is not available for this patient and an alternative route must therefore be considered
- Impaired renal function: This will mean slower excretion of opiate metabolites, increasing the likelihood of opiate toxicity. Prescribe opiate analgesia with caution. Consider oxycodone instead of MST
- Regular medications: Always review and consider the patient's regular medications

COMPLICATIONS OF ABDOMINAL SEPSIS

- Septic shock
- Multi-organ failure
- Disseminated intravascular coagulation (DIC)
- Perforation
- VTE

❓ QUESTIONS AND ANSWERS FOR CANDIDATE

What are the SIRS criteria?
- Two or more of:
  - Pulse > 90 bpm
  - RR > 20 or $PaCO_2 < 4.3$ kPa
  - WCC $> 12 \times 10^9$/L or $< 4 \times 10^9$/L
  - Temperature > 38.0°C or < 36.0°C

Which groups of bacteria are commonly implicated in sepsis with presumed abdominal source?
- Gram-negatives
- Anaerobes

Which haematological abnormalities might you see in a patient with DIC?
- Prolongated prothrombin time (PT)
- Prolonged activated partial thromboplastin time (APTT)
- Low fibrinogen level
- Thrombocytopenia

Prescription and Administration Record

Prescription and Administration Record

Name: JENNIFER WILLIAMS	Weight: 70 KG	Known allergies:
DOB: 12/05/1977	Age: 42 YEARS	ERYTHROMYCIN (RASH)
		Signature: Date:
Hospital number: 0706401225	Consultant: MHS	**M. Slack** 20/11/2019
		MATT SLACK

Once-Only Medications

Date	Time	Medicine (approved name)	Dose	Route	Prescriber – sign and print	Time given	Given by
20/11/19	1430	MORPHINE (TITRATE TO PAIN)	1–10 MG	IV	**M. Slack** MATT SLACK		
20/11/19	1430	CYCLIZINE	50 MG	IV	**M. Slack** MATT SLACK		
20/11/19	1430	PARACETAMOL	1 G	IV	**M. Slack** MATT SLACK		
20/11/19	1430	PIPERACILLIN AND TAZOBACTAM	4.5 G	IV	**M. Slack** MATT SLACK		

Oxygen Therapy

Start		Route				Stop	
Date	Time	Mask (%)	Prongs (L/min)	Prescriber – sign and print	Administered by	Date	Time
20/11/19	1430	VENTURI (60)		**M. Slack** MATT SLACK			

VTE Prophylaxis

VTE risk assessment:	Comment: AWAITING POSSIBLE SURGERY
Yes [ ]	Signature: **M. Slack** MATT SLACK
Prophylaxis not required [ ]	Date: 20/11/19
Contraindicated [X]	

Continued

Prescription and Administration Record—cont'd

Regular Medications

			Date: →	20/11							
			Time: ↓								
Drug: SERETIDE 250 (SALMETEROL 25MCG/FLUTICASONE 250MCG)			02								
Dose:	Freq:	Route:	(06)								
2 PUFFS	BD	INH	10								
Start: 20/11/19		Stop/review:	(14)								
Signature: M. Slack MATT SLACK			18								
Indication: ASTHMA			22								
Drug: DESOGESTREL			02								
Dose:	Freq:	Route:	06								
75 MCG	OD	ORAL	(10)								
Start: 20/11/19		Stop/review:	14								
Signature: M. Slack MATT SLACK			18								
Indication: CONTRACEPTION			22								
Drug: SIMVASTATIN			02								
Dose:	Freq:	Route:	06								
10 MG	ON	ORAL	10								
Start: 20/11/19		Stop/review:	14								
Signature: M. Slack MATT SLACK			18								
Indication: HYPERCHOLESTEROLAEMIA			(22)								

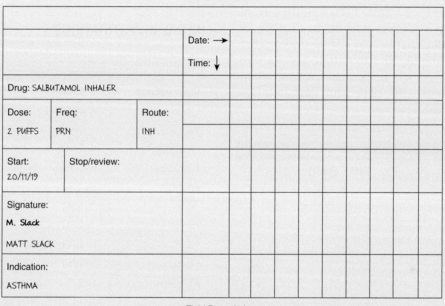

Drug: TAZOCIN	02						
Dose: 4.5 G / Freq: TDS / Route: IV	06						
	10						
Start: 20/11/19 / Stop/review:	14						
Signature: **M. Slack** MATT SLACK	18						
Indication: INTRA-ABDOMINAL SEPSIS	(22)						

PRN Medications

		Date: → Time: ↓									
Drug: SALBUTAMOL INHALER											
Dose: 2 PUFFS / Freq: PRN / Route: INH											
Start: 20/11/19 / Stop/review:											
Signature: **M. Slack** MATT SLACK											
Indication: ASTHMA											

Fluid Prescriptions

Date	Fluid	Additive	Volume	Route	Rate	Signature	Given	Batch
20/11/19	0.9% SODIUM CHLORIDE	NONE	500 ML	IV	Over 20 min	**M. Slack** MATT SLACK		

Fluid boluses should be prescribed one at a time, with immediate reassessment after each.

🐘 A Case to Learn From

Whilst working in general surgery I was asked to review an unwell patient. The man had a background of chronic abdominal pain secondary to diverticular disease and had been admitted the previous day with a fever and an episode of abdominal pain. He had been commenced on amoxicillin and metronidazole for presumed intra-abdominal source of sepsis. When I reviewed him, he was pyrexial, tachycardic and rigoring. His abdominal pain had settled. His chest was clear on auscultation and his abdomen was soft and non-tender. CXR was unremarkable and urinalysis was negative.

His CRP had increased from 50 mg/L on admission to 250 mg/L. I went on to examine his skin for evidence of infection and when I rolled up his trouser legs, I discovered that he had an area of erythema, swelling and increased heat over his right knee. Clinically this was cellulitis rather than abdominal sepsis. We changed his antibiotics to flucloxacillin and benzylpenicillin and within a day the cellulitis had improved, he was afebrile and his inflammatory markers had improved. This experience reinforced the need for a thorough search for a source of infection in a septic patient.

Top Tip

Sepsis guidance states that antibiotics should be given within the first 60 min of presentation. This is proven to reduce morbidity and mortality in patients with sepsis.

STATION 11.8: ACUTE UPPER GASTROINTESTINAL BLEED

SCENARIO

You are the junior doctor on call and are bleeped to see Steve Smith, a 65-year-old patient, who is having haematemesis. He was admitted directly from the medical outpatient clinic yesterday as he 'was yellow' and had a scan of his abdomen yesterday. He has never vomited blood before and he does not get indigestion. You see him as he is vomiting frank blood into a sick bowl. He is alert but is slurring his speech, and tells you that he was sitting in bed when he vomited 30 min ago. He has vomited repeatedly since then. Please review the patient, formulate an appropriate management plan and complete the drug chart provided.

Patient Details

NAME:	STEVE SMITH
DOB:	01/03/1955
Hospital number:	0103551252
Weight:	65 kg
Height:	1.73 m
Consultant:	MJK
Hospital/ward:	RIE/209
Current medications:	Atorvastatin, lactulose
Allergies:	Nil
Admission date:	13/09/2019

INITIAL ASSESSMENT

AIRWAY
- Patent

BREATHING
- RR 25 breaths/min
- SpO₂ 96% on air
- Chest is clear on auscultation

CIRCULATION
- HR 120 bpm
- BP 78/40 mmHg
- Cool peripheries with a CRT of 3 s
- Heart sounds are normal with no added sounds

DISABILITY
- Temperature 37.8°C
- GCS 14/15
- Capillary glucose level 7.1 mmol/L

EXPOSURE
- He is covered in crusted and fresh blood
- His abdomen is soft and non-tender
- Bowel sounds are present
- PR examination reveals no masses, melaena or fresh blood

INITIAL INVESTIGATIONS

Bloods

COMPONENTS	RESULTS	REFERENCE RANGES
Hb	66↓	130–170 g/L
WCC	16.5↑	3.7–11.1 × 10⁹/L
Neutrophils	14.9↑	1.5–7.4 × 10⁹/L
Platelets	126↓	150–400 × 10⁹/L
Bilirubin	145↑	0–21 μmol/L
ALT	164↑	0–41 IU/L
ALP	431↑	40–129 IU/L
GGT	170↑	6–42 IU/L
Sodium	129↓	136–145 mmol/L
Potassium	3.7	3.5–5.1 mmol/L
Urea	14.8↑	2.1–7.1 mmol/L
Creatinine	101	62–106 μmol/L
CRP	195↑	0–10 mg/L
Amylase	63	28–100 IU/L
Lactate	3.8↑	0.5–2.2 mmol/L
Albumin	27↓	35–52 g/L
International normalised ratio (INR)	3.0↑	0.8–1.2
APTT	50↑	35–45 s
PT	12	11.0–13.5 s
Thrombin	17↑	10–15 s
Fibrinogen	3.2	2.0–4.0 g/L

ABG		
COMPONENTS	**RESULTS**	**REFERENCE RANGES**
pH	7.35	7.35–7.45
PaO_2	14.1	> 8 kPa
$PaCO_2$	4.8	4.7–6.0 kPa
HCO_3^-	20↓	22–26 mmol/L
Base excess	–1.0	–2.0–2.0 mEq
Lactate	1.8↑	0.5–1.0 mmol/L

ERECT CXR

- Clear lung fields, no evidence of pneumoperitoneum

IMPRESSION

- This patient shows features of severe bleeding with hypovolaemic shock. He is peripherally shut down, with tachypnoea, tachycardia >100 bpm, hypotension and reduced conscious level

INITIAL MANAGEMENT

- Activate major haemorrhage protocol: Refer to local trust policy, but it can consist of: Tranexamic acid, packed red blood cells, fresh frozen plasma, cryoprecipitates and platelets
- Nil by mouth: This patient may require surgical intervention. He should be nil by mouth until the senior review
- Oxygen: Maintain oxygen saturations > 94%
- IV fluids: Obtain IV access with two wide-bore cannulae. Rapid IV fluid resuscitation is required. Give 500-mL boluses of 0.9% sodium chloride and reassess after each bolus. If features of circulatory compromise persist after initial boluses of fluids, commence blood transfusion. If available, use type-specific or cross-matched blood. If not, use O-negative blood. Use O-negative blood if patient is exsanguinating or unable to keep BP above 100 mmHg systolic, after more than 1 L of fluid given. Also consider prescribing vitamin K, also known as phytonadione, to reverse the effects of any anticoagulation process

PLUS

- Catheter: Urinary catheter is definitely required in an acute upper GI bleed, to monitor urine output, look out for other sites of bleeding and help assess fluid balance
- Escalate: Contact the GI registrar and critical care areas (HDU/ITU) for definitive management of the bleed and further support. Early endoscopy should be performed for all large bleeds and suspected varices, but the patient must be adequately resuscitated first

DRUG CHART

The important aspects to consider when prescribing for this patient are:
- Allergies: Should be considered in all cases
- IV fluids: The patient is in hypovolaemic shock and is likely to require large volumes of fluid. Clearly indicate on the drug chart if two bags of fluid should be given simultaneously
- Oxygen therapy: Should be considered in all cases. When prescribing oxygen therapy, indicate the device, desired oxygen flow and target saturations
- Blood transfusion: This is often prescribed on a separate prescription chart. If the patient has capacity then you should gain their consent, but if they do not have capacity, you may act in their best interests in this life-threatening situation
- Regular medications: Although not important during the resuscitation effort, the patient's regular medications should be reviewed. Consider stopping any medications that increase the risk of bleeding; for example anticoagulants, antiplatelet agents, NSAIDs and selective serotonin reuptake inhibitors (SSRIs)
- Impaired liver function: This may alter the metabolism of some drugs
- Thromboprophylaxis: Withhold currently until patient is stable

ADDITIONAL MANAGEMENT FOR VARICEAL BLEEDING

- This patient has possible variceal bleeding secondary to chronic liver disease
- Where possible, avoid the use of sodium chloride in patients with liver disease, as this will lead to accumulation of fluid; for example, as ascites, use albumin instead
- Terlipressin 2 mg IV can be given, followed by 1–2 mg IV every 6 h until the bleeding is controlled, for up to 72 h. Caution in ischaemic heart disease and peripheral vascular disease
- Antibiotics should be given. The choice will depend on local antibiotic policies. The British Society of Gastroenterology guidelines suggest 1 g ceftriaxone IV orally. Another option is 4.5 g piperacillin and tazobactam IV TDS
- Transjugular intrahepatic portosystemic shunt may be considered if endoscopic treatment fails

Prescription and Administration Record

Prescription and Administration Record

Name: STEVE SMITH	Weight: 70 KG	Known allergies:
		NO KNOWN DRUG ALLERGIES
DOB: 01/03/1955	Age: 65 YEARS	
Hospital number: 0103551252	Consultant: MJK	Signature: Date:
		M. Khan 13/09/2019
		MATT KHAN

Oxygen Therapy

Start		**Route**				**Stop**	
Date	Time	Mask (%)	Prongs (L/min)	Prescriber – sign andprint	Administered by	Date	Time
13/09/19	2100	NASAL CANNULA	2 L/min	**M. Khan** MATT KHAN			

VTE Prophylaxis

VTE risk assessment:	Comment: ONGOING BLOOD LOSS
Yes [ ]	Signature: **M. Khan** MATT KHAN
Prophylaxis not required [ ]	Date: 13/09/19
Contraindicated [X]	

Prescription and Administration Record—cont'd

Fluid Prescription

Date	Fluid	Additive	Volume	Route	Rate	Signature	Given	Batch
13/09/19 VENFLON 1	0.9% SODIUM CHLORIDE	NONE	500 ML	IV	OVER 15 MIN	M. Khan MATT KHAN		
13/09/19 VENFLON 2	0.9% SODIUM CHLORIDE	NONE	500 ML	IV	OVER 15 MIN	M. Khan MATT KHAN		

> After 1L of 0.9% saline, the patient begins to develop central chest pain and ischaemic changes on the ECG. HR 110bpm, BP 95/50 mmHg. This implies significant bleeding and associated cardiac ischaemia. Red cells should be prescribed as below:

Date	Fluid	Additive	Volume	Route	Rate	Signature	Given	Batch
13/09/19 VENFLON 1	RED CELL CONCENTRATE	NONE	1 UNIT	IV	OVER 15 MIN	M. Khan MATT KHAN		
13/09/19 VENFLON 2	RED CELL CONCENTRATE	NONE	1 UNIT	IV	OVER 15 MIN	M. Khan MATT KHAN		

> Further fluid prescriptions will be determined by the patient's response to this fluid challenge. Reassess before prescribing further fluids.

QUESTIONS AND ANSWERS FOR CANDIDATE

What is the role of terlipressin in variceal bleeding?
- Terlipressin is a vasopressin analogue that targets the splanchnic circulation and causes vasoconstriction, thereby decreasing portal pressure

Describe one mechanism by which alcohol excess leads to coagulopathy.
- Poor nutritional content of alcohol leads to dietary vitamin K deficiency and therefore decreased synthesis of vitamin K-dependent clotting factors
- Cirrhosis secondary to alcohol excess leads to impaired hepatocyte function and decreased synthesis of clotting factors
- Cirrhosis leads to portal hypertension which can in turn cause splenomegaly, with increased consumption of platelets in the enlarged spleen
- Alcohol can cause bone marrow toxicity, resulting in pancytopenia

Name three causes of haematemesis.
- Peptic ulcer (these account for 50% of upper GI bleeds)
- Variceal bleed (5–10%)
- Oesophagitis (10%)
- Mallory–Weiss tear (5%)
- Vascular malformation (5%)
- Gastritis (5%)
- Haemoptysis

A Case to Learn From

A 43-year-old woman described vomiting large quantities of blood, associated with severe epigastric pain, following a 2-day alcohol binge. She had known cirrhosis secondary to alcohol excess and my initial thought was that this could be a variceal bleed. Bloods showed a stable macrocytic anaemia with the Hb level at 102 g/L, raised inflammatory markers and an amylase of 3000 IU/L. The surgeons requested a CT scan of her abdomen, which showed acute pancreatitis. She continued to vomit in the department, but it wasn't blood; it was the red wine she'd been binging on.

If you are asked to review a patient with haematemesis, it is always useful to see the evidence. Although unpleasant, it can give you a lot of information – is it large or small? Fresh blood or coffee-ground vomit? Or has your patient been eating beetroot, drinking wine, or consuming large quantities of red food colouring?

Top Tip

Patients with GI bleeds can bleed suddenly and catastrophically, but don't miss those who are bleeding slowly or occultly. Repeat the FBC or take a venous blood gas a few hours after the bleed to see if the Hb level is dropping.

STATION 11.9: DIABETIC KETOACIDOSIS (DKA)

SCENARIO

You are the junior doctor on the medical admissions unit and are seeing Janet Smith, an 18-year-old woman, who has come in with shortness of breath, abdominal pain and vomiting. She is too confused to give you much history, but her mother tells you that she has recently been unwell with diarrhoea and has been passing large amounts of urine. Please review the patient, formulate an appropriate management plan and complete the drug chart provided.

Patient Details

NAME:	JANET SMITH
DOB:	01/04/2001
Hospital number:	0104920045
Weight:	64 kg
Height:	1.70 m
Consultant:	CAP
Hospital/ward:	WGH/53
Current medications:	Nil
Allergies:	Penicillin (rash)
Admission date:	06/12/2019

INITIAL ASSESSMENT

AIRWAY

- Patent

BREATHING

- RR 30 breaths/min
- SpO$_2$ 99% on air
- Chest is clear on auscultation

CIRCULATION

- HR 128 bpm
- BP 104/68 mmHg
- Cool peripheries with a CRT of 3 s
- Heart sounds are normal with no added sounds

DISABILITY

- Temperature 38.2°C
- GCS 14/15
- Capillary glucose level 31.0 mmol/L

EXPOSURE

- She looks dehydrated and is taking deep rapid breaths. There is an unusual smell on her breath

INITIAL INVESTIGATIONS

BLOOD GLUCOSE LEVEL

- 24 mmol/L

Urine Dip

Leukocytes	–
Nitrites	–
Ketones	+++
Glucose	++++

Beta hCG negative.

STOOL SAMPLE

- Sent for virology and culture

Bloods

COMPONENTS	RESULTS	REFERENCE RANGES
Hb	143	120–150 g/L
WCC	13.4↑	3.7–11.1 × 10^9/L
Neutrophils	11.1↑	1.5–7.4 × 10^9/L
Platelets	324	150–400 × 10^9/L
Bilirubin	18	0–21 µmol/L
ALT	20	0–33 IU/L
ALP	43	35–104 IU/L
Sodium	136	136–145 mmol/L
Potassium	5.0	3.5–5.1 mmol/L
Urea	5.4	2.1–7.1 mmol/L
Creatinine	101↑	44–80 µmol/L
CRP	29↑	0–10 mg/L
Amylase	54	28–100 IU/L
Lactate	1.2	0.5–2.2 mmol/L

ABG

COMPONENTS	RESULTS	REFERENCE RANGES
pH	7.28↓	7.35–7.45
PaO$_2$	18.1	> 8 kPa
PaCO$_2$	2.8↓	4.7–6.0 kPa
HCO$_3^-$	14.2↓	22–26 mmol/L
Base excess	–2.9↓	–2.0–2.0 mEq
Lactate	1.1↑	0.5–1.0 mmol/L

IMPRESSION

- This patient has DKA, which has caused severe dehydration. Her blood gas shows metabolic acidosis
- Differential diagnoses include: Infection (which is a cause of DKA in patients with type 1 diabetes), sepsis (which can cause a raised blood glucose, but not to the degree seen here)

INITIAL MANAGEMENT

- Oxygen: Aim for $SpO_2 > 94\%$
- IV access: At least two cannulae will be required, one for fluids and one for insulin

MONITORING

- ECG: Monitor for arrhythmias due to severe electrolyte imbalance; for example, hypokalaemia
- Bloods: Hourly laboratory glucose is initially required. Monitor the serum potassium level closely
- Catheter: Consider urinary catheterisation to allow monitoring of urine output

INSULIN AND FLUID REPLACEMENT

- Aim for blood glucose 9–14 mmol/L by the end of the first 24 h
- Make up an infusion of 50 units soluble insulin, for example, Actrapid in 50 mL 0.9% NaCl (1 unit/mL), and infuse using a syringe driver
- Start DKA management with a fixed-rate insulin infusion, usually 0.1 unit/kg/h. The prescription mainly amended is the amount and rate of IV fluid infusion
- Fluid initially should be 0.9% sodium chloride – starting with a stat bag (over 1 h) then gradually slowing down the rate of fluids. Often potassium needs to be added to these slower fluids – each trust will have a DKA protocol to follow about what to prescribe in the local healthcare setting. Care needs to be taken that potassium is not added too fast – the maximum rate of potassium infusion outside of HDU/ITU is 10 mmol/h
- When blood glucose falls below 14 then 10% dextrose should be added as a separate infusion, not instead of the 0.9% NaCl. This is usually done at a rate of 125 mL/h
- If capillary blood gas level falls to < 4 mmol/L, then treat as hypoglycaemia and reduce the insulin rate by 25%
- Avoid Hartmann's solution as it contains glucose
- Once the DKA has resolved (pH >7.3 and ketones <0.6), then there are two options:

- If the patient is eating and drinking, then she can be converted straight on to subcutaneous insulin with her next meal, and the fixed-rate IV insulin stopped an hour after the meal
- If the patient is not eating and drinking, then switch to a variable-rate insulin infusion. The term 'sliding scale' is confusing and therefore not used in most DKA protocols
- It is vital that, if a patient is known to be a type 1 diabetic and on insulin, their long-acting insulin is given as usual when they are being treated for DKA

Electrolyte Replacement

- Aim for potassium 4.0–5.0 mmol/L. Potassium will fall following commencement of insulin and should be closely monitored throughout the treatment of DKA, as hypokalaemia can be fatal

Correction of Acidosis

- Volume resuscitation and insulin infusion will correct metabolic acidosis in most patients. IV sodium bicarbonate is not used routinely and should certainly not be given without discussion with a senior doctor

PLUS

- Identify precipitating factors: For example, infection
- Thromboprophylaxis: As per local protocol. This is extremely important in patients with DKA as they are at a significantly higher risk of VTE due to a degree of dehydration and hyperosmolarity
- Contact: Diabetes registrar and/or medical registrar. Contact critical care if organ support or invasive monitoring is required

DRUG CHART

The important aspects to consider when prescribing for this patient are:

- Allergies: Should be considered in all cases
- Oxygen therapy: Should be considered in all cases. When prescribing oxygen therapy, indicate the device, desired oxygen flow and target saturations
- IV fluids: Always check all prescription charts. The patient may already have a separate fluid chart
- Regular medications: Regular medication should be reviewed every time the medication chart is looked at
- Insulin: Known type 1 diabetic patients should never have their long-acting insulin omitted whilst being treated for DKA. If there are any concerns, a diabetes specialist should be consulted

Prescription and Administration Record

Prescription and Administration Record

Name: JANET SMITH	Weight: 64 KG	Known allergies:
DOB: 01/04/2001	Age: 18 YEARS	PENICILLIN (RASH)
Hospital number: 0104920045	Consultant: CAP	Signature: Date: C. Price 06/12/19 CATHERINE PRICE

VTE Prophylaxis

VTE risk assessment: Yes [X] Prophylaxis not required [ ] Contraindicated [ ]	Comment: Signature: C. Price CATHERINE PRICE Date: 06/12/19

	Date: →	06/12/19						
	Time: ↓							
Drug: ENOXAPARIN		1800						
Dose: 20 MG	Freq: OD	Route: SC						
Start: 06/12/19	Stop/review:							
Signature: C. Price CATHERINE PRICE								

Once-Only Medications

Date	Time	Medicine (approved name)	Dose	Route	Prescriber – sign and print	Time given	Given by
06/12/19	2000	50 UNITS ACTRAPID IN 50ML 0.9% NACL	SEE SLIDING SCALE CHART	IV INFUSION	C. Price CATHERINE PRICE		

Insulin Prescription

Blood glucose (mmol/L)	Insulin infusion rate	Route	Prescriber – sign and print	Time given	Given by
	(unit/h = mL/h)				
> 13	6	IV	Signature: C. Price Print name: CATHERINE PRICE		
≤ 13	3				
≤ 10	2				

Prescription and Administration Record—cont'd

Fluid Prescriptions

Date	Fluid	Additive	Volume	Route	Rate	Signature	Given	Batch
06/12/19	0.9% SODIUM CHLORIDE	NONE	1 L	IV	250 mL/h	C. Price CATHERINE PRICE		

> Reassess fluid status and continue with fluid rehydration if indicated. Send U&Es and replace potassium if required. Do not give potassium faster than 10 mmol/hour.

Date	Fluid	Additive	Volume	Route	Rate	Signature	Given	Batch
06/12/19	0.9% SODIUM CHLORIDE	40 MMOL POTASSIUM CHLORIDE	1 L	IV	250 mL/h	C. Price CATHERINE PRICE		

> Again, reassess fluid status before prescribing further fluids. A venous blood gas can give information about the effectiveness of treatment and a serum potassium level to guide further treatment.

Date	Fluid	Additive	Volume	Route	Rate	Signature	Given	Batch
06/12/19	0.9% SODIUM CHLORIDE	20 MMOL POTASSIUM CHLORIDE	500 ML	IV	250 mL/h	C. Price CATHERINE PRICE		

> Add dextrose 5% at 100mL/hour once blood glucose is <14 mmol/L, as shown below. Continue fixed rate insulin and consider further electrolyte replacement. When the DKA has resolved, the insulin may be switched to sliding scale insulin. SC insulin can commence when the patient is eating and drinking and should be administered 30 minutes before IV insulin is stopped.

Date	Fluid	Additive	Volume	Route	Rate	Signature	Given	Batch
06/12/19	5% DEXTROSE	NONE	500 ML	IV	250 mL/h	C. Price CATHERINE PRICE		

HOW DKA OCCURS

DKA is an abbreviation for 'diabetic ketoacidosis'. This is primarily because it happens in diabetic patients and is a life-threatening problem. When the patient's insulin level in the body is low, it means that the body cannot effectively utilise the blood glucose and the body will be lacking a fuel source. Under these circumstances, the body will begin to break down fat, in order for the products to be used as a source of energy. The liver processes the fat into ketones, which in high levels, are toxic and acidotic. So, in the name of DKA, 'diabetic' refers to a high blood glucose level and 'ketoacidosis' refers to a high ketone level, so high that it has caused an acidosis.

COMPLICATIONS OF DKA

- Cerebral oedema
- AKI
- Adult respiratory distress syndrome
- Aspiration pneumonia

❓ QUESTIONS AND ANSWERS FOR CANDIDATE

Name two factors that may precipitate DKA.
- Insufficient insulin therapy: Missed doses, changed regimen
- Infection
- MI or stroke
- Pancreatitis
- Drugs

Which cells produce insulin?
- Insulin is produced by beta cells in the islets of Langerhans in the pancreas

Name two causes of hypoglycaemia in diabetic patients.
- Oral hypoglycaemic agents
- Excessive insulin therapy
- Liver disease: For example, hepatitis, cirrhosis
- Alcohol
- Insulinoma

A Case to Learn From

An 11-year-old boy, who had no past medical history, presented to his primary care physician with a 6-week history of weight loss and feeling generally unwell. On admission, his capillary glucose level was unrecordable and laboratory glucose was 26 mmol/L. Capillary blood gas showed a metabolic acidosis and urine dip showed ketones +++. With a clear diagnosis of DKA, we were able to commence treatment and transfer the patient to our specialist centre. The patient was terrified of the needles and medicines he would require for the type 1 diabetes, while his parents were heartbroken by this 'life sentence'. There were three learning points here. Firstly, always check a capillary glucose level, including at presentation in primary care. Secondly, the onset of type 1 diabetes and DKA can be insidious, as this patient had been unwell for at least 6 weeks before diagnosis. Thirdly, be sensitive to the devastation that a diagnosis like diabetes can cause to a young patient and family. Many areas have excellent diabetes services that can provide psychological as well as physical support for patients and their families.

💡 **Top Tip**

IV access is essential for the treatment of DKA but can be very difficult to obtain due to dehydration. Don't be afraid to ask for senior support. Ultrasound may be required to find a vein or the patient may need a central line.

STATION 11.10: DISCHARGE PRESCRIBING

SCENARIO

George Smith is a 50-year-old man who was admitted to hospital recently with a right lower-lobe pneumonia. He is now fit for discharge but requires 'to take out' (TTO) prescriptions of his medications. On admission he was septic with hypotension and an AKI, and his ramipril was withheld. His systolic BP has been 110–120 mmHg throughout admission and ramipril has not been restarted yet. He needs a further 3 days of antibiotics following discharge. He is also requiring paracetamol and MST modified-release (MR) for pain, with Oramorph for breakthrough pain. Please complete the TTO form below using Mr Smith's drug chart and the BNF if necessary.

Patient Details

NAME:	GEORGE SMITH
DOB:	22/12/1970
Hospital number:	2212660994
Weight:	81 kg
Height:	1.74 m
Consultant:	RHM
Hospital/ward:	RIE/207
Current medications:	Levothyroxine, aspirin, omeprazole, ramipril
Allergies:	Nil
Admission date:	13/01/2018

It is possible to pass this station and do very well if you are methodical in your approach and know the specific information that is required for certain drugs. The best source of information is the BNF, which also has information on the prescribing of controlled drugs.

PART 1: PRESCRIBING REGULAR MEDICATIONS

- Look at the regular medications section of the drug chart. The patient will need to continue the majority of these drugs once they leave the hospital (see Table 11.2 for an example)
- Do not continue drugs such as enoxaparin (unless specifically indicated and arrangements have been made for it to be given in the community)
- Antibiotics should only be given for the prescribed course; for example for 3 more days. If you do have to prescribe antibiotics on a TTO, you should know how long they need to be continued and if you are unsure, check with a senior colleague
- Regular medications may have been stopped during admission. Review the pre-admission drugs to make sure they have been restarted, if indicated. If they have been permanently stopped, ensure that the reason is documented clearly for the primary care physician in the discharge letter

Do not fill in the pharmacy box on the right. This is for the pharmacy staff to fill in when they dispense the drug.

On the discharge letter, document the reasons for changes to medication (Table 11.3).

 Table **11.2** **Example of Regular Medications Prescribed on a TTO**

DRUG	DOSE & FREQUENCY	DURATION	PHARMACY
ASPIRIN	75 mg OD	28 DAYS (CONTINUE LONG-TERM)	
OMEPRAZOLE	40 mg OD	28 DAYS (CONTINUE LONG-TERM)	
LEVOTHYROXINE	125 mcg ORALLY	28 DAYS (CONTINUE LONG-TERM)	
PARACETAMOL	1 g QDS	14 DAYS (SHORT-TERM)	
AMOXICILLIN	500 mg TDS	THREE DAYS REMAINING (7-DAY COURSE TO FINISH ON 20/01/18)	

PART 2: PRESCRIBING AS-REQUIRED (PRN) MEDICATION

- Decide whether the patient will require regular or PRN analgesia
- PRN analgesia is usually prescribed for 7–14 days after discharge (as opposed to 28 days for regular medication)
- In order to decide which medications to prescribe, you need to look at how many times these drugs have been required in the time leading up to discharge and use your common sense
- If the drug has not been given for a number of days, you may not need to prescribe it

EXAMPLE

- Mr Smith has been taking paracetamol 1 g QDS and MST MR 10 mg BD during his admission for pleuritic chest pain
- He has also required 20–30 mg Oramorph daily for breakthrough pain
- Assuming his pain is improving, it would be sensible to send him home with 7 days' worth of 20 mg Oramorph. Oramorph is distributed as 10 mg/5 mL MST in 100-mL and 300-mL bottles
- 20 mg/day = 10 mL/day, which adds up to 70 mL in 7 days. Therefore you could prescribe a 100-mL bottle, leaving slightly extra in case more analgesia is required

  The prescription might look something like Table 11.4

PART 3: PRESCRIBING CONTROLLED DRUGS

When prescribing controlled drugs, the prescription must state:
- The name and address of the patient
- The form and strength of the drug (as appropriate)
- Either the total quantity or the number of dosage units of the drug, written in both words and figures
- The dose of the drug

  The prescription must then be signed and contain the prescriber's hospital address. Without this information, the pharmacy will not dispense the drug.

EXAMPLE

Mr Smith's morphine MR would be prescribed as shown in Table 11.5.

❓ QUESTIONS AND ANSWERS FOR CANDIDATE

A 65-year-old man is admitted for pneumonia and is started on treatment with IV amoxicillin and oral clarithromycin. His usual medications are aspirin, bisoprolol, simvastatin, co-codamol 30/500 and ranitidine. Which one of his usual medications should be withheld while he is taking the antibiotics?

Simvastatin should be withheld while he is taking clarithromycin. Clarithromycin is a macrolide antibiotic. Macrolides inhibit CYP3A4, an enzyme involved in the metabolism of simvastatin. This can lead to a large increase in levels of simvastatin, increasing the risk of adverse effects; for example, myopathy and rhabdomyolysis.

Which of the following is not required on a prescription for a controlled drug? (1) Name of patient; (2) age of patient; (3) address of patient; (4) quantity to be supplied in words and figures; or (5) date of prescription.

The age of the patient is not required, but the DOB should instead be written. The prescription must also state the route and dose and must be signed and dated by the prescriber.

Table 11.3	Examples of Reasons for Changes to Medications
MEDICATION	CHANGE
RAMIPRIL 5 mg OD	CURRENTLY WITHHELD DUE TO AKI AND HYPOTENSION. PRIMARY CARE PHYSICIAN PLEASE RECHECK THE RENAL FUNCTION AND BP IN 1 WEEK AND RESTART RAMIPRIL IF REQUIRED
AMOXICILLIN 500 mg TDS	FOR COMMUNITY-ACQUIRED PNEUMONIA. SEVEN-DAY COURSE TO FINISH 20/01/18
PARACETAMOL 1 g QDS	FOR PLEURITIC CHEST PAIN (SHORT-TERM)

Table 11.4 Example Prescription of Oramorph

DRUG	DOSE AND FREQUENCY	DURATION	PHARMACY
ORAMORPH (MORPHINE SULPHATE) 10 mg/5 mL. PLEASE SUPPLY 100 mL	10 mg MAXIMUM 2-HOURLY AS REQUIRED	7 DAYS	

Table 11.5 Example Prescription of MST

DRUG	DOSE AND FREQUENCY	DURATION	PHARMACY
MST (MORPHINE SULPHATE MODIFIED-RELEASE) 10-mg TABLETS. PLEASE SUPPLY 56 (FIFTY-SIX) TABLETS	10 mg BD	28 DAYS	

Which two of the following are not controlled drugs? (1) Tramadol; (2) Oramorph (MST immediate-release oral suspension 10 mg/5 mL); (3) Zomorph (MST MR); (4) oxybutynin; or (5) alfentanil.

Oramorph and oxybutynin are not controlled drugs. Oramorph is immediate-release morphine and is available in 10 mg/5 mL and 100 mg/5 mL strengths. In clinical practice, you will be prescribing 10 mg/5 mL, and this is not a controlled drug. The stronger preparation is rarely used. Oxybutynin is an anticholinergic drug used to treat symptoms of overactive bladder and is also not a controlled drug.

 A Case to Learn From

For a patient taking long-term warfarin for AF, I had drafted the discharge letter and prescription for the expected discharge date and called the primary care physician to arrange for an INR check 3 days later. However, the patient then developed a urinary tract infection and required a further few days in hospital before being discharged. I quickly updated the discharge letter and prescription with his new antibiotics but forgot to rearrange the INR check. The appointment at the primary care practice was wasted and I had an anxious patient on the phone to me asking what he should do about his warfarin dosing. It was an unfortunate oversight on a busy day on a very busy ward and thankfully the patient came to no harm. When prescribing a medication that requires monitoring, it is important to think about how this will be continued in the community.

 Top Tip

Communication is key! Clearly document the reasons for stopping and starting drugs in the discharge letter for the primary care physician. If the reason is not clear, try to find out why changes have been made in case they were mistakes or accidental omissions. Similarly, always document your reasons for making changes on the drug chart.

STATION 11.11: ANALGESIA

SCENARIO

You are a junior doctor working in the ED and have been asked to see Peter Robinson, a 20-year-old man, who has suffered a traumatic injury to his left leg while playing rugby. He is complaining of severe pain and is unable to weight-bear. The orthopaedic surgeon is in theatre and will come to review the patient when he is finished. Please review the patient, formulate an appropriate management plan and complete the drug chart provided.

Patient Details

NAME:	PETER ROBINSON
DOB:	10/12/1990
Hospital number:	1012908911
Weight:	83 kg
Height:	1.86 m
Consultant:	MJR
Hospital/ward:	WGH/SAU
Current medications:	Nil
Allergies:	Nil
Admission date:	30/05/19

INITIAL ASSESSMENT

AIRWAY

- Patent

BREATHING

- RR 18 breaths/min
- SpO$_2$ 99% on air
- Chest is clear on auscultation

CIRCULATION

- HR 80 bpm
- BP 114/70 mmHg
- Warm peripheries with a CRT of <2 s
- Heart sounds are normal with no added sounds

DISABILITY

- Temperature 36.1°C
- GCS 15/15
- Capillary glucose 4.9 mmol/L

EXPOSURE

- The left lower leg is deformed. There is extensive bruising, but the skin is intact. The leg is exquisitely tender to palpation

INITIAL INVESTIGATIONS

Bloods

COMPONENTS	RESULTS	REFERENCE RANGES
Hb	158	130–170 g/L
WCC	8.9	3.7–11.1 × 10^9/L
Neutrophils	6.2	1.5–7.4 × 10^9/L
Platelets	320	150–400 × 10^9/L
Sodium	142	136–145 mmol/L
Potassium	4.5	3.5–5.1 mmol/L
Urea	4.9	2.1–7.1 mmol/L
Creatinine	94	62–106 µmol/L
INR	1.0	< 1.1

A group-and-save sample has been sent in case an operation is required.

X-RAY LEFT LEG

- There is a displaced fracture of the tibial mid-shaft
- The knee and ankle joints are normal
- No other fractures are evident

IMPRESSION

- This man has a closed displaced fracture of his tibia and is likely to require surgery

INITIAL MANAGEMENT

ANALGESIA

The patient is in severe pain and requires immediate analgesia while awaiting orthopaedic review.

Analgesia should be prescribed using the WHO analgesic ladder as a guide. Start at the step most appropriate for the patient's pain. If the pain is not controlled, avoid changing one drug for another of equal potency in the same class. For example, do not change codeine to dihydrocodeine; instead move up the ladder until adequate analgesia is reached.

- Non-opioids: Paracetamol (1 g QDS oral/IV) is an effective painkiller and should (invariably) be prescribed regularly to every patient who has pain
- Weak opioids: If the pain is not controlled with regular paracetamol alone, a weak opioid should be added. Options include codeine phosphate (30–60 mg up to 4-hourly oral, maximum 240 mg/24 h) and dihydrocodeine (30 mg up to 4-hourly oral/SC/IM)
- Strong opioids: If pain continues despite maximum doses of non-opioids and weak opioids, the weak opioid should be stopped and a trial of strong opioids (morphine) commenced. Morphine has serious side effects and needs to be prescribed with care (see below)
- Adjuvants: These include NSAIDs (for bony metastases, liver pain), corticosteroids (for nerve compression, liver pain, raised intracranial pressure), gabapentin and amitriptyline (for neuropathic pain). The nature of the pain will determine which adjuvant is appropriate and these should be considered with any step in the analgesic ladder. It is best to discuss the use of these drugs with a senior and/or the pain team. In this case, if the patient is confirmed to have had a fracture which needs reducing in the ED, then you could consider prescribing nitrous oxide, also known as Entonox, as a form of analgesia during the reduction

Prescribing Morphine

- Morphine can either be immediate-release, short-acting or controlled-release, long-acting
- It can be administered orally, IV, IM, SC or topically, and dosing changes depending on the route
- For acute severe pain, short-acting morphine should be prescribed. This takes about 20 min to work and lasts approximately 4 h. It is difficult to predict how much morphine a patient will need. Therefore, it is best to prescribe it initially as an 'as-required' medication; for example, 'morphine, 5 mg PRN, maximum frequency 4-hourly, oral'. The dose and frequency can then be adjusted
- Long-acting morphine takes longer to have an effect but lasts 12 h. It is prescribed twice a day, after titration with short-acting morphine has demonstrated the adequate analgesia cover for the patient. The dose of long-acting morphine is calculated by taking the total amount of short-acting morphine used in 24 h and giving this in divided doses
- 'Breakthrough' short-acting morphine should also be prescribed. The usual dose is one-sixth of the total morphine requirement (in a 24-h period)
- Avoid 'mixing' opiates. Use short- and long-acting morphine together, and short- and long-acting oxycodone together. Avoid, for example, using OxyContin (long-acting oxycodone) with breakthrough Oramorph (short-acting morphine)

DRUG CHART

The important aspects to consider when prescribing for this patient are:

- Allergies: Should be considered in all cases
- Oxygen therapy: Should be considered in all cases, even if your primary aim is to manage pain. When prescribing oxygen therapy indicate the device, desired oxygen flow and target saturations
- IV fluids: Always check all prescription charts. The patient may have a separate fluid chart and it is vital that this is also reviewed
- Regular medications: Regular medication should be reviewed every time the medication chart is looked at
- Renal and liver impairment: Check that renal function and liver function are normal in all patients before prescribing opiate analgesia. Morphine is renally excreted and patients with renal impairment are more likely to accumulate morphine and become opiate-toxic. Oxycodone may be a better choice in these patients as it is partially excreted by the liver. However, caution is needed if there is liver impairment
- Thromboprophylaxis: Needs to be considered in all patients and is especially important in those who are not mobile

Prescription and Administration Record

Prescription and Administration Record

Name: PETER ROBINSON	Weight: 93 KG	Known allergies:
		NO KNOWN DRUG ALLERGIES
DOB: 25/03/1990	Age: 20 YEARS	
Hospital number: 1012.908911	Consultant: MJR	Signature: Date:
		M. Ross 30.5.19
		MARTHA ROSS

Once-Only Medications

Date	Time	Medicine (approved name)	Dose	Route	Prescriber – sign and print	Time given	Given by
30/05/19	1700	PARACETAMOL	1 G	ORAL	**M. Ross** MARTHA ROSS		
30/05/19	1700	ORAMORPH (MST) 10 MG/5 ML	10 MG	ORAL	**M. Ross** MARTHA ROSS		
30/05/19	1745	ORAMORPH (MST) 10 MG/5 ML	10 MG	ORAL	**M. Ross** MARTHA ROSS		

VTE Prophylaxis

VTE risk assessment:			Comment:							
Yes [X]			Signature: **M. Ross** MARTHA ROSS							
Prophylaxis not required [ ]			Date: 30/05/19							
Contraindicated [ ]										
		Date: → Time: ↓	30/05							
Drug: Enoxaparin			1800							
Dose: 20 MG	Freq: OD	Route: SC								
Start: 13/09/19	Stop/review:									
Signature: **M. Ross** MARTHA ROSS										

QUESTIONS AND ANSWERS FOR CANDIDATE

Side effects of paracetamol are very rare. Can you name any?

- Thrombocytopenia
- Neutropenia

Name three side effects of opiate analgesia.

- Itch
- Nausea and vomiting
- Constipation
- Drowsiness
- Respiratory depression
- Dry mouth
- Difficulty micturating

Suggest an opiate that may be used where morphine and oxycodone are not tolerated due to renal impairment.

- Fentanyl
- Alfentanil

A Case to Learn From

As a surgical junior doctor, I was involved in the care of an elderly man who was being treated palliatively for pancreatic cancer and was waiting for a hospice bed. One weekend he developed severe pain which was not controlled by his usual paracetamol and codeine. We gave him a small dose of Oramorph, which quickly settled the pain. However, over the next half-hour he became increasingly drowsy until he was unresponsive. We treated him with naloxone to reverse the morphine, which was effective but unfortunately, left him with severe pain. His renal function was very poor with a creatinine of 320 mmol/L and this was why he had become opiate-toxic so quickly. We spoke to the palliative care consultant on call, who suggested commencing alfentanil in a syringe driver, with extra alfentanil breakthrough. Alfentanil has a very short half-life and therefore does not accumulate and cause toxicity. His pain was effectively controlled, and he remained alert. He passed away peacefully and comfortably 2 days later. Always seek expert advice when necessary, and the palliative care team are great with pain management.

Top Tip

Patients who already take opiate analgesia long-term are likely to require larger doses of morphine for acute pain. I have seen a tiny 80-year-old woman, who was taking 140 mg MST BD with 50 mg Oramorph breakthrough – and her pain was well controlled! Similarly, patients who take methadone are likely to require larger doses of opiate analgesia to control their pain.

STATION 11.12: PRESCRIBING FOR PAEDIATRICS

SCENARIO

You are a junior doctor working in the ED and have been asked to see James Taylor, a 7-year-old boy who has presented with wheeze and shortness of breath. This is on a background of a sore throat, runny nose, fever and cough. He has a history of asthma and eczema. His medications are Seretide 250, salbutamol inhalers and montelukast. Review the history and examination taken by your colleague, formulate an appropriate management plan and complete the drug chart provided.

Patient Details

NAME:	JAMES TAYLOR
DOB:	22/03/2012
Hospital number:	2203090334
Weight:	28 kg
Height:	1.30 m
Consultant:	PHR
Hospital/ward:	SJH/Children's ward
Current medications:	Seretide 250, salbutamol, montelukast
Allergies:	Nil
Admission date:	26/05/2019

INITIAL ASSESSMENT

AIRWAY

- Patent

BREATHING

- RR 32 breaths/min
- SpO_2 86% on air
- Increased work of breathing, use of accessory muscles
- Struggling to speak
- Quiet breath sounds with audible wheeze throughout

CIRCULATION

- HR 140 bpm
- BP 100/60 mmHg
- Peripheries warm with CRT < 2 s
- Heart sounds are normal with no added sounds

DISABILITY

- Temperature 39.2°C
- GCS 15/15
- Blood glucose level 4.9 mmol/L

EXPOSURE

- Fine maculopapular rash across the chest
- Red throat and runny nose
- Pink tympanic membranes bilaterally

INITIAL INVESTIGATIONS

Peak Flow

PEFR	50	L/MIN
Predicted PEFR	170	L/min

Bloods

COMPONENTS	RESULTS	REFERENCE RANGES
Hb	140	115–155 g/L
WCC	20.1↓	4.5–14.5 × 10^9/L
Neutrophils	16.4↑	1.5–8.0 × 10^9/L
Platelets	250	150–400 × 10^9/L
CRP	32↑	0–10 mg/L
Sodium	136	133–143 mmol/L
Potassium	3.8	3.3–5.5 mmol/L
Urea	2.6	2.5–6.5 mmol/L
Creatinine	40	25–60 µmol/L
Lactate	1.4↑	0.5–1.0 mmol/L

Capillary Blood Gas

COMPONENTS	RESULTS	REFERENCE RANGES
pH	7.44	7.35–7.45
PaO_2	4.5↓	> 8 kPa
$PaCO_2$	3.1↓	4.7–6.0 kPa
HCO_3^-	28.1↑	22–26 mmol/L
Base excess	1.2	–2.0–2.0 mEq
Lactate	1.4↑	0.5–1.0 mmol/L

CXR

- Lung fields are clear
- Hyperinflated chest
- No pneumothoraces

IMPRESSION

- This is a life-threatening exacerbation of asthma with hypoxia
- The patient has features consistent with viral infection which may have precipitated the attack
- Differential diagnosis includes: Inhaled foreign body (which is more common in children than in adults), pneumonia or pneumothorax. You should consider structural heart disease as a differential in children with shortness of breath, although this is unlikely in a 7-year-old with no previous history

INITIAL MANAGEMENT

- Oxygen: Give high-flow oxygen via a non-rebreathe mask, aiming for oxygen saturations > 94%
- Bronchodilators: Give nebulised bronchodilators (salbutamol and ipratropium bromide), adding nebulised magnesium if there is poor response to salbutamol, according to local policy. Reassess after each nebuliser
- Steroids: Give prednisolone 40 mg OD. If he is too unwell to take oral medication, give hydrocortisone 200 mg IV for the first dose
- Obtain IV access: Remember that the patient is a child and this may cause distress to the point of worsening his breathing. Apply local anaesthetic cream if time permits and take bloods and a venous blood gas simultaneously
- Antipyretics: Give paracetamol for fever if fever is causing distress
- Senior review: This patient is very unwell and needs an early senior review as IV therapy with salbutamol, magnesium or aminophylline may be indicated. If he is not improving, he may require intubation and ventilation

DRUG CHART

The important aspects to consider when prescribing for this patient are:

- Allergies: Should be considered in all cases
- Bronchodilators: This child is presenting with a life-threatening exacerbation of asthma and is hypoxic. Give three back-to-back nebulisers with salbutamol 5 mg, ipratropium bromide 500 mcg and magnesium sulphate 150 mg
- Oxygen therapy: Should be considered in all cases. When prescribing oxygen therapy, indicate the device, desired oxygen flow and target saturations
- Steroids: The dose is based on weight and severity. Usually 1–2 mg/kg (maximum dose 40 mg) prednisolone orally or consider IV steroids if oral medications are not tolerated. A 3-day course is usually sufficient, but it may be extended to 5 days
- Antipyretics: A fever may make a child seem more unwell as they are more tachycardic and tachypnoeic than they would otherwise be. Give paracetamol 5 mg/kg, 4–6-hourly, four times a day if unwell with it. Avoid ibuprofen in sensitive asthmatics
- Local anaesthetic spray: Topical anaesthetic sprays, for example benzydamine, are very useful in children with sore throats, particularly where this is contributing to decreased oral intake. This would not be a priority in the acute setting but could be considered once the child is stable
- Regular medications: Regular inhalers should be withheld while he is being treated with nebulisers

Prescription and Administration Record

Prescription and Administration Record

Name: JAMES TAYLOR	Weight: 28 KG	Known allergies:
DOB: 22/03/2012	Age: 7 YEARS	NO KNOWN DRUG ALLERGIES
Hospital number: 2203090334	Consultant: MHS	Signature: Date: **M. Slack** 26/5/19 MATT SLACK

Once-only medications

Date	Time	Medicine (approved name)	Dose	Route	Prescriber – sign and print	Time given	Given by
26/5/19	1400	SALBUTAMOL (DRIVEN WITH OXYGEN)	5 MG	NEB	**M. Slack** MATT SLACK		
26/5/19	1400	IPRATROPIUM BROMIDE (DRIVEN WITH OXYGEN)	500 MCG	NEB	**M. Slack** MATT SLACK		
26/5/19	1400	MAGNESIUM SULPHATE (DRIVEN WITH OXYGEN)	150 MG	NEB	**M. Slack** MATT SLACK		
26/5/19	1430	PREDNISOLONE	40 MG	ORAL	**M. Slack** MATT SLACK		
26/5/19	1430	PARACETAMOL	140 MG	ORAL	**M. Slack** MATT SLACK		

Oxygen Therapy

Date	Time	Route		Prescriber – sign and print	Administered by	Stop	
		Mask (%)	Prongs (L/min)			Date	Time
26/5/19	1400	NON-REBREATHE MASK	15 L/MIN	**M. Slack** MATT SLACK			

Continued

Prescription and Administration Record—cont'd

Regular Medications

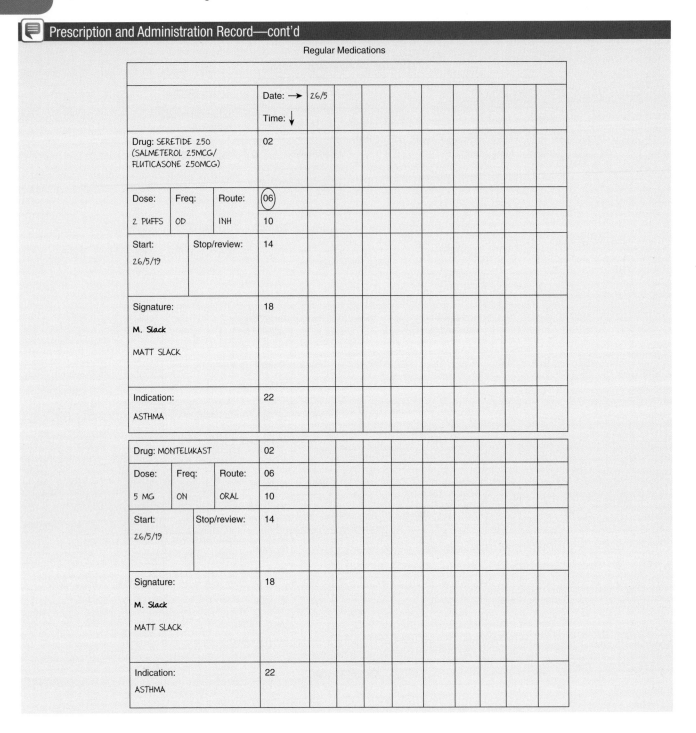

		Date: →	26/5							
		Time: ↓								
Drug: SERETIDE 250 (SALMETEROL 25MCG/ FLUTICASONE 250MCG)		02								
Dose: 2 PUFFS	**Freq:** OD	**Route:** INH	(06)							
			10							
Start: 26/5/19	**Stop/review:**	14								
Signature: *M. Slack* MATT SLACK		18								
Indication: ASTHMA		22								
Drug: MONTELUKAST		02								
Dose: 5 MG	**Freq:** ON	**Route:** ORAL	06							
			10							
Start: 26/5/19	**Stop/review:**	14								
Signature: *M. Slack* MATT SLACK		18								
Indication: ASTHMA		22								

VIRAL-INDUCED WHEEZE VERSUS ASTHMA

In children, it can be difficult to distinguish asthma from viral-induced wheeze. In viral-induced wheeze, there are no chronic changes to the lungs. Asthma is more likely if there is a family history of atopy, if there is a nocturnal cough and if there are recurrent wheezy episodes after the age of 5.

❓ QUESTIONS AND ANSWERS FOR CANDIDATE

Which other conditions are often present in children with asthma?
- Eczema
- Hay fever
- Allergies

How might increased work of breathing present in an infant?
- Nasal flaring
- Head bobbing
- Subcostal and intercostal recession
- Grunting
- Increased RR
- Cyanosis
- Inability to feed

A 5-month-old baby should not in general be treated for wheeze with salbutamol. Why?

- Beta receptors in the lungs are not fully developed in infants and therefore are unlikely to respond to salbutamol

 A Case to Learn From

While working in paediatrics, I went to review a 6-year-old boy who had presented with wheeze, cough, coryzal symptoms and fever, on a background of asthma. He was tachycardic and tachypnoeic, with poor peripheral perfusion and he appeared lethargic and unwell. However, even after his fever settled, he remained tachycardic, tachypnoeic and lethargic. His wheeze responded well to salbutamol inhalers, at which point, re-examination of his chest revealed right basal crackles, which had previously not been audible over his widespread wheeze. A CXR showed right basal consolidation which was treated with oral amoxicillin. By the next day he was back to his bright and happy self, playing with toy trains in the corner of the bay. This was a useful reminder that if patients do not respond as expected to treatment, you should revisit your differential in case you have missed a diagnosis.

 Top Tip

Children are easier to assess when they are afebrile. Fever may cause tachycardia, tachypnoea and poor peripheral perfusion. Treat a fever in a child that is unwell with it with paracetamol. Ibuprofen is also an excellent antipyretic in children, although it should be avoided in sensitive asthmatics.

Content Outline

Writing any official documentation can be daunting and is often not taught at medical school.

It requires an in-depth understanding of an inpatient episode and the ability to summarise the clinically relevant information, pertinent investigations, results and follow-up.

It is useful to consider what you would like to know if you were asked to take over the care of a patient. Depending on the clinical scenario, different information will be required; however, having a standard framework for approaching letters will enable you to ensure a good handover of care.

Death certification is usually a role that is carried out by junior doctors. However, the decision regarding what should be written as the cause of death should be made by the clinical consultant and consultant pathologist, if required.

Study Action Plan

- Prepare a basic structure that makes sense to you and that you can follow for writing each type of letter
- Practise summarising cases succinctly. Write drafts for letters on the wards for patients who are being discharged and ask the junior doctors to check them. Most doctors will be very grateful for this – it helps them out! Try and understand any changes that they make to your draft letter
- Get experience at interpreting letters. Whilst on a primary care placement, read the hospital discharge summaries of patients. This is a great way to learn what relevant information is commonly missed and sought

STATION 12.1: TRANSFER LETTER

SCENARIO

Mr Jenson, a 38-year-old man, presented to the emergency department (ED) 5 days ago with chest tightness and sounding wheezy. Over time he became increasingly cyanosed and exhausted and peak expiratory flow (PEF) < 33% best or predicted. An arterial blood gas (ABG) was taken and $PaCO_2$ came back raised. He was diagnosed with near-fatal asthma and was treated appropriately in the intensive care unit (ICU). He is now clinically stable and ready to go to a respiratory ward. Please write an appropriate transfer letter for his step down to the respiratory ward, ward 15.

CORE CONCEPT

- A transfer letter is required when a patient's care is to be transferred from one location to another
- The transfer can be within the same hospital, within the same trust but across different hospital sites or between different trusts. Sometimes the transfer can be from one end of the country to the other
- It is vital that all of the important information is included for the receiving team, to ensure a safe transfer for the patient

Common Concerns

Who needs to be informed about this transfer?	Always inform the patient in advance of transfer and explore if they have any concerns or expectations. Make all relevant members of the medical and nursing team aware of the circumstances so that the most appropriate care is provided. On the day, the hospital porters may need to assist in the transfer
What if the patient does not seem well enough for a transfer?	The decision for the patient to be transferred was most likely made by a senior doctor; for example, a consultant, and they will have taken the whole clinical picture into account. However, if you feel that a transfer is unsafe, then it is your duty to voice your concerns and it could be a good learning point for yourself as well
Whose care is the patient under while awaiting the transfer?	While the patient is waiting to be transferred, it is important that the patient is still receiving care from the organising team, at least until the patient has been safely transferred. Even after a transfer, a patient may require follow-up care at the new location from the parent team

EXAMPLE LAYOUT

[Insert address of receiving hospital]   [Insert address of doctor sending the letter]

[Insert date of letter]

Dear: [Insert doctor's name]
Re: [Insert name and identification details of patient]

Admission Date: Transfer date:
Ward:
Consultant:

[Insert main text: Refer to the 'Key Information' section of this station below]
Yours sincerely

[Insert name of referring doctor]

[Insert designation of referring doctor and consultant; for example, Foundation Year 1 to Dr Jones]
[Insert contact details of referring doctor]

KEY INFORMATION

DIAGNOSIS

- Name all diagnoses that the patient has been given, including any given before this hospital admission. Try to list them in order of clinical importance and with the new conditions first
- The conditions should be as specific as possible; for example, 'left lower-lobe pneumonia' rather than 'chest infection'

REASON FOR TRANSFER

- State clearly what your expectations are of the unit receiving the patient. For example, whether the patient is being transferred for an operation, rehabilitation or optimisation of medical management post-surgery
- Clarify whether any additional investigations are required while the patient is in their unit

PROGRESS

Try to provide some details on the following points:
- Presenting complaint: Include any other relevant associated symptoms. Depending on the case, it may be relevant to include past medical, drug, family and/or social history
- Mode of admission: Elective or emergency
- Treatment: Initial treatment that the patient has undergone and whether there were any complications

- Other healthcare professionals: Whether other services have been involved; for example, liaison psychiatry, physiotherapy
- Current circumstances: Whether the patient is clinically stable or if extra assistance or equipment is required

KEY INVESTIGATIONS

- It is not necessary to include every single investigation result; however, clinically relevant results that it would be useful to be aware of should be provided. For example, computed tomography (CT) and magnetic resonance imaging (MRI) scans, or if recent blood tests have been abnormal, these are likely to be particularly relevant as well
- Even if investigation results were unremarkable, they may be relevant; for example, an electrocardiogram (ECG) showing normal sinus rhythm for a patient being investigated for heart palpitations
- Highlight any tests that have been ordered but are yet to be carried out, and any tests that have been performed but are awaiting results
- Remember to include the dates of the investigations

DRUGS ON TRANSFER

- State the drugs that are to be continued at transfer
- Remember to include the following key points:
  - Generic name of drug
  - Dose

- Frequency of administration
- Route of administration
- Length of treatment
- Any special instructions; for example, if a patient is taking gentamicin, state whether blood tests need to be done and if so, when
- It may be helpful to state which medications were newly commenced on this hospital admission and which were already being taken at home
- Highlight any drugs that have been discontinued and whether recommencement needs to be considered. For example, 'simvastatin has been permanently discontinued due to proximal myopathy' and 'lisinopril was discontinued due to renal failure; please consider restarting when renal function is appropriate'
- Clearly state information about allergies or adverse reactions to drugs
- Some very unwell patients may be receiving infusions so this would also need to be detailed

FOLLOW-UP

- Clarify if the patient needs to be seen in clinic after discharge from hospital and if so, whether an appointment has already been made. Given that the patient will have received care from two different places, it is important

to clarify where the follow-up will take place – at the organising hospital or at the receiving unit
- State if the patient will also be followed up by other services; for example, occupational therapy

INFORMATION GIVEN TO PATIENT AND FAMILY

Communication, especially with the patient and the family, plays an extremely important role during the transfer of a patient. Understandably, the patient and family are perhaps anxious about the transfer and it is our duty to ensure that they have been provided with all of the information they may need. Some key points to cover include:
- Reason behind the transfer
- Information about the receiving unit
- Estimated time and date of transfer
- Further ongoing follow-up care
- Any other concerns that they may have

OVERNIGHT TRANSFERS

In general, try to avoid step-down transfers overnight. There has been evidence to show that patients who are transferred out of ICU at night do worse than those transferred during the day. Some trusts would regard an overnight transfer as an adverse incident and this should be reported accordingly.

EXAMPLE TRANSFER LETTER

Ward 15
Borders District Hospital
Queen Elizabeth Road
Ambrose
Armshire
TD6 5AT

ITU
Royal Victoria Infirmary
Queen Victoria Road
Melrish
Armshire
TD8 3AB

13.9.19

Dear Dr Joseph Gray
Re: Harry Jenson
DOB: 15/06/1989 (38 years old)
NHS Number: 0568 7849

Admission date: 10/02/2019
Ward: ITU
Consultant: Dr Waltz

Transfer date: 13/02/2019

Diagnosis: Near-fatal asthma attack

Many thanks for accepting Mr Jenson on to your ward after his stay in ICU, where he was treated for a nearfatal asthma attack for 3 days but is now ready to be stepped down to ward-level care.

Mr Jenson originally presented to the ED with chest tightness and wheeziness. At this point his peak expiratory flow rate was 60% but he was tachypnoeic at 30 breaths/min and tachycardic at 130 bpm, so he was managed as severe acute asthma. He was given nebulised salbutamol and ipratropium bromide but over time he became increasingly cyanosed, exhausted and PEF < 33% best or predicted. An ABG showed $PaCO_2$ 7.1 kPa and the patient had begun to show signs of exhaustion, at which point he had been quickly transferred to ICU.

We also gave him a single intravenous dose of 2 g magnesium sulphate over 20 min and started him on a 5-day course of 50 mg prednisolone PO. He required bilevel positive airway pressure for 3 days, stopped yesterday. Mr Jenson is now self-ventilating in air; his PEF is 56%, with a normal $PaCO_2$. Since he has been managed accordingly and has been stable for the past 24 h, his most recent PEF was 80%, showing no signs of respiratory distress. He has been seen by physiotherapy and had a hyperinflated chest X-ray at presentation.

Apart from asthma, he has no other significant past medical history. He has no known allergies. He is currently on:
Prednisolone 50mg OD PO (2 days remaining of 5)
Salbumatol 5mg 2 hourly NEBS
Ipratropium bromide 500 micrograms 6 hourly NEBS

Drugs on Transfer

DRUG	DOSE	FREQUENCY	ROUTE	LENGTH OF TREATMENT
Prednisolone	50mg	OD	PO	2 days (3 doses given)
Salbumatol	5mg	2 hourly	NEBS	Wean as able
Ipratropium bromide	500	micrograms 6 hourly	NEBS	Wean as able

Please could you continue with his management as prescribed and continue to monitor Mr Jenson's condition for at least another 24 h. Wean the nebulisers as able. Once he is ready for discharge, please can you ensure that Mr Jenson is reviewed by his GP 2 days post-discharge and is under the surveillance of the respiratory team.

The patient and his partner, Lisa, have both been fully aware of the events so far. If you have any further questions, please do not hesitate to contact me or another member of the ICU team.

Yours sincerely
Dr Ahmed Arif
FY2 to Dr Sarah Waltz, ICU Consultant
Tel extension: 56161
Secretary: Miss Helen Bradshaw (54718)

CRITICAL CARE OUTREACH

It is not uncommon for the critical care outreach nurse on duty to pay a follow-up visit to patients who have recently been stepped down from critical care.

❓ QUESTIONS AND ANSWERS FOR CANDIDATE

Name three signs and symptoms of acute severe asthma.
- PEF 33–50% best or predicted
- Respiratory rate ≥ 25 breaths/min
- Heart rate ≥ 110 bpm
- Inability to complete sentences in one breath

Name the six parameters that are taken into consideration for calculating the National Early Warning Score (NEWS).
- Respiratory rate
- Oxygen saturation
- Heart rate

- Systolic blood pressure
- Temperature
- Level of consciousness

How many critical care levels exist?
- Four:
  - Level 0: Ward-based care
  - Level 1: Patients who are at risk of deterioration, or those who have recently been relocated from higher levels of care and whose current needs can be met on a ward but require additional input; for example, more regular monitoring, continuous oxygenation
  - Level 2: Patients who require support for a single failing organ system, postoperative care or more detailed observations
  - Level 3: Patients who require advanced respiratory support alone or support for two or more organ systems

 A Case to Learn From

A patient was receiving antenatal care at hospital A but wanted to be transferred to hospital B to deliver her baby. She wasn't seen at hospital B until 38 weeks' gestation, when she arrived in labour! It was initially a challenge to plan her care and birth, as no delivery plan had been made in her notes from hospital A. For pregnant women, it is always good to have a more definitive plan earlier on so that we're not cutting too close to the estimated due date. You can't document a plan that hasn't been made in a transfer letter, but you can clarify whether one needs to be made.

 Top Tip

Bear in mind that the actual transfer could be longer than expected so make sure that the patient is still being reviewed regularly. Give the patient and family regular updates as to what is happening instead of leaving them in the dark.

STATION 12.2: REFERRAL LETTER

SCENARIO

You are a junior doctor working in a family care practice. Mrs Sharp, a 72-year-old woman, presents with vaginal bleeding. This was the fourth episode in the past month, her last menstrual period was 15 years ago and she has never given birth. She also has a background history of asthma and diabetes. Given the symptom of postmenopausal bleeding, you would like Mrs Sharp to be seen by a gynaecologist to be investigated for endometrial cancer. Please write an appropriate referral letter for her to be seen in a specialist clinic.

CORE CONCEPT

- A referral letter may be required when you want a patient to be reviewed by another healthcare professional. This situation usually arises when you feel that others are more equipped with the knowledge or facility to provide the appropriate care to the patient
- It is most commonly used as a means of communication between primary and secondary care
- Some examples of the receiving department include: Social services, dieticians, reproductive medicine, anaesthetists or any other medical or surgical (sub) specialties

 Common Concerns

How much detail do I need to provide?	There is no minimum amount of information that you need to provide in the referral letter; however, the more relevant information you offer, the better it is for the other clinician to assess the situation
What if I do not have a diagnosis?	Sometimes you will be referring a patient back to the care of a team that has already seen the patient. At other times, you will be making a new referral based on a symptom complex and in these situations, it is appropriate to refer the patient with details of the presenting complaint only
	Try to provide as much detail as possible anyway. It would be useful if you could provide a differential diagnosis, but don't worry if you can't
Do I need to contact someone personally to make them aware of the referral?	This can vary depending on where you work, so check local policies. For example, if you are referring to an acute assessment unit such as an early pregnancy unit, it may be a good idea to give them a ring before sending the patient to the hospital. If you are referring for a patient to be seen in a specialist clinic, a letter should suffice

EXAMPLE LAYOUT

[Insert address of corresponding hospital]   [Insert address of doctor sending the letter]

[Insert date of letter]

Dear: [Insert doctor's name]
Re: [Insert name and identification details of patient]

[Insert main text: Refer to the 'Key Information' section of this station below]
Yours sincerely

[Insert name of referring doctor]

[Insert designation of referring doctor and senior doctor if relevant]
[Insert contact details of referring doctor]

KEY INFORMATION

DIAGNOSIS

- List all major health conditions that the patient has been diagnosed with, preferably with those most relevant to this referral first

INTRODUCTION TO THE REFERRAL

- Try to begin with a polite introduction; for example, 'I would be grateful if you could review [insert name of the patient] regarding her [insert name of condition]'
- If you are unsure what the diagnosis or condition is, then it is acceptable to write down a symptom complex but ensure that you specify exactly what you would like to be assessed. For example, 'breast lump for further investigation'
- Whether you give a diagnosis or a symptom complex, it is important to provide more information on the current issue as outlined below

CURRENT PROBLEM

- Describe the issue for which the patient has presented today as you have seen her in your clinic
- Explore why the patient has decided to present with her problem now and the course of progression since her first presentation. For example, aim to cover duration of symptoms, worsening symptoms or if there has been a new symptom
- Give details on the relevant symptoms and find out if there was a known cause

KEY INVESTIGATIONS

- Only the most relevant investigations need to be mentioned; for example, CT and MRI scans, or if recent blood tests have been abnormal, these are likely to be particularly relevant as well
- Highlight any tests that have been ordered but are yet to be carried out, and any tests that have been performed but are awaiting results
- Remember to include the dates of the investigations

TREATMENT TO DATE

- Give details on how this problem has been managed to date; for example, previous referrals to other relevant specialties, investigations undertaken and current treatment as well as previous treatment trials
- It is worth documenting other relevant history that is not directly linked to the current problem

CURRENT MEDICATION

- State the drugs that the patient is currently taking
- Remember to include the following key points:
  - Generic name of drug
  - Dose
  - Frequency of administration
  - Route of administration
  - Length of treatment
- Clearly state information about allergies or adverse reactions to drugs

SOCIAL HISTORY

- Smoking status and alcohol intake (if relevant)
- State the patient's home and work circumstances
- Explore how the problem is affecting the patient's life
- Find out the patient's impression of their current problem and what it is that they are particularly concerned about

INFORMATION GIVEN TO PATIENT AND FAMILY

- Explain what has been communicated to the patient and if there is any important information; for example, a cancer diagnosis, that they may be unaware of

CONCLUSION TO THE REFERRAL

- Clearly state what you would like from the consultation. For example, 'I would like your opinion with regard to the most likely diagnosis' or 'I would like advice on further management options for this patient's eczema'

EXAMPLE REFERRAL LETTER

Gynaecology Outpatients
Harrogate District Hospital
Long Road
Hoarrogate
HG1 5EE

Harrogate Medical Practice
Harrogate Road
Harrogate
HG3 1XP

16 June 2019

Dear Colleague,
Re: Jennifer Sharp
DOB: 04/05/1948 (72 years old)
NHS Number: 0874 5311

Diagnosis
1. Postmenopausal bleeding
2. Asthma
3. Type 2 diabetes

Dear colleague

I would appreciate it if you could see this patient in your 2-week-wait gynaecological cancer clinic.

Mrs Sharp is a 72-year-old woman who had presented to my GP surgery complaining of postmenopausal bleeding. Her last menstrual period was 15 years ago and over the past 4 weeks she has had four episodes of vaginal bleeding – minimal in volume, described as 'spotting'. Otherwise she is well in herself, denies any blood in her urine or stools. She has never given birth before and her body mass index (BMI) is 31.

She also has a past medical history of asthma and type 2 diabetes, for which she is currently taking a salbutamol inhaler as required and 500 mg metformin tablets once a day. At the moment, the symptoms are not significantly affecting her life, but she is worried they might get worse. She has never smoked and drinks approximately 1 unit per week. She is a retired teacher and is married to Clark.

I have explained to Mrs Sharp that her symptoms of postmenopausal bleeding could be a sign of endometrial cancer and that is why we have referred her to you on a 2-week waiting list.

Many thanks for seeing this patient and please do not hesitate to contact me for more information. I look forward to hearing from you.

Yours sincerely
Dr Samuel Smith
GP Trainee
Tel extension: 01423 549 667

- Try to end with something like, 'If you would like any more information, do not hesitate to contact me. I look forward to hearing from you'

SPECIAL REQUIREMENTS

If you know that the patient will be requiring any special assistance; for example, transportation aid, interpretation or advocate, then mention it in your letter, making sure that this is in place for when they see the corresponding healthcare professional

 QUESTIONS AND ANSWERS FOR CANDIDATE

How do you refer a patient with a suspicion of malignancy?

- In these cases, you can refer the patient to a 2-week-wait clinic, where they must be seen within 2 weeks from the date of the referral so that they can be assessed sooner rather than later, to rule out sinister causes

Name three red-flag symptoms of cauda equina syndrome.

- Saddle anaesthesia
- Bladder disturbance
- Bowel disturbance
- Sexual problems
- Nerve root pain

Name three risk factors for endometrial cancer.

- Increasing age
- Use of oestrogen-only hormone replacement therapy
- High parity
- Early menarche
- Late menopause

 A Case to Learn From

A patient had been referred to radiology for a cystogram and she was given an appointment with a specific radiologist. However, it turned out that this radiologist does not perform cystograms and so that appointment slot was unused, and the patient had made an unnecessary trip to the hospital. With specialist radiological imaging, it is a good idea to check with the department if only certain members of the team can carry them out or if you are aware that only certain clinicians perform such investigations, then state their names in the referral letter.

 Top Tip

If possible, try to give a guideline for how long the patient may be waiting to hear back from the corresponding team. This will give the patient a more realistic expectation and they won't be left anxious thinking that they might have been lost in the system. It will also let them know when it might be appropriate to chase things up.

STATION 12.3: DISCHARGE LETTER

SCENARIO

Mrs Finn, a 50-year-old woman, was admitted to hospital due to haematemesis. This morning after she had woken up, she had vomited up a teaspoon amount of blood and passed melaena. For the past few months she has also been experiencing heartburn and intermittent abdominal discomfort. She takes regular non-steroidal anti-inflammatory drugs (NSAIDs) and sulfasalazine for rheumatoid arthritis and drinks approximately 19 units of alcohol per week. A diagnosis of peptic ulcer disease was given, the appropriate treatment was started and she is now ready to go home. Please write her discharge letter.

CORE CONCEPT

- A discharge letter, also known as a discharge summary, is essentially a report of what has happened to a patient from the moment they stepped into the unit to the moment they were discharged
- It is a common means of communication from secondary to primary care
- It is considered a legal document
- The skill is to pick out key pieces of information that the primary care physician needs to know without having to read every single note entry

Common Concerns

When should you begin discharge planning?	It is best practice to begin the process of discharge planning as soon as a patient is admitted to hospital. This allows time for the relevant teams to get everything in place that the patient will need upon returning to the community, thereby avoiding delays
Who receives a copy of the discharge letter?	The discharge letter should be aimed at giving primary care physicians a concise overview of what happened to their patient while they were in hospital. Usually, the patient will also receive a copy of the discharge letter and often, there is a section that is specifically used to summarise the hospital stay for the patient using non-medical jargon. For complex patients, key specialists should also get copies
Does the discharge letter always have to be written by the patient's responsible doctor?	Ideally, the discharge letter should be written by a doctor who was involved in the patient's care during the stay in hospital. However, if this is not possible, the doctor writing the discharge letter should obtain as much information as they can from the patient's medical notes to give the most accurate picture of what had happened. Medical notes should in theory always be good enough to write a summary

EXAMPLE LAYOUT

[Insert address and name of receiving doctor]   [Insert address of hospital and ward]

[Insert date of letter]

Dear: [Insert doctor's name]
Re: [Insert name and identification details of patient]

Admission date: Discharge date:
Ward:
Consultant:

[Insert main text: Refer to the 'Key Information' section of this station, below]
Yours sincerely

[Insert name of referring doctor]

[Insert designation of referring doctor and senior doctor if relevant]
[Insert contact details of referring doctor]

KEY INFORMATION

DIAGNOSIS

- Name all diagnoses that the patient has been given, including any given before this hospital admission. Try to list them in order of clinical importance, and with the new conditions first
- The conditions should be as specific as possible; for example, 'anterior ST elevation myocardial infarction' rather than 'heart attack'

PROGRESS

- State the date of admission, mode of admission (elective or emergency) and the symptoms the patient presented with
- Explain the procedures and main treatments that the patient has undergone, medical and surgical. Mention any complications as well
- Clarify the involvement of other services; for example, social work, physiotherapy
- Depending on the case, it may be relevant to include key factors in the past medical and social history. For example, if the patient is admitted in neutropenic sepsis, it may be worthwhile mentioning the dates of recent chemotherapy treatments
- Record the state of the patient on discharge; for example well versus unwell. If the patient is now very frail and expected to die at home, not only should this be stated but the primary care physician should be contacted directly as well

KEY INVESTIGATIONS

- It is not necessary to include every single investigation result; however, clinically relevant results that it would be useful to be aware of should be provided. For example, ultrasound contrast scans; or if recent blood tests have been abnormal, these are like to be particularly relevant as well
- Even if investigation results were unremarkable, they may be relevant; for example, a chest X-ray showing normal lung fields for a patient being investigated for breathlessness
- Remember to include the dates of the investigations

DRUGS ON DISCHARGE

- State the drugs that will be continued on discharge
- Remember to include the following key points:
  - Generic name of drug
  - Dose
  - Frequency of administration
  - Route of administration
  - Length of treatment
- Mention any drug monitoring that may be required; for example, if the patient is on warfarin, give the date the next drug level is due to be measured
- Clearly state information about allergies or adverse reactions to drugs, including the route it was given

CHANGES TO MEDICATION

- Highlight any drugs that have been discontinued and whether recommencement needs to be considered. For example, 'propranolol has been permanently discontinued because of low blood pressure' and 'furosemide was discontinued due to low sodium; please consider restarting when sodium normalises if still oedematous'
- Also highlight any changes in drug doses, either increased or decreased
- It may be helpful to state which medications were newly commenced on this hospital admission and which were on admission. For the new drugs, state their indication, the duration of therapy and whether they need to be reviewed; for example, 'for 7-day course of oral co-amoxiclav for a lower respiratory tract infection'

CHANGES MADE TO CARE ARRANGEMENTS

- Mention any changes that have been made to community care. For example, arrangements for district nurses to administer low-molecular-weight heparin or social work arranging a package of care in the community

OUTSTANDING TESTS/RESULTS

- Highlight any tests that have been ordered but are yet to be carried out, and any tests that have been performed but are awaiting results. Of these, state whether these are being chased by the hospital team or are to be chased by the primary care team

FOLLOW-UP

- Clarify if the patient needs to be seen in clinic after discharge from hospital and if so, whether an appointment has already been made and where it is
- Clarify if any follow-up investigations have been arranged for the patient as an outpatient
- Clarify if follow-up is required from other services; for example, dieticians, physiotherapy
- It is important to be clear on what is expected of the primary care physician; for example, 'please could the primary care practice arrange for [insert name of patient] to have repeat urea and electrolytes (U&Es) checked in 1–2 weeks'. It is equally vital to be clear on what is being arranged by the hospital; for example, 'Dr Smith's team will arrange for a follow-up chest X-ray in 4–6 weeks' time'

GP TO PLEASE CONSIDER THE FOLLOWING...

- Include information that is particularly important for the primary care physician to be aware of with regard to the patient's ongoing care. For example, if the patient had gone home with a Do Not Attempt Cardiopulmonary Resuscitation (DNACPR) form
- Other vital information to include are the criteria that will require a more urgent reassessment; for example, on discharge from a cardiology ward, 'if [insert name of patient] has any further angina, please re-refer her for consideration of further percutaneous coronary intervention to her right coronary artery'

INFORMATION GIVEN TO PATIENT/FAMILY

- Find out whether the patient and family have been counselled and debriefed about the admission and current problem(s), reason for discharge and any further follow-up or contact with the admitting unit

EXAMPLE DISCHARGE LETTER

Central London Medical Practice
Franklin Road
London
EN7 4FR

Queen's College Hospital
Queen Road
London
SE5 3WQ

1 October 2019

Dear Dr Bethany Khan
Re: Rebecca Finn
DOB: 19/11/1970 (50 years old)
NHS Number: 0983 0114

Admission date: 28/09/2019   Discharge date: 01/10/2019
Ward: 7, Gastroenterology ward
Consultant: Dr Tipp

Diagnosis:
1. Haematemesis secondary to gastric ulcers
2. Rheumatoid arthritis

I am writing this discharge letter to provide you with a summary of Miss Rebecca Finn's stay in hospital, during which she has been given a diagnosis of gastrointestinal (GI) bleed secondary to gastric ulcer.

   She was admitted on 28 September due to haematemesis. There was a teaspoon amount of fresh red blood and she reported an episode of melaena. For the past few months she has also been experiencing heartburn and intermittent abdominal discomfort. She denied any haemoptysis and bleeding from elsewhere. She admits to taking regular ibuprofen over the counter for rheumatoid arthritis.

   An inpatient endoscopy was performed and this confirmed GI bleeding secondary multiple gastric ulcers, all of which had been treated endoscopically and the bleeding stopped (please see the attached report for more detail). Rebecca has remained haemodynamically stable throughout her stay, without needing any blood transfusion. Her stool sample was negative for Helicobacter pylori infection.

   She normally smokes 10 cigarettes a day and drinks 19 units a week. Her BMI is currently 33. She has been given weight loss, alcohol intake and smoking cessation advice, as well as asked to stop taking ibuprofen and to avoid trigger foods such as coffee and spicy or fatty food. Please note the patient's admission and medication changes. She has been started on omeprazole 20 mg OD for 8 weeks; please kindly review this and the appropriateness of continuation if the patient is still having symptoms.

Drugs on Discharge

DRUG	DOSE	FREQUENCY	ROUTE	LENGTH OF TREATMENT
Omeprazole	20 mg	OD	PO	8 weeks
Sulfasalazine	500 mg	OD	PO	–

Rebecca will be followed up by the gastroenterologists in clinic post-discharge (in 6 weeks). She also has a rheumatology clinic review as previously scheduled in January next year. She has been fully updated with regard to her diagnosis and management plan. Please do not hesitate to contact me for more information.

Yours sincerely
Dr Bethany Tipp
Consultant Gastroenterologist
Tel. extension: 96558
Secretary: Miss Susan Bradbury (96777)

OTHER SECTIONS THAT MAY BE INCLUDED IN A DISCHARGE LETTER

- Clinical tools: For example, record the Medical Research Council (MRC) Dyspnoea Scale score used in chronic obstructive pulmonary disease
- Social context: Who they have for support, the type of housing they live in, their independence with activities of daily living
- Research participation: Identifies patients involved in a clinical trial

QUESTIONS AND ANSWERS FOR CANDIDATE

Name the risk-scoring system used at the first presentation of an upper GI bleed.
- The Blatchford score is used to consider if an adult patient should be admitted to hospital due to an upper GI bleed, alongside the clinical presentation. The total score varies from 0 to 23, with a higher score being associated with greater mortality

Name the risk-scoring system used when there is a suspicion of an upper GI bleed post-endoscopy.
- The Rockall score is used to estimate mortality in patients who have undergone endoscopy and present with symptoms of an upper GI bleed. It considers both clinical information and endoscopy results

Name three teams that may need to be involved in preparing for discharge a patient who has had a stroke and a prolonged stay in hospital.
- Speech and language therapy
- Physiotherapy
- Occupational therapy
- Rehabilitation
- Dietician
- District nurses

A Case to Learn From

I was writing a discharge letter for a child who had been admitted for sepsis. As part of the process, I reviewed all the lab results on the computer system and identified that the child was neutropenic. This hadn't been picked up initially as the child was very well, and there was no reason to suspect the child would be neutropenic. I discussed it with the consultant, and we spoke to haematology; it turned out that three people in the family had neutropenia, and it was a familial condition. Writing a discharge letter is an opportunity for one final review of the patient's notes, and it can pick up things that would otherwise be missed.

Top Tip

When you are writing the discharge summary, try and put yourself in the position of the primary care physician and think about the most important details that you want to take away from the patient's admission into hospital.

STATION 12.4: DEATH CERTIFICATION

SCENARIO

Mr Phillip Jones, a 75-year-old man, was admitted to hospital last week due to a severe headache and his CT scan showed an intracerebral haemorrhage, which was secondary to his cerebral metastases from squamous cell carcinoma of the left main bronchus, which were both diagnosed six months ago. He also had Parkinson's disease, (4 years) and unstable angina (3 years). Unfortunately, he died on the ward 8 days after he was admitted. You have been called to complete the death certificate for Mr Jones.

CORE CONCEPT

- The death certificate is an important legal document
- It enables the death to be formally registered, so that the family can make arrangements for disposal of the body
- The Births and Deaths Registration Act 1953 in the UK requires you, as a registered medical practitioner, to certify the cause of death to the best of your knowledge and belief
- You must identify the underlying cause of death, which must be a specific disease rather than a mechanism of death
- The death certificate also provides epidemiological information from which mortality data are derived

Common Concerns

What if I am unsure of the cause of death?	This scenario may arise and if it does, there are plenty of people around to ask for advice. You could have a look through the notes to see the reason for admission and try to deduce the cause of death from the notes thereafter. Alternatively, approach the consultant to whom the patient was assigned for advice
Can I fill out a death certificate if I had not confirmed the death?	Even if you had not verified the death, you are still able to complete the death certificate. Just remember to circle the correct detail; for example, 'Seen after death by another medical practitioner but not me'
What if I do not know whether the patient requires a postmortem examination?	Do not be afraid to ask your consultant for advice. Staff working in the bereavement office are also extremely helpful. If required, you can also call the coroners to ask them for advice

EXAMPLE LAYOUT (FIG. 12.1)

KEY INFORMATION

PATIENT DETAILS

- Name of deceased: Write out the patient's full name

- Date of death as stated to me: The date must be stated as the number of day(s) of that month for example, second day of July 2019, unless stated otherwise on the form
- Age as stated to me: Record as complete years, or if under 1 year old, as complete months. This number should be written in words

---

Medical certificate of cause of death

Name of deceased Phillip Jones

Date of death:	Day	Month	Year		
	0 3	0 7	2 0 1 9

Time of death	Hour	Min
	1 4	3 0

Age as stated to me: Seventy Five

Place of death: Manchester Royal Infirmary, Ward 15

Last seen alive by me   **3rd** day of **July 2019**

Cause of death

I hereby certify that to the best of my knowledge and belief, the cause of death was as stated below:

		Approximate interval between onset and death
		Years Months Days

1. Disease or condition directly leading to death

Antecedent causes
Morbid conditions, if any, giving rise to above cause, stating the underlying condition last

		Years	Months	Days
a.)	Intracerebral haemorrhage	0	0	8
b.)	Cerebral metastasis	0	6	0
c.)	Squamous cell carcinoma of left main bronchus	0	6	0
d.)				

2. Other significant conditions contributing to the death, but not related to the disease or condition causing it

	Years	Months	Days
Parkinson's disease,	4	0	0
Unstable angina	3	0	0

Please tick the relevant box

Post mortem

PM1 ☐ Post mortem has been done and information is included above

PM2 ☐ Post mortem information may be available later

PM3 ☒ No post mortem is being done

Procurator fiscal/coroner

PF ☐ This death has been reported to the procurator fiscal/coroner

Extra information for statistical purposes

X ☐ I may later be able to supply the registrar general with additional information

Attendance on deceased

A1 ☒ I was in attendance upon the deceased during last illness

A2 ☐ I was not in attendance upon the deceased during last illness: the doctor who was is unable to provide the certificate

A3 ☐ No doctor was in attendance on the deceased

Signature	E.Walter	Date: 4th July 2019
Name in BLOCK CAPITALS	ELENA WALTER	**For a death in hospital**
Official address	Ward 15, Manchester Royal Infirmary, M13 9WL	Name of the consultant responsible Dr. Walsh Qualifications MBBS (Medicine and Surgery) GMC 546753

Counterfoil – Medical certificate of cause of death

Name of deceased Phillip Jones

Date of death 3rd July 2019

Place of death Manchester Royal Infirmary, Ward 15

Please circle as appropriate			
Post mortem	PM1 or PM2 or (PM3)
Procurator fiscal/coroner	PF
Extra information	X
Attendance on deceased	(A1) A2 A3

Cause of death

I (a) Intracerebral haemorrhage
 (b) Cerebral metastasis
 (c) Squamous cell carcinoma of left main bronchus
 (d)

II

Date of certificate   4th July 2019

Fig. 12.1 A filled-out example of the death certificate for the patient in this case, Mr Jones. Note design may vary.

- Place of death: Aim to record a precise place of death; for example, Ward 15, Leeds General Infirmary, or provide a private address if the patient died in his own home

CIRCUMSTANCES OF DEATH CERTIFICATION

- Last seen alive by me: Record the date that you last saw the patient alive. Again, similarly to the date of death, the date must be stated as the number of day(s) of that month; for example, twenty-fourth day of June 2019
- Information from postmortem: In the column on the left, there are four potential options regarding postmortem and you need to circle the one that is most applicable to the patient. The options are listed below:
    1. 'The certified cause of death takes account of information obtained from postmortem'.
    2. 'Information from postmortem may be available later'.
    3. 'Postmortem not being held'.
    4. 'I have reported the death to the coroner for further action'.
- Seen after death: In the column on the right, there are three potential options regarding who the patient was seen by after death, and this person most likely will have performed the death confirmation. The most applicable option needs to be circled. The options are listed below:
    - 'Seen after death by me'
    - 'Seen after death by another medical practitioner but not me'
    - 'Not seen after death by a medical practitioner'

CAUSE OF DEATH

The section regarding the cause of death is divided into two sections, I and II. Section I is further divided into a, b and c, as applicable.

Section I

- This section considers the main causal conditions leading to death:
    - I(a): Disease or condition that led directly to death
    - I(b): Other disease or condition, if any, leading to (a)
    - I(c): Other disease or condition, if any, leading to (b)
- Fill in I(a) by identifying the disease or condition that led directly to death. Then, backtrack to see if there are other diseases or conditions that may have led to this; for example, Parkinson's disease may have caused an aspiration pneumonia
- Aim to be as specific as possible; for example, 'adenocarcinoma of the left main bronchus', rather than 'lung cancer'
- I(a) must be filled in; however I(b) and I(c) can be left blank if nothing had contributed to it; for example, subarachnoid haemorrhage is acceptable alone
- Beware of certain phrases that should be avoided in I(a), as they are considered to be modes of death

rather than causes of death. Among others, these include:
- Heart/kidney/liver/respiratory failure
- Cardiac arrest
- Asphyxia
- Coma
- Exhaustion
- Old age/frailty as the sole cause of death. It is also useful to note that this phrase can only be used for those over the age of 80

Section II

- This section considers all other significant conditions that contributed to the death but are not related to the diseases nor the conditions directly causing it. For example, asthma in a patient who had died of adenocarcinoma of the left main bronchus
- Do not list the patient's entire past medical history; for example, something like mild eczema is unlikely to be relevant, unless the eczema becoming infected was the cause of death

APPROXIMATE INTERVAL BETWEEN ONSET AND DEATH

Provide an approximation of the length of time between the onset of the disease or condition directly leading to death and the time of death.

PERSONAL DETAILS

- Signature: Sign and print your name in block capital letters
- Qualifications: List your higher-education qualifications; for example, 'MbCHB Medicine and Surgery'
- Residence: State the address of the hospital where you are working. Do not provide your own address
- Date: The date when the death certificate is completed
- Consultant responsible for the above-named patient: If the patient died in hospital, state the consultant responsible for the deceased patient when he was alive

COUNTERFOIL

To the left of the death certificate, there is a counterfoil that you need to remember to fill in. The information that you need to cover includes: Deceased patient's name, section I and II of the cause of death and your personal details. This will remain in the death certificate book.

BACK OF THE DEATH CERTIFICATE

There are two boxes, box A and B, at the back of the death certificate that may be relevant to you. Put your initials against the box if the following is the case:
- Box A: The death has been referred to the coroner. A simple discussion with the coroner will not require this to be filled in

• Box B: If further information about this death may be required at a later stage; for example, if awaiting histology results. In these scenarios, the deceased patient's responsible consultant will be contacted for more information when required

QUESTIONS AND ANSWERS FOR CANDIDATE

What additional forms are required if the deceased patient is to be cremated?

• You would need to complete a death certificate as well as another medical certificate, known as Cremation Form 4

Name three reasons for referring to coroners.

• The cause of death is unknown
• The deceased was not seen by the certifying doctor either after death or within 14 days of death
• The death was violent or unnatural or suspicious
• The death may be due to an accident (whenever it occurred)
• The death may be due to self-neglect or neglect by others
• The death may be due to an industrial disease or related to the deceased's employment
• The death may be due to an abortion
• The death occurred during an operation or before recovery from the effects of anaesthetic

• The death may be suicide
• The death occurred during or shortly after detention in police or prison custody

How is death confirmed (note requirements vary)?

• No palpable pulses felt after 1 min of checking
• No breath or heart sounds on auscultation after 5 min of checking
• Both eyes fixed and dilated

 A Case to Learn From

A patient came into hospital because of progressive deterioration of his known heart failure. It was evident that he was coming to the end of his life, at which point he revealed that he wanted to die at home. However, at this point, he was already too unwell and there was not enough time to put things in place for him at home. Sadly, he passed away in the hospital soon after. It is important to have these discussions with patients sooner rather than later, so that healthcare professionals can accommodate patients' wishes as much as possible.

Top Tip

When I was a medical student, as part of a mandatory skill, I had to show competency in completing a death certificate and therefore I wrote one with a junior doctor before I graduated. Getting the practice in while you're a medical student will allow you to be more confident when you actually have to do it as a junior doctor.

Index

Note: Page numbers followed by *f* indicate figures and *t* indicate tables.